W9-AGP-419

Basic Maternal/Pediatric Nursing

Basic Maternal/Pediatric Nursing

PAMELA J. SHAPIRO
WITH CONTRIBUTORS

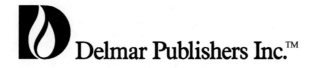

I(T)P™

NOTICE TO THE READER

Publisher does not warrant or guarantee any of the products described herein or perform any independent analysis in connection with any of the product information contained herein. Publisher does not assume, and expressly disclaims, any obligation to obtain and include information other than that provided to it by the manufacturer.

The reader is expressly warned to consider and adopt all safety precautions that might be indicated by the activities described herein and to avoid all potential hazards. By following the instructions contained herein, the reader willingly assumes all risks in connection with such instructions.

The publisher makes no representations or warranties of any kind, including but not limited to, the warranties of fitness for particular purpose or merchantability, nor are any such representations implied with respect to the material set forth herein, and the publisher takes no responsibility with respect to such material. The publisher shall not be liable for any special, consequential, or exemplary damages resulting, in whole or in part, from the readers' use of, or reliance upon, this material.

Cover Illustration, Bob Crofut
Cover Design, Juan Vargas, Vargas Williams Design

Delmar Staff
David C. Gordon, Publisher
Marion Waldman, Sponsoring Editor
Helen Yackel, Developmental Editor
Mary Robinson, Senior Project Editor
Mary Siener, Art and Design Coordinator
Megan DeSantis, Art and Design Coordinator
Barbara A. Bullock, Production Coordinator

For information, address Delmar Publishers Inc.
3 Columbia Circle
Box 15015
Albany, NY 12212-5015

Printed in the United States of America
Published simultaneously in Canada
by Nelson Canada,
a division of the Thomson Corporation

10 9 8 7 6 5 4 3 2 xxx 01 00 99 98 97 96 95
ISBN 0-8273-4993-9

Library of Congress Cataloging-in-Publication Data
Shapiro, Pamela J.
Basic maternal/newborn nursing/Pamela J. Shapiro with contributors.
p. cm.
Includes bibliographical references and index.
ISBN 0-8273-4993-9
1. Maternity nursing. 2. Pediatric nursing. I. Title.
[DNLM: 1. Obstetrical Nursing. 2. Maternal-Child Nursing.
3. Pediatric Nursing. WY 157 S529b 1994]
RG951.S455 1995
610.73'67—dc20
DNLM/DLC
for Library of Congress

94-19097
CIP

Contributors

AUTHORS

Molly Allison, MSN, RN
Assistant Professor
Department of Nursing
Angelo State University
San Angelo, Texas
(Chapter 31 — The Pediatric Surgical Patient)

Ruth Bindler, MS, RNC
Associate Professor
Intercollegiate Center for Nursing Education
Washington State University
Spokane, Washington
(Chapter 23 — Developmental Stages; co-author)

Donna Marie Frassetto
Senior Developmental Editor
Cracom Corporation
Maryland Heights, Missouri
(Chapter 22 — Physical Growth; co-author)
(Chapter 23 — Developmental Stages; co-author)
(Chapters 26, 28, 30, 34–36, 39, 40; co-author)

P. K. Holmes
Advising Coordinator
Department of Nursing
University of South Dakota
Vermillion, South Dakota
(Chapter 24 — Basic Nutrition)

Peggy Larsen, MS, RN
Assistant Professor
Nursing Department
University of South Dakota
Vermillion, South Dakota
(Chapter 41 — Musculoskeletal Conditions; primary author)

June Peterson Larson, MS, RN
Associate Professor, Assistant Director, Department of Nursing
Director, Vermillion Campus
University of South Dakota
Vermillion, South Dakota
(Chapter 29 — The Hospitalized Child; primary author)
(Chapter 32 — Caring for the Dying Child)

Stephanie G. Metzger, MS, RN, C
Clinical Nurse Specialist
Children's Hospital
Richmond, Virginia
(Chapter 42 — Neurological Conditions)

Barbara Ellen Norwitz, BSN, RN, PNP
Publisher and Editorial Director
Cracom Corporation
Maryland Heights, Missouri;
formerly Pediatric Nurse Practitioner
Johns Hopkins Hospital
Baltimore, Maryland
(Chapter 22 — Physical Growth)
(Chapter 23 — Developmental Stages; primary author)
(Chapter 26 — Child Safety)
(Chapter 28 — Assessment)
(Chapter 30 — Routine Pediatric Procedures)
(Chapter 34 — Communicable and Infectious Diseases)
(Chapter 35 — Integumentary Conditions)
(Chapter 36 — Conditions of the Eyes and Ears)
(Chapter 39 — Digestive and Metabolic Conditions)
(Chapter 40 — Genitourinary Conditions)

Nancy O'Donnell, BSN, MS, RN
Associate Professor
J. Sargeant Reynolds Community College
Richmond, Virginia
(Chapter 43 — Conditions of the Blood and Blood-forming Organs)

Joann F. Pieronek, PhD, RN
Director of Nursing
Wayne County Community College
Detroit, Michigan
(Chapter 27 — Preparing for Hospitalization)

Carla Ries
Assistant Professor
Department of Nursing
University of South Dakota
Vermillion, South Dakota
(Chapter 29 — The Hospitalized Child; co-author)
(Chapter 41 — Musculoskeletal Conditions; co-author)

Ann G. Ross, MN, ARNP, CS
Professor of Nursing
Health Occupations Division
Shorelines Community College
Seattle, Washington
(Chapter 44 — Emotional and Behavioral Conditions)

Mary Ann Scoloveno, EdD, RN
Associate Professor
Rutgers, The State University of New Jersey
College of Nursing
Newark, New Jersey
(Chapter 21 — Principles of Growth and Development)
(Chapter 25 — Immunizations)

Pamela J. Shapiro, BSN, ARNP
OB-GYN Nurse Practitioner
Kirkland, Washington
(Chapters 1–20 — Maternal/Newborn Chapters)

Lisa Shaver
Assistant Professor
J. Sargeant Reynolds Community College
Richmond, Virginia
(Chapter 37 — Cardiovascular Conditions)

Rosemarie C. Westberg, MSN, RN
Associate Professor, Nursing
Northern Virginia Community College
Annandale, Virginia
(Chapter 33 — Sudden Infant Death Syndrome)
(Chapter 38 — Respiratory Conditions)

Preface

The health care delivery system in the United States is undergoing a dynamic change. Our society is faced with several issues that will have long-term effects on the quality of our lives.

Consumers have begun to demand control of their own health care. They expect health care providers to be open and honest about treatment options and to include them in the decision-making process. Sensitivity toward cultural differences is expected. If these needs are not met, consumers exercise their right to choose another health care provider. For these reasons, all health care professionals in direct contact with patients need to be expert communicators. We see therapeutic communications as the key to the success of the licensed practical nurse who often works as a first line manager as well as a primary care giver. Communicating effectively in all of these roles is essential for success in the nurse/patient/family relationship.

The licensed practical nurse is in a unique position. Few professions provide so much responsibility and challenge so soon after graduation. The licensed practical nurse who serves as a first line manager must exert leadership and management skills. The licensed practical nurse must be able to make decisions and accept responsibility. He or she will be expected to provide hands-on care, performing a variety of functions.

Licensed practical nurses are found in every setting. The role of the licensed practical nurse as a leader and educator in patient care is emphasized throughout this text. We stress the nursing process and care of the whole family as integral steps in delivering quality nursing care.

In preparing this textbook, we followed the premise that complicated material can be presented in a straightforward and friendly manner. Chapters are short and readable. Each chapter includes learning objectives and key terms. Charts and tables highlight important information, and extensive use of photographs support and illustrate textual content. Detailed nursing care sections, including nursing care plans, emphasize the nursing process. Review questions and suggested activities reinforce learning.

The first half of the textbook focuses on maternal-newborn nursing. The second half presents common pediatric problems using a growth and development approach. The maternal-newborn section discusses the reproductive system, conception, and fetal development. Sections on nutrition, prenatal screening tests, and risk factors for fetal development are presented. Alternative birthing methods and cultural differences are emphasized.

The pediatric section presents common pediatric disorders of each body system. Health maintenance and prevention, including anticipatory guidance, are emphasized. Developmental considerations in caring for the hospitalized child are incorporated throughout and highlighted in specific chapters. A separate chapter discusses psychosocial aspects of caring for the dying child.

Use of the accompanying student study guide is recommended. The study guide contains numerous exercises as well as procedures and additional activities. An instructor's manual containing answers to all review questions also is available.

Acknowledgments

A special thanks to Barabara Ellen Norwitz, BSN, RN, PNP, and Donna Marie Frassetto for their contributions to the pediatric section of this textbook.

Thanks and appreciation also are extended to the following people and facilities:

Colleen Booth, RN, MSN, Assistant Professor of Nursing, Westchester Community College, for her invaluable help and expertise during the photography session for the maternal/newborn chapters.

Veronica Casey, RNC, MA, Nursing Department Head; Maureen Maher, RN; and the students of the J. M. Wright Technical School, Stamford, Connecticut, who coordinated and participated in the photography sessions for the pediatric procedures chapters.

Photographers Michael Gallitelli and George Dodson, whose sensitive photographs illustrated the maternal/newborn and pediatric chapters, respectively.

Uniform Village, Inc., Crossgates Mall, Albany, New York, for providing many of the uniforms for the maternal/newborn photography session.

The authors would like to acknowledge the contributions of the following reviewers throughout the development of this project.

Carolyn Banks, MSN, RN
Director of Nursing Education
Nursing Department
Pratt Community College
Pratt, Kansas

Ann C. Barbara
Jefferson Vocational Technical Center
Watertown, New York

Cynthia A. Bean, MS, RN
Coordinator Health Occupations
Erie 1 BOCES
Lancaster, New York

Colleen Booth, RN, MSN
Westchester Community College
Valhalla, New York

Shirley J. Cashio, MSN, RN
Associate Professor of Nursing
Division of Nursing
Northwestern State University
Shreveport, Louisiana

Marcia Costello, MS, RD
Assistant Professor
College of Nursing
Villanova University
Villanova, Pennsylvania

Joan Darden, PhD
Darton College
Albany, Georgia

Joann Dever, MSNEd, RN
Department Chairperson
Health and Human Services Division
Indiana Vocational Technical College — 03
Fort Wayne, Indiana

Janet M. Dicke, RN
Instructor
Department of Practical Nursing
Rochester Community College
Rochester, Minnesota

Catherine Jenner, RN
Pediatric Instructor
Erie 1 BOCES
Lancaster, New York

Janet L. Joost, BA, RNC
Instructor
Boulder Technical Educational Center
Boulder, Colorado

Katherine R. Kneist, MSN, RN
Assistant Professor
William Rainey Harper College
Palatine, Illinois

Jennifer Lahl, BSN, RN
Children's Hospital-Oakland
Oakland, California

Mary S. Lewin
Health Occupations Educator
New York State BOCES
Lockport, New York

Marlene H. Loebig, MSN, RN, PNP
Professor of Nursing
Community College of Rhode Island
Warwick, Rhode Island

David K. Miller
Indiana Vocational Technical College
Columbus, Indiana

Jane Powhida
Hocking College
Nelsonville, Ohio

Donna Roddy
Chattanooga Technical Community College
Chattanooga, TN

Carol Ann Stacy
State of Michigan, Department of Education
Health Occupations Educator
Portage, Michigan

Barbara Strande, MSN, RN
Assistant Professor
Western Kentucky University
Department of Nursing
Bowling Green, Kentucky

Donna B. Vaughn, MS, RN
Professor
Department of Vocational Nursing
Del Mar College
Corpus Christie, Texas

Contents

UNIT TWO PREGNANCY AND PRENATAL CARE

UNIT THREE LABOR AND DELIVERY

UNIT

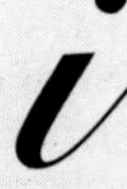

The Beginning of Life

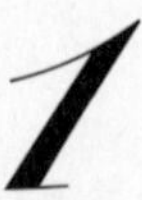

CHAPTER 1

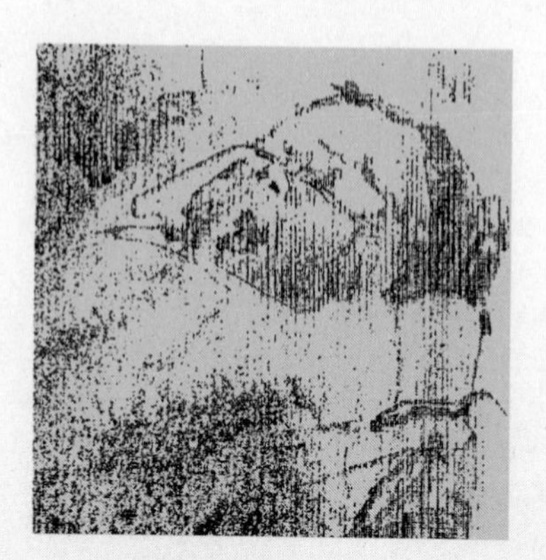

The History of Maternal/Newborn Nursing

Objectives

After studying this chapter, the student should be able to:

- Define *nursing* in general terms.
- Describe the training given to midwives throughout history.
- List factors that have influenced changing trends in obstetrics.
- Explain the role of the obstetrical nurse.

Key Terms

Nutricius
Granny Midwives
Hill-Burton Act
Family-Centered Units
OB-GYN
NAACOG/AWHONN
Rooming-In
Lamaze, Dick-Read, Bradley
Alternative Birthing Center (ABC)
Neonatal Period

Nursing has been defined in many ways. Its meaning varies with the times and the customs. The term *nursing* is derived from the Latin term **nutricius** meaning to nourish, to conserve energy, to protect, or to foster. Mothers were the first nurses. As an art, nursing requires a sympathetic heart and willing hands. Clara Barton (1821–1912) is an excellent example of one of the first practitioners of the art of nursing, Figure 1–1. She organized the American Red Cross, which is concerned with the alleviation of human suffering and the promotion of public health. She also has been called the angel of the battlefield for her work in the army camps and on battlefields during the Civil War. The chief purpose of nursing today is to help the individual attain or maintain health. Emphasis is now also on prevention and education. The nurse of today is not merely an attendant in the sickroom; she is a teacher of health and a symbol of hope.

Nursing also has been defined as a science. A science is a body of knowledge based on carefully collected facts that have been arranged and classified in such a way as to establish certain laws and principles. Nursing today involves knowledge not only of biological and physical sciences, but also of social and behavioral sciences. The ability to understand and adjust to other people will have more influence than any other on the nurse's success.

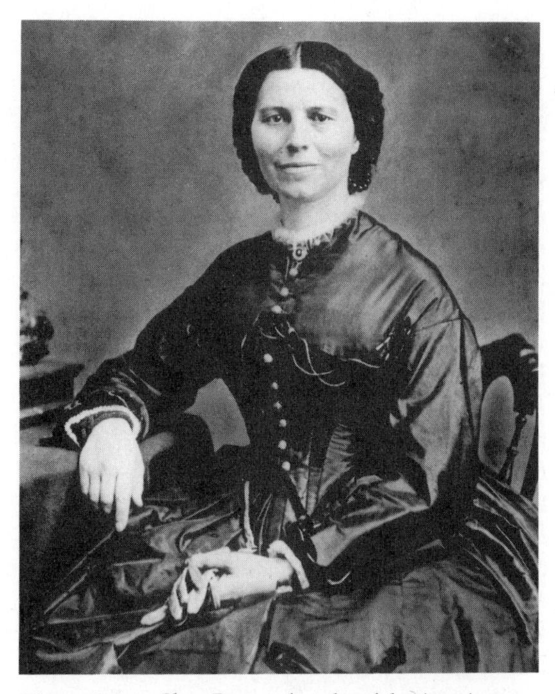

Figure 1–1 *Clara Barton, founder of the American Red Cross (Photo courtesy American Red Cross)*

MIDWIFERY AND MIDWIVES

From the earliest recorded time and in every culture women have attended other women in childbirth. In the fifth century B.C. the first formal training for midwives was instituted by Hippocrates. For centuries thereafter, however, efforts toward education were rare. Basic obstetrical knowledge for midwives was contained in two books: one published in 1513 by a surgeon named Rodienm, the other written by Jacob Rueff in 1554. Self-taught or instructed by older midwives, most midwives remained anonymous and ignorant of simple principles of obstetrics.

A few European midwives of the seventeenth and eighteenth centuries did achieve renown for their skill, writing, and devotion. Loyse Boursier (1563–1636) was a midwife to the French court and royal family for 27 years. Elizabeth Nihell (1723–?) was a famous English midwife who wrote *A Treatise on the Art of Midwifery* in 1760. During the seventeenth century, physicians did not participate in delivery. Their role was limited to writing prescriptions for drugs that a midwife wished to administer. As late as the eighteenth century, caring for pregnant women was considered beneath the dignity of physicians (usually men), who were summoned only in complicated or neglected cases.

The first known instance of midwifery in the New World occurred in 1621 when Mrs. Bridget Lee Fuller, with knowledge acquired from experience, helped in a delivery on the *Mayflower*. Anne Hutchinson, America's best remembered midwife, practiced in the mid-seventeenth century. In addition to her involvement as a midwife, she also was active in religious work. In 1637 she was condemned in Boston for her interpretations of the Bible. She was accused of witchcraft after she helped Jane Hawkins deliver a terribly deformed baby. Anne Hutchinson was massacred by Indians in the late summer of 1643. The Hutchinson River Parkway near New York City was named after this notable midwife.

Throughout the eighteenth and nineteenth centuries most labors were still attended by midwives, although the role of the physician was gradually increasing. Some midwives were called **granny midwives** or granny women; these women were untrained, often illiterate, and superstitious. Most were foreign-born or black and served in cities of the Northeast or on plantations of the South. The inept practices of the granny midwives were reflected in the maternal and infant mortality statistics, and the countless cases of gonorrheal ophthalmia resulting in blindness of the newborn.

REGULATION OF STANDARDS

By the sixteenth century, rules and regulations were being drawn up in many countries in order to improve the work of the midwives. In the seventeenth century, many cities required prospective midwives to work under a recognized and experienced midwife before being allowed to practice.

Legal regulation of midwifery standards began earlier in Western Europe than in the United States. The first formal edicts governing obstetrical practice were so general that they were virtually without effect. New York's ordinance of July 16, 1716, was more specific but dealt mainly with the midwife's ethical conduct and ignored her professional qualifications.

During the nineteenth century, medical licensure came under state control, but there was little regulation. A significant beginning toward effective regulation came in 1907 with the enactment of the State Midwifery Law, which transferred control of midwives in New York City to the city's board of health. The city's midwives were required to register annually, to demonstrate their ability to read and write, to be of good moral character, and to have attended a minimum of 20 cases of labor under the supervision of a licensed and registered physician. Enforcement of this law, however, was difficult, and many women continued to practice midwifery without training.

In 1910 about 50% of all births in the United States were reported by midwives. But a commissioned study made by New York State revealed that midwifery practices in the state were essentially medieval and very different from European midwifery. This study resulted in the tightening of existing legislation. A new institution was created with licensing and supervisory authority. That institution eventually became the Bellevue School of Midwives. In the early 1900s, it was the midwife's duty to assist in labor and delivery and to keep the household running normally. The midwife's training consisted of at least six months to a year of instruction on pregnancy, asepsis, care during labor, and care after delivery. Above all, the midwife was taught to recognize any condition that indicated a doctor was needed.

A commendable revival of educating midwives has taken place in the United States. Since 1915, the Maternity Center Association in New York City has been teaching midwifery. Also, training has taken place in several obstetrical centers such as Yale and Johns Hopkins Medical Center. Moreover, a revival of lay midwifery in the United States began in the mid-1970s with the renewed interest in childbirth in the home. By the end of 1977, lay midwives were licensed in 14 states, mostly in the South. Today, formal midwifery training is available nationwide and has stringent licensing requirements. Many hospitals are accepting licensed midwives to offer total care to the expectant mother, including delivery.

Even though the number of home births has increased, the American College of Nurse Midwives prefers the hospital or maternity home as the site for childbirth; these institutions can provide better for the physical welfare of both the mother and the infant. The college encourages members of the obstetrics team to provide for the personal needs of the family by combining a family-centered atmosphere with the safety of readily available obstetrical care, including the services of a physician.

HOSPITAL BIRTHS

During the period from 1930 to 1960 the proportion of births in hospitals increased from 36.9% (1935) to 88% (1950) to 96% (1960). During this period the campaign to hospitalize birth was supported by obstetricians, public health officials, upperclass women, and insurance companies. In 1946 the **Hill-Burton Act** provided funds for the construction of hospitals in rural areas, thereby creating the possibility of hospital birth for women who previously had no choice but to give birth at home, Figure 1–2.

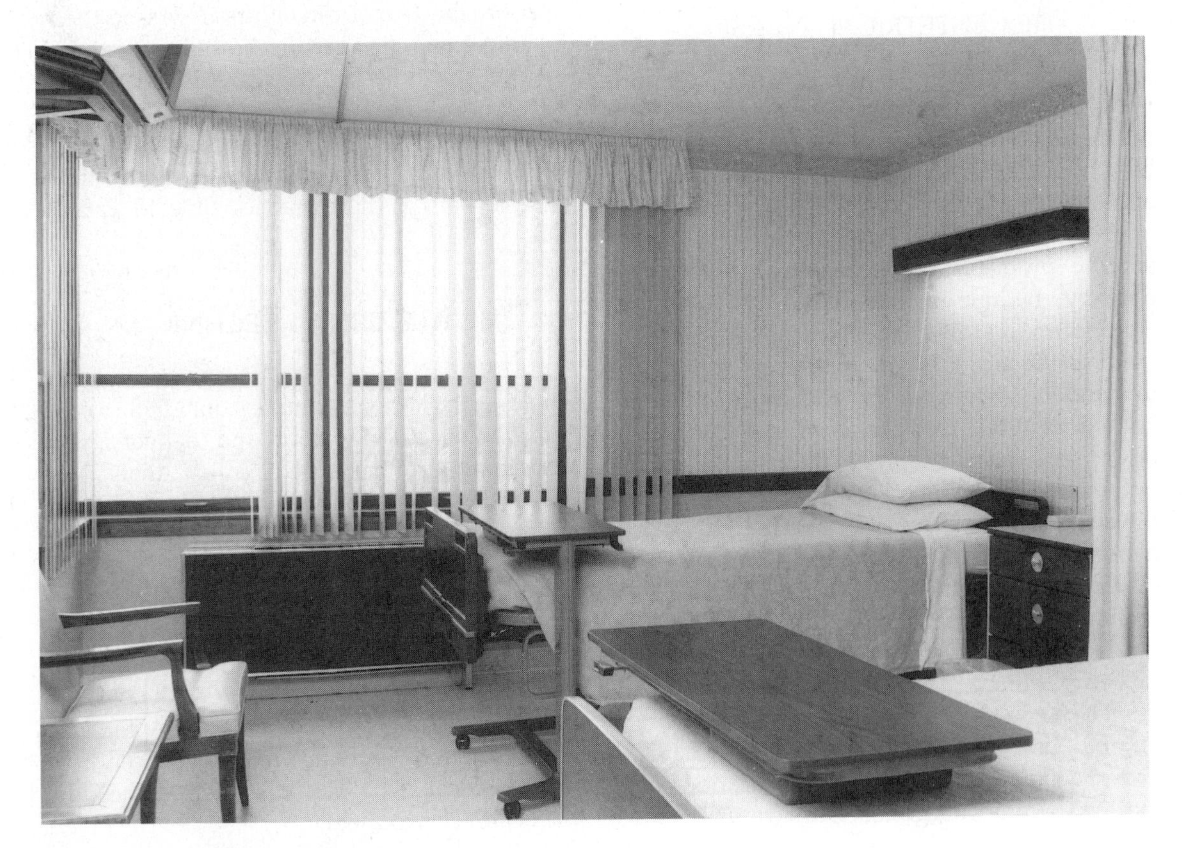

Figure 1–2 *Standard hospital room*

In the 1930s, when about 50% of deliveries in the United States were at home, the maternal mortality rate was 60 per 10,000 live births. In 1975, when more than 99% of deliveries were in hospitals, maternal mortality was less than 3 per 10,000 live births. This decrease is not a coincidence

Since the early 1980s, there has been a significant change in the hospital environment of obstetrical patients. There is a trend toward **family-centered maternity units**. Women are given a nicely decorated, homelike room. They labor, deliver their babies, recover, and remain in the same room throughout their hospital stay. This practice combines many of the benefits of a home delivery with the safety of a hospital birth.

THE OBSTETRICAL NURSE

Special obstetrical training for nurses began in the United States with the founding of maternity hospitals in the late nineteenth century and the establishment of separate departments of obstetrics in general hospitals. Instruction in specific problems of pregnancy, labor, and delivery became a standard part of the curriculum in nurses' training schools. As U.S. medical practice grew in complexity, nursing demanded greater skills. Maternity nurses known as **OB-GYN** (obstetrics and gynecology) nurse practitioners were trained to carry out many of the functions of the obstetrical physician. These nurses (1) take the patient's history, (2) perform the physical examination, (3) make an obstetrical evaluation, (4) manage and support the patient through labor up to the time of delivery, and (5) recognize obstetrical complication.

The most significant source of support for the obstetrical nurse in the United States and Canada is the Nurses Association of the American College of Obstetricians and Gynecologists **(NAACOG)**. The association was formed in 1969 and is committed to the goal of improving the health of women and newborn babies. In 1993, the organization was renamed Association of Women's Health, Obstetric, and Neonatal Nurses (AWHONN). The AWHONN conducts educational programs in obstetrical and gynecological nursing, and publishes the bimonthly *Journal of Obstetric, Gynecologic and Neonatal Nursing*.

To stimulate and recognize excellence in obstetrical and gynecological nursing, the association has formed the AWHONN Certification Corporation. This corporation has organized a voluntary joint certification program in maternal-gynecological-neonatal nursing in conjunction with the Division on Maternal and Child Health Nursing Practice of the American Nurses' Association. Examinations for certification were offered for the first time in 1976 to registered nurses who have been engaged in obstetrical-gynecological nursing for at least two consecutive years and who are currently devoting at least half of their practice time to patient care.

THE MATERNAL TECHNICIAN

The drastic shortage of nurses qualified to care for women during labor and delivery was apparent more than a decade ago. Analysis of the problem showed that an obstetrical technician could fill the need, just as the surgical technician fills a role in the operating room. The nursing shortage is apparent in all fields of nursing. With a basic understanding of the physiological principles related to pregnancy and birth, a technical knowledge of the process of normal labor, awareness of the symptoms of abnormal labor, and knowledge of procedures, an obstetrical technician fills a definite need in the health-service field.

CONSUMER INFLUENCE

The practice of obstetrics has changed radically since 1920 with the introduction of blood transfusions, knowledge of the Rh factor, the advent of antibiotics, progress in anesthesiology, and other new knowledge. Since the 1960s, maternity care has improved rapidly not only because of advances in technology and better trained nurses, but also because of a continued emphasis on educating consumers. This phenomenon has been very visible in the health field, particularly in the area of obstetrics.

The pregnant woman is involved in a natural process and does not have an illness or disease. However, prenatal health care is essential to prevent complications. With increased information and support from physicians and nurses, prepared childbirth classes, and an increasing abundance of literature for the expectant mother, women have more knowledge to take an active part in their own health care.

Consumers have already had a great effect on changing policies in obstetrics. Fathers now actively participate in labor and delivery, and babies are allowed to stay with their mothers during the hospital stay **(rooming-in)** rather than being viewed behind glass in the nursery, Figure 1–3. Other medical practices such as positions for delivery (semi-sitting, squatting, or side-lying), enemas on admission, and walking during labor have been influenced by the consumer.

Prepared childbirth classes have become a recommended choice by many expectant parents and allow the couple to participate more actively in the birth of their baby. **Lamaze**, **Dick-Read**, and **Bradley** are the three best known methods of childbirth preparation. All use special breathing and relaxation techniques and all attempt to educate participants about the physiology of childbirth. The methods differ mainly in the specific breathing patterns and the specific comfort-producing behaviors taught to couples for use during labor. All prepared childbirth philosophies have the common goal of making the birth experience personally satisfying and safe. Some of these groups and organizations are listed in Figure 1–4.

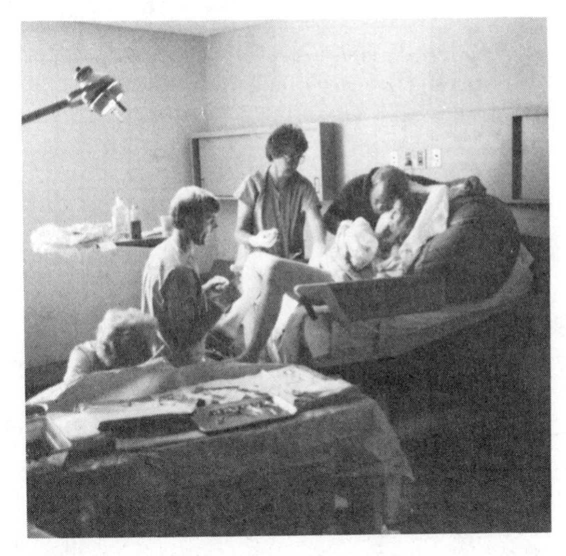

Figure 1–3 *Teamwork in action*

Hospitals and personnel are attempting to meet the desires of consumers. Many hospitals today have birthing rooms with cheerful wallpaper, dressers, sitting areas, and other amenities to create a more comfortable and homelike atmosphere, see Figure 1–5. Variations of the birthing room concept are found across the country. Some are a compromise between traditional delivery rooms and **alternative birthing centers (ABC)**, which began to open between 1976 and 1982. ABCs provide homelike accommodations for low-risk deliveries, but they are not in a hospital.

The concept underlying birthing rooms is that of humanizing the birth experience and emphasizing the individual. Traditionally the

RESOURCE GROUPS AND ORGANIZATIONS

American Academy of Husband Coached Childbirth
P.O. Box 5224
Sherman Oaks, CA 91413
(Teaches the Bradley method and has lists of local chapters.)

American Academy of Pediatrics
P.O. Box 1034
Evanston, IL 60204
(Has literature for parents and families.)

The American College of Home Obstetrics
664 North Michigan Avenue, Suite 600
Chicago, IL 60611

The American College of Nurse Midwives
1522 K Street, N.W., Suite 1120
Washington, D.C. 20005

American College of Obstetricians and Gynecologists
Suite 2700, Resource Center
1 East Wacker Drive
Chicago, IL 60601
(Has resource publication.)

American Foundation for Maternal and Child Health
30 Beekman Place
New York, NY 10022

American Society for Psychoprophylaxis in Obstetrics (ASPO)
1411 K Street, N.W.
Washington, D.C. 20005
(Teaches Lamaze technique, offers literature, and has lists of local chapters.)

Association for Childbirth at Home, International
Box 1219
Cerritos, CA 90701

Cesarean/Support, Education, and Concern
22 Forest Road
Framingham, MA 01701

Cooperative Birth Center Network (CBCN)
Box 1, Route 1
Perkiomenville, PA 18074

Coping with the Overall Pregnancy Experience (COPE)
37 Clarendon Street
Boston, MA 02116

The Farm
156 Drakes Lane
Summertown, TN 39483

Frontier Nursing Service
Wendover, KY 41775

Holistic Childbirth Institute
1627 10th Avenue
San Francisco, CA 94122

Home-Oriented Maternity Experience (HOME)
511 New York Avenue
Tacoma Park
Washington, D.C. 20010

Informed Home Birth, Inc.
P.O. Box 788
Boulder, CO 80306

International Childbirth Education Association (ICEA)
Box 20048
Minneapolis, MN 55420

La Leche League International, Inc.
9616 Minneapolis Avenue
Franklin Park, IL 60131
(Provides support for nursing mothers, list of local chapters, and a pattern for making a baby carrier.)

MANA (Midwives' Alliance of North America)
℅ Concord Midwifery Service
30 So. Main St.
Concord, NH 03301

Maternity Center Association, Inc.
48 East 92nd Street
New York, NY 10028
(Brochure on free publications.)

National Association of Parents and Professionals for Safe Alternatives in Childbirth (NAPSAC)
P.O. Box 267
Marble Hill, MO 63764
(Extensive directory of home-birth organizations throughout the world.)

U.S. Government Printing Office
Washington, D.C. 20402
(Information and publications on pregnancy.)

Figure 1–4

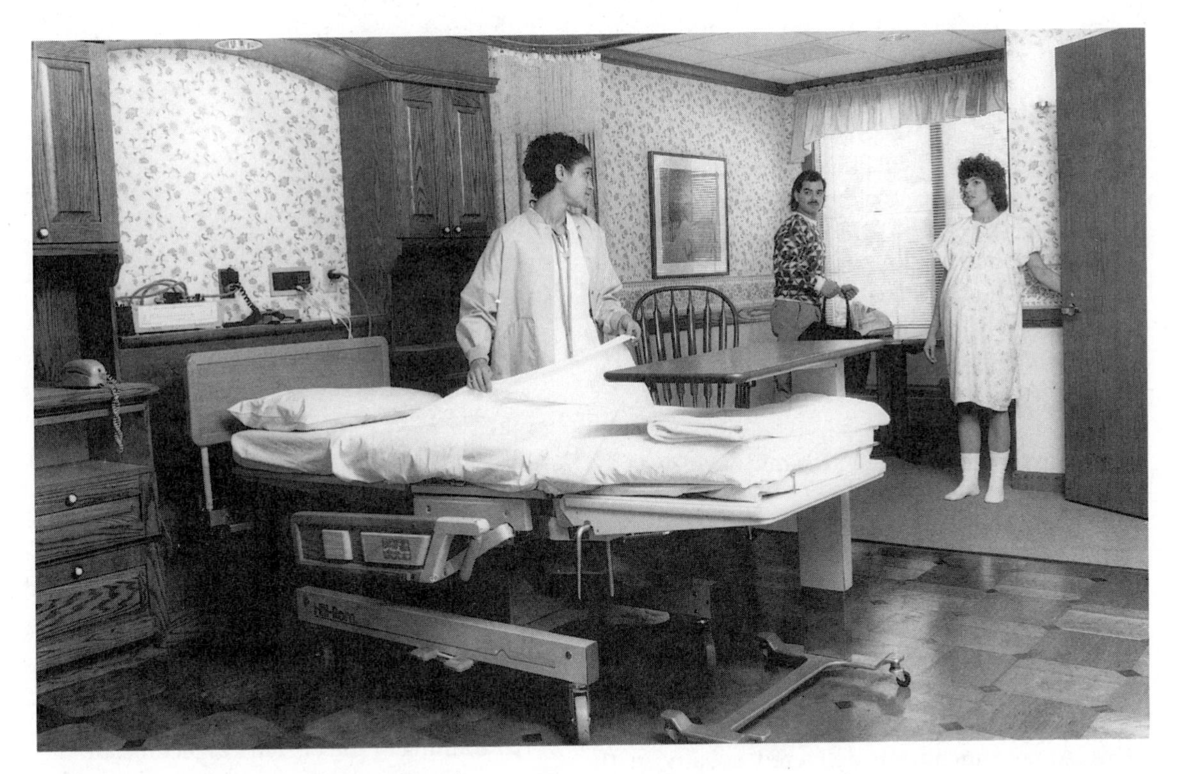

Figure 1–5 *Family-centered maternity unit*

mother has been moved to a postpartum unit after delivery. But birthing rooms provide a single unit for labor, delivery, and recovery of both mother and baby. These units are often referred to as LDRs (labor, delivery, recovery). LDRs minimize nursing staff and prevent disruption of the family unit during hospitalization. Advantages of a birthing room are:

- The nurse does not have to decide when to move the mother.
- No second room needs to be set up and cleaned.
- Cost in staff, linen, and equipment is reduced.
- Client satisfaction is increased.

ABCs have a crib for the newborn, private bathroom facilities, and lounge area. Many also provide a place for the father to sleep in the same room with the new mother and their baby. The philosophical difference between the ABC concept and a birthing room is based on screening criteria. ABCs should be used only by low-risk mothers. The nurse encourages couples to explore the birthing alternatives available to them so that they can make a responsible informed decision.

REVIEW QUESTIONS

A. Multiple choice. Select the best answer.

1. The factor that will have more influence than any other on the nurse's success will be
   a. a firm body of knowledge
   b. knowing how to educate others
   c. having the ability to understand, care for, and adjust to other people
   d. being licensed in her field

2. The first formal training for midwives was instituted in
   a. the fourteenth century
   b. the fifth century B.C.
   c. the seventeenth century
   d. the nineteenth century

3. The first known instance of midwifery in the United States occurred when
   a. Anne Hutchinson delivered a baby in New York City
   b. Bridget Lee Fuller helped in a delivery on the *Mayflower*
   c. Elizabeth Nihell wrote a book on midwifery
   d. Loyse Boursier came to the United States from France to practice midwifery

4. During the seventeenth century, the physician's role in obstetrics was to
   a. deliver the baby only
   b. attend the labor and delivery
   c. supervise the midwife
   d. write prescriptions for drugs that a midwife wished to administer

5. After 1935, the trend toward hospital births
   a. decreased the maternal mortality rate
   b. increased the infant mortality rate
   c. was limited only to upperclass women
   d. all of the above

6. The American College of Nurse Midwives recommends
   a. home deliveries
   b. strict laws governing midwives
   c. hospital or maternity-home deliveries
   d. prohibiting the licensing of lay midwives

7. During 1935, hospital births in the United States occurred at the rate of
   a. 36.9 percent
   b. 50 percent
   c. 88.4 percent
   d. 96 percent

8. The Hill-Burton Act of 1946 provided for
   a. tuition for education of midwives
   b. better regulation and licensing of midwives
   c. construction of hospitals in rural areas
   d. training of the obstetrical technician

9. Factors that have influenced the changing trends in obstetrics since 1960 include
   a. advances in technology
   b. better trained nurses
   c. consumer education
   d. all of the above

10. Midwife training in the early 1900s consisted of instruction in
    a. pregnancy, asepsis, and care during labor
    b. care of the mother and child after delivery
    c. recognizing conditions that require a doctor
    d. all of the above

11. Duties of the midwife during the early 1900s included
    a. notifying the physician when the delivery was about to occur
    b. assisting in labor and delivery and keeping the household running normally
    c. providing self-care instruction to the mother
    d. providing postnatal care for the newborn

B. Match the term in column II to the correct statement in column I.

Column I

1. homelike atmosphere where labor, delivery, and recovery take place
2. conducts educational programs in obstetrics and gynecology
3. first practitioners in the art of nursing
4. babies stay with their mothers during the hospital stay
5. carries out many of the functions of the obstetric physician
6. transferred control of midwives in New York City to the board of health
7. untrained, illiterate, superstitious midwives
8. influence the factors that determine physical, mental, and emotional pattern of each child
9. helps out in the obstetrical unit
10. wrote a basic obstetrics text in 1513
11. method of childbirth preparation
12. wrote *A Treatise on the Art of Midwifery*
13. to nourish, conserve energy, protect, and foster
14. notable American midwife of the seventeenth century
15. teaches midwifery

Column II

a. OB-GYN nurse practitioner
b. obstetrical technician
c. granny midwives
d. Anne Hutchinson
e. Rodienm
f. Dick-Read
g. Elizabeth Nihell
h. State Midwifery Law
i. Maternity Center Association
j. Nurses Association of the American College of Obstetricians and Gynecologists
k. birthing room
l. rooming-in
m. parents
n. *nutricius*
o. mothers

SUGGESTED ACTIVITIES

- Describe the setting and the style of care a patient might expect in:
  - a hospital
  - an alternative birthing center
  - a home birth with midwife
- Describe ways in which the prenatal period may affect the newborn and beyond toward adolescence. List ways the nurse could be helpful to the family in influencing a positive outcome.

BIBLIOGRAPHY

Cianfrani, T. *A Short History of Obstetrics and Gynecology*. Springfield, IL: Charles C. Thomas, 1960.

Simkin, P., Whalley, J., and A. Keppler. *Pregnancy, Childbirth and the Newborn*. Deephaven, MN: Meadowbrook Books, 1991.

CHAPTER

2

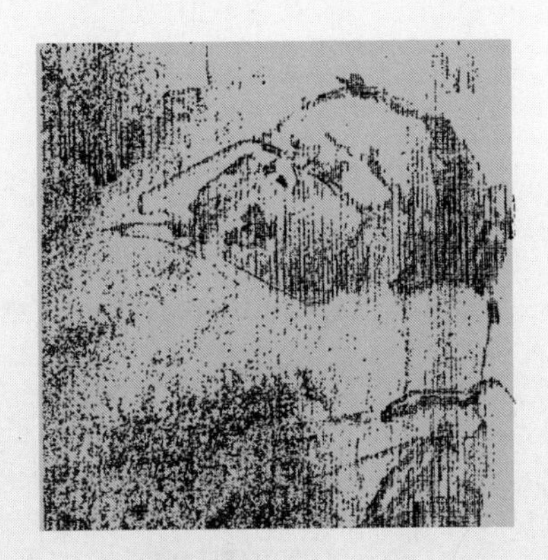

The Female Reproductive System

Objectives

After studying this chapter, the student should be able to:

- State the primary functions of the female reproductive system.
- Identify the primary parts of the female reproductive system.
- Explain the function of each of the primary parts of the female reproductive system.
- Explain the interrelated processes of menstruation and ovulation.
- List the functions of estrogen, progesterone, FSH, and LH.

Key Terms

- OBSTETRICS
- OVUM
- FERTILIZATION
- VULVA
- LABIA MAJORA
- MONS PUBIS
- LABIA MINORA
- PREPUCE
- CLITORIS
- BARTHOLIN'S GLANDS
- URINARY MEATUS
- HYMEN
- PERINEUM
- ANUS
- VAGINA
- UTERUS
- ENDOMETRIUM
- MYOMETRIUM
- PERIMETRIUM
- CERVIX
- INTERNAL OS
- EXTERNAL OS
- UTERINE LIGAMENTS
- FALLOPIAN TUBES
- OVARIES
- OVULATION
- MENSTRUATION
- FOLLICULAR (PREOVULATORY) PHASE
- ESTROGEN
- PROLIFERATIVE PHASE
- CORPUS LUTEUM
- LUTEAL PHASE
- PROGESTERONE
- SECRETORY PHASE
- CHORIONIC GONADOTROPIN
- AMENORRHEA
- MENORRHAGIA
- METRORRHAGIA
- DYSMENORRHEA
- ANOVULATORY MENSTRUATION
- INNOMINATE BONES
- GYNECOID PELVIS
- ANDROID PELVIS
- ANTHROPOID PELVIS
- PLATYPELLOID PELVIS
- LEVATOR ANI
- AREOLA
- GLANDS OF MONTGOMERY
- ALVEOLI
- ACINI
- PUBERTY
- MENARCHE
- MENOPAUSE

Obstetrics is the branch of medical science that deals with childbirth and that which precedes and follows it. The nurse must understand the reproductive process in order to administer nursing care to the obstetrical patient before and during childbirth. A knowledge of this process is also essential to caring for the mother and child after delivery.

Human life begins with the union of two cells: one from the female, called the **ovum,** and one from the male, called the sperm. This union of male and female cells, known as **fertilization** or conception, takes place within the female. She is responsible, both directly and indirectly, for the growth and development of the fertilized ovum that eventually results in the birth of a child. A beginning study should first examine the female reproductive system to discover how it is specially adapted for this purpose.

The female reproductive system has four basic functions:

- to produce ovarian hormones, which are responsible for female sex characteristics and reproductive functions;
- to produce the ovum and a favorable environment for conception to occur and to deliver the ovum to the uterus;
- to nurture and sustain the developing fertilized ovum until birth; and
- to accomplish delivery of the product of conception.

The female reproductive system includes the external genitals, internal organs, the pelvis and related pelvic structures, and the breasts.

EXTERNAL GENITALS

The external genitals are adjacent to but outside the entrance to the vagina, Figure 2–1. They protect the vagina and provide access for the male reproductive organ.

THE VULVA

The **vulva** consists of two heavy lips called the **labia majora** and the external structures contained within them. The outside surface of the labia majora is composed of skin and fat and covered with pubic hair. The inner surface resembles mucous membrane. The labia extend from the **mons pubis**, a pad of fat covering the pubic area, to the perineum. The function of the labia majora is to cover and protect the vaginal entrance.

Inside the labia majora are two smaller lips called the **labia minora**. These thinner lips meet to form a partial hood called the **prepuce**, which covers a tiny erectile structure, the **clitoris**. This structure is a small elongated mass of tissue, nerves, and muscle richly supplied with blood vessels and covered with

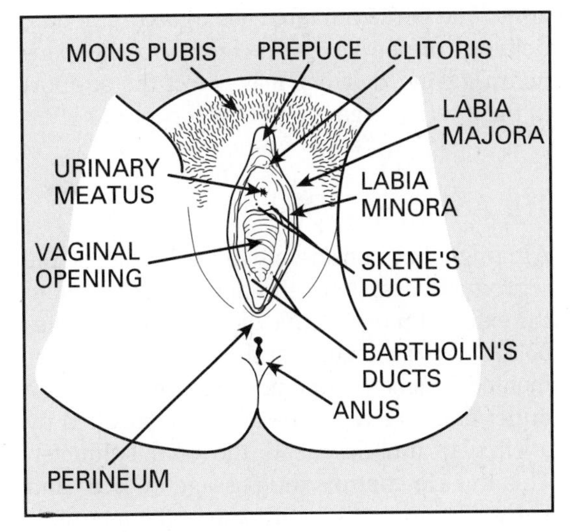

Figure 2–1 External genitals

mucous membrane. The clitoris is like the penis in that it is extremely sensitive and responds to sexual excitation. **Bartholin's glands** secrete a mucoid, lubricating substance during sexual intercourse. One gland is located on each side of the vaginal opening. Below the clitoris are two raised ridges with an opening, called the **urinary meatus**, between them. Urine is voided through this opening. On either side of this opening of the urethra are the paraurethral ducts, or Skene's ducts.

Just below the meatus is a fold of mucous membrane called the **hymen**, which protects the vaginal opening. The hymen partly (and occasionally completely) closes the outlet of the vagina. Contrary to popular belief, rupture of the hymen is not necessarily an indication of sexual activity. It could occur from injury, surgery, use of tampons for menstruation, active sports, or gynecological examination.

THE PERINEUM

The area of skin, connective tissue, and muscle between the vulva and the anus is known as the **perineum**. The muscle tissues affect the opening and closing of the vagina and the anus. The perineum stretches to accommodate delivery of the newborn. Injury to the perineum during delivery may affect the support of the internal organs and bowel control.

THE ANUS

Although not considered to be a part of the reproductive system, the anus is adjacent to the external reproductive organs. The **anus** lies below the perineum and is a deeply pigmented, puckered opening that serves as the outlet of the rectum. The anus is controlled by a circular muscle called the anal sphincter. This muscle controls the passage of feces and flatus. The mucous membrane of the rectum is very sensitive and easily injured. Because of its anatomical position, the rectum is sometimes used for examining procedures during pregnancy and labor.

INTERNAL ORGANS

The internal reproductive organs lie within the pelvic cavity. They consist of the vagina, uterus, fallopian tubes, and ovaries. Also included are the supporting structures, Figure 2–2.

THE VAGINA

The **vagina** is a curved tubelike passage 8–12 cm (centimeters) long that leads from the vulva to the uterus. The lower portion of the uterus, called the cervix, protrudes into it. The vagina is internally situated between the bladder and rectum. The vagina is made up of muscle and connective tissue and is capable of great distention during childbirth. It is lined with mucous membrane containing many folds called rugae. The secretion observed in the vagina is derived largely from glands of the cervix. The vagina serves three important functions as a passage: (1) introduction of the penis and reception of semen (fluid in which sperm is carried), (2) discharge of menstrual flow and uterine secretions, and (3) delivery of the product of conception.

THE UTERUS

The **uterus** is the organ that holds the fetus during pregnancy. It is a hollow, pear-shaped organ with thick muscular walls, and is 6 cm–7½ cm (2½–3 in.) long and ≈ 2 cm (¾ in.) thick. It occupies the middle of the pelvis between the bladder and the rectum (see Figure 2–3) and consists of the fundus (rounded top part), the body (middle part), and a narrow lower portion (the cervix, or neck). The fundus and body make up the cor-

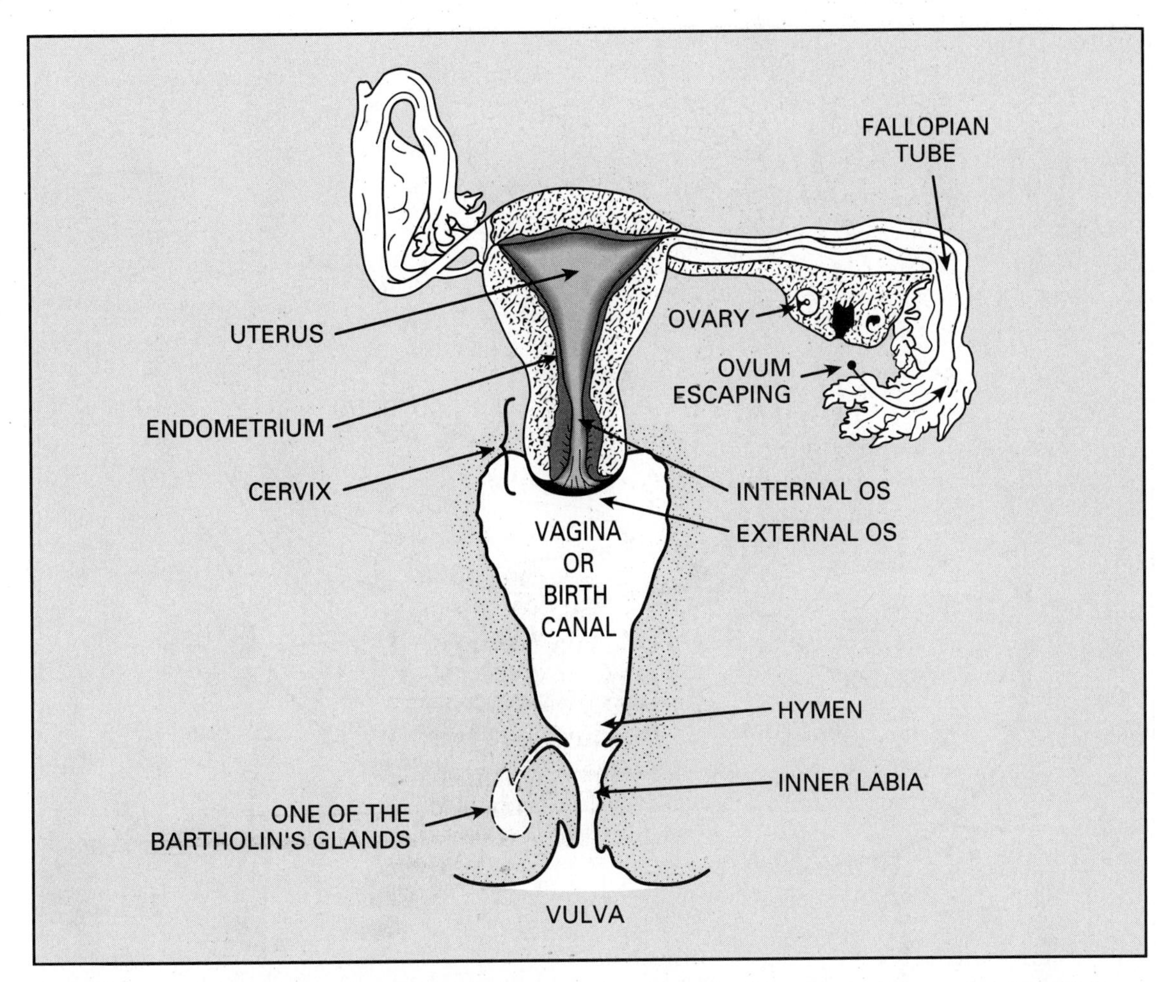

Figure 2–2 *Internal female reproductive organs (Adapted from Educational Department, Tampax, Inc., New York)*

pus of the uterus. The lining of the uterus is called the **endometrium**. The muscular substance of the uterus is called the **myometrium**, and the connective tissue around the muscle is the **perimetrium**, Figure 2–4a. The endometrium receives and nourishes the fertilized egg. During pregnancy, the uterus grows very soft and increases greatly in size to hold the growing fetus. By the end of pregnancy, the uterus becomes a thin, soft-walled muscular sac that yields to the movement of the fetus.

About half the length of the **cervix** projects into the vagina where the vaginal walls are attached to it. The cervix has a small round passageway called the cervical canal; the **internal os** (mouth, or opening) of the canal opens into the uterus, and the **external os** opens into the vagina. Uterine secretions, the menstrual flow, the unfertilized ovum, the fetus during labor, and the lochial discharge (vaginal drainage during the six-week period following delivery) pass through the cervix to the vagina. The cervix also is instrumental in helping the process of fertilization by producing a mucus that aids sperm's movement through this passageway on their journey to find the ovum.

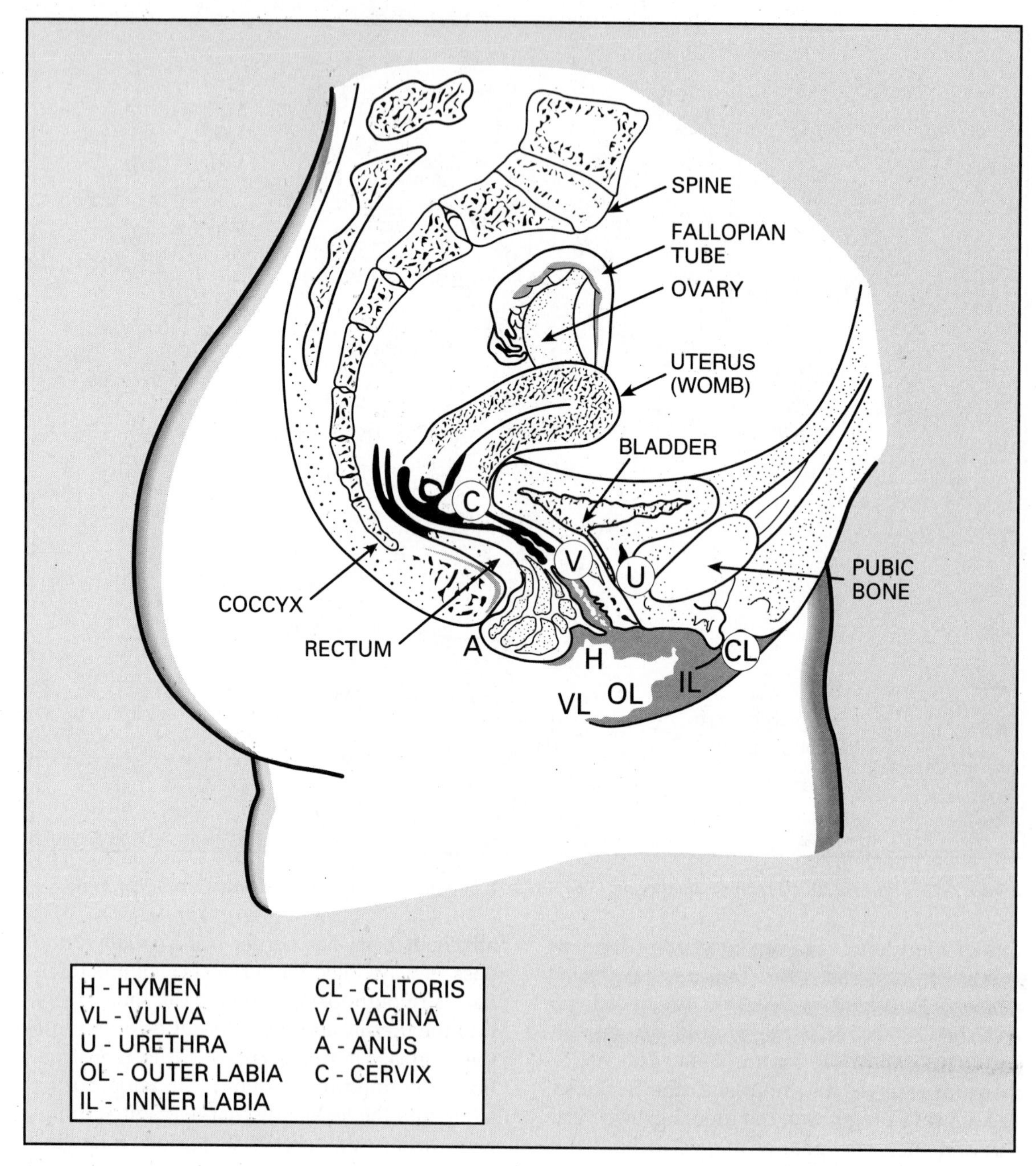

Figure 2–3 *Side view of the female pelvic organs (Adapted from Educational Department, Tampax, Inc., New York)*

THE UTERINE LIGAMENTS

The broad **uterine ligaments** are two structures that extend from the side walls of the uterus to the pelvic walls. The ovaries and fallopian tubes are attached to these ligaments. The round ligaments of the uterus, attached to the

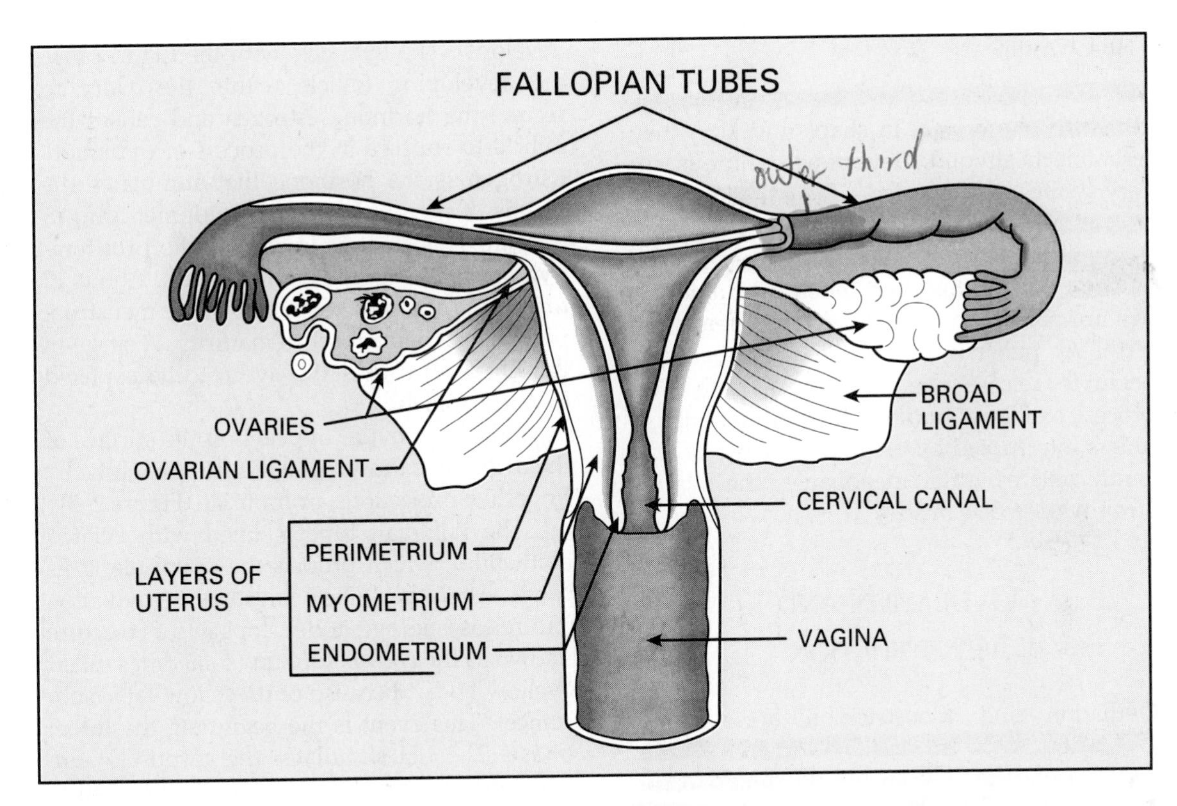

Figure 2–4a

side walls of the uterus, pass through the broad ligaments to reach the mons pubis. These ligaments help to support the pelvic organs. The uterosacral ligaments extend from the posterior cervical portion of the uterus to the sacrum and support the cervix, Figure 2–4b.

THE FALLOPIAN TUBES

The two **fallopian tubes**, or oviducts, extend outward from the upper corners of the uterus to the abdominal cavity. They are about the diameter of a drinking straw and are largely muscular structures. The distal portion of the tube curves around the ovary in such a way that the fingerlike projections (called fimbriae) cup over the ovary but are not actually attached to it. Their function is to carry the ovum along the canal by peristaltic action from the ovary to the uterus. Conception normally takes place in the outer third of a fallopian tube.

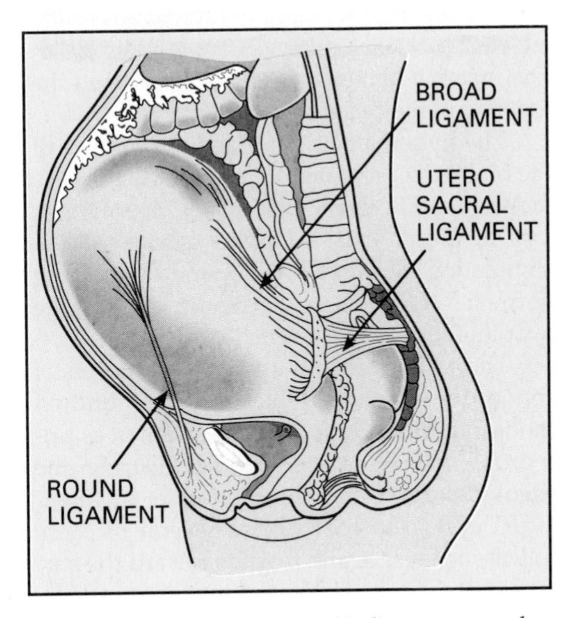

Figure 2–4b *Uterus suspended by ligaments; round, broad, and uterosacral*

THE OVARIES

The two **ovaries** are also known as the sex glands of the female. In shape and size, they resemble an almond; they are hard, fibrous, silvery white, and dimpled. Their functions are to mature and discharge ova and to produce hormones necessary to the process of reproduction. Several hundred thousand immature ova are present in the ovaries of the female at birth. At puberty, the ovaries systematically begin to release one ovum at a time. The process continues until the time of menopause unless interrupted by pregnancy or use of oral contraceptives. After menopause, the ovaries atrophy (decrease in size).

OVULATION AND MENSTRUATION

Ovulation and menstruation are related. **Ovulation** is the process by which a mature ovum is released and the uterus is made ready to receive the fertilized ovum. **Menstruation** is the process of shedding the unnecessary uterine lining when conception does not occur. The first day of menstruation is considered the first day of the cycle.

The hypothalamus, a gland at the base of the brain, releases gonadotropin-releasing hormone (GnRH). GnRH stimulates the anterior lobe of the pituitary gland to secrete follicle-stimulating hormone (FSH) and luteinizing hormone (LH). These hormones control the ovarian function in the female.

The interior of the ovary is composed of connective tissue in which several hundred thousand microscopic structures known as primordial follicles are embedded. During the **preovulatory**, or **follicular, phase** of the menstrual cycle, the FSH causes several of these follicles to enlarge and migrate toward the surface of the ovary. Under the influence of FSH, one of these follicles develops into a graafian follicle (microscopic sac in which the ovum develops). The FSH acts with the LH to cause the developing follicle within the ovary to secrete the hormone estrogen and causes the follicle to rupture in the process of ovulation. **Estrogen** is the hormone that stimulates the glands of the uterine lining (endometrium) to thicken. This stage is known as the **proliferative phase** within the endometrium. About 12 to 16 days after the beginning of the menstrual period, the ovum reaches maturity. A surge in the LH level causes the ovum to be expelled from the follicle.

When the ovum appears on the surface of the ovary, it is drawn into the fallopian tube by fingerlike projections, or fimbriae (Figure 2–5).

The fallopian tube is lined with ciliated epithelium, which propels the ovum along its route. After the follicle ruptures in ovulation and releases its egg, it develops into a structure known as the **corpus luteum** (sometimes called "yellow body" because of its yellow fatty substance). This event is the beginning the **luteal phase**. The LH stimulates the corpus luteum (contained within the ovary) to secrete another hormone, **progesterone**, which increases the number and length of the blood vessels in the endometrium and causes uterine secretions. The endometrium is now in the **secretory phase**, see Figure 2–6. These changes prepare the uterus to receive the fertilized ovum. At this point, the uterine lining is engorged with blood and is thick and spongy. If conception does not occur, the corpus luteum disintegrates, the secretion of hormones decreases, and a portion of the endometrium is discharged through the vagina as the menstrual flow. The menstrual flow consists of mucous secretions, tissue fragments, and blood. After menstruation, the endometrium of the uterus is very thin, as shown in Figure 2–7.

If the ovum is fertilized, menstruation does not occur. After implantation, the fertilized ovum secretes a hormone called human **chorionic gonadotropin** hormone that enables the corpus luteum to continue to secrete progesterone during the first three months of

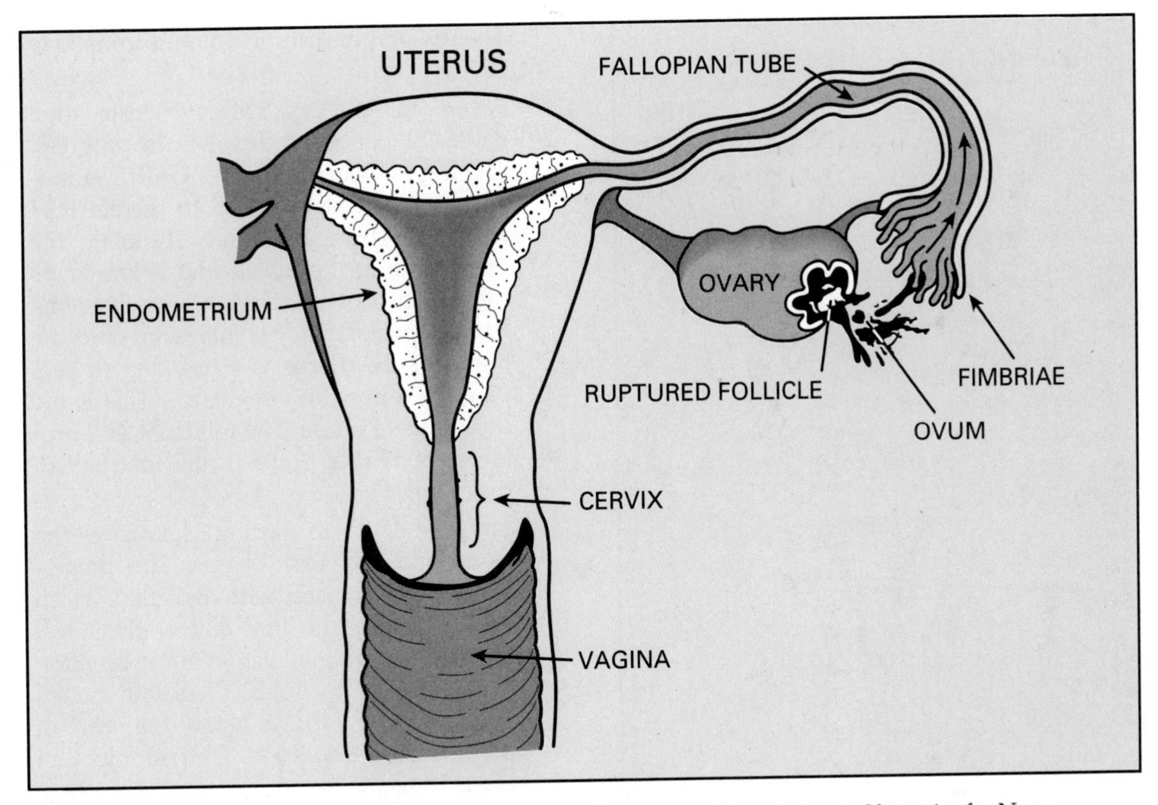

Figure 2–5 *Ovulation. The release of the ovum from the follicle (Adapted from* DeLee's Obstetrics for Nurses, *W. B. Saunders)*

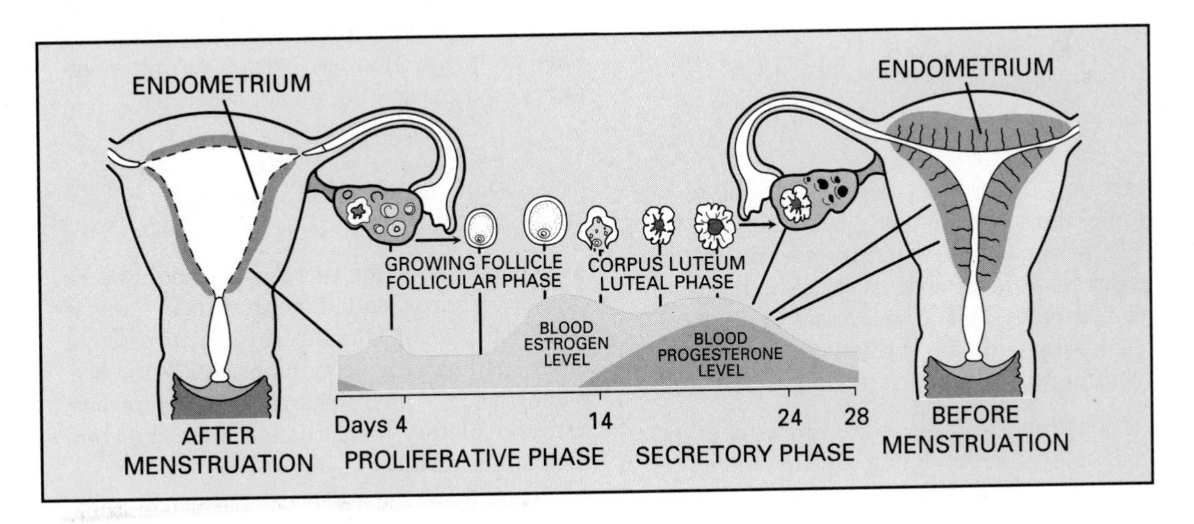

Figure 2–6 *Hormones regulate the reproductive organs.*

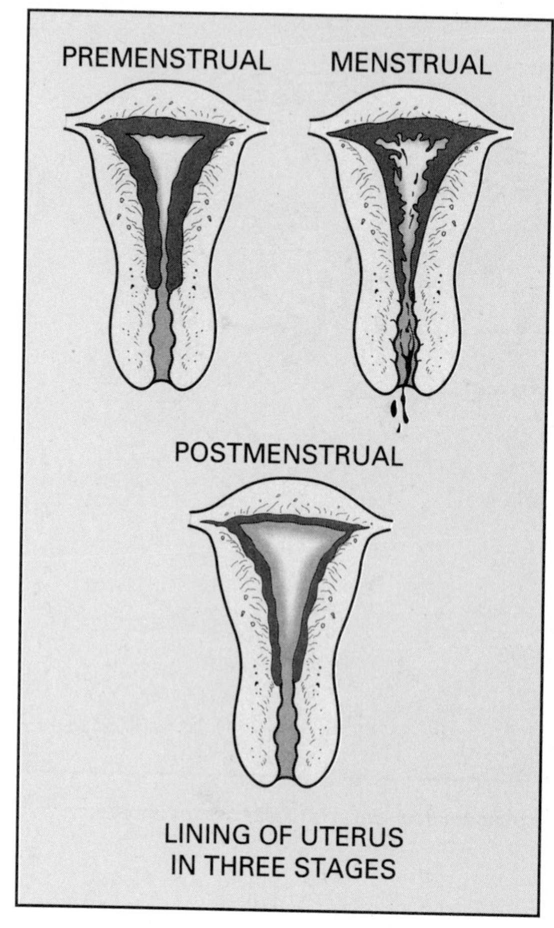

Figure 2–7 *The uterus changes during the menstrual cycle. (Adapted from Educational Department, Tampax, Inc., New York)*

pregnancy. After this period, the placenta assumes the secretion of progesterone.

In summary, the menstrual cycle begins with menstruation and is usually repeated every 28 days. This approximate cycle, however, varies with the individual. The events that occur during the cycle are:

- Menstruation lasts from three to seven days while the lining of the uterus is expelled. The onset of menses is considered the beginning of the menstrual cycle. The discharge varies in amount from 30 to 200 mL.
- Seven to 10 days after menstruation begins, a period of repair is in progress. The hypothalamus releases GnRH, stimulating the pituitary gland to secrete FSH and LH. These hormones stimulate the maturation of the follicle and is known as the follicular phase. The estrogen hormone level from the ovary is increasing and the lining of the uterus is thickening to prepare for a possible pregnancy. This is the proliferative phase. The follicular and proliferative phases occur in the first half of the cycle.
- The next 12 to 16 days are known as the luteal and secretory phases. The progesterone level increases with ovulation, which occurs around the first day of the luteal phase. It is during ovulation that conception is most likely to occur. Ovulation occurs approximately 14 days before the onset of the next expected period. The endometrium is made ready during this secretory phase either to accept the fertilized ovum or to be released as menstrual flow.

The cycle begins again and continues at regular intervals. Variations of the menstrual cycle occur in the follicular and proliferative phases. This process continues, except during pregnancy, and ceases after menopause.

ABNORMAL CONDITIONS RELATED TO MENSTRUATION

Abnormalities in the menstrual cycle may be caused by stress, endocrine dysfunction, overwork, change of climate, chronic disease, or other pathological conditions. Amenorrhea, menorrhagia, metrorrhagia, dysmenorrhea, and anovulatory menstruation are some common abnormalities.

- **Amenorrhea** is a permanent or temporary suppression of menstruation. It occurs as a normal condition before puberty, during pregnancy, between periods, sometimes during lactation, and after menopause. The absence of menstruation may be congenital, or it may be due to the removal of the uterus. It may also be caused by an obstruction of the cervix or vagina, which prevents external flow. A debilitating disease, severe anemia, thyroid imbalance, psychical upsets, and excessive exercise can also cause amenorrhea.

- **Menorrhagia** is prolonged or excessive bleeding during the menstrual period.
- **Metrorrhagia** is vaginal bleeding at a time other than the normal menstrual period.
- **Dysmenorrhea** is painful menstruation.
- **Anovulatory menstruation** is menstruation that takes place even though the ovary has failed to expel or discharge the egg. Without ovulation, fertilization cannot occur; failure to ovulate is one cause of infertility.

THE PELVIS

The pelvis, illustrated in Figure 2–8, is formed by three **innominate bones** (the ilium, the ischium, and the pubis), the sacrum, the coccyx, and the ligaments connecting them. The innominate bones form the lateral and anterior boundaries of the pelvis. The sacrum, a large, wedge-shaped bone composed of five consolidated sacral vertebrae, forms the posterior wall of the pelvis. The coccyx is a small, triangular bone made up of four vertebrae fused together, located at the end of the spine. It is connected to the sacrum by a hinge-type joint and forms part of the posterior boundary of the pelvis. The coccyx helps support the pelvic floor.

The pelvis is further separated into the false pelvis and the true pelvis. The upper flaring part is termed the false pelvis. The false pelvis is seldom involved in the problems of labor. The true pelvis is the lower part of the pelvis. It forms the bony canal through which the baby must pass during delivery. The pelvic inlet, sometimes referred to as the pelvic brim, divides the false pelvis from the true pelvis.

The male pelvis is heavier, narrower, and deeper than the female pelvis. A female pelvis can be gynecoid, android, anthropoid, or platypelloid in shape, Figure 2–9. About 50%

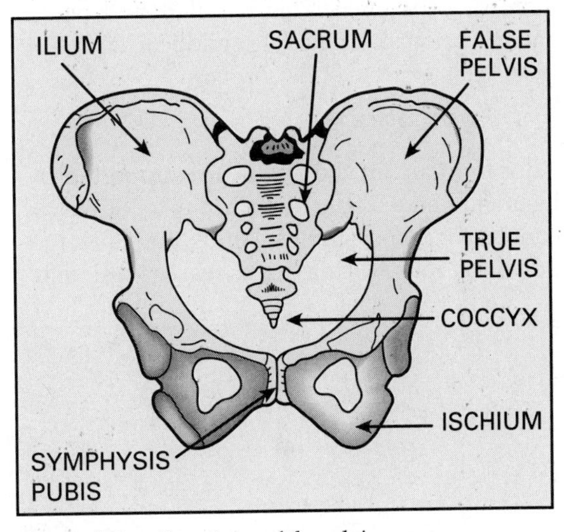

Figure 2–8 *Structures of the pelvis*

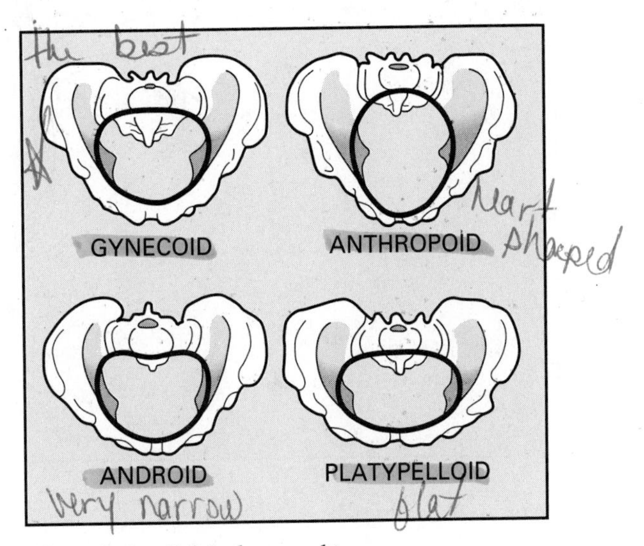

Figure 2–9 *Pelvis shapes and types*

of women have a **gynecoid pelvis**. This is a round or transverse oval pelvis and is good for childbearing. An **android pelvis** is heart- or wedge-shaped and is less suitable for childbearing. The **anthropoid pelvis** has a greater anteroposterior diameter and is narrower in its transverse plane. This pelvis is also well suited for vaginal delivery. The **platypelloid pelvis** is the least common of shapes, occurring in less than 5% of women. This is a flattened pelvis and does not accommodate childbearing well.

THE PELVIC FLOOR

All the organs in the pelvis are supported by ligaments and fascias, which are made up of connective tissue, strands, bands, and layers. A powerful muscle called the **levator ani** reinforces the pelvic ligaments and fascias. The levator ani forms a "hammock," which extends from the side walls of the pelvis and meets in the middle line around the anus and vagina. The vagina, rectum, bladder, and uterus are suspended by ligaments and fascias above the levator ani, Figure 2–10.

The internal reproductive organs, which form a canal for the passage of the ovum and sperm, contain muscle and connective tissue completely lined with mucous membrane. They are partly covered by the peritoneum, a transparent membrane that lines the abdominal cavity. Characteristics of the mucous membrane vary according to the function required by the part. The membrane of the vulva is very sensitive; in the vagina it is rough and strong; the membrane lining the cervix and uterus is

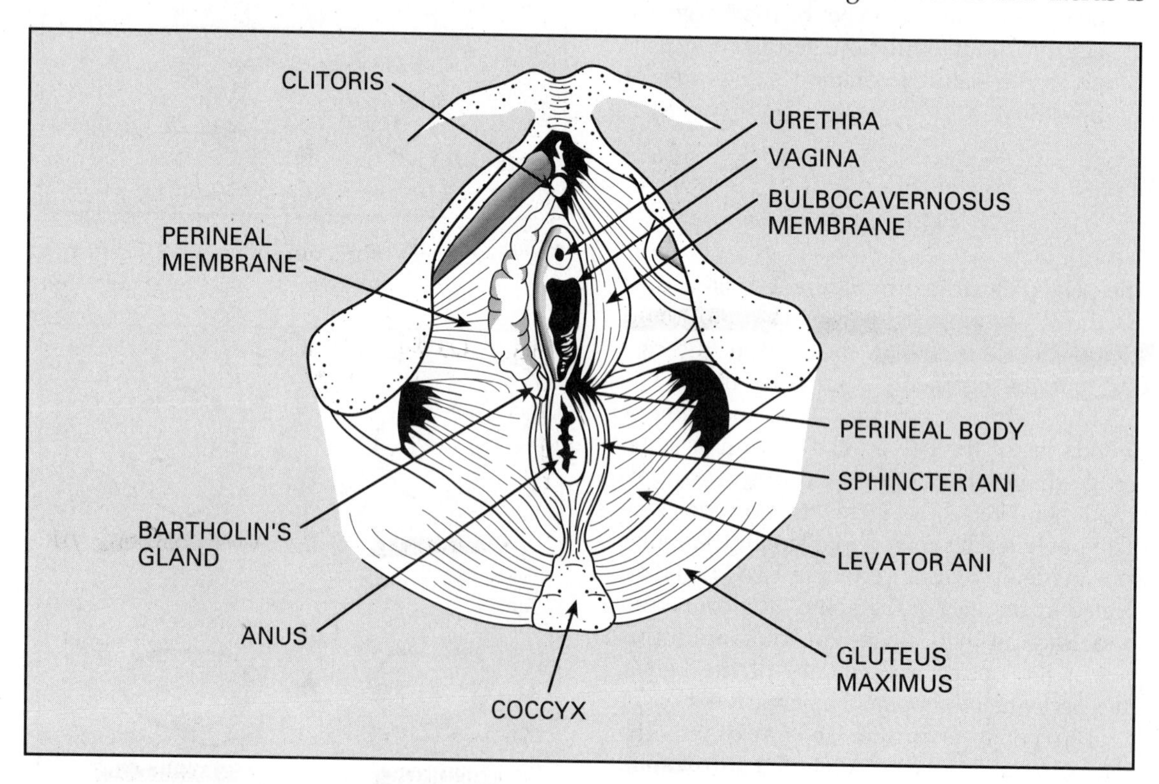

Figure 2–10 *Perineum*

very vascular and strong. The epithelium is a layer of cells forming the surface layer of mucous membrane of the fallopian tubes and uterus. In the fallopian tubes, it is covered with microscopic "hairs," or cilia, which, by their waving action, assist in transporting the ovum.

RELATED STRUCTURES OF THE PELVIS

Related pelvic structures are the ureters, bladder, urethra, and rectum. The ureters convey the urine from the kidneys to the bladder. The bladder lies behind the pubis and in front of the uterus. It is a storage space for urine. The urethra leads from the bladder to the urinary meatus. Bladder distention delays the progress of labor.

The rectum is the terminal portion of the bowel. It opens externally to the anus and lies behind the uterus in the pelvic cavity.

THE BREASTS

The breasts are considered to be accessory reproductive organs since they play an important part in pregnancy and lactation. They are located over the anterior part of the chest. The external breast is divided into three portions: (1) the soft area of skin; (2) the **areola**, which surrounds the nipple and contains the **glands of Montgomery**; and (3) the nipple.

Internally, each breast contains 15 to 20 lobes of glandular tissue (the mammary glands) and fat. The mammary glands are responsible for the production of milk (lactation). The lobes of the mammary gland consist of several lobules arranged in clusters around tiny ducts. These clusters are called **alveoli** and are lined with milk-producing cells called **acini**. As the ducts lead from the alveoli to the lobes and from the lobes to the nipple, they dilate to form little reservoirs in which milk is stored, Figure 2–11. The size of the breasts varies with the amount of fat deposited in them, but there is no relationship between size and the ability to produce milk. As pregnancy progresses, the breasts undergo physiological changes to make them ready for the demands of nursing the newborn infant.

THE CYCLE OF CHANGE: PUBERTY TO MENOPAUSE

The female reproductive system undergoes great changes during the life cycle of the individual. Even before birth, the reproductive organs are undergoing growth and development as the fetus grows and develops. The reproductive organs generally reach maturity during puberty. **Puberty** is the period between ages 12 and 18 during which the individual becomes capable of reproduction. In women, the production of a mature ovum (ovulation) usually occurs several months after the first menstrual period **(menarche)**. During puberty, the size of the external and internal genitals increases, pubic hair develops, and the breasts enlarge, primarily because increasing amounts of the hormone estrogen are secreted. Although mammary glands are present in both sexes, they normally develop and function only in the female. At puberty, female breasts are influenced to develop by the hormones estrogen and progesterone. The childbearing years extend from the onset of ovulation to menopause.

Menopause is the permanent physiological cessation of the menstrual flow. The ovaries atrophy as do the uterus, breasts, and external genitals. Ovulation ceases, and childbearing is no longer possible.

Menopause, sometimes referred to as the "change of life," is a normal physiological process; it is not an illness. Like menarche, the time it occurs varies with the individual.

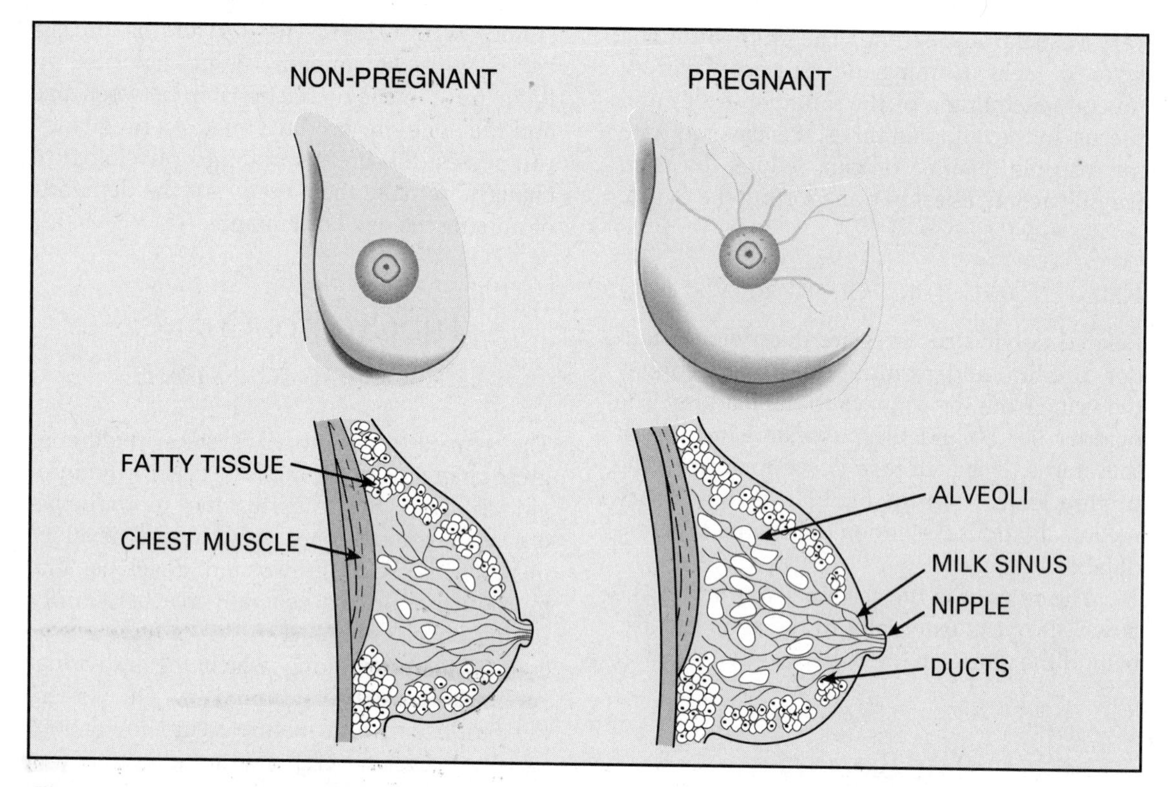

Figure 2–11 The mammary glands prepare the breasts for nursing the newborn. (Adapted from Nursing Education Aid, No. 10, Courtesy Ross Laboratories)

last about 18 mths

Menopause occurs between the ages of 45 and 55 in about 50% of all females. Surgical removal of the ovaries also causes menopause. Between the ages of 35 and 55 years, there are approximately 10,000 ova remaining in the ovaries; more than 400,000 are present at birth.

The tendency to gain weight during menopause is common. Nervous disturbances, hot flashes, and sweating may occur because of the decreased level of sex hormones. Women may also report difficulty sleeping well and complain of vaginal dryness during this time. Anxiety and irritability may also be symptoms. Women may experience these symptoms before menses stops entirely; however, most will note a change in their menstrual pattern. Hormone treatment may be ordered by the physician to relieve these conditions. Hormone therapy also has been shown to be effective in decreasing the risks of osteoporosis and cardiovascular disease, and is therefore recommended by many physicians for general health maintenance.

REVIEW QUESTIONS

A. Multiple choice. Select the best answer.

1. At the opening of the vagina is a fold of mucous membrane called the
   a. urinary meatus
   b. hymen
   c. clitoris
   d. perineum

2. Ova travel from the ovaries to the uterus through the
   a. internal os
   b. external os
   c. fallopian tubes
   d. fascia

3. The union of the sperm and ovum is called
   a. gestation
   b. coitus
   c. intercourse
   d. conception or fertilization

4. The labia majora extend from the perineum to the
   a. clitoris
   b. vagina
   c. urinary meatus
   d. mons pubis

5. The lining of the uterus is called the
   a. labia majora
   b. endometrium
   c. cilia
   d. myometrium

6. The organ of sexual excitation in the female is the
   a. cervix
   b. vagina
   c. clitoris
   d. labia majora

7. The basic functions of the female reproductive system are to
   a. produce ovarian hormones, which are responsible for the female sex characteristics and reproductive functions
   b. produce the ovum and deliver it to the place where conception may take place
   c. nurture and sustain the product of conception until birth and accomplish delivery of the product of conception
   d. all of the above

8. The organs of the pelvis are supported by
   a. fascias and ligaments
   b. muscle
   c. the levator ani
   d. cilia

9. The function of the ovaries is to
   a. mature and discharge ova
   b. produce hormones
   c. neither of the above
   d. a and b

10. The part of the pelvis that is most involved with childbirth is the
    a. coccyx
    b. sacrum
    c. true pelvis
    d. false pelvis

11. The area of skin, connective tissue, and muscle between the vulva and anus is called the
    a. perineum
    b. urinary meatus
    c. labia
    d. fascia

12. Conception usually takes place in the
    a. uterus
    b. fallopian tube
    c. ovary
    d. cervix

13. The neck of the uterus is called the
    a. vagina
    b. perineum
    c. cervix
    d. labia majora

14. Located on each side of the labia minora and responsible for secreting a mucoid, lubricating substance during sexual intercourse is (are) the
    a. cilia
    b. Bartholin's glands
    c. hymen
    d. prepuce

15. Gonadotropic hormones are secreted by the
    a. graafian follicle
    b. pituitary gland
    c. corpus luteum
    d. hypothalamus

16. Failure to ovulate is termed
    a. anovulatory menstruation
    b. menorrhagia
    c. dysmenorrhea
    d. amenorrhea

17. The reproductive system becomes capable of functioning
    a. during adolescence
    b. in adulthood
    c. during puberty
    d. before birth

18. The first menstrual cycle is known as
    a. metrorrhagia
    b. menarche
    c. dysmenorrhea
    d. amenorrhea

B. Match the function in column I to the correct hormone in column II.

	Column I		Column II
D 1.	increases the number and length of the blood vessels in the endometrium and stimulates uterine secretions	a.	estrogen
C 2.	stimulates the corpus luteum to secrete female sex hormones	b.	FSH
A 3.	stimulates the glands of the endometrium to thicken	c.	LH
B 4.	stimulates development of the graafian follicle; causes rupture of the follicle	d.	progesterone

---

C. Briefly answer the following questions.

1. What physical changes occur during puberty?
2. How are the processes of ovulation and menstruation related?
3. What events occur during a normal 28-day menstrual cycle, and when do they occur?
4. At what time during the menstrual cycle is a woman most likely to conceive?

5. Of what does the menstrual flow consist?
6. Name three causes of irregular menstrual cycles.
7. Where does the ovum mature in the ovary? What is this structure called after ovulation?

SUGGESTED ACTIVITIES

- Using a diagram of the female reproductive system, identify each part and explain its role in reproduction.
- Define the following:
  - menstruation
  - ovulation
  - ovarian hormones
  - gonadotropins
  - follicular phase
  - luteal phase
  - proliferative phase
  - secretory phase
- Prepare a panel discussion for class presentation on the causes and treatment of menorrhagia, metrorrhagia, and dysmenorrhea. Refer to textbooks on gynecological nursing.
- Prepare a detailed written report on one of the following. Document your report with reading references.
  - ovulation
  - changes in the uterine lining during the menstrual cycle
  - hormones that regulate the female reproductive organs
- Describe the feedback mechanism of the hypothalamic-pituitary-ovarian axis

BIBLIOGRAPHY

Bates, B. *Guide to the Physical Exam and History Taking*, 5th ed. Philadelphia: J. B. Lippincott, 1991.

Crouch, J. E. *Functional Human Anatomy*, 4th ed. Philadelphia: Lea and Febiger, 1985.

Guyton, A. C. *Textbook of Medical Physiology*, 8th ed. W. B. Saunders, 1991.

Pritchard, J. A., Paul C. MacDonald, and Norman F. Grant. *Williams Obstetrics*, 17th ed. E. Norwalk, CT: Appleton-Century-Crofts, 1985.

CHAPTER

3

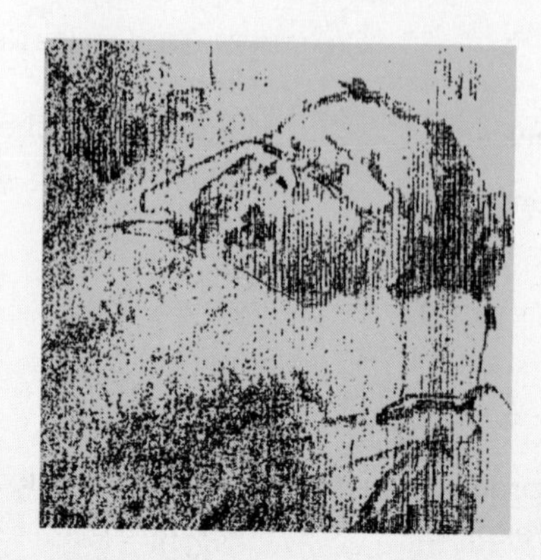

Conception

Objectives

After studying this chapter, the student should be able to:

- Explain the primary function of each part of the male reproductive system.
- List the functions of testosterone.
- Describe the process of conception.
- Explain how traits are inherited in terms of sex-linked and sex-limited traits.
- Explain how traits are inherited in terms of dominant and recessive traits.
- Distinguish between identical and fraternal twins.
- State some of the reasons for male and female infertility.

Key Terms

PENIS
GLANS PENIS
PREPUCE (FORESKIN)
SCROTUM
DARTOS
SUPERFICIAL FASCIA
SEMINAL DUCTS
TESTIS

SPERMATOZOA (SPERM)
SEMINIFEROUS TUBULES
EPIDIDYMIS
SEMEN
VAS DEFERENS
PROSTATE GLAND
SEMINAL VESICLE GLANDS
BULBOURETHRAL GLANDS
GONADOTROPIC HORMONES
TESTOSTERONE
COITUS
EJACULATION
ZYGOTE
CLEAVAGE
BLASTOMERE
MORULA
BLASTOCYST
TROPHOBLAST
PLACENTA
CHORION
AMNION
CHORIONIC VILLI
BLASTODERM
ECTODERM
ENDODERM
MESODERM
CHROMOSOME
DNA
GENE
GENETICIST
RNA
DIFFERENTIATION
SEX-LINKED CHARACTERISTICS
DOMINANT TRAIT
HETEROZYGOTE
RECESSIVE TRAIT
HOMOZYGOTE
STERILITY
IMPOTENT

Modern obstetrics concerns itself with more than just the growth and delivery of a baby. It incorporates a sharing by both man and woman from the time of conception and includes the hereditary and environmental influence they will both have on their child. It is, therefore, important for nurses to understand the father's function and role in the creation of his baby so that they can provide information to the family unit.

MALE EXTERNAL REPRODUCTIVE ORGANS

The external organs of reproduction in the male are the penis and the scrotum, Figure 3–1. The reproductive cells and their accompanying secretions are produced and carried to the outside by these organs.

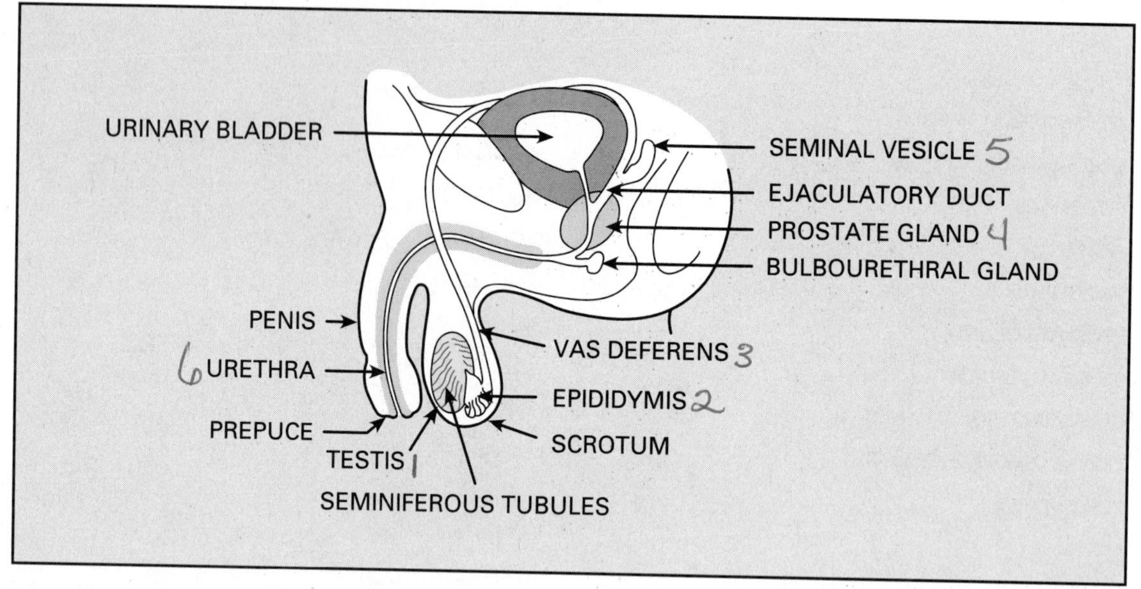

Figure 3–1 *Male reproductive organs*

The **penis** is the male organ of copulation. It consists of erectile parts known as cavernous bodies and a urethra, through which semen is released. The cavernous bodies contain spaces that are usually empty, allowing the penis to be flaccid (limp). When these spaces fill with blood, the penis becomes enlarged, turgid (swollen), and erect. The flow of blood is controlled by the autonomic nervous system and varies with psychical and physical stimulation. The slightly enlarged structure at the end of the penis, which contains the orifice of the urethra, is called the **glans penis**. It is enclosed by a fold of skin called the **prepuce**, or foreskin.

The **scrotum** is a pouch of loose skin and superficial fascia that is divided into two lateral portions. Involuntary muscle fibers called **dartos** lie within the superficial fascia. The dartos and the **superficial fascia** divide the scrotum internally into right and left compartments; each compartment contains a testis, epididymis, and associated structures. The dartos are subject to temperature conditions. Heat causes the dartos to relax, allowing the scrotum to elongate and become flaccid. This relaxation keeps the sperm away from the heat of the body. Sperm must be kept approximately 6°F cooler than body temperature or they cannot survive. Cold causes the dartos to contract, pulling the scrotum upward and closer to the body for warmth. The contracting-and-relaxing mechanism allows sperm to remain at the most satisfactory temperature.

MALE INTERNAL REPRODUCTIVE ORGANS

The male's internal reproductive organs are: (1) the testes, which contain the seminiferous tubules; (2) **seminal ducts** for transporting the sperm from the testes; (3) seminal vesicle glands; (4) the prostate gland; and (5) the bulbourethral (Cowper's) glands. Semen is a mixture of secretions from the testes, the prostate gland, the seminal vesicles, and the bulbourethral (Cowper's) glands.

The **testes** are the primary sex organs of the male; they produce **spermatozoa (sperm)** and the male sex hormone testosterone. The testes are suspended in the scrotum by spermatic cords. They average 4–5 cm (1½ to 2 in.) in length and 10.5–14 g (⅓–½ oz) in weight. Each testis is divided into lobes. Each lobe contains **seminiferous tubules**. The lining of these tubules consists of spermatogenic (sperm-producing) cells. Millions of sperm are produced in each testis. Spermatozoa production begins at puberty and continues throughout the life of the male. The seminiferous tubules join repeatedly to form the epididymis.

The **epididymis** is a single, coiled tube, 396–610 cm (13–20 ft) long, located on and beside the posterior surface of each testis. It is the principal storehouse for sperm. It also adds an essential secretion to the **semen** (fluid in which spermatozoa are activated and stored). Starting in the epididymis, secretions are added to the semen as the sperm travel.

From the epididymis, the semen passes through the ductus deferens, or vas deferens. The **vas deferens** is a slim muscular tube, approximately 45.7 cm (18 in.) long, that carries the semen to the urethra. The urethra serves two purposes in the male — as a passage for semen and as a passage for urine.

Surrounding the urethra at the base of the bladder is the **prostate gland**, which adds a milky secretion to the semen. This milky fluid is highly alkaline and neutralizes the acidic fluid from the testes in a way that stimulates the sperm to action. Sperm are immobile in acidic media but very active in alkaline media.

Behind the prostate gland are two **seminal vesicle glands**; they also produce fluid. Their ducts join the vas deferens to form ejaculatory ducts. The two ejaculatory ducts then empty the semen (containing sperm) into the urethra.

The two **bulbourethral glands,** or Cowper's glands, lie below the prostate on either side of the urethra. They also add secretions to the semen through ducts that open into the urethra. The urethra carries the sperm and secretions to the outside.

The secretions of the various glands help to lubricate the penis; this lubrication allows the vagina to massage the penis and create the necessary sexual stimulation to cause a release of the semen (ejaculation). Without this lubrication, there is a painful, abrasive effect, which inhibits sexual desire and blocks completion of the sexual act.

HORMONE REGULATION

The testes of a male remain dormant until they are stimulated by **gonadotropic hormones** from the pituitary gland. This stimulation occurs between the ages of 12 and 14 at puberty. The pituitary gland begins to secrete both the follicle-stimulating hormone (FSH) and the luteinizing hormone (LH), which are responsible for testicular growth and function. Testicular growth and function stimulate the release of the primary male sex hormone, **testosterone**. Testosterone is derived from the interstitial cells of the testes and is secreted directly into the bloodstream. Testosterone contributes to:

- development of secondary sex characteristics such as hair distribution and growth, changes in body contour, and voice changes;
- sex urge and behavior; and
- development, maintenance, and function of accessory sex organs, such as the seminal ducts, seminal vesicles, and prostate gland.

Adolescence is the name given to this time of change; it extends from puberty to maturity. The reproductive organs of the male continue to function throughout life. They do, however, diminish in activity to varying degrees in old age, as do all body systems.

SPERMATOZOA

The testes of the male produce billions of spermatozoa, or sperm. Sperm is the mature sex cell of the male. Each sperm is a single cell made up of a head, a midsection, and a tail, Figure 3–2. The head is composed chiefly of the nucleus. It carries the genes that are responsible for transmitting traits of the male (father) and the chromosome that determines the sex of the baby. The tail of the sperm (flagellum) is responsible for motility. As long as the sperm remains alive, the tail moves back and forth, propelling the sperm forward at a velocity of about 7½ cm (3 in.) per hour.

CONCEPTION

Copulation, or **coitus**, is the sexual act; sperm are delivered to the cervix by the erect penis. **Ejaculation** is the forcible release of semen from the penis. The amount of semen may vary from 1.5 to 4 mL (milliliters) per ejaculation. The microscopic sperm, often numbering more than 150 million per ejaculation, are propelled by their tails from the vagina to the uterus and then to the fallopian tube in search of an ovum, Figure 3–3. In spite of the excessive number of sperm, only one sperm fertilizes one egg. Once a sperm has penetrated an ovum, the chemical composition of the ovum's outer wall changes. The ovum shuts tight, preventing any other sperm from entering. The ovum and the sperm each contribute exactly half of the baby's total hereditary qualities.

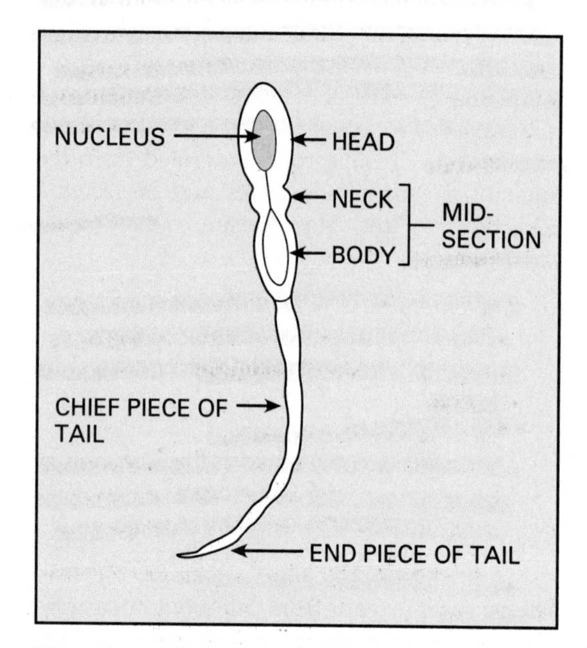

Figure 3–2 *Each sperm consists of a head, a midsection, and a tail.*

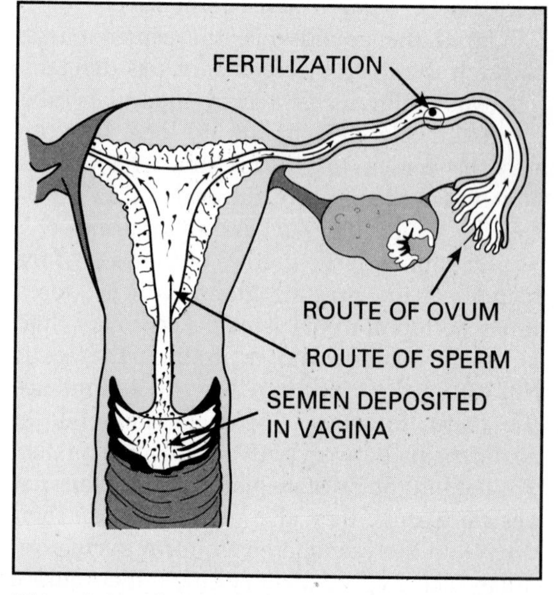

Figure 3–3 *Conception usually occurs in the fallopian tube. (Adapted from* DeLee's Obstetrics for Nurses, *W. B. Saunders)*

Multiple births occur when more than one egg is fertilized or when one fertilized egg divides into more than one embryo.

The human life cycle begins when the head and neck of the sperm enter the ovum, Figure 3–4. Entry usually takes place in the outer third of the fallopian tube. The resulting fertilized egg is called a **zygote,** Figure 3–5. The zygote is one cell with one nucleus, containing all the necessary elements for the future development of the offspring.

CLEAVAGE

Soon after the nucleus of the sperm has merged with the nucleus of the ovum, a series of cell divisions begins as shown in Figure 3–6. This process of cell division is called **cleavage** and usually starts while the fertilized egg is in the fallopian tube.

The first division of the fertilized ovum results in two cells called **blastomeres.** Before the division, each chromosome doubles its hereditary material. It then splits lengthwise to provide two equal half-chromosomes that regroup into two distinct nuclei, one of which goes with each half of the divided egg. Thus, right from the beginning, each cell of the developing baby contains an equal number of chromosomes from each of the parents. It is these chromosomes that carry genes.

The first cleavage takes about 36 hours; each succeeding division takes slightly less

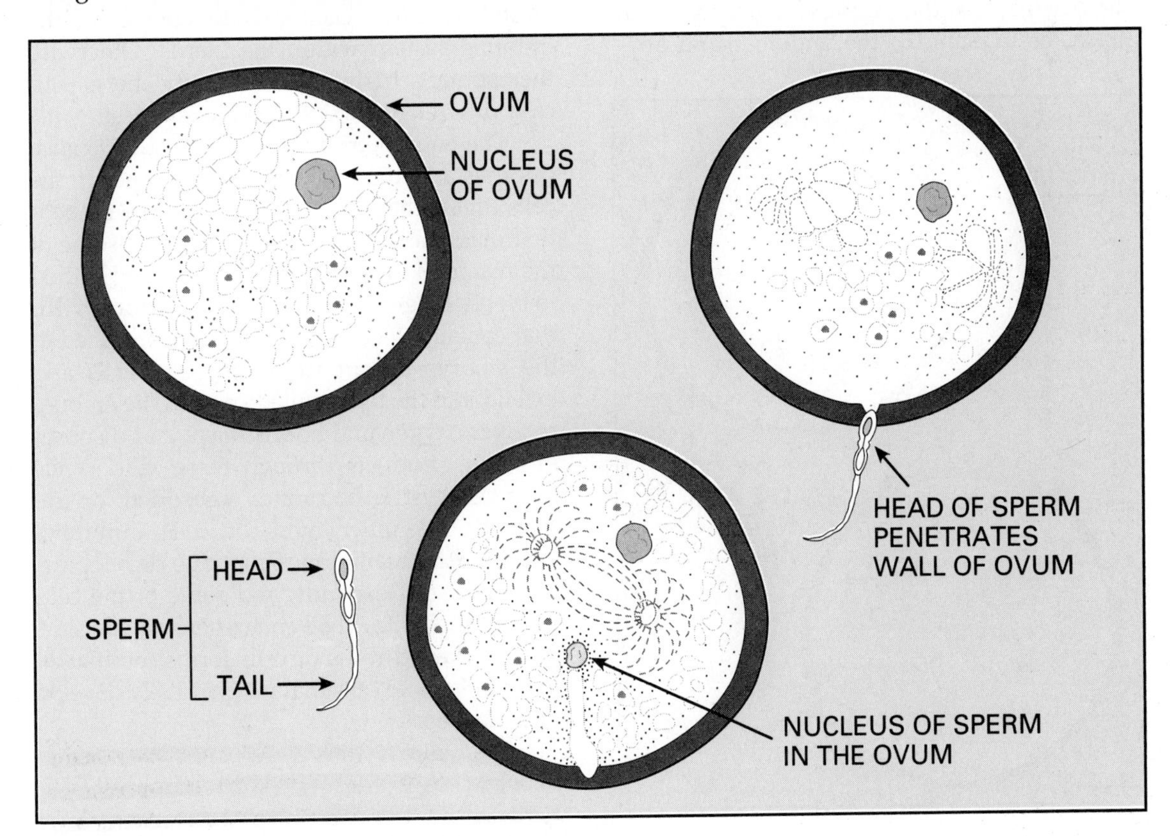

Figure 3–4 *Fertilization. Sperm unites with ovum.*

time. The multiplying continues at a fairly constant rate. The egg does not increase in size (bulk) as the cell division and multiplication continue.

The fertilized ovum gradually takes on the appearance of a mulberry and is called a **morula**. During cell division, the fertilized ovum is traveling down the fallopian tube to the uterus; this passage takes about four days. By the time the cells reach the end of the fallopian tube, there will be more than 100. The morula now takes on the shape of a sphere with a hollow center and is called a **blastocyst**.

IMPLANTATION

The blastocyst is the primitive embryo. It can attach, or implant, to the endometrium anywhere in the uterus, but usually implants near the uterine ceiling, Figure 3–7. The blastocyst implants into the uterine mucosa, which has been prepared for it. The discs of the cells near the outer rim develop into the embryo; the rim itself forms the fetal membrane. The rim, called the **trophoblast**, becomes the **placenta** and the covering **(chorion)**. The placenta nourishes, and the chorion protects the developing fetus. The chorion, the placenta, and the **amnion** (bag of waters) play an important role but are not physically part of the fetus.

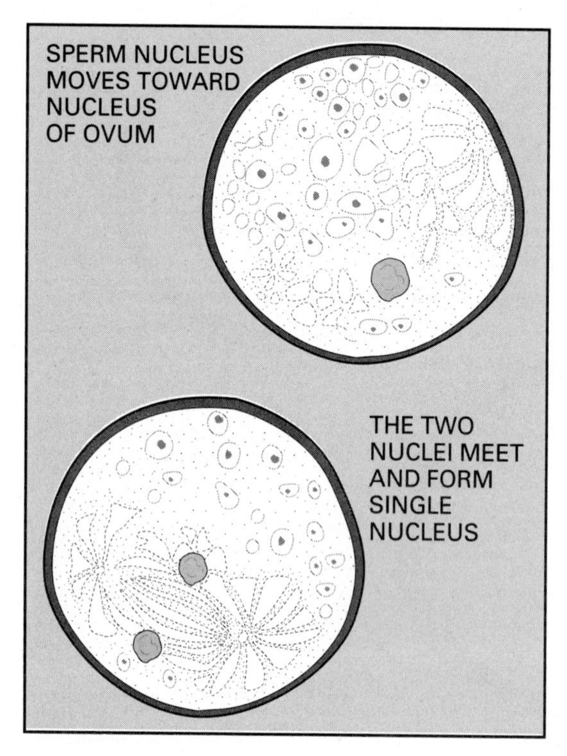

Figure 3–5 *Formation of the zygote*

The blastocyst begins producing a hormone that signals the ovaries to make progesterone. The progesterone tells the pituitary gland that the woman is pregnant and that no menstruation should take place. At the same time, the blastocyst emits chemicals to counteract the immune system within the uterus. Otherwise the mother's body would identify the genetically different growth as foreign and destroy it.

The endometrium, now called the *decidua*, thickens and the cells enlarge. Enzymes in the cells digest the uterine tissue until the embedded mass has broken into the walls of some of the maternal vessels; strands of cells are bathed in blood. Fingerlike projections **(chorionic villi)** that contain blood vessels and are connected to the embryo sprout from the outer cells and extend into the blood-filled spaces. The embryo receives oxygen and nourishment and disposes of waste products through these villi. While the blastocyst is becoming embedded, or implanted, the inner mass of cells multiplies and the fetal membranes continue developing. The blastocyst expands, and some of the cells around the hollow ball congregate on one side. This thickened mass of cells forms the **blastoderm**. It is these cells that progressively develop into the fetus.

The blastoderm is made up of two distinct layers of cells. The original outer and thicker layer, called the **ectoderm,** develops into the brain, the spinal cord, all the nerves and sensory

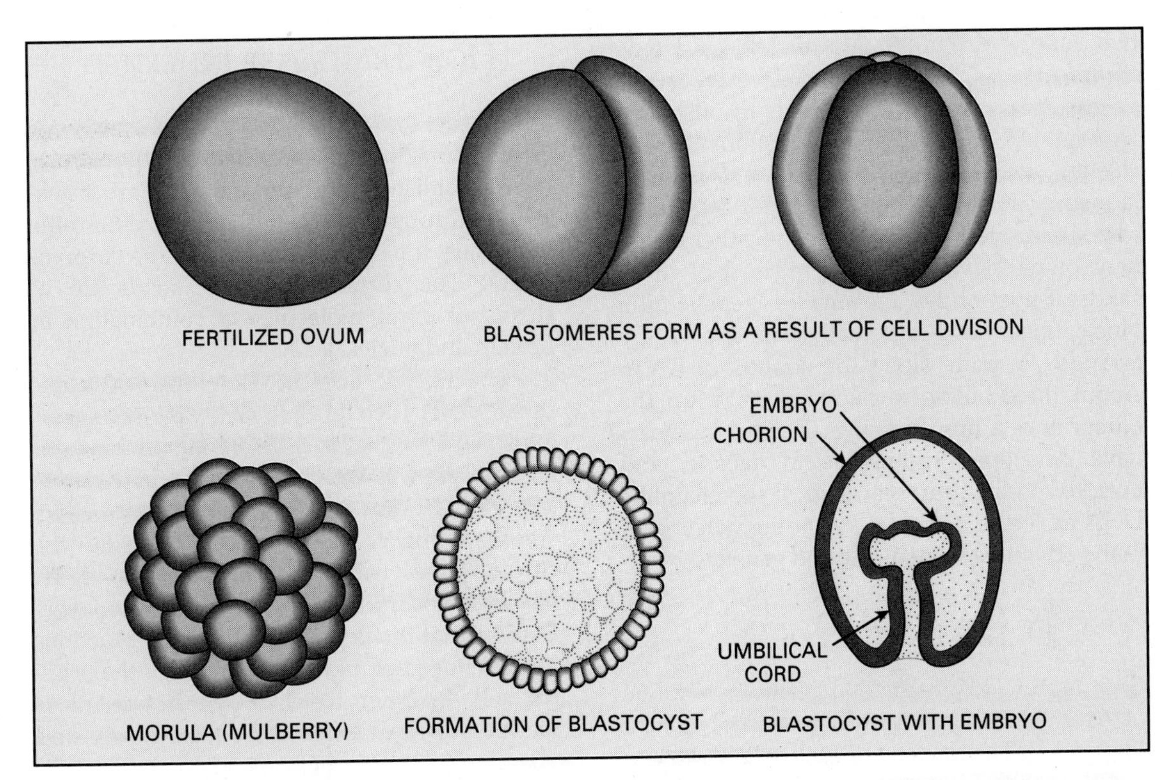

Figure 3–6 *Stages in embryonic development*

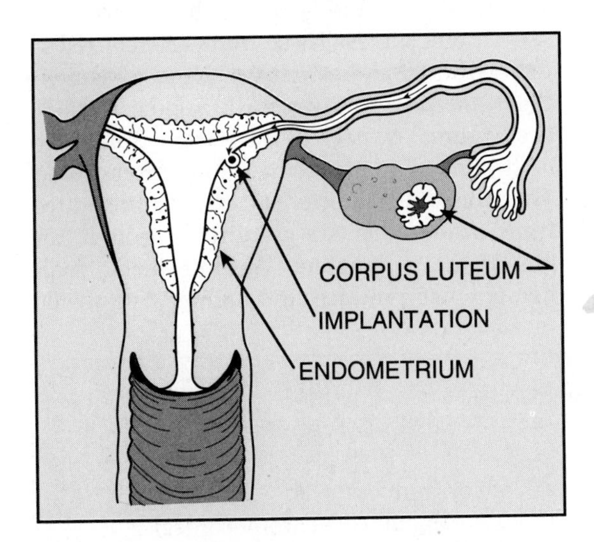

Figure 3–7 *Implantation. The blastocyst attaches to the endometrium. (Adapted from* DeLee's Obstetrics for Nurses, *W. B. Saunders)*

organs, and the skin. The newer and innermost layer, called the **endoderm**, becomes the lining of the entire digestive tract from the pharynx down through the esophagus, stomach, liver, and intestines to the anus. The intermediate layer, called the **mesoderm**, appears later and gives rise to the skeleton, muscles, and many internal organs. These three layers of cells appear in the development of all higher animals.

THE GENETIC CODE

The human body consists of about 10 trillion cells. Large molecules called proteins determine the structure and function of each cell. A cell nucleus contains 23 pairs of chromosomes. The **chromosomes** control the manufacture of proteins by the cell. A chromosome consists of two long, twisted strands of **DNA** (deoxyribonucleic acid), the chemical that carries genetic information from parents to offspring. Human DNA is divided into about 100,000 clusters called genes. A **gene** determines a human characteristic such as height, eye color, or resistance to disease. Genes are either dominant or recessive and are composed of thousands of nucleotides, the smallest genetic unit. Nucleotides have different shapes and are arranged in pairs along the strands of DNA. About three billion nucleotides make up the blueprint of a human being. Genetic engineers have developed techniques to decode, and even to modify, tiny segments of the chainlike DNA molecule. This understanding will enable many advances in medicine and genetics.

DETERMINATION OF SEX

Each mature ovum has 23 chromosomes, one of which is the X, or female sex factor, refer to Figure 3–8. The nucleus of each mature sperm also contains 23 chromosomes, one of which is either the Y (male sex factor) or the X (female sex factor). Usually equal numbers of each type of sperm are produced in the testes.

The zygote resulting from conception contains 46 chromosomes: 23 chromosomes (includes a sex factor) from each parent. If the ovum has been fertilized by a sperm carrying the X (female) sex factor, the resulting offspring is female. If the sperm carried the Y (male) sex factor, the offspring is male.

HOW TRAITS ARE INHERITED

Geneticists (scientists who are concerned with the phenomena of heredity and its variations) have established that certain traits are transmitted through the genes. Genes determine hereditary traits and are found in the chromosomes. The chromosomes are made up of chains of giant molecules, a combination of protein and nucleic acid.

The nucleic acid in the chromosomes is called DNA (deoxyribonucleic acid) and contains the full genetic information needed for the formation of the human body. DNA could be called the master template for cell building. Another nucleic acid, present outside the chromosomes, is **RNA** (ribonucleic acid). RNA has a major function in cell differentiation. **Differentiation** is the acquiring of functions that do not resemble the functions of the original cell. In other words, RNA is needed to make a bone cell different from a lung cell and so on.

It is known that some physical traits are associated with the genes in the X and Y, or sex, chromosomes. These traits are referred to as **sex-linked characteristics**. Hemophilia and color blindness are two sex-linked characteristics, Figure 3–9. Each of these traits is believed to be linked to the female (X) chromosome. Therefore, the characteristic can be transmitted from grandfather to grandson through the grandfather's daughter. Assume that a male hemophiliac produces a daughter. She would

Female Child: 22 chromosomes + X factor from ovum +
22 chromosomes + X factor from sperm = 44 + 2X factors (23 chromosomes)

Male Child: 22 chromosomes + X factor from ovum +
22 chromosomes + Y factor from sperm = 44 + X + Y factors (23 chromosomes)

Figure 3–8 *How sex is determined*

XX = Female	Hemophiliac X_hY	=	Grandfather, Hemophiliac
			↓
XY = Male	Not Hemophiliac X_hX	=	Daughter, Not Hemophiliac
			↓
X_h = Hemophiliac Chromosome	Hemophiliac X_hY	=	Grandson, Hemophiliac

Figure 3–9 *Transmission of hemophilia*

carry one normal X chromosome from her mother and one hemophiliac X chromosome from her father. She would not be a hemophiliac since the healthy X chromosome would mask the hemophiliac chromosome. If, however, she had a son, he could receive either a normal or a hemophiliac X chromosome from his mother. If he received a hemophiliac chromosome, he would be a hemophiliac (since he has no healthy X chromosome to mask the hemophiliac chromosome). A female would be a hemophiliac only if she inherited a hemophiliac chromosome from both her mother and her father. These sex-linked characteristics often are limited to the male and are therefore called sex-limited characteristics. Genes for certain traits other than sex are located on the X chromosome. When a male offspring inherits such a trait on his X chromosome, there is no matching gene on the Y chromosome. Therefore, that trait will invariably be shown. A female offspring, on the other hand, has two X chromosomes. Therefore, even if she inherits a trait, it may be masked by another more dominant gene for the same trait on the other X chromosome. For this reason, certain sex-linked characteristics appear more often in men than in women. Red-green color blindness, blood-clotting disorder, hemophilia, and baldness in men belong in this category, Figure 3–10.

Traits and genes are said to be dominant or recessive. A **dominant trait** (carried by a dominant gene) requires only a single gene to produce an offspring with the trait because it can mask another (recessive) trait. The product of a dominant and a recessive gene is a **heterozygote**. A **recessive trait** appears only when a pair of recessive genes is present, Figure 3–11. The product of two like genes (either dominant or recessive) is a **homozygote.** Some dominant traits include dark hair, brown eyes, farsightedness, astigmatism, curly hair, glaucoma, and cataracts. Among the recessive traits are blue or gray eyes, myopia, light hair, Rh-negative blood type, diabetes mellitus, sickle cell anemia, and congenital deafness. Diabetes and hemophilia are transmitted by lethal genes, so named because their effect interferes with life.

MULTIPLE BIRTHS

Twins are described according to their origin. Identical twins result from the union of one sperm and one ovum; fraternal twins result when two ova are fertilized by two sperm. In identical twins the fertilized egg divides into two embryos. There is one placenta and two amniotic sacs, see Figure 3–12. The twins are always the same sex. Fraternal twins may or

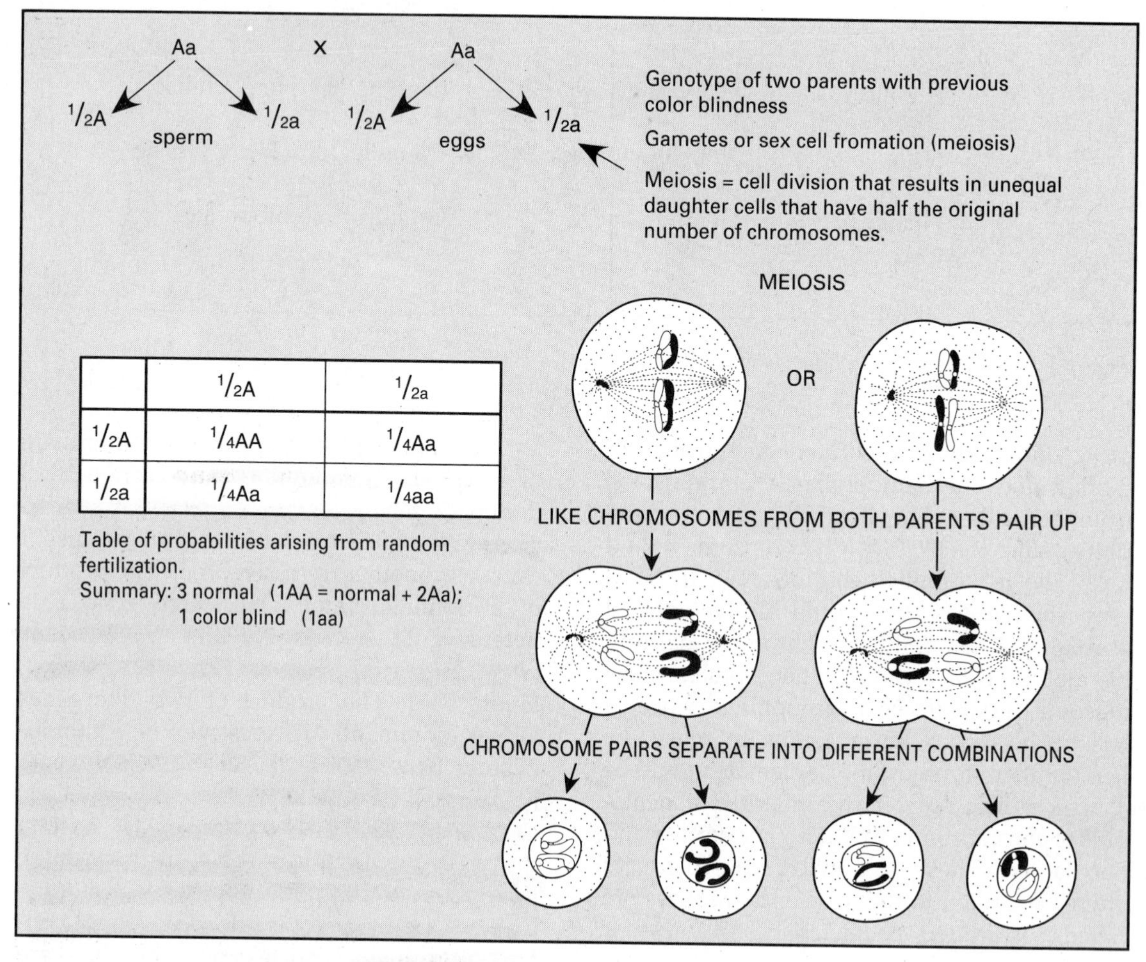

	1/2A	1/2a
1/2A	1/4AA	1/4Aa
1/2a	1/4Aa	1/4aa

Figure 3–10 *Transmission of color blindness*

may not be of the same sex. They have two amniotic sacs and separate or fused placentas, Figure 3–13.

The frequency of identical twins appears to be relatively constant throughout the world at approximately one set of identical twins per 250 births. It is largely independent of race, heredity, age, parity, and therapy for infertility. The incidence of fraternal twins is influenced remarkably by race, heredity, maternal age, parity, and, especially, fertility drugs. The likelihood of fraternal twins increases with both parity and maternal age. White women are more likely to deliver twins than black women. Twinning among Asians is less common than among whites or blacks.

INFERTILITY

Inability to become pregnant after one year of regular intercourse is considered infertility. It affects an estimated 15 percent of American

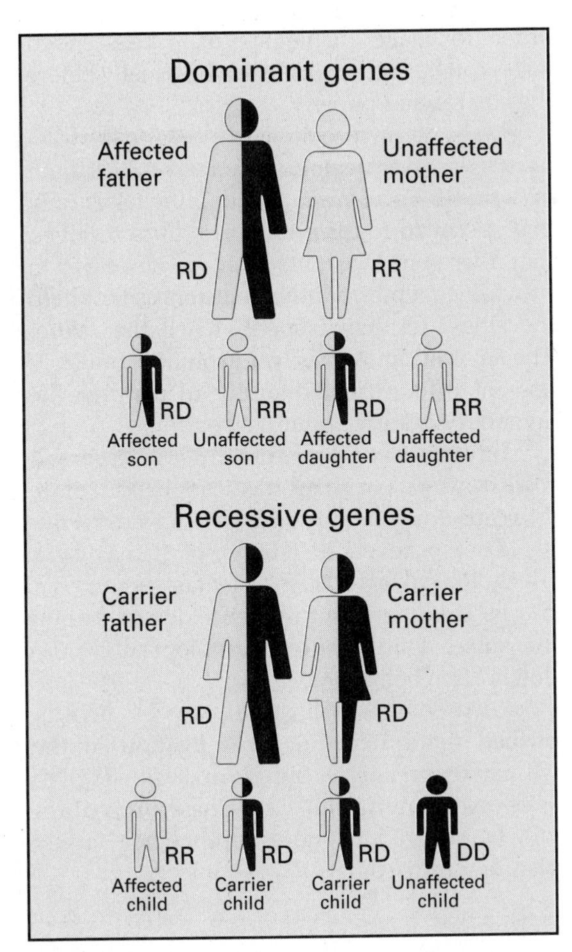

Figure 3–11 *Genes are passed in pairs, one from each parent.*

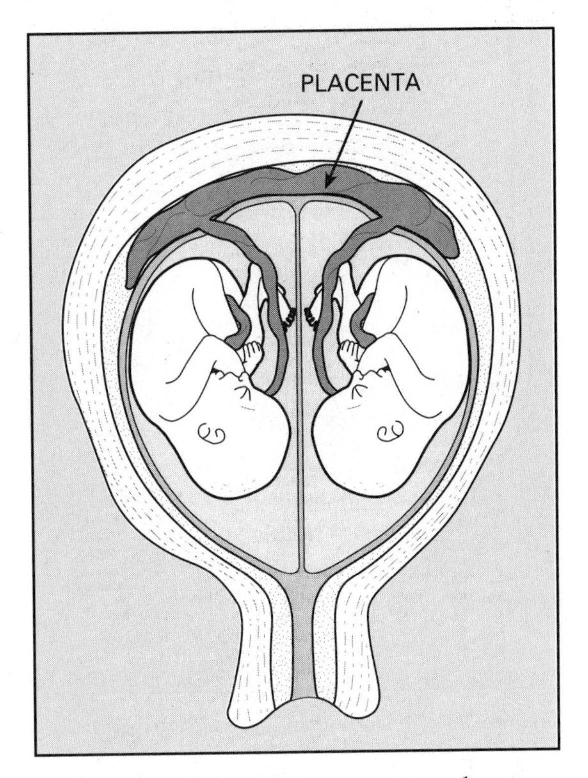

Figure 3–12 *Identical twins: two sacs, one placenta*

couples. In primary infertility there has been no preceding pregnancy; secondary infertility follows one or more pregnancies. In approximately 40 percent of cases the cause lies in the woman; in about 40 percent of the cases the cause lies in the man and most often is poor sperm production; and in the remaining 20 percent the cause is either a combination of factors in both or is never determined.

Infertility in women is usually due to several factors rather than a single cause. Systemic, local, nutritional, glandular, and emotional factors can affect a woman's ability to conceive. Failure to ovulate, obstructions in the genital tract, especially in the cervix or fallopian tubes, or disturbances in the development of the uterus and its lining that interfere with the implantation and growth of a fertilized ovum are a few causes of infertility in women. Research is continuing into both physical and psychological causes of infertility. New techniques in diagnosis and treatment have enabled many "infertile" women to conceive.

About one out of every 30 males is sterile. **Sterility** may be defined as the lack of viable (capable of growing and developing) sperm; this lack results in the inability to bring about conception. The most frequent cause of sterility is infection of the genital ducts. A few men have congenitally deficient testes that are incapable of producing normal sperm. Undescended testicles produce sterility because the spermatogenic

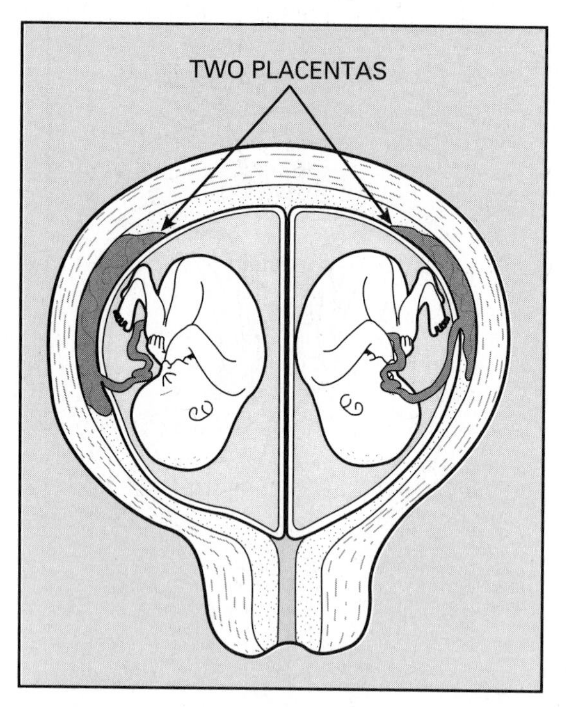

Figure 3–13 *Fraternal twins: two sacs, two placentas*

(sperm-producing) cells cannot live at body temperature. The testes must descend into the scrotum, which is at a cooler temperature, in order to make viable sperm. Undescended testes can be corrected surgically, usually before the boy reaches puberty.

Male sterility can also occur when the number of viable sperm falls below 20 million in a single ejaculation. Although it takes only one sperm to fertilize an ovum, it is believed that a large number of sperm are necessary to provide enzymes or other substances that help the single fertilizing sperm reach the ovum. The enzyme, known as hyaluronidase, must be present in sufficient quantity to dissolve the layer of cells surrounding the ovum.

Impotent is a term used when the adult male cannot have an erection or an ejaculation. The cause may be physical, such as a debilitating disease, fever, or fatigue, or it may be a psychological factor such as fear, stress, or psychosis. Treatment for impotence depends upon the cause. A medical or psychological evaluation is often beneficial.

Purposeful sterilization can be accomplished by a bilateral tubal ligation in the woman or a relatively simple operation known as a vasectomy in the man. These procedures will be covered in more depth when family planning is discussed.

REVIEW QUESTIONS

A. Multiple choice. Select the best answer.

1. Fertilization usually takes place in the
   a. uterus
   b. vagina
   c. ovary
   d. fallopian tubes
2. The number of chromosomes contained in the zygote is
   a. 46 and 2 sex factors
   b. 48 and 2 sex factors
   c. 44 and 2 sex factors
   d. 42 and 2 sex factors
3. The process of cell division that takes place soon after fertilization is called
   a. DNA
   b. RNA
   c. cleavage
   d. chromosomes
4. DNA is believed to be in the
   a. tail of the sperm
   b. nucleus of the cell
   c. cytoplasm of the cell
   d. wall of the ovum

5. An example of a recessive trait is
   a. dark hair
   b. astigmatism
   c. diabetes mellitus
   d. glaucoma

6. After fertilization, implantation takes place in the uterus in approximately
   a. 24 hours
   b. 2–3 days
   c. 6–7 days
   d. 14 days

7. During puberty, the testes of the male are stimulated to produce male sex hormones by
   a. gonadotropic hormones
   b. estrogen
   c. testosterone
   d. progesterone

8. The seminiferous tubules are located within the
   a. ejaculatory ducts
   b. bulbourethral glands
   c. prostate gland
   d. testes

9. The thin muscular tube that carries the semen to the urethra is the
   a. epididymis
   b. vas deferens
   c. seminal duct
   d. seminal vesicle

10. Inherited traits of the father and sex of the baby are determined by
    a. genes in the sperm nucleus
    b. female ovum
    c. body of the sperm
    d. neck of the sperm

11. The most frequent cause of sterility in the male is
    a. low sperm count
    b. congenitally deficient testes
    c. undescended testes
    d. infection of the genital ducts

12. The function of testosterone is that
    a. it contributes to the development of secondary sex characteristics
    b. it contributes to the sex urge and sexual behavior
    c. it contributes to the development, maintenance, and functioning of accessory sex organs
    d. all of the above

13. The mature sex cell of the male is called
    a. seminal vesicle
    b. sperm
    c. testosterone
    d. bulbourethral gland

B. Label the parts of the male reproductive system on the following diagram.

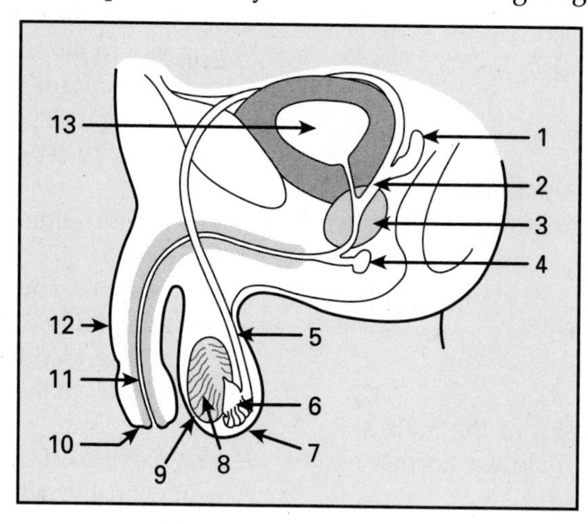

C. Match the description in column I to the correct term in column II.

Column I	Column II
1. contains genes	a. chromosome
2. two sperm + two ova	b. fraternal twins
3. develop in the testes	c. identical twins
4. one sperm + one ovum	d. male sex chromosomes
5. fertilized ovum	e. sperm
6. determines sex of child	f. zygote

D. Briefly answer the following questions.

1. Define sex-linked characteristics and give an example.
2. How many amniotic sacs and placentas are there for identical twins? For fraternal twins?
3. Birth of fraternal twins depends largely upon what factors?

SUGGESTED ACTIVITIES

- Prepare a report on the history of genetics. How can genetics contribute to the health of the generations of the future?
- Construct pedigrees and analyze them for inheritance patterns.
- Explain the importance of preventive genetics in the areas of preconception, prenatal, and postnatal periods.
- Prepare a written report on the causes of male and female infertility.
- Describe the physiology of the male reproductive system.

BIBLIOGRAPHY

Bates, B. *Guide to the Physical Exam and History Taking*, 5th ed. Philadelphia: J.B. Lippincott, 1991.

Crouch, J. E. *Functional Human Anatomy*, 4th ed. Philadelphia: Lea and Febiger, 1985.

Guyton, A. C. *Textbook of Medical Physiology*, 8th ed. W. B. Saunders, 1991.

Page, E. W., Claude A. Villee, and Dorothy B. Villee. *Human Reproduction*, 3rd ed. Philadelphia: W. B. Saunders, 1981.

Pritchard, J. A.; Paul C. MacDonald, and Norman F. Grant. *Williams Obstetrics*, 17th ed. E. Norwalk, CT: Appleton-Century-Crofts, 1985.

Time-Life Education Materials. *Life before Birth*, 1965.

CHAPTER

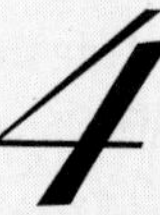

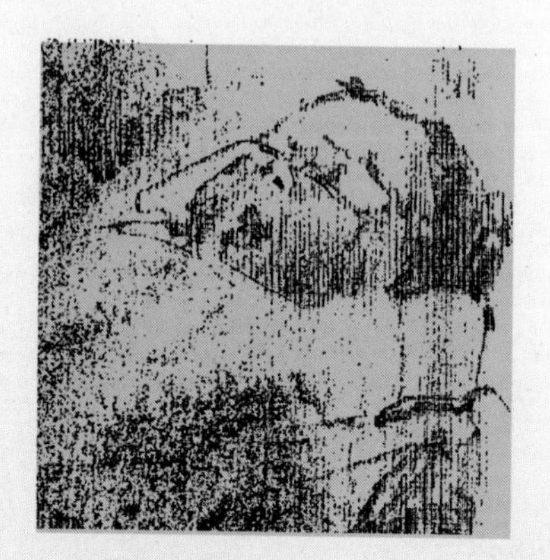

Fetal Development

Objectives

After studying this chapter, the student should be able to:

- State how the placenta is formed.
- Explain the function of the amniotic sac and amniotic fluid.
- Name the functions of the placenta.
- Identify the means by which nutrients and gases pass through the placenta.
- Trace the flow of blood through fetal circulation.
- Identify changes that take place in fetal circulation at birth.
- Trace the development of the zygote from the first through the tenth lunar month.
- Identify factors detrimental to the development of the embryo and fetus.

Key Terms

DECIDUA BASALIS
CHORIONIC VILLI
UMBILICAL CORD
PLACENTA
HUMAN CHORIONIC GONADOTROPIN (hCG)
CHORIONIC SOMATOTROPHIN
COTYLEDONS
AMNIOTIC MEMBRANE
CHORIONIC MEMBRANE
OSMOSIS
DIFFUSION
AMNIOTIC SAC
HYDRAMNIOS
OLIGOHYDRAMNIOS
WHARTON'S JELLY
VENA CAVA
DUCTUS VENOSUS
FORAMEN OVALE
AORTA
DUCTUS ARTERIOSUS
OSSIFICATION
FETUS
QUICKENING
VERNIX CASEOSA
MECONIUM
ALKALOIDAL COCAINE
FETAL ALCOHOL SYNDROME (FAS)
SYPHILIS
GONORRHEA
CHLAMYDIA
OPHTHALMIA NEONATORUM
ENDOMETRITIS
CYTOMEGALOVIRUS (CMV)
HERPES SIMPLEX
ACQUIRED IMMUNE DEFICIENCY SYNDROME (AIDS)
HUMAN IMMUNODEFICIENCY VIRUS (HIV)
RUBELLA
SCARLET FEVER
MULTIPLE PREGNANCY

During the first to second week after conception, the fertilized ovum forms a blastocyst while traveling down the fallopian tube. The embryo enters the uterus and becomes implanted in the endometrium and the rapid growth of the embryo begins. The period of the embryo is considered to be from the second to the eighth week after fertilization. Full-term pregnancy (38–42 weeks) is broken into trimesters. The full term is calculated from the first day of the woman's last normal menstrual period. Each trimester is one-third of the pregnancy.

EMBRYONIC DEVELOPMENT

By the 28th day after conception (the first lunar month), traces of all organs have become differentiated; rudiments of the eyes, ears, nose, and limb buds are present, Figure 4–1. The embryo is about 7.5–10 mm (millimeters), or less than ½ inch, long. Development proceeds from head to tail. Although the sex is determined at conception by the genes of the sperm and ovum, it cannot yet be distinguished.

During the next 28 days, or second lunar month, the head becomes larger because of the development of the brain. The features appear relatively small. The external genitals appear toward the end of this month, and the embryo is now about 2.5–3 cm, or about 1 inch, long. The circulatory system between the mother and the embryo is established through the umbilical cord attached to the embryo at the navel. The cord varies from 7 in. to 4 feet long (18–122 cm), averaging about 20 in. (50 cm). Blood rushing through the cord keeps it taut in utero (in the uterus). The blood travels at a rate of about four miles per hour by the end of the pregnancy. The cord contains two arteries, which take waste products from the fetus to the placenta to be excreted by the mother, and one vein, which carries nourishment and oxygen to the fetus.

MATERNAL AND FETAL CIRCULATION

Early in pregnancy, the portion of the endometrium that lies directly beneath the embedded ovum becomes thicker. This portion of the endometrium is called the **decidua basalis**. The **chorionic villi** are fingerlike projections that have developed from fetal tissue at the base of the implanted fertilized ovum. They contain blood vessels, which unite to form larger blood vessels communicating with the fetus. By the end of the third month, the placenta has been formed from the decidua basalis and chorionic villi. Through these villi, oxygen and nourishment are received from the mother and passed to the fetus by way of the umbilical cord. The **umbilical cord** connects the fetus to the placenta. Waste products of the fetus are discharged through the umbilical cord to the placenta.

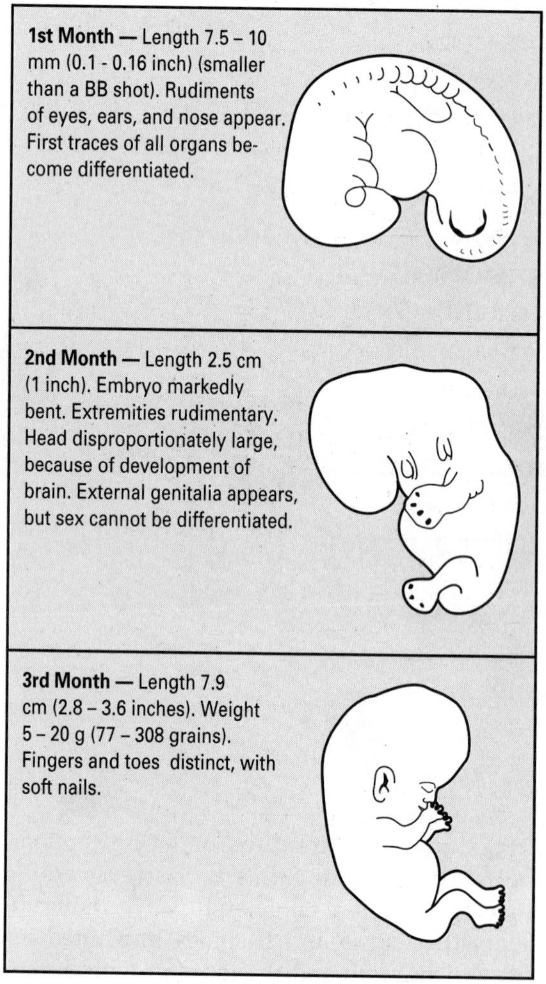

1st Month — Length 7.5 – 10 mm (0.1 - 0.16 inch) (smaller than a BB shot). Rudiments of eyes, ears, and nose appear. First traces of all organs become differentiated.

2nd Month — Length 2.5 cm (1 inch). Embryo markedly bent. Extremities rudimentary. Head disproportionately large, because of development of brain. External genitalia appears, but sex cannot be differentiated.

3rd Month — Length 7.9 cm (2.8 – 3.6 inches). Weight 5 – 20 g (77 – 308 grains). Fingers and toes distinct, with soft nails.

Figure 4–1 *The first trimester of pregnancy (Adapted from* Pelvic Anatomy for the Patient, *Shering Corp.)*

THE PLACENTA

The **placenta**, also known as the "afterbirth," is a highly specialized organ that connects the fetus to its mother and enables the exchange of soluble, blood-borne nutrients, oxygen, and secretions. The placenta acts as a respiratory, nutritive, and executory organ for the developing fetus; it connects the developing fetus to the uterine wall. The placenta develops from both embryonic and maternal tissue; that is, from the outer rim of the blastocyst and the inner lining of the uterus (endometrium), Figure 4–2.

The placenta usually lies at the top of the uterus and is connected to the fetus by the umbilical cord. The development of the placenta is stimulated by the hormone progesterone, which is secreted by the corpus luteum within the ovary. After the placenta has developed, it secretes estrogen and progesterone, which are needed to sustain the pregnancy. In addition to estrogen and progesterone, the placenta produces at least two other hormones, **human chorionic gonadotropin (hCG)** and **chorionic somatotrophin**, associated with fetal growth. Estrogen promotes the growth of the uterine muscle and blood vessels that supply oxygen to this muscle; progesterone delays uterine contractions, so that the baby is not pushed out prematurely.

The placenta is a fleshy organ, which at term measures about 8 inches (20 cm) in diameter, is 1 inch (2½ cm) thick, and weighs about one-sixth of the baby's weight, or slightly over one pound (454 g). The side of the placenta that implants in the uterine wall is rough and bloody, and it is divided into lobes called **cotyledons**. As the placenta ages, calcium deposits begin to appear in this side. The fetal side of the placenta is smooth, pale, and shiny and is covered by the **amniotic membrane**. The amniotic and **chorionic membranes** extend from the edge of the placenta to form the sac (or bag of waters), which contains the amniotic fluid and fetus. Branches of the umbilical vein and arteries can be seen on the fetal side of the placenta spreading out from the umbilical cord. The placenta resembles a plant sending roots into the earth for nourishment. When the plant is pulled up, particles of earth cling to the roots, see Figure 4–3. Likewise, a thin layer of the uterine wall clings to the chorionic villi when the placenta detaches after delivery.

PLACENTAL TRANSFER

Intensive studies of the transfer of nourishment from maternal to fetal circulation have been made. It appears that nourishing materials pass from the maternal side of the placenta (the decidua basalis) to the fetal side (the chorionic villi) by **osmosis**; osmosis is the passage of a solvent through a semipermeable membrane into a more concentrated solution, which tends to equalize the concentrations on both sides of the membrane. Waste products pass from the fetus to the mother's bloodstream in the same manner. The layer of cells separating the fetal placenta from the maternal tissue and maternal blood vessels prevents intermixing of maternal and fetal blood. It is believed that calcium, phosphorus, amino acids, glucose, fats, and certain bacteria, viruses, drugs, and antibodies pass through this layer of cells into the fetal circulation.

The blood circulating in the fetus is never as rich in oxygen as the blood in the adult. The oxygen and carbon dioxide pass through the placenta by **diffusion**; that is, when the solutions of two gases at different concentrations are separated by a permeable membrane, the gas molecules pass through the membrane in both directions until the concentrations on both sides are equal. In this way, the oxygen from the maternal side passes through the placenta to the fetal side; carbon dioxide and

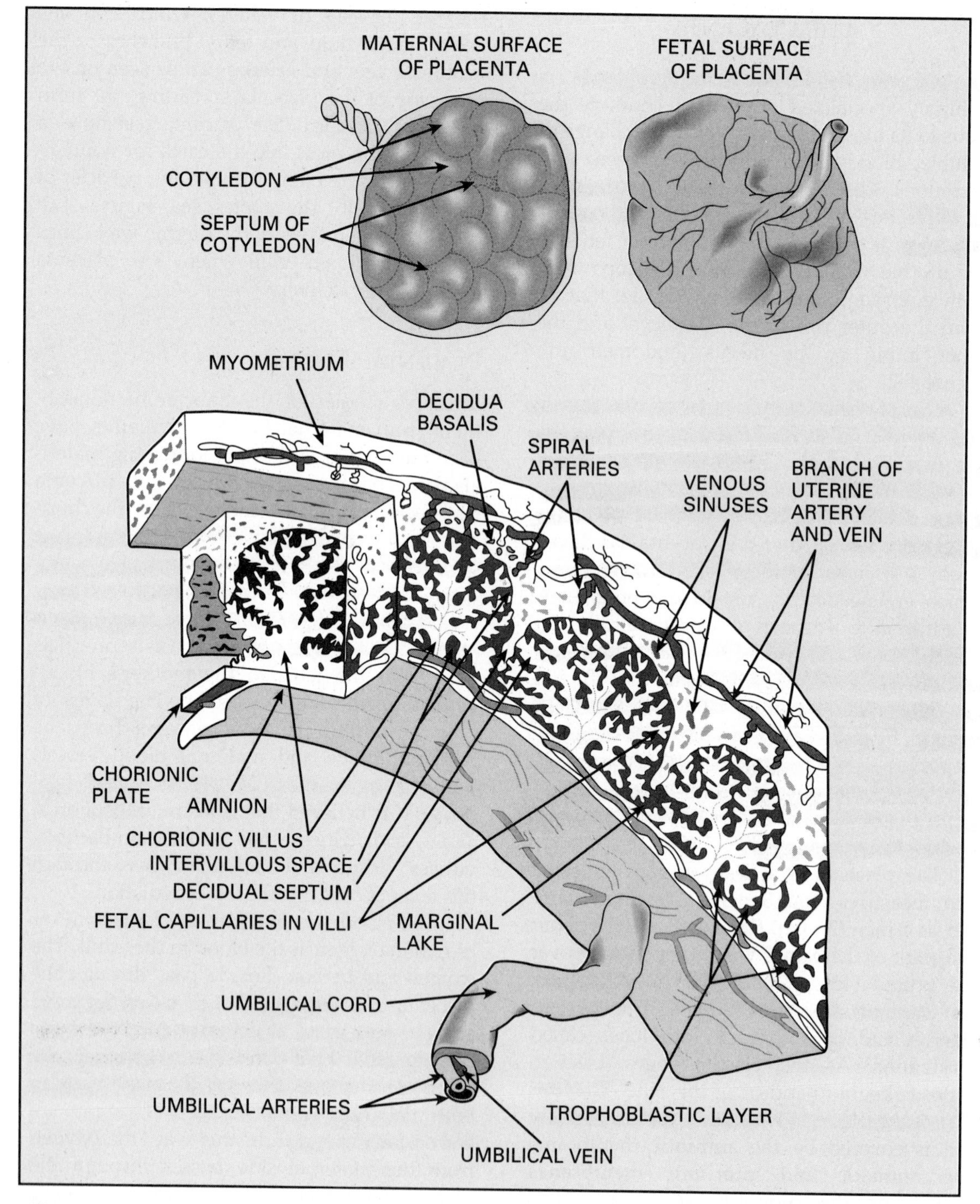

Figure 4–2 *Wall of the placenta (Adapted from Clinical Education Aid, No. 2, Ross Laboratories)*

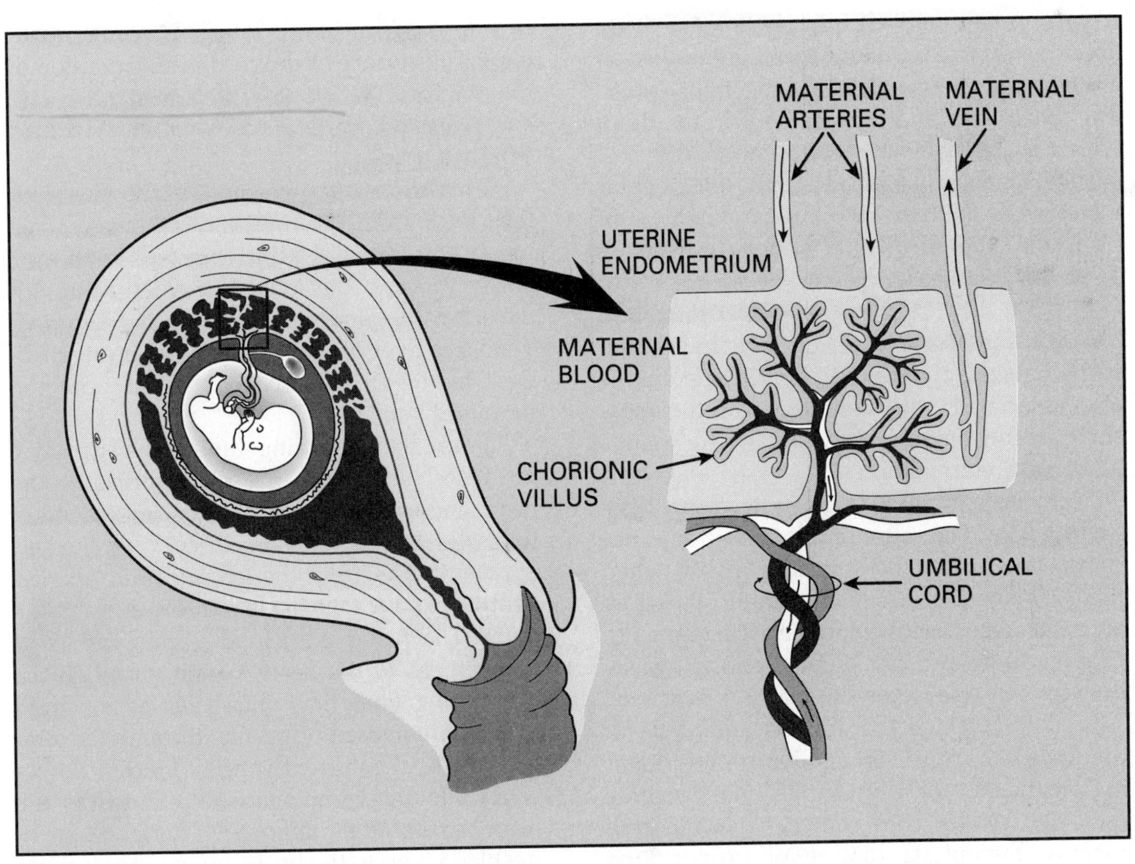

Figure 4–3 *The placenta carries oxygen and nutrients to the fetus and transports waste from the fetus.*

waste products pass from the fetal side to the maternal side.

The new life within the mother needs increased amounts of oxygen to grow from one cell to billions of cells in just nine months. The placenta feeds the fetus. It also filters out harmful substances such as bacteria. However, it cannot filter out all harmful material. For example, smoking can increase the risk of spontaneous abortion and premature birth. Nicotine in the mother's bloodstream can impair the heart rate, blood pressure, oxygen supply, and acid balance and may cause the placental blood vessels to narrow and diminish the supply of nourishment to the unborn baby.

THE AMNIOTIC SAC

A fluid-filled sac that develops around the embryo is called the **amniotic sac**. This sac is formed by the amnion which is a smooth, transparent, inner fetal membrane.

The amnion grows rapidly, and by the end of the eighth week it fuses with the outer fetal membrane (the chorion). The chorion forms the outer walls of the blastocyst. The fusion of the amnion and the chorion forms the amniochorionic sac, which is more commonly known as the "bag of waters." The embryo is suspended in this sac in the amniotic fluid.

Amniotic fluid is slightly alkaline and about 98% water. It equalizes the pressure around the fetus and keeps the fetus moist. The fetus floats and moves about in the fluid, which keeps it at an even temperature and cushions it from injury. The amount of fluid increases as the fetus develops. At the time of birth, the amount of fluid varies from 500 to 1,000 mL. Amniotic fluid in amounts greater than 2,000 mL (1¾ qt) at term is a condition called **hydramnios**. It is common in women with diabetes and cardiac conditions and is also associated with conditions of the fetus such as congenital heart defects and gastrointestinal abnormalities.

Too little amniotic fluid is termed **oligohydramnios**. The cause of this condition is not completely understood. It may occur when there is an obstruction of the fetal urinary tract or renal agenesis (incomplete development). Oligohydramnios can have serious consequences for the fetus. In early pregnancy, adhesions between the amnion and parts of the fetus can cause serious deformities. Later in pregnancy, other complications include increased risk of cord compression and pulmonary hypoplasia (failure of proper lung development).

Fetal Circulation

Certain fetal capillaries transfer waste products to the maternal circulation while others accept nourishment into the fetal circulation. The capillaries merge in the fetal side of the placenta, eventually meeting to form the umbilical vein and arteries, which communicate with the fetus. The arteries transport waste materials from the fetus, and the vein supplies oxygen and nutrients to the fetus, see Figure 4–4.

The two arteries and one vein are enclosed in the umbilical cord, which is about 20 in. long. The surface of the cord is an extension of the amnion. The blood vessels inside the cord are protected by a mucoid substance called **Wharton's jelly**.

The arterial (oxygenated) blood flows up the cord through the umbilical vein and passes into the ascending (inferior) **vena cava** partly through the liver, but chiefly through the special fetal structure the **ductus venosus**. The large liver of the newborn has been attributed to the supply of fresh blood from the umbilical vein.

From the ascending (inferior) vena cava, the blood flows into the right auricle of the heart and passes through another fetal structure, the **foramen ovale**, directly to the left auricle. It goes from the left auricle to the left ventricle and leaves the fetal heart through the **aorta**. The blood goes to the arms and head and returns to the heart, passing through the descending (superior) vena cava to the right auricle. But instead of passing through the foramen ovale, the current is now directed downward into the right ventricle and leaves the heart through the pulmonary arteries. Some of the blood goes to the lungs, but most of it flows through another fetal structure, the **ductus arteriosus**, into the aorta. See Figure 4–5.

Because the fetus receives oxygen from the placenta, its lungs do not function. The blood must be shunted around its lungs; a small amount goes through them to nourish the tissues, not to secure oxygen.

The blood in the aorta, except that which supplies the head and arms, passes downward to supply the trunk and lower extremities. The greater part of this blood flows through the hypogastric arteries and back through the umbilical arteries of the cord to the placenta, where it is again oxygenated. A small amount passes back into the ascending vena cava to mingle with fresh blood from the umbilical vein and again makes the circuit of the fetal body.

foramen ovale didn't close properly → heart murmur

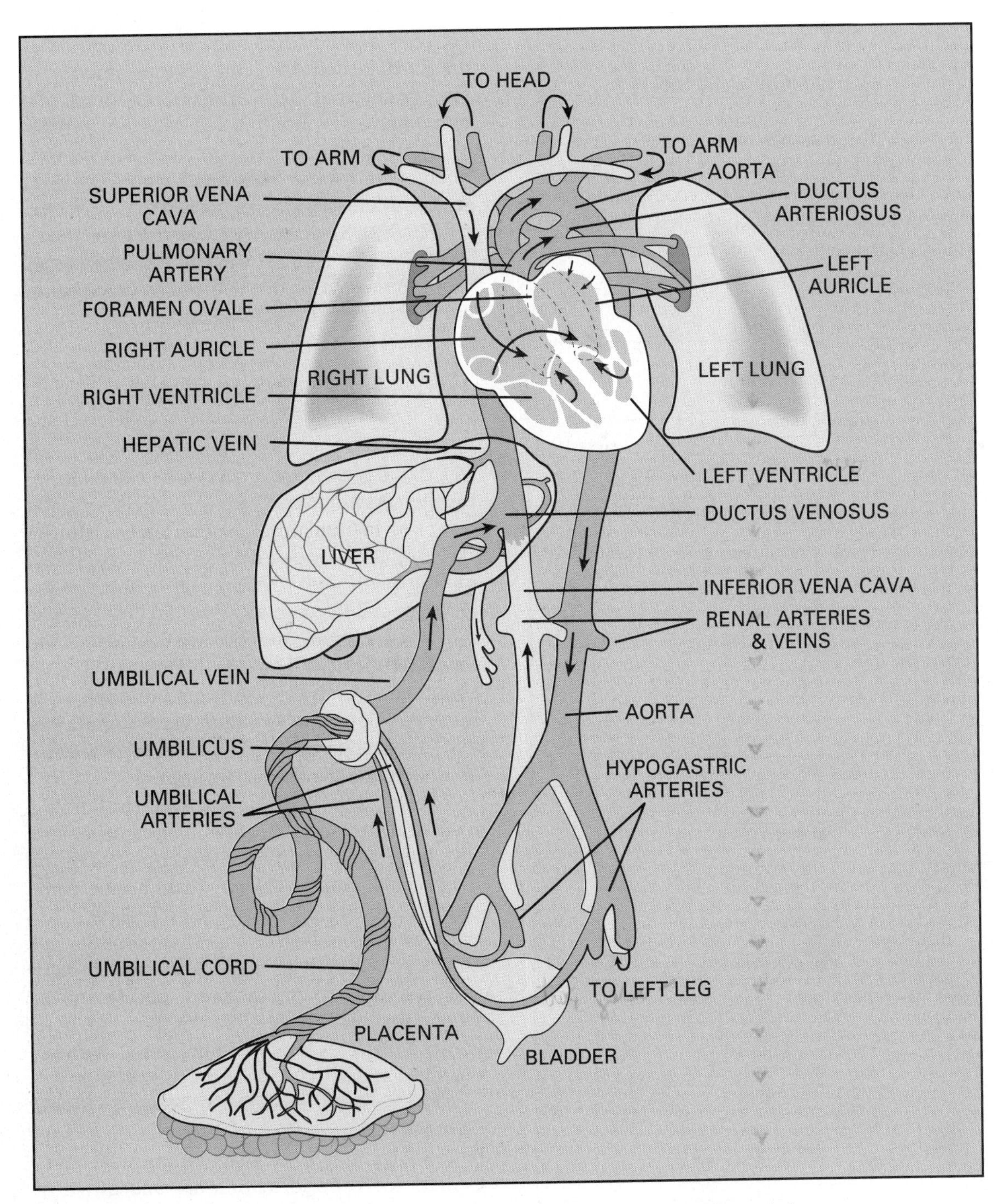

Figure 4–4 *Fetal circulation (Adapted from Nursing Education Aid, No. 1, Ross Laboratories)*

CIRCULATION CHANGES AT BIRTH

At birth, the infant's lung function is established; several of the vessels are no longer of use. The umbilical arteries become filled with clotted blood and are converted into fibrous cords. The umbilical vein in the baby's body becomes a round ligament of the liver. After the cord is tied and cut, a large amount of blood returns to the heart from the lungs. The more or less equal pressure in the auricles causes the foramen ovale to close and it eventually disappears. The ductus venosus and ductus arteriosus shrivel up and are converted to fibrous ligaments within two to three months. The closure of the foramen ovale changes the course of the blood flow to that of normal adult human circulation.

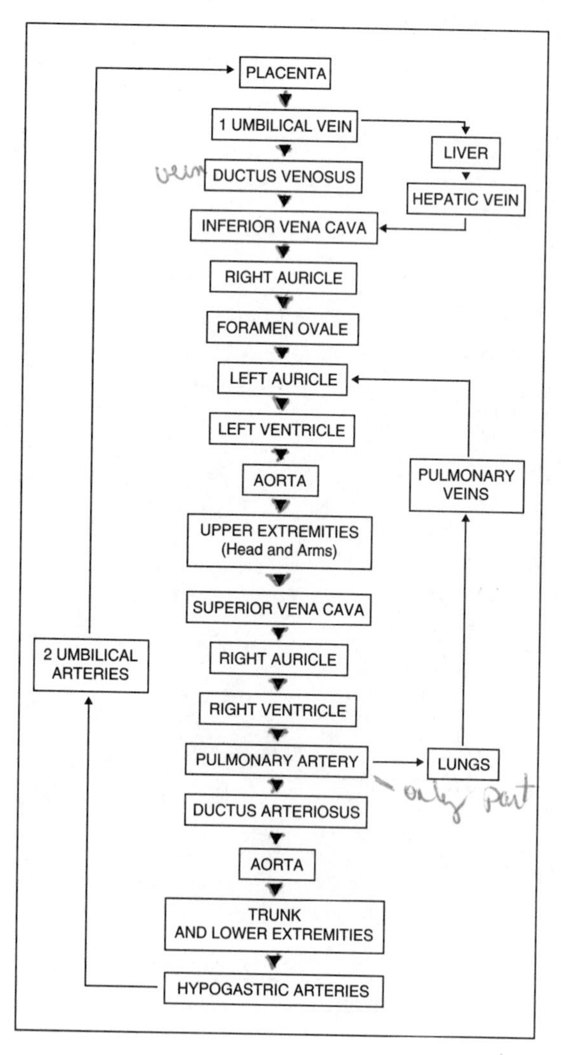

Figure 4–5 *Flow chart of fetal circulation*

FETAL DEVELOPMENT

In a four-week embryo, the spine, arms, and legs are all present but in underdeveloped form. By the seventh week the skeleton is virtually complete in miniature. At this early date the skeleton is made of cartilage, not bone. Much more growth and development of the various parts are still to come about before birth, Figure 4–6. **Ossification**, the transformation of the tough, elastic cartilage into hard bone, begins about the seventh week and continues into adolescence. For example, almost all of the 26 bones that eventually make up the skeleton of the adult foot are still cartilage at birth.

The muscles that are involved in standing erect and in using the arms, hands, legs, and feet have their beginning structures early in the prenatal period. They increase in size, complexity, and strength as gestation proceeds. No mother needs to be told that these muscles get an active workout in utero. The unborn baby can and does perform many bodily movements that are impossible for the newborn because the fetus floats within the sac of amniotic fluid and is thereby rendered weightless.

The embryo becomes a **fetus** at around eight weeks gestation, when the first true bone cells replace cartilage in the skeleton. Centers for bone formation are laid down in the long bones during the third lunar month, and the fingers and toes can be distinguished.

The nails begin to form and the external genitals show some sex distinction. The fetus resembles a human form, weighs from 5 to 20 g (about ½ ounce) and is now about 9 cm (3½ inches) long.

If the fetus were expelled from the uterus at this time, it would not survive. Expulsion of the fetus at this stage is called a miscarriage or an early spontaneous abortion. A large number of miscarriages that occur in the early months of pregnancy are believed to be caused by imperfect implantation or embryonic formation. Miscarriage could be nature's way of handling the problem of a possibly defective offspring.

At the beginning of the second trimester of pregnancy, the fetus looks like a baby with its eyes closed, Figure 4–7. The arms and legs are short; the fingers and toes are well formed. Fingernails are beginning to grow, and the deciduous, or temporary, teeth are developing in the gums. During the second trimester (fourth through sixth month) the lanugo or downy hair begins to appear on the shoulders and back. The skin is wrinkled.

The fetal heartbeat can be heard as early as the 12th week with a fetone (a very sensitive instrument that uses sound waves to detect the heartbeat). By the 20th week, the fetal heartbeat can be heard with a fetoscope. At about this time the mother-to-be notices movement of the fetus. This first movement is known as **quickening**.

By the end of the fifth lunar month the fetus weighs about 10 ounces (285 g) and is 10–13 inches (25–33 cm) long. It is previable

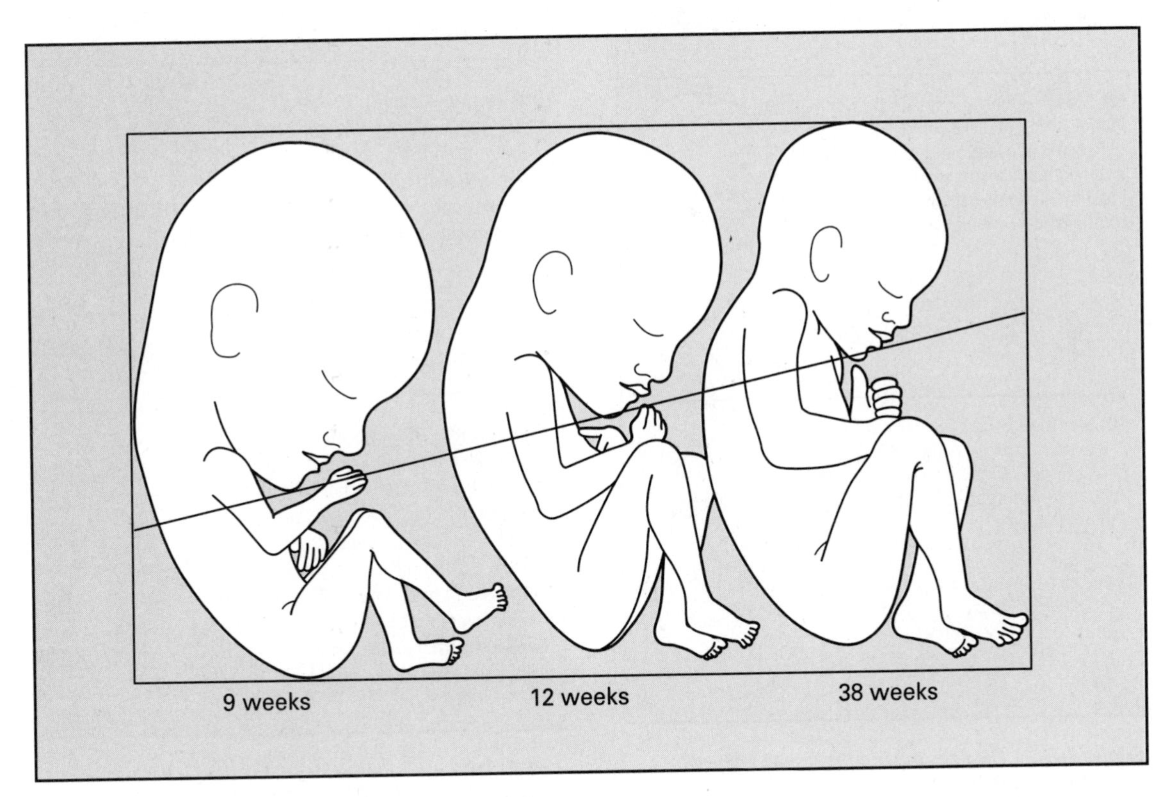

Figure 4–6 *Fetal proportion changes throughout the pregnancy*

(not sufficiently developed to live outside the uterus). If it were born at this time, it would be extremely frail. Its expulsion from the uterus could be called a late abortion. Most states require a fetal death certificate if the fetus is expelled at this time. If the fetus showed any signs of life, a birth certificate is also issued.

During the third trimester (7th through 10th lunar month) the fetus becomes covered

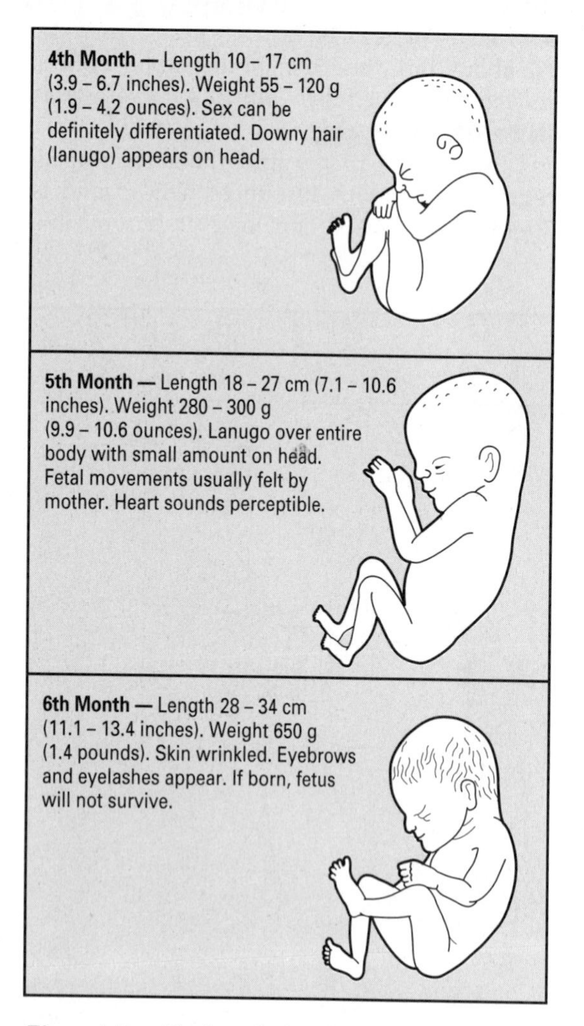

4th Month — Length 10 – 17 cm (3.9 – 6.7 inches). Weight 55 – 120 g (1.9 – 4.2 ounces). Sex can be definitely differentiated. Downy hair (lanugo) appears on head.
5th Month — Length 18 – 27 cm (7.1 – 10.6 inches). Weight 280 – 300 g (9.9 – 10.6 ounces). Lanugo over entire body with small amount on head. Fetal movements usually felt by mother. Heart sounds perceptible.
6th Month — Length 28 – 34 cm (11.1 – 13.4 inches). Weight 650 g (1.4 pounds). Skin wrinkled. Eyebrows and eyelashes appear. If born, fetus will not survive.

Figure 4–7 The fetus during the second trimester (Adapted from Pelvic Anatomy for the Patient, *Shering Corp.)*

7th Month — Length 35 – 38 cm (13.8 – 15.0 inches). Weight 1200 g (2.6 pounds). Skin red and covered with vernix. Pupillary membranes disappear from eyes. If born, fetus breathes, cries, moves but usually dies.

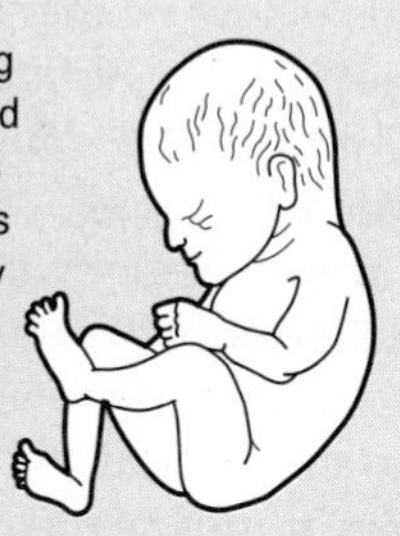

8th Month — Length 38 – 43 cm (15.0 – 17.0 inches). Weight 1600 – 1900 g (3.5 – 4.2 pounds). Appearance of "little old man." If born, may live with proper care.

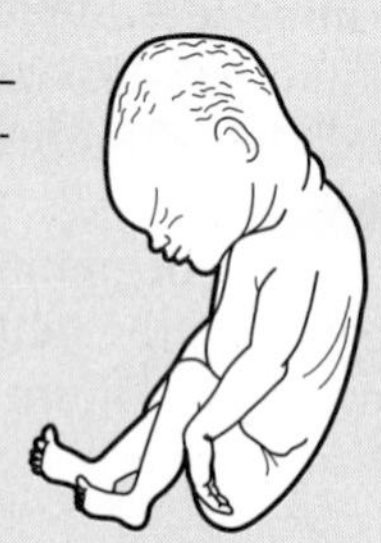

9th Month — Length 42 – 48 cm (16.6 – 18.9 inches). Weight 1700 – 2600 g (3.7 – 5.7 pounds). Face loses wrinkled appearance due to subcutaneous fat deposit. If born, good chance to survive.

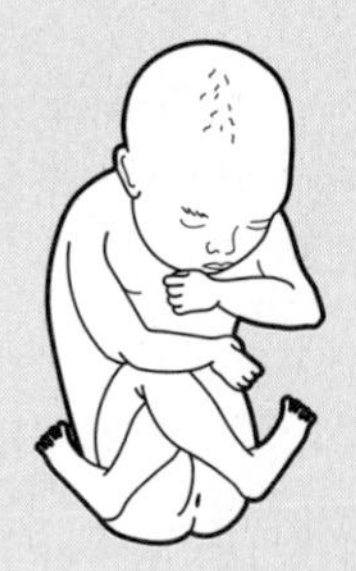

10th Month — Length 48 – 52 cm (18.9 – 20.5 inches). Weight 3000 – 3600 g (6.6 – 7.9 pounds). Skin smooth, without lanugo (except about shoulders), covered with vernix. Scalp hair usually dark. Fingers and toes with well-developed nails projecting beyond their tips. Eyes uniformly slate colored; impossible to predict final hue.

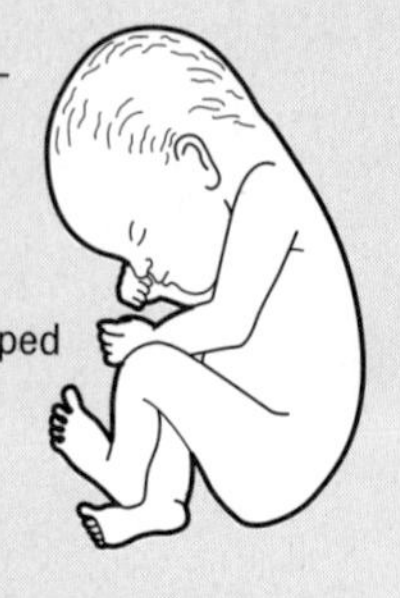

Figure 4–8 The fetus during the final trimester (Adapted from Pelvic Anatomy for the Patient, *Shering Corp.)*

with vernix caseosa, see Figure 4–8. **Vernix caseosa** is a cheeselike, greasy substance secreted probably by the sebaceous glands. It protects the skin of the fetus from softening (maceration) that might be caused by the surrounding amniotic fluid. Deposits of fat begin to form under the tissue-paper-thin skin.

The bowel of the fetus contains a thick, dark green tenacious substance called **meconium**. Meconium is made from bile, mucus, and desquamated (peeled off) epithelial cells. It will be the neonate's (newborn) first bowel movement.

The eighth lunar month can be called the month of storage. At this time the supplies of iron, calcium, phosphorus, and nitrogen needed for continuing development and immediate use in the neonatal period are being stored. The fetus is now fully developed and weighs nearly 3 pounds (1,360 g). The baby should be able to survive a premature delivery. The amount of care required is still very great if a premature baby is to live.

In the ninth and tenth lunar months, the fetus gains weight rapidly, approximately 8 ounces (227 g) per week, because of subcutaneous (under the skin) fat deposits. The hair and nails are fairly long. The fetus begins to shed the lanugo and may even suck its thumb. Breathing movements can be noted on ultrasound as the fetus prepares for the outside environment. The fetus born at nine lunar months has an excellent chance of survival.

DETRIMENTS TO DEVELOPMENT

Certain factors may influence fetal development during the first trimester of pregnancy. Frequently, the mother-to-be is unaware of her pregnancy. She may contract infectious diseases, have x-ray studies done, or take drugs that could affect the developing embryo. Figure 4–9 contains information regarding medications harmful to prenatal development. Thalidomide is an example of a drug that affects the embryo.

In several surveys of American and British pregnant women, nearly one-third of the women took some kind of mood-changing drug: sedatives, hypnotics, or appetite suppressants. Babies born to drug-dependent women are found to have breathing trouble, pneumonia, brain hemorrhage, blood disease, infection, and jaundice. Approximately 75% to 95% of babies born to heroin-addicted mothers are addicted themselves. Withdrawal symptoms begin within 24 hours after the umbilical cord is cut and the baby is deprived of its supply of heroin. Withdrawal can last from several days to six months.

Cocaine use has increased dramatically in the United States since 1980. An estimated 20 million Americans have tried the drug at least once. The availability, low cost, and highly addictive nature of **alkaloidal cocaine**, also referred to as "crack," have caused health care providers mounting concerns about the effects of the drug on exposed fetuses. It has been estimated that nearly 1 in 10 pregnant women use cocaine. The rate is significantly higher in some urban areas. Available information indicates that the drug has the potential to be more hazardous to the fetus than any other illicit drug; it is fat-soluble and of relatively low molecular weight, so it can readily pass the blood-brain barrier, as well as move across the placenta to the fetus by diffusion. The incidence of spontaneous first-trimester abortions due to placenta vasoconstriction is higher among women who use cocaine than among nonusers. Increased uterine irritability, maternal anorexia, and subsequent fetal malnutrition have widely been accepted as causes of increasing fetal morbidity. Abruptio placenta (premature separation of placenta from uterine wall) is also more common among cocaine users, and studies suggest that the damage done to placental and uterine vessels in early

EFFECT OF MEDICATIONS ON FETUS

Medication	Effect on Fetus or Neonate
Cortisone	Anomalies; cleft plate
Oral progestogens, Androgens, Estrogens	Masculinization and advanced bone age
Potassium iodide, Propylthiouracil	Goiter and mental retardation
Dicumarol, Coumadin	Fetal death; hemorrhage
Salicylates (large amounts)	Neonatal bleeding
Streptomycin	Possible eighth-nerve deafness
Sulfonamides	Kernicterus
Chlormycetin	"Gray" syndrome (anemia); death
Erythromycin	Liver damage
Furadantin	Hemolysis
Vitamin K preparations	Hyperbilirubinemia
Ammonium chloride	Acidosis
Reserpine (Serpasil)	Stuffy nose; respiratory obstruction
Heroin and morphine	Neonatal death
Phenobarbital (in excess)	Neonatal bleeding; death
Smoking	Birth of small babies
Sulfonylureas (oral antidiabetic drugs)	Anomalies
Meprobamate (Equanil, Miltown)	Retarded development
Thalidomide	Phocomelia; death; hearing loss
Vaccination; influenza	Increased titers of A and B strain antibodies in mothers
Antihistamines	Anomalies

Figure 4–9

gestation places these pregnancies at continued risk, even if cocaine use ceases.

Cocaine affects the fetal heart, causing tachycardia and decreased beat-to-beat variability. Cocaine use in the third trimester results in increased fetal activity, abrupt onset of uterine contractions, and preterm labor. Additional complications of maternal cocaine use include increased incidence of premature rupture of membranes, precipitous delivery, and fetal meconium passage, indicating distress.

Formal neurobehavioral evaluations performed on three-day-old babies, using the Brazelton neonatal behavioral assessment scale (NBAS), have revealed that many infants exposed to cocaine have difficulty responding to the human voice and face and exhibit depressed interactive behaviors and poor responses to environmental stimuli. These babies have difficulty maintaining alert states, alternate between periods of sleep and agitation, and respond poorly to comforting by caregivers.

Although not illegal, alcohol is also a drug that can have harmful effects on the fetus. Alcohol quickly passes through the placenta and enters the baby's bloodstream. **Fetal alcohol syndrome (FAS)** is a serious consequence that can occur if the mother consumes too much alcohol during her pregnancy. FAS will be discussed in more detail in Chapter 6.

Syphilis is another infectious condition that may affect the development of the embryo. In some states, mandatory premarital serological testing for venereal disease has reduced the incidence of deformities due to syphilis. A fetus infected before the fifth month probably will die.

If syphilis is contracted by the mother in the later months of pregnancy and inadequately treated, it may cause congenital syphilis affecting the heart, long bones, skin, and respiratory system of the fetus. It may also cause premature delivery or a stillborn infant.

Gonorrhea is a sexually transmitted disease that may be chronic or may be acquired by the mother at time of conception. It is generally confined to her lower genital tract, particularly the vagina and cervix. If the cervical plug has formed before the mother is infected, the gonococci may not reach the fetus. However, if a baby is born through an infected birth canal, the gonococci can cause blindness in the newborn infant unless its eyes are treated with an antibiotic or (less commonly used today) silver nitrate. Gonorrhea is generally treated with an antibiotic and can be cured.

Chlamydia is thought to be the most prevalent sexually transmitted disease in the United States. In the pregnant woman, the causative organism (*Chlamydia trachomatis*) has been linked with an increased risk for prematurity, stillbirth, and **ophthalmia neonatorum** (eye infection in the newborn). It is also thought to be responsible for **endometritis** (infection within the uterus) in the postpartum mother. Because many women who harbor the organism do not display any symptoms, routine prenatal screening cultures for *Chlamydia* are taken in many clinics. Erythromycin is the treatment of choice in pregnancy. Treatment of the male partner at the same time with tetracycline is also important so that the woman is not reinfected.

Cytomegalovirus (CMV) infection can be passed to the baby through the placenta, the vagina, or the breast milk. The risk of the fetus becoming infected is greatest during the primary (first) infection in the mother. Symptoms of CMV in the infant exposed in utero include jaundice, microcephaly (small head and often mentally retarded), deafness, and eye problems. There is no treatment for CMV infection, and it is not known exactly how CMV is spread. It is thought to be passed from close person-to-person contact through saliva, urine, or sexual contact.

Herpes simplex virus is sexually transmitted and highly contagious. Herpes infections, which are viral in origin, have been called the fastest growing sexually transmitted disease in the United States. Herpes is a lifelong disease that has a tendency to recur. Genital herpes causes blisterlike sores on and around the genital organs. Pregnant women who have genital herpes should be especially careful because a baby can become infected during delivery. A pregnant woman who has herpes should tell her doctor about it even if sores are not visible, as there may be sores inside the body. If tests show that the woman is infectious at the time of delivery, the baby can be delivered by cesarean section to avoid the possibility of infecting the infant. If an infection is present, the fetus almost always becomes infected by virus that was shed from the cervix or lower genital tract. Frequently, neonatal herpes simplex viral infections prove lethal. Serious eye and central nervous system damage has been identified in at least one-half of survivors. If tests show that the infection is not active, the mother may be able to deliver vaginally without infecting the infant.

Acquired immune deficiency syndrome (AIDS), first identified in 1979, is now well recognized as a serious health problem. The Centers for Disease Control define a case of AIDS as "a reliable diagnosed disease that is at least moderately indicative of an underlying cellular immunodeficiency in a person who has had no known underlying cause of reduced resistance reported to be associated with that disease." In 1986, the virus that causes AIDS, the third human T-lymphocyte virus (HTLV III\LAV), was renamed the **human immunodeficiency virus (HIV)**. Individuals exposed to HIV can generally be divided into three categories: HIV antibody reactive but who develop no symptoms; AIDS-related complex (ARC), who develop certain physical symptoms but who do not have AIDS; and those with AIDS. AIDS appears to be transmitted by intimate sexual contact or through direct contact with blood or blood products of someone with AIDS. Women in the following categories are at risk: intravenous drug users; recipients of blood or blood products; sex partners of hemophiliacs, intravenous drug users, or homosexual or bisexual men; and women who have undergone artificial insemination with sperm from a donor who may be at risk. AIDS may be passed to the newborn either in utero or shortly afterward. A woman who has been exposed to the HIV virus has a 50% chance of producing a child infected with the virus. The woman with AIDS may not be able to complete the emotional tasks of pregnancy and may have mixed feelings about delivering an infant that might be affected with this disease syndrome. AIDS brings with it a mortality rate of 80% within two years of diagnosis.

German measles **(rubella)** contracted during the first trimester may cause cataracts, mental retardation, deafness, and abnormalities of the heart in the developing embryo. How the virus affects the developing embryo is not clear. It is suggested that young girls be vaccinated against rubella before their reproductive years to prevent deformities in a future embryo. In June 1969, live rubella virus vaccine was licensed for use in the United States. However, rubella vaccine should not be given to pregnant women; attenuated rubella vaccine virus can infect the embryo and result in damage to the embryo.

Scarlet fever is another infectious disease that may interfere with normal embryonic development if contracted by the mother-to-be. Immediate treatment of streptococcal sore throats reduces the possibility of harm to the embryo.

During development of the fetus, serious problems arise if the nourishment of the mother or oxygen level of her blood is deficient. The common cold, heavy smoking, pneumonia, extreme anemia, and heart failure are dangerous since they interfere with the circulation of adequately oxygenated blood to the placenta. If the brain of the fetus does not receive sufficient oxygen, brain damage may result. Such damage is manifested by disturbances of the central nervous system.

If the mother's diet is deficient in protein, vitamins, or minerals during pregnancy, the child's future mental and physical development may be retarded, and he or she may have a predisposition to rickets, scurvy, anemia, tetany, or dental caries.

If the mother has diabetes, there is an increased possibility of spontaneous abortion, stillbirth, and congenital defects. Babies born to diabetic mothers usually are larger than normal, and hydramnios is common, Figure 4–10.

Another factor that may adversely affect the fetus is a **multiple pregnancy**. Because of intrauterine crowding, premature birth may result. One of the fetuses may not receive adequate supplies of minerals and vitamins. Therefore, it is likely to be less developed and smaller than the other fetus. Sometimes one survives at the cost of the other's life.

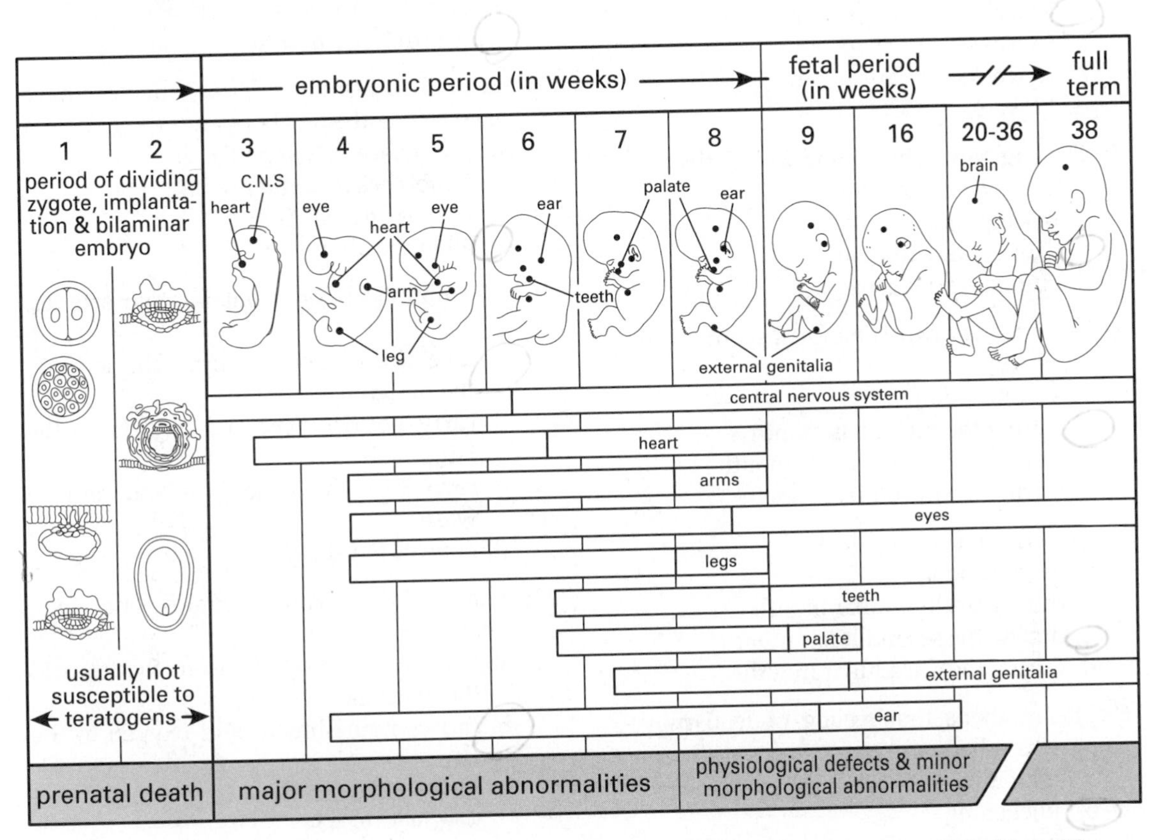

Figure 4–10 *Sensitive periods in fetal development are affected by environmental insults. (From Keith Moore.* The Developing Human, *4th ed. © 1988 by the W. B. Saunders Company, Philadelphia, PA)*

REVIEW QUESTIONS

A. Multiple choice. Select the best answer.

1. The sex of the embryo is determined at
   a. two weeks
   b. two months
   c. two days
   d. conception
2. The embryo becomes a fetus after
   a. 8 weeks
   b. 4 weeks
   c. 16 weeks
   d. 12 weeks
3. The bag of waters is composed of the
   a. amnion and placenta
   b. placenta and uterus
   c. chorion and amnion
   d. amnion and uterus
4. The organs of the embryo become differentiated
   a. at conception
   b. during the first lunar month
   c. during the second lunar month
   d. during the third lunar month
5. Circulation is established
   a. at conception
   b. during the first lunar month
   c. during the second lunar month
   d. during the third lunar month
6. The mother's first feeling of fetal movement is called
   a. lightening
   b. quickening
   c. fluttering
   d. conception
7. A thick, dark green tenacious substance that is the newborn's first bowel movement is called
   a. bile
   b. desquamated epithelial
   c. meconium
   d. vernix caseosa
8. The month in which the fetus stores iron, calcium, phosphorus, and nitrogen for continuing development and immediate use in the neonatal period is the
   a. ninth lunar month
   b. seventh lunar month
   c. sixth lunar month
   d. eighth lunar month
9. Sexually transmitted diseases that can have an effect on the newborn are
   a. gonorrhea and syphilis
   b. gonorrhea and chlamydia
   c. herpes and AIDS
   d. all of the above
10. The umbilical cord contains two arteries, which
    a. take waste products from the fetus to the placenta
    b. carry nourishment and oxygen to the fetus
    c. carry oxygen to the fetus and remove waste
    d. none of the above
11. The umbilical cord contains one vein, which
    a. takes waste products from the fetus to the placenta
    b. carries nourishment and oxygen to the fetus
    c. carries nourishment to the fetus and removes wastes
    d. none of the above
12. Hydramnios is a condition where
    a. the amniotic fluid is slightly alkaline
    b. amniotic fluid is in amounts greater than 2,000 mL at term
    c. the fetus has congenital heart defects and gastrointestinal abnormalities
    d. amniotic fluid is in amounts less than 500 mL

13. If the mother's diet is deficient in protein, vitamins, and minerals during pregnancy, the newborn may have a predisposition to
    a. rickets and scurvy
    b. anemia and tetany
    c. dental caries
    d. all of the above

14. There is a greater chance of spontaneous abortion, stillbirth, and congenital defects if the mother
    a. smokes
    b. has pneumonia during her pregnancy
    c. has diabetes
    d. has syphilis

15. The amniotic fluid
    a. equalizes the pressure around the fetus and keeps it moist
    b. cushions the fetus from injury
    c. keeps the fetus at an even temperature
    d. all of the above

16. Too little amniotic fluid
    a. causes no deformities
    b. develops small gestational age babies
    c. has no effect
    d. develops infants with pulmonary problems

17. At birth, the course of fetal blood circulation is changed to normal adult human circulation by the closing of the
    a. foramen ovale
    b. ductus venosus
    c. ductus arteriosus
    d. aorta

18. The transfer of nutrients from the maternal side of the placenta to the fetal side occurs by
    a. intermixing of maternal and fetal blood
    b. diffusion
    c. osmosis
    d. umbilical cord

19. Oxygen and carbon dioxide pass through the placenta by means of
    a. osmosis
    b. diffusion
    c. fetal lungs
    d. umbilical cord

20. The umbilical cord contains
    a. one vein and two arteries
    b. two veins and one artery
    c. one artery and one vein
    d. two veins and two arteries

21. In the umbilical cord, nourishment and oxygen are carried from the placenta to the fetus by
    a. one vein
    b. two arteries
    c. two veins
    d. one artery

B. Match the description in column I to the correct structure in column II.

Column I

1. a short blood vessel between the pulmonary artery and aorta of the fetus
2. special fetal structure for passing fetal blood from the umbilical vein into the inferior vena cava
3. thickened portion of the endometrium lying directly beneath the embedded ovum
4. opening between the right and left auricles of the fetal heart
5. fingerlike projections that have developed from the outer wall of the fertilized egg

Column II

a. chorionic villi
b. decidua basalis
c. ductus arteriosus
d. ductus venosus
e. foramen ovale

C. Briefly answer the following questions.

1. What is the function of the placenta?
2. How is the placenta formed?
3. Trace the flow of fetal blood from the placenta through the fetal circulation and back to the placenta.

SUGGESTED ACTIVITIES

- Write a report describing the effect of smoking on the developing fetus. Document your report with a bibliography.
- Describe the (a) approximate weight, (b) length, and (c) developmental milestones of the fetus at the following gestational ages.
  - 8–12 weeks
  - 13–16 weeks
  - 17–20 weeks
  - 21–25 weeks
  - 26–29 weeks
  - 30–38 weeks
- Discuss the effects of known teratogens (substances or processes that cause fetal malformation) on the developing fetus.
- Describe the fetal development in terms that can be used for patient education.
- Prepare a diagram showing the difference between fetal circulation and adult circulation.

BIBLIOGRAPHY

Benson, R. C. *Current Obstetric and Gynecologic Diagnosis and Treatment*, 5th ed. Los Altos, CA: Lange Medical Publications, 1984.

Page, E. W., Villee, C. A., and D. B. Villee. *Human Reproduction*, 3rd ed. Philadelphia: W. B. Saunders, 1981.

Pritchard, J. A., MacDonald, P. C., and N. F. Grant. *Williams Obstetrics*, 17th ed. E. Norwalk, CT: Appleton-Century-Crofts, 1985.

Scott, J. R., et al. *Danforth's Obstetrics and Gynecology*, 6th ed. Philadelphia: J. B. Lippincott, 1990.

UNIT

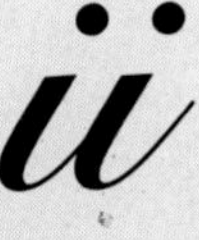

Pregnancy and Prenatal Care

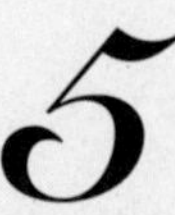

CHAPTER 5

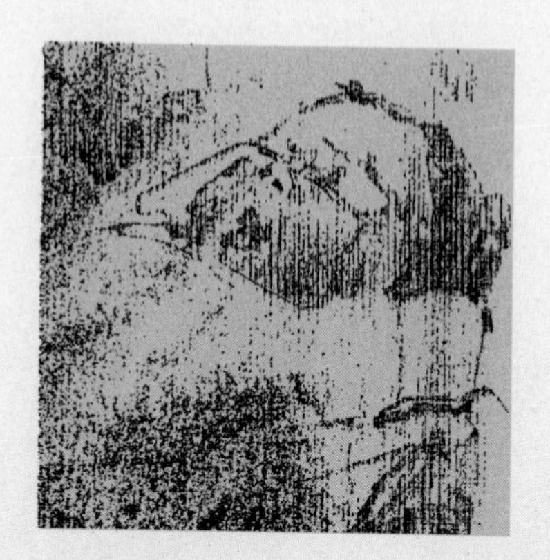

Signs and Symptoms of Pregnancy

OBJECTIVES

AFTER STUDYING THIS CHAPTER, THE STUDENT SHOULD BE ABLE TO:

- IDENTIFY THE PHYSIOLOGICAL CHANGES OF PREGNANCY.
- DEFINE PRIMIGRAVIDA, MULTIGRAVIDA, PRIMIPARA, AND MULTIPARA.
- STATE HOW THE INCREASED BLOOD VOLUME AFFECTS HEART ACTION.
- DISTINGUISH BETWEEN THE PRESUMPTIVE, PROBABLE, AND POSITIVE SIGNS OF PREGNANCY.

KEY TERMS

PRIMIGRAVIDA
MULTIGRAVIDA
NULLIPARA
PRIMIPARA

MULTIPARA
ANTEFLEXED
HEGAR'S SIGN
GOODELL'S SIGN
CHADWICK'S SIGN
BRAXTON-HICKS CONTRACTIONS
BALLOTTEMENT
LINEA NIGRA
CHLOASMA GRAVIDARUM
STRIAE GRAVIDARUM
VARICOSE VEINS
ALBUMINURIA
PREECLAMPSIA
CYSTITIS
PYELITIS
HEARTBURN
OXYTOCIN
PRESUMPTIVE, PROBABLE, AND POSITIVE SIGNS OF PREGNANCY
ULTRASONOGRAPHY
RADIOGRAPHY
FUNIC SOUFFLE
PLACENTAL SOUFFLE

This unit investigates the changes that affect the body systems of the pregnant woman. The signs of pregnancy, which are classed as presumptive, probable, and positive, are also described.

Early in the obstetrical nursing program, the student should learn the following definitions because these terms are used constantly in the obstetrical field.

primigravida: a woman pregnant for the first time

multigravida: a woman who has been pregnant several times

nullipara: a woman who has not borne children

primipara: a woman in labor with or having borne her first child (or children in the case of multiple gestation)

multipara: a woman in labor with or having borne her second child and subsequent children

PHYSIOLOGICAL CHANGES

A woman's body undergoes many physical changes during pregnancy. It is important for the nurse working with obstetrical patients to be aware of these changes.

REPRODUCTIVE SYSTEM

During the first three months of pregnancy the uterus changes in size and shape, see Figure 5–1. It becomes more **anteflexed** (bent forward) than usual. It eventually increases to 500 times larger than its original size. Its weight increases

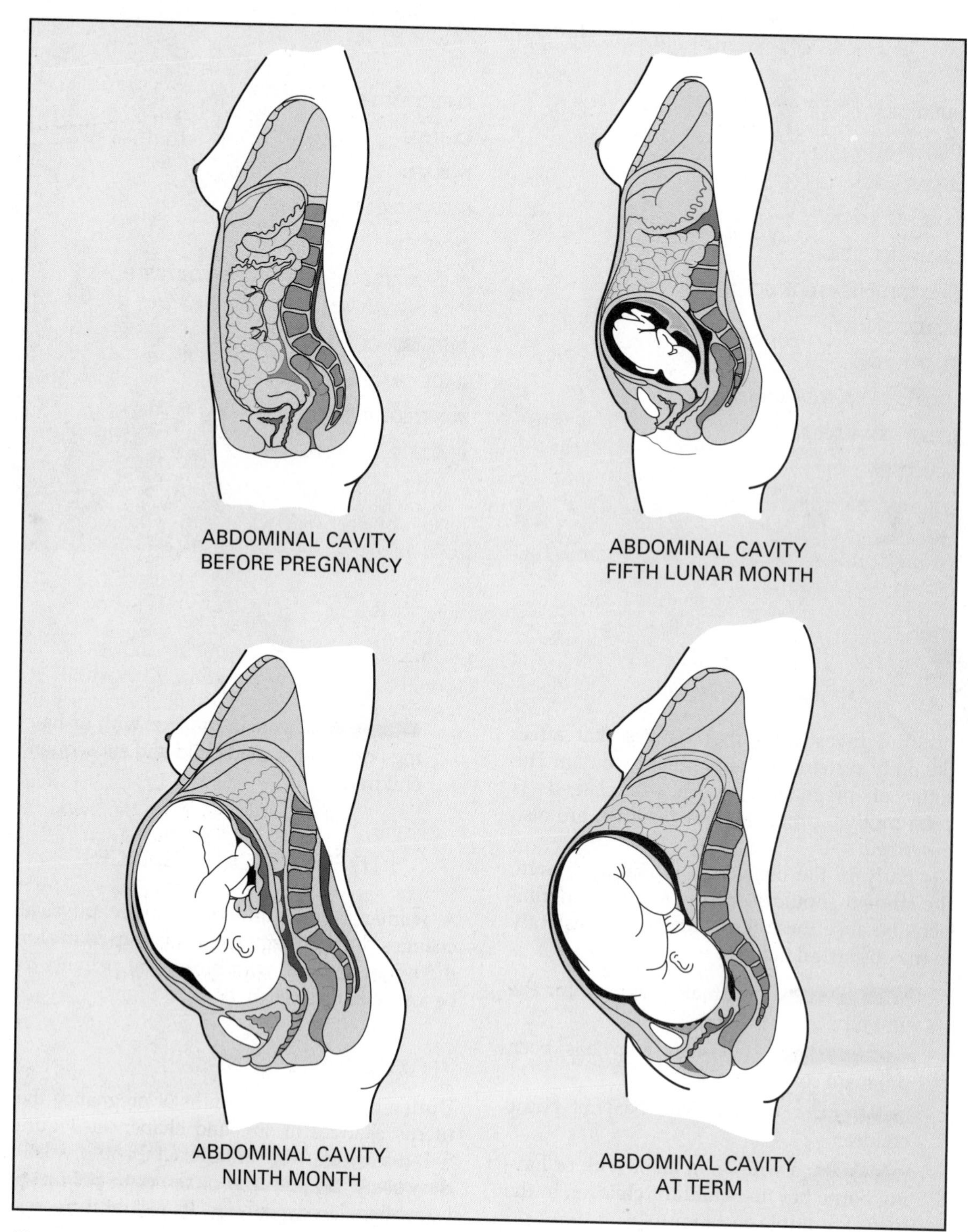

Figure 5–1 *Changes in abdominal cavity (Courtesy of Maternity Center Association)*

from 2 ounces to 2 pounds (56½–908 g). At about the sixth week of pregnancy, Hegar's sign is perceptible. **Hegar's sign** is the softening of the lower portion of the uterus above the cervix. This is one of the most indicative signs of early pregnancy.

A second sign noted by vaginal examination is Goodell's sign. **Goodell's sign** is softening of the cervix, which occurs early in pregnancy.

Another early indication of pregnancy is known as **Chadwick's sign**. The tissue around the vagina and external genitals becomes thicker and softer. It takes on a bluish purple color due to the increase in blood supply to that area. During the first trimester, vaginal secretions increase and consist of a thick, white discharge.

Uterine contractions begin in the early weeks of pregnancy and continue throughout the entire period of gestation. They are painless, and the patient is usually not conscious of them. These painless, intermittent contractions of the uterus are known as **Braxton-Hicks contractions**. The uterine muscles contract and relax, thereby enlarging the uterus to accommodate the growing fetus and developing power to expel the baby.

Between the fourth and fifth month of pregnancy, the fetus is small in relation to the amount of amniotic fluid. At this time ballottement can be performed. **Ballottement** is the rebounding of the floating fetus in the uterus when the fetus is lightly tapped during a vaginal examination. A gentle tap makes the fetus rise in the amniotic fluid; it then returns to its original position, tapping the examining finger. Ballottement can be done only after the fetus has grown large enough to be felt and before it becomes too large to move about freely. It is not a positive sign of pregnancy, as a tumor could produce the same effect.

THE BREASTS

In the early months of pregnancy, the breasts become larger, firmer, and more tender. The nipple is elevated and the areola (pigmented area around nipple) becomes darker. The weight of the breasts increases approximately 1½ pounds (680 g) because of the increased growth and activity of the glandular tissues and a richer blood supply.

SKELETAL AND MUSCULAR SYSTEMS

The skeletal system responds to pregnancy by producing a greater blood supply in the bone marrow. The ligaments holding the pelvis together at the pubic symphysis and sacroiliac articulation soften because of hormonal changes during pregnancy. This softening allows the pelvis to spread out, allowing more room for the passage of the baby. General muscle tone decreases.

THE SKIN

During pregnancy, the skin shows many changes throughout the body. In addition to increased pigmentation around the nipples of the breasts, other pigmentary changes are common in pregnancy. The **linea nigra** is a dark color line running from the umbilicus to the mons pubis. **Chloasma gravidarum**, a frecklelike pigmentation of the face, often occurs during pregnancy. This pigmentation is sometimes referred to as the "mask of pregnancy"; it usually disappears after delivery. However, pigmentation of the breasts and the **striae gravidarum** (streaks on the sides of the abdomen, breasts, and thighs caused by stretching of the skin) never entirely disappear.

CIRCULATORY SYSTEM

During pregnancy, blood volume in the body increases about 30%; this means that 500 to 1,000 mL (1–1¾ pt) of blood is added to the circulatory system. The increase in blood volume is due mostly to an increase in its water content. Because the blood is diluted, the hemoglobin is slightly lower in pregnant women, but it is not a true anemia. If the hemoglobin goes below 70%, however, the woman has a true anemia, often due to an inadequate iron supply in her diet. The increased blood volume makes it necessary for the heart to pump about 50% more blood per minute than it did prior to pregnancy.

Blood volume reaches its peak during the seventh and eighth months of pregnancy and declines during the last weeks of gestation. Women with normal hearts carry this extra load without difficulty. For the woman with heart disease, however, this increase in blood volume can be of grave concern.

Palpitation of the heart is not uncommon during this period; shortness of breath may occur also. The enlarged uterus causes increased pressure on the diaphragm and lungs. The thoracic cage widens to compensate for the uterine changes. Varicose veins are common during pregnancy, particularly in the legs, vulva, and rectum. A **varicose vein** is a vein that has become extremely painful and swollen as a result of prolonged increased pressure.

URINARY SYSTEM

The urinary system changes during pregnancy; therefore, urine tests are important throughout pregnancy. During the course of pregnancy, the amount of urine increases and its specific gravity decreases. Sugar is sometimes found in the urine because of a decreased kidney threshold for glucose. It is likely to appear in the urine after a meal. Further testing is needed to determine whether diabetes is present. Transitory **albuminuria** (presence of albumin, a simple protein, in the urine) sometimes occurs in normal pregnancy, but it can also be an indication of preeclampsia. **Preeclampsia**, which in past years was termed toxemia, refers to a disorder during gestation characterized by hypertension, albuminuria, excessive weight gain, and edema (swelling). If left untreated, eclampsia (convulsion and coma) may occur. **Cystitis** (bladder infection) often occurs in pregnancy, as does **pyelitis** (inflammation of the kidney pelvis). The ureters become dilated in pregnancy because the enlarging uterus exerts pressure on the ureters as they cross the pelvic brim and the ureteral walls soften as a result of endocrine influences. The ureters lose much of their muscular tone, and with the pressure of the enlarging uterus, are unable to expel the urine as satisfactorily as before.

RESPIRATORY SYSTEM

A pregnant woman must inhale much more air than a nonpregnant woman, because she must oxygenate her own blood as well as that of the fetus. In the later months of pregnancy, the diaphragm can be displaced upward as much as one inch (2½ cm). The lungs are subjected to pressure from the expanding uterus, and shortness of breath occurs. The lung capacity is not decreased, however, because of the slight widening of the thoracic cage.

NERVOUS SYSTEM

The effect of pregnancy on the nervous system varies. The more emotionally unstable the woman is, the more likely the nervous system will be affected. Some women escape emotional upsets entirely, while other women become sensitive and irritable. Instances of actual psychosis do occur, but they are rare.

Pregnancy is not incompatible with most diseases of the nervous system (i.e., epilepsies, Bell's palsy, multiple sclerosis), but the diseases or their treatment may adversely affect the pregnancy.

DIGESTIVE SYSTEM

The digestive system often is taxed throughout pregnancy. During the early months, nausea is common, and sometimes vomiting occurs. These symptoms generally diminish by the end of the first trimester. The appetite may be either decreased, if nausea is present, or increased in the early months. The digestive system seems to become accustomed to its new role and accept the job it has to do to nourish the baby as well as the mother. Constipation is common, due in part to the nervous control of the bowels, hormonal influences, and the pressure of the expanding uterus on the sigmoid and the rectum. It may also be a result of medication, such as ferrous sulfate (iron). Constipation is often accompanied by flatulence (excessive gas in the gastrointestinal tract). Emptying time of the stomach is also changed because of pressure from the diaphragm and diminished tone of the stomach.

Heartburn often occurs in the second trimester. **Heartburn** is the regurgitation of acid liquid from the stomach into the esophagus, which causes a burning sensation in the esophagus. It has nothing to do with the heart. Heartburn may be caused by nervous tension, worry, fatigue, or improper diet. It can be lessened by eliminating most of the fat from the diet and eating smaller, more frequent meals.

ENDOCRINE SYSTEM

The anterior lobe of the pituitary gland secretes hormones that act on the breasts, ovaries, thyroid, and growth process. The posterior lobe of the pituitary gland secretes **oxytocin**, a hormone that stimulates uterine contractions. The pituitary gland is an important link in the endocrine network of pregnancy. The thyroid tends to enlarge, and as it does, its function declines, resulting in fatigue and lethargy.

WEIGHT GAIN

In the early months of pregnancy the woman may lose a little weight. This weight loss is later made up by a gain varying from 25 to 30 pounds, which usually is lost after delivery. The body stores up albumin and fat to provide for the growth of the fetus, to supply energy during labor, and to furnish materials for milk in the breasts.

The average weight gain in pregnancy is 25–30 pounds. It is distributed as follows: fetus 7½ pounds, placenta 1 pound, amniotic fluid 2 pounds, increased uterine weight 2 pounds, increased blood volume 2½ pounds, and increased breast weight 1½ pounds. The remaining pounds are fat accumulation and increased amount of tissue fluid, see Figure 5–2. The Committee on Maternal Nutrition of the National Research Council and the American College of Obstetricians and Gynecologists recommend a weight gain of 25 to 30 pounds as ideal for the pregnant woman.

SIGNS AND SYMPTOMS

Signs of pregnancy are generally well defined; in most instances, diagnosis by the physician is

Weight Gain During Pregnancy	
Fetus	7½ lb
Placenta	1 lb
Amniotic fluid	2 lb
Uterus	2 lb
Breasts	1½ lb
Blood volume	2½ lb
Fat	5 lb
Tissue fluid	6 lb
Total	27½ lb

Figure 5–2

not difficult, Figure 5–3. These signs are classified as:

- **presumptive** (presumed but not proven)
- **probable** (likely but not definite)
- **positive** (no doubt regarding pregnancy)

PRESUMPTIVE SIGNS

1. Cessation of menses. In a woman who has been menstruating regularly, the abrupt cessation of the periods is usually caused by pregnancy. Cessation of menstruation is called amenorrhea.
2. Changes in the breasts. Early in pregnancy the breasts enlarge, and usually there is some tingling in the region of the nipple, which grows and becomes more erectile and darker.
3. Chadwick's sign. The mucous membrane of the vagina just below the urethral orifice is a violet color after the fourth week of pregnancy.
4. Pigmentation. The breast nipples turn darker and occasionally chloasma (mask of pregnancy) will appear as irregular brownish patches on the face. The linea nigra

PREGNANCY SIGNS AND SYMPTOMS

Trimester	Presumptive	Probable	Positive
First **1–3 months**	Amenorrhea; tender, fuller breasts; nausea and vomiting after 1st month for 6–8 weeks in 50% of women; discoloration of the vaginal mucosa; Chadwick's sign; frequency of urination; abdominal distention; increased appetite; fatigue; loss of weight; headache; constipation; increase in vaginal discharge	Enlargement of uterus; change in shape, size, and consistency of the uterus; changes in female reproductive system: Goodell's sign, Hegar's sign, positive hormone tests; Braxton-Hicks sign	Ultrasound image of fetus
Second **4–6 months**	Colostrum expressed; quickening; pigmentation of skin (chloasma, linea nigra, areola of breast); heartburn, flatulence; weight gain; feeling of well-being	Ballottement	Hear fetal heart tones; feel fetal movement; see skeleton by x-ray, placental souffle; funic souffle

Figure 5–3

(pigmentation change, midline, from the umbilicus to the mons pubis) appears.

5. Morning sickness. Nausea and vomiting, particularly upon awakening in the morning, may begin soon after the first menstrual period is missed and usually disappear by the third month of pregnancy as the woman's body adjusts. Nausea and vomiting that last beyond the fourth month or affect general health are considered a complication of pregnancy.
6. Frequency of urination (micturition). During early pregnancy, frequency occurs because the enlarging uterus presses against the bladder. In mid-pregnancy, pressure is relieved as the uterus rises into the abdominal cavity.
7. Striae gravidarum. Shining, reddish lines on the abdomen, thighs, and breasts caused by the stretching of tissue.
8. Quickening. The first sensation of fetal life, usually felt by the mother between the 18th and 20th weeks.
9. General symptoms. During the first month of pregnancy, the woman may have a vague feeling of fatigue. She may find she requires more rest and sleep than usual; 12 hours or more is not uncommon. She may also have a dull headache, although this could be caused by reasons other than pregnancy.

PROBABLE SIGNS

1. Changes in the abdomen. The abdomen gradually increases in size. As it increases the gait and carriage of the woman change. Any enlargement of the abdomen, however, whether due to tumor or fluid, may produce the same results.
2. Hegar's sign. Softening of the lower uterine segment.
3. Ballottement. Gently tapping the fetus, which moves away and rebounds within the uterus. The movement can be felt with experienced hands.
4. Braxton-Hicks sign. Painless uterine contractions occurring periodically throughout pregnancy, enlarging the uterus to accommodate the growing fetus.
5. Outlining the fetus. The fetal body may be palpated through the maternal abdominal wall by the second half of pregnancy.
6. Hormone tests. Various tests, such as Friedman, Aschheim-Zondek, agglutination, and hCG (human chorionic gonadotropin). With newly developed monoclonal antibody technology, hCG can be detected in a woman's bloodstream or urine as early as 7–10 days after conception. Thus early determination of pregnancy is possible in the office or clinic setting even before a missed period, Figure 5–4. hCG can also be quantitatively measured in the mother's blood suggesting how advanced the pregnancy might be. Today there are several over-the-counter home pregnancy kits. To date there has been a fair percentage of false negative results. These results may be due to the test itself, incorrectly following the test steps, or misinterpreting the end results. This false negative reading often causes a delay in seeking prenatal care.

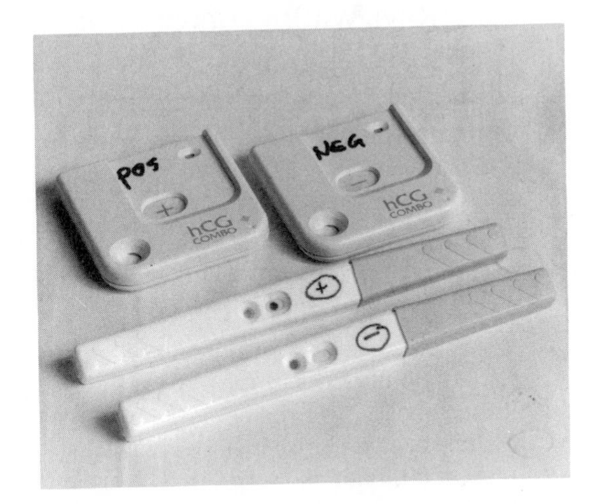

Figure 5–4 *Urine pregnancy tests can make early pregnancy determination fast and reliable.*

POSITIVE SIGNS

1. Fetal heart beat. The fetal heart tones can be heard from the third month with a fetone, see Figure 5–5.
2. **Ultrasonography**. An outline of the baby, placenta, and other structures can be seen when high-frequency sound waves scan the mother's abdomen and transmit a picture to a video screen. An embryo can be identified as early as the fourth week using ultrasound.
3. **Radiography**. After the fourth month, the fetal skeleton can be seen by x-ray examination. This type of examination is used less frequently since the development of ultrasound.
4. **Funic souffle**. A soft murmur produced by the blood flowing through the umbilical arteries.
5. **Placental souffle**: A soft murmur produced by the blood flow in the placenta.
6. Fetal movements. The movement of the fetus can be felt by the physician or nurse around the 20th week of pregnancy.

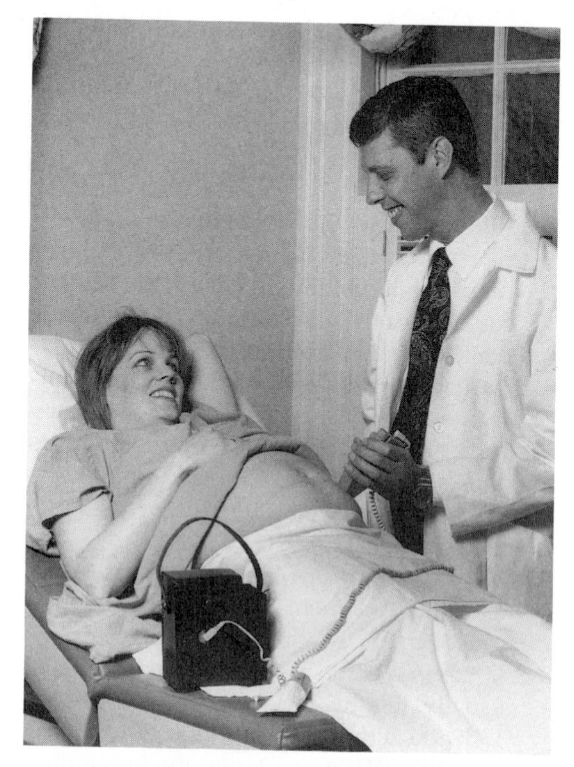

Figure 5–5 *Listening for fetal heart tones*

REVIEW QUESTIONS

A. Multiple choice. Select the best answer.

1. During pregnancy, the uterus increases in size as much as
   a. 20%
   b. 50%
   c. 500%
   d. 100%

2. A positive diagnosis of pregnancy can be made with ultrasonography about the end of the
   a. first six weeks
   b. second month
   c. third month
   d. fourth month

3. A presumptive sign of pregnancy is
   a. cessation of menses
   b. Hegar's sign
   c. funic souffle
   d. Braxton-Hicks contractions

4. Movement of the fetus can usually be felt by the physician about the
   a. fourth week
   b. eighth week
   c. third month
   d. fourth month

5. A probable sign of pregnancy is
   a. quickening
   b. detectable hCG levels
   c. amenorrhea
   d. morning sickness

6. A primigravida is a woman
   a. in labor with or having borne her first child
   b. pregnant for the first time
   c. in labor with or having borne her second or subsequent child
   d. who has been pregnant several times

7. A multipara is a woman
   a. in labor with or having borne her first child
   b. pregnant for the first time
   c. in labor with or having borne her second or subsequent child
   d. who has been pregnant several times

8. Painless, intermittent contractions of the uterus that begin in the early weeks of pregnancy and continue throughout the entire period of gestation are called
   a. Goodell's sign
   b. ballottement
   c. Braxton-Hicks contractions
   d. Hegar's sign

9. The recommended weight gain for most pregnant women is
   a. 18–20 pounds
   b. 30–34 pounds
   c. 24–28 pounds
   d. 25–30 pounds

10. Skin changes that occur during pregnancy are
    a. linea nigra and striae gravidarum
    b. chloasma gravidarum
    c. Hegar's sign
    d. a and b
    e. all of the above

11. During pregnancy, blood volume in the body increases about
    a. 3%
    b. 10%
    c. 30%
    d. 70%

12. Changes in the urinary system that might occur during pregnancy are
    a. sugar in the urine in trace amounts
    b. transitory albuminuria
    c. nitrites in the urine
    d. a and b

13. Preeclampsia is characterized by
    a. hypertension
    b. sugar in the urine
    c. albuminuria and excessive weight gain and edema
    d. a and c

14. Heartburn, which frequently occurs during pregnancy, can be lessened by all the following except
    a. eliminating most of the fat from the diet
    b. eliminating most of the sugar from the diet
    c. eliminating large meals and eating small, frequent meals
    d. lessening nervous tension, worry, and fatigue

SUGGESTED ACTIVITIES

- Demonstrate the ability to clinically diagnose pregnancy by use of historical signs, physical exam, and laboratory data.
- List the probable, presumptive, and positive signs of pregnancy.
- Describe Goodell's, Hegar's, and Chadwick's sign according to time of occurrence. Also describe why the change occurs.
- Outline a care plan for a primigravida in her first trimester.

BIBLIOGRAPHY

Hamilton, P. M., *Basic Maternity Nursing*, 6th ed. St. Louis, MO: C. V. Mosby, 1989.

Hawkins, J. W., and L. Pierfedeici. *Maternity and Gynecological Nursing*. New York: J. B. Lippincott, 1981.

Jenson, M. D., Benson, R., and I. Bobsk. *Maternity Care: The Nurse and the Family*, 3rd ed. St. Louis, MO: C. V. Mosby, 1985.

McNall, L. K. *Obstetric and Gynecologic Nursing*. St. Louis, MO: C. V. Mosby, 1980.

Niswander, K. R. *Manual of Obstetrics, Diagnosis and Therapy*, 3rd ed. Boston: Little, Brown and Co., 1987.

Oxorn, H. *Oxorn-Foote Human Labor and Birth*, 5th ed. E. Norwalk, CT: Appleton-Century-Crofts, 1986.

Pillitteri, A. *Maternal-Newborn Nursing: Care of the Growing Family*, 2nd ed. Boston: Little, Brown and Co., 1981.

Pritchard, J. A., MacDonald, P. C., and N. F. Grant. *Williams Obstetrics*, 17th ed. E. Norwalk, CT: Appleton-Century-Crofts, 1985.

Reeder, S., Mastroianni, L., Jr., and L. Martin. *Maternity Nursing*, 16th ed. New York: J. B. Lippincott, 1987.

Scott, J. R., et al. *Danforth's Obstetrics and Gynecology*, 6th ed. Philadelphia: J. B. Lippincott, 1990.

CHAPTER

6

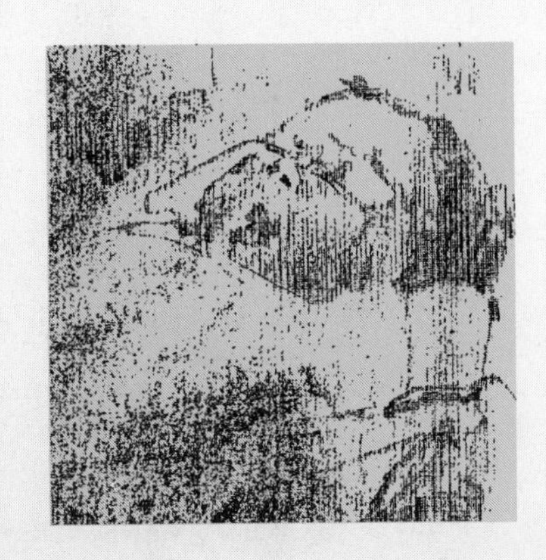

Nursing Care and Medical Supervision

Objectives

After studying this chapter, the student should be able to:

- Identify the components of the nursing process and their application to patient care.
- Describe how to prepare a pregnant patient for a physical and obstetrical examination.
- Calculate the expected date of confinement using Naegle's rule.
- Explain the reasons for procedures and laboratory tests related to prenatal medical care.
- List the danger signals that the patient should immediately report to the physician.
- Identify medications and other substances that, if taken during pregnancy, can affect the fetus or neonate.

Key Terms

- ANTEPARTUM
- NURSING PROCESS
- NURSING CARE PLAN
- SOAP NOTES
- LMP
- EDC
- NAEGLE'S RULE
- LUNAR MONTH
- PAP SMEAR
- LITHOTOMY POSITION
- FUNDUS
- LEOPOLD'S MANEUVERS
- FLOATING
- ENGAGED
- FETAL ALCOHOL SYNDROME (FAS)

Care of the pregnant woman before delivery of the infant is called prenatal or **antepartum** care. Prenatal care is the foundation for the general good health of the mother and her infant. The guidance and supervision help the woman pass through pregnancy with a minimum of mental and physical discomfort and a maximum of mental and physical fitness. In the area of prenatal care, the nurse can be of great assistance to the mother-to-be and the unborn child.

This chapter deals with early medical supervision and care of the uncomplicated pregnancy. Complications that may threaten the life of the child or the mother are addressed in Chapter 8.

The Nursing Process in Maternity Care

The **nursing process** is the framework upon which nursing care of the childbearing family is based. It involves the application of a logical problem-solving method in order to meet the needs of individual patients. The nursing process is composed of four separate but related steps: assessment, planning, implementation (or intervention), and evaluation. It is not a static process, but one that changes as the needs of the patient change.

Assessment

Assessment of the obstetrical patient involves a systematic and orderly identification of the patient's needs or problems. To identify these needs or problem areas, the nurse must first gather information about the patient. The data gathered are based on both subjective and objective observations. The data may be obtained from various sources, including the patient, other family members, significant others, members of the health care team, and the patient's chart. Methods of collecting the data include direct observation, interviewing, and examination.

Observation involves both objective and subjective data collection. Objective data are measurable and include observations made by the nurse, without benefit of interpretation. For example, the nurse might observe that her patient was taking short, frequent breaths and wringing her hands during a prenatal office visit. This observation would be considered objective data because it is a statement of what is perceived by the senses. If the patient tells the nurse, "I can't seem to catch my breath sometimes and I'm afraid something's wrong," it is a subjective observation because it is based on information given by the patient. From both of these observations, the nurse can draw certain conclusions about the patient's physiological and emotional status.

Interviewing may be both formal and informal. Asking the patient for background information on her health in order to obtain a personal history is an example of formal interviewing. This health history helps the nurse understand the patient and define her individual needs.

Informal interviewing occurs when the nurse talks with the patient while giving nursing care. This interaction is often the beginning of a therapeutic relationship between the nurse and the patient. Important information about the patient's feelings and problems may result from this informal exchange. Although informal, this information needs to be included in nursing process documentation.

The third component of data collection is the examination. During a physical examination of the patient, the nurse obtains additional facts about the patient, such as weight, temperature, pulse, respiration rate, and blood pressure. These observations are recorded on the patient's chart as part of the objective data obtained.

PLANNING

The data collected during the assessment phase are then organized, usually according to basic human needs, so that a **nursing care plan** can be developed. Maslow has identified these needs, in order of priority, as physiological needs and the need for safety and security, love and belonging, self-esteem, and self-actualization. The needs of highest priority, such as the physiological needs of air, food, drink, and rest, must be met before needs such as self-actualization can be fulfilled. The nurse usually considers the patient's developmental level, too, in organizing the data collected. The patient's mastery of certain developmental "tasks" will greatly influence the goals established for nursing care.

As data are collected, the nurse usually becomes aware of certain patient problems. In the case of the mother who was wringing her hands and experiencing shortness of breath, the nurse might identify anxiety as a possible problem. This identification of a problem would be considered a nursing diagnosis.

A part of the planning process is the writing of a nursing care plan. Outlining a plan of care for the patient is beneficial because the nurse can then see the care process in terms of the "total patient." A written care plan also enables a nurse to take over the care of a patient from another nurse without losing continuity of care. The nurse may derive a sense of satisfaction from the fact that specific long- or short-term goals of patient care have been achieved. The nursing care plan ensures that the best possible nursing care is delivered. It also provides a tool by which future related problems may be identified and resolved.

The physician's orders and recommendations, together with the nurse's assessments, form the basis for the care plan. The following should be considered in the development of a nursing care plan:

- nursing responsibilities
- problems that may affect the method of carrying out a nursing technique or fulfilling a nursing responsibility

- problems concerning the information to be given to a patient or family members
- problems that may affect interpersonal relationships between the patient and members of the health care team
- suggestions for approaches to problems geared specifically for individual patients

The nursing care plan includes a statement of specific, prioritized patient problems, the approach to be used to resolve the problems, the rationale of the planned nursing care, and the means by which the health care team can evaluate whether these goals have been reached.

IMPLEMENTATION

Implementation (or intervention) is the nursing action that is taken to resolve a patient problem. Implementing the nursing care plan can take the form of various nursing activities: performing a nursing procedure, offering physical or emotional comfort, counseling, or instructing a patient in some aspect of self-care. Nurses must always bear in mind the underlying rationale of whatever nursing action they take. In terms of the patient described previously, the partial nursing care plan shown in Figure 6–1 might be appropriate.

EVALUATION

The evaluation phase of the nursing process involves obtaining continuous feedback to determine whether the goals outlined in the nursing care plan were reached. This feedback helps determine whether the nursing care plan should be modified, depending on the degree to which the goals were met. The patient has both an active and a passive role in this process. Does she feel that her needs have been met? Are there observable signs that her anxiety has been allayed? On the basis of the observations of other members of the health care team, have the patient's needs been met? Answering these questions will help the nurse determine the effectiveness of the nursing care plan and will guide the nurse in modifying it, if necessary. If the goals have not been met, or if they have been met only partially, the nursing process is used again to revise the care plan. This care plan too, will be evaluated for its effectiveness. The cycle of assessment, planning, implementation, and evaluation will be an ongoing process throughout the course of the patient's care.

SOAP NOTES

In some hospitals, doctors may chart in **SOAP note** (subjective information, objective information, assessment, and plan) form to devise a plan of care.

SUBJECTIVE

- Describe the patient's complaint with a short quote.
- Be aware of the patient's medical history and current condition. It may be related to the present complaint.
- Give a description of the symptoms with regard to:

  onset
  character
  location
  radiation
  duration
  frequency
  severity
  associated phenomena
  aggravating or alleviating factors
  history or prior treatment of the same symptom

OBJECTIVE

- Vital signs
- Exam appropriate to system involved
- Lab data if available or indicated

PARTIAL NURSING CARE PLAN

Patient Problem	Goal(s)	Nursing Intervention	Rationale
Shortness of breath with resulting increased anxiety	By the end of her office visit, the patient will express the knowledge that her shortness of breath can be a normal and expected discomfort associated with pregnancy. She will also understand the need to report any other associated symptoms or an abnormal persistence of the problem.	Explain to the patient, in terms she can understand, the usual cause for shortness of breath in pregnancy and its effects, if any, on her baby.	Knowledge of the cause of her breathlessness (usually pressure exerted on the diaphragm by the growing uterus) should alleviate the mother's anxiety about her condition and its effect on her baby.
		Instruct the patient to sleep in a semi-Fowler's position, supported by two or three pillows.	A semi-upright position reduces the pressure of the uterus on the diaphragm, thereby making the patient more comfortable and promoting rest.

Figure 6–1 *Process for formulating a nursing care plan*

ASSESSMENT

List the findings from the subjective and objective observations at your level of understanding. Include the patient's complaint, pertinent physical findings, and important incidental findings such as history of drug allergy, high blood pressure, family history of heart disease, and health risk factors such as smoking or drug use.

PLAN

Document and give rational reasons concerning what you plan to do for each problem. Your plan should include:

- information gathering — lab or other diagnostic tests
- treatment — medical and nonmedical therapeutic modalities
- patient education
- follow-up

The following is an example of SOAP charting.

EVALUATION AND TREATMENT OF MILD IRON DEFICIENCY ANEMIA

Definition of Problem

Anemia in pregnancy is defined as a hemoglobin level of less than 10.0 g/dL or a hematocrit level of less than 30%–31%. Anemia in the nonpregnant woman is defined as a hemoglobin level of less than 12.0 g/dL: the difference in values is due to the expansion of plasma volume in pregnancy. Hemoglobin and hematocrit levels reach their lowest point during the second trimester. Then they stabilize or increase slightly near term. Iron deficiency anemia occurs not only because the amount of iron required in pregnancy exceeds what can be provided by the maternal iron stores, but also because of increased absorption of iron from the maternal GI tract.

Subjective observation (patient's own words)

- History of closely spaced pregnancies.
- Poor dietary intake of iron or failure to take prescribed iron supplementation.
- Patient may be symptomatic or asymptomatic.
- Possible fatigue, dizziness, headache, and palpitations.
- Patient complains of mouth soreness.

Objective observation (nurse's comments)

- Patient shows possible pallor and pale conjunctiva.
- Tachycardia.
- Hemoglobin (Hb) level below 10.0 g/dL or hematocrit (Hct) below 31%.

Assessment

A presumptive diagnosis is based on clinical data, in the absence of other pathology.

Plan

- Diagnostic tests
  1. Hemogram to be done on all initial prenatal visits.
  2. Hemogram routinely repeated at 30–32 weeks' gestation.
- Treatment
  1. If hematocrit is 37% or greater
     a. no treatment required
     b. repeat at 30–32 weeks' gestation
  2. If hematocrit is 31%–36%
     a. review diet
     b. encourage the intake of daily prenatal vitamin with Fe and folic acid
     c. repeat Hct at 30–32 weeks' gestation
  3. If the hematocrit is 30% or below
     a. review diet
     b. treat with ferrous sulfate 300 mg tid, and prenatal vitamins as above
     c. repeat Hct in 2–4 weeks. If Hct is not responding to treatment, consult with physician
     d. obtain indices: CBC, serum iron reticulocyte count
     e. check for bleeding parasites
- Patient Education
  1. Inform patient of foods high in iron and folic acid.
  2. Stress importance of good nutrition.
  3. Encourage patient to take prenatal vitamin supplements daily.
  4. Advise patient to avoid milk and milk products when taking Fe supplement, as calcium interferes with the absorption of iron.
  5. Explain reason for iron or folic acid deficiency in late pregnancy.

A nursing care plan assesses the patient's problem, formulates goals and a plan of action, and states the rationale for the expected outcome. Nursing care plans appear throughout the text.

The next three chapters deal with prenatal care; medical supervision; normal care, diet, and exercise; and complications of pregnancy. These aspects should be considered connected to each other, since each affects the others. The patient's initial visit to the physician is discussed here, since this is generally the time when prenatal care begins.

FIRST VISIT TO THE PHYSICIAN

The pregnant woman usually visits the doctor after she has missed one or two menstrual periods. It is likely that some probable signs of pregnancy have been noticed. The nurse can do much to allay any fears or embarrassment of the patient. The attitude must be one of helpful care and understanding. As the patient proceeds through the examinations and tests of this first visit, the nurse should explain the procedures to help put the patient at ease.

MEDICAL AND OBSTETRICAL HISTORY

The purpose of the medical and obstetrical history is to provide the doctor with an accurate record of the patient's past and present health. After a brief, but friendly, introduction, questioning should be carried out in an orderly, systematic manner. The patient's personal, medical, and social history is recorded, and inquiries are made regarding family history with special reference to any condition likely to affect childbearing, see Figure 6–2.

ABBREVIATIONS

AIDS: Acquired immune deficiency syndrome
BCP: Birth control pills
BP: Blood pressure
BR: Breech
CVS: Chorionic villus sampling
DIL: Dilation
EDD: Estimated date of delivery
EFF: Effacement
FHT: Fetal heart tones
FHR: Fetal heart rate
GA: Gestational age
GC: Gonococcal (gonorrhea)
GTT: Glucose tolerance test
HB S Ag: Hepatitis B surface antigen
hCG: Human chorionic gonadotropin
Hct: Hematocrit
HEENT: Head, eyes, ears, nose, and throat
HGB: Hemoglobin
HIV: Human immunodeficiency virus
HPV: Human papillomavirus
LMP: Last menstrual period
MCV: Mean corpuscular volume
MSAFP: Maternal serum alphafetoprotein
OTC: Over-the-counter
Rh: Rhesus blood factor
RhIG: Rhesus immunoglobulin
Rx: Treatment, prescription
STA: Station
STD: Sexually transmitted disease
TB: Tuberculosis
TPAL: term, premature, abortions, living
UTI: Urinary tract infection
VBAC: Vaginal birth after cesarean
VDRL: Venereal Disease Research Laboratory (syphilis test)
VTX: Vertex

Figure 6–2 *Abbreviations commonly used in the prenatal record*

Personal History

- Patient identification (name, age, sex, race, height, weight, appearance)
- Reason for visit
- Present symptoms, such as common discomforts of pregnancy or bleeding problems

Medical History

- illness
- hospitalizations
- surgeries
- childhood illness
- medication (include OTC and street drugs)
- tobacco use
- alcohol use
- allergies
- exposures (occupational, travel, home)
- contraceptive history
- immunizations
- transfusions
- trauma
- GYN and menstrual history (menarche, frequency, duration, flow, LMP, pain)
- pregnancy history (TPAL; complications during pregnancy, delivery, or abortion)

Social History

- cultural and religious background
- financial (income, resources, insurance)
- living situation, martial status, family support system
- occupation (satisfaction, stress, exposure risk)
- education
- hobbies, interests, and exercise
- typical day (sleep patterns, diet)

Family History

- health of parents, siblings, and grandparents
- chronic diseases of family members
- genetic history (congenital diseases, twins, etc.)

After the information needed has been obtained the interview can be brought to a close by giving the patient a chance to express any concerns or questions.

If the patient is taking any medications, this fact should be brought to the doctor's attention. The doctor will decide whether the medication should be continued during pregnancy.

Regulations require that all prescription drugs be labeled to indicate their effect on fetal development. The labels must also indicate the short-term and long-term effects the drugs have on the mother and child. Physicians should advise the woman about any potential hazards associated with taking a particular drug. All drugs, even simple over-the-counter (OTC) drugs, should not be taken without permission from the physician.

Until the early 1960s, it was assumed that the placenta screened all harmful substances for the fetus. The thalidomide tragedy of the sixties, however, dramatically altered that assumption. Many babies whose mothers had used the drug were born with serious deformities. It is difficult to trace the connection between drugs and birth defects because animals, not humans, are used as experimental subjects. Although information obtained from animal studies is valuable, it cannot always be applied to humans. It is also difficult to isolate a single drug used during pregnancy. Most women use more than one OTC drug as well as prescription medications during a pregnancy. The issue is further complicated by the fact that a drug may be harmful only when used at a particular time during a pregnancy or only in conjunction with other drugs.

Despite the difficulties and complexities of tracing the specific effects of particular drugs, we do know that virtually all drugs and medications cross the placenta and reach the fetus. If any medication is administered during pregnancy, the advantages gained must outweigh any risk associated with its use.

The Food and Drug Administration (FDA) has established five categories of drugs based on their potential for causing birth defects (teratogenicity) in infants born to women who use the drug during pregnancy. By law, the label must supply all available information on the teratogenicity. These categories are as follows:

Category A. Well-controlled human studies have not disclosed any fetal risk.

Category B. Animal studies have not disclosed any fetal risk, but have suggested some risk to women. That risk, however, has not been confirmed in controlled studies of women. There are no adequate studies concerning pregnant women.

Category C. Animal studies have revealed adverse fetal effects, but again, there are no adequate controlled studies of pregnant women.

Category D. There is some fetal risk, but the benefits may outweigh the risk (e.g., control life-threatening illness or no safer effective drug). Patients should be warned.

Category X. Fetal abnormalities in animal and human studies confirm that the risk is not outweighed by the benefit. Drugs in this category are contraindicated during pregnancy.

An important part of the health record involves the patient's menstrual cycle. The following information should be recorded about the patient:

- At what age did menstruation begin (menarche)?
- What is her normal menstrual cycle?
- Are her periods regular?
- Are her periods painful?
- How heavy is her menstrual flow?
- How many days does her period last?
- When was the first day of her last menstrual period **(LMP)**?
- Was that last period normal in cycle and flow?

The doctor needs the date of the last menstrual period (LMP) to estimate the expected date of confinement **(EDC)**. **Naegle's rule** is used for calculating the EDC: Add 7 days to the first day of the LMP; subtract 3 calendar months from the new date, and add 1 calendar year (9 calendar months = 10 lunar months, 1 **lunar month** is about 28 days). Obviously, the result will be only an approximation, and the error may be as much as 2 weeks in either direction. Figure 6–3 shows another means of determining the EDC. The top line in each block refers to the date of menstruation. The second line in each block indicates the expected date of confinement. For example, if the date of menstruation is June 1, the baby may be expected to be born on March 8 (or one day earlier during a leap year).

The normal length of pregnancy varies greatly from 240 days to 300 days. The average duration is 9½ lunar months, or 38 weeks, or 266 days from the time of conception. From the first day of the last normal menstrual period, it is 10 lunar months, or 40 weeks, or 280 days. Some fetuses seem to require slightly longer and some slightly shorter times in the uterus for full development.

PHYSICAL EXAMINATION

After obtaining the patient's medical and obstetrical history, the nurse prepares the patient for the physical examination by the doctor. The patient is weighed, her blood pressure is taken, and both results are recorded. A urine specimen is then obtained and saved for evaluation. The nurse accom-

---

For more specific information regarding individual drug effects on the mother and fetus, refer to: Richard L. Berkowitz, M.D.; Donald R. Coustan, M.D.; and Tara K. Mochizuke, Pharm D., J.D., *Handbook for Prescribing Medications during Pregnancy*, 2d edition (Boston/Toronto: Little, Brown and Company, 1986).

January	1	2	3	4	5	6	7	8	9	10	11	12	13	14	15	16	17	18	19	20	21	22	23	24	25	26	27	28	29	30	31	Nov.
October	8	9	10	11	12	13	14	15	16	17	18	19	20	21	22	23	24	25	26	27	28	29	30	31	1	2	3	4	5	6	7	
February	1	2	3	4	5	6	7	8	9	10	11	12	13	14	15	16	17	18	19	20	21	22	23	24	25	26	27	28				Dec.
November	8	9	10	11	12	13	14	15	16	17	18	19	20	21	22	23	24	25	26	27	28	29	30	1	2	3	4	5				
March	1	2	3	4	5	6	7	8	9	10	11	12	13	14	15	16	17	18	19	20	21	22	23	24	25	26	27	28	29	30	31	Jan.
December	6	7	10	9	10	11	12	13	14	15	16	17	18	19	20	21	22	23	24	25	26	27	28	29	30	31	1	2	3	4	5	
April	1	2	4	4	5	6	7	8	9	10	11	12	13	14	15	16	17	18	19	20	21	22	23	24	25	26	27	28	29	30		Feb.
January	6	7	8	9	10	11	12	13	14	15	16	17	18	19	20	21	22	23	24	25	26	27	28	29	30	31	1	2	3	4		
May	1	2	3	4	5	6	7	8	9	10	11	12	13	14	15	16	17	18	19	20	21	22	23	24	25	26	27	28	29	30	31	Mar.
February	5	6	7	8	9	10	11	12	13	14	15	16	17	18	19	20	21	22	23	24	25	26	27	28	1	2	3	4	5	6	7	
June	1	2	3	4	5	6	7	8	9	10	11	12	13	14	15	16	17	18	19	20	21	22	23	24	25	26	27	28	29	30		April
March	8	9	10	11	12	13	14	15	16	17	18	19	20	21	22	23	24	25	26	27	28	29	30	31	1	2	3	4	5	6		
July	1	2	3	4	5	6	7	8	9	10	11	12	13	14	15	16	17	18	19	20	21	22	23	24	25	26	27	28	29	30	31	May
April	7	8	9	10	11	12	13	14	15	16	17	18	19	20	21	22	23	24	25	26	27	28	29	30	1	2	3	4	5	6	7	
August	1	2	3	4	5	6	7	8	9	10	11	12	13	14	15	16	17	18	19	20	21	22	23	24	25	26	27	28	29	30	31	June
May	8	9	10	11	12	13	14	15	16	17	18	19	20	21	22	23	24	25	26	27	28	29	30	31	1	2	3	4	5	6	7	
September	1	2	3	4	5	6	7	8	9	10	11	12	13	14	14	16	17	18	19	20	21	22	23	24	25	26	27	28	29	30		July
June	8	9	10	11	12	13	14	15	16	17	18	19	20	21	22	23	24	25	26	27	28	29	30	1	2	3	4	5	6	7		
October	1	2	3	4	5	6	7	8	9	10	11	12	13	14	15	16	17	18	19	20	21	22	23	24	25	26	27	28	29	30	31	Aug.
July	8	9	10	11	12	13	14	15	16	17	18	19	20	21	22	23	24	25	26	27	28	29	30	31	1	2	3	4	5	6	7	
November	1	2	3	4	5	6	7	8	9	10	11	12	13	14	15	16	17	18	19	20	21	22	23	24	25	26	27	28	29	30		Sept.
August	8	9	10	11	12	13	14	15	16	17	18	19	20	21	22	23	24	25	26	27	28	29	30	31	1	2	3	4	5	6		
December	1	2	3	4	5	6	7	8	9	10	11	12	13	14	15	16	17	18	19	20	21	22	23	24	25	26	27	28	29	30	31	Oct.
September	7	8	9	10	11	12	13	14	15	16	17	18	19	20	21	22	23	24	25	26	27	28	29	30	1	2	3	4	5	6	7	

Figure 6–3 *To calculate the period of uterogestation, from the top row of a block, select the month and day when the last menstrual period began. The month and day immediately below that date is the estimated date of confinement.*

panies the patient to the dressing room and explains the need for the patient to undress completely. The nurse shows the patient how to wear the examination gown.

The nurse is expected to remain with the patient during the examination to provide support as well as to assist the doctor. The patient is given a complete physical examination, with special attention to the heart, lungs, pelvis, breasts, and nipples.

OBSTETRICAL EXAMINATION

The purposes of the internal examination are to examine the vagina and pelvic organs for signs of pregnancy; to take a cervical smear **(Pap smear)** for a cancer cytology test; to detect abnormalities such as cysts or infections; and to determine if the true pelvis is large enough to allow the baby to pass through at birth.

Before an internal examination is made, the patient should be asked to empty her bladder. The nurse then helps the patient onto the examination table; the patient is placed in the **lithotomy position** (on her back, with buttocks at end of table and feet in stirrups) and draped to minimize immediate exposure. The equipment to be used should be ready for the doctor, Figure 6–4.

LABORATORY TESTS

During prenatal care, the urine is checked for albumin and sugar and in some clinics, nitrites and leukocytes. Also, the blood is examined for hemoglobin, blood type, Rh factor, rubella antibodies, and syphilis. In many areas, the blood specimen is also screened for hepatitis. A urine specimen is required at each visit to the doctor. Blood pressure and weight are also recorded each time the patient is seen.

Other laboratory tests are performed as the pregnancy progresses. Between the 15th

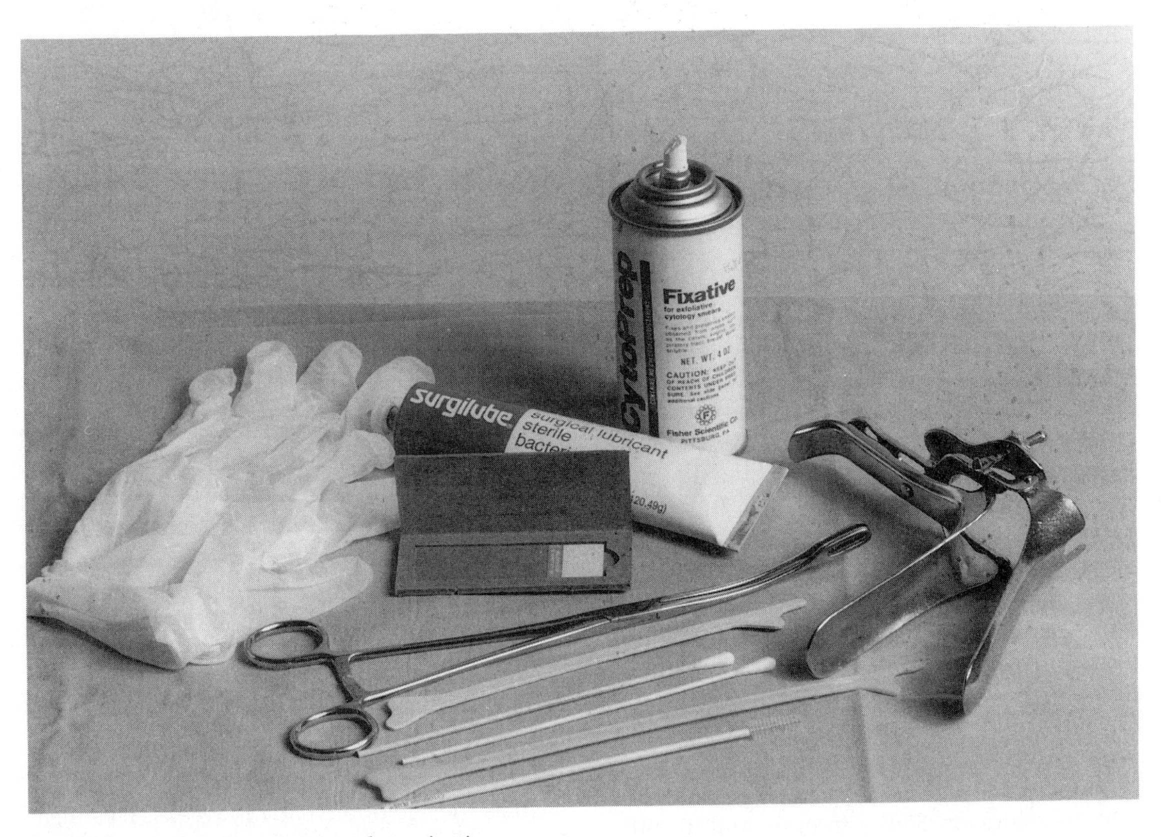

Figure 6–4 *Equipment for internal examination*

and 20th week of pregnancy, another sample of mother's blood is drawn to measure the amount of alphafetoprotein (a substance made by the fetal liver). A measure of alphafetoprotein (AFP) may be used for prenatal detection of neural-tube defects (spina bifida, anencephaly). Recent research has also shown an association between low alphafetoprotein values and an increased risk for Down syndrome. If the test shows an abnormal value, a repeat test may be suggested. If necessary, additional diagnostic procedures such as ultrasound or amniocentesis will be used to evaluate the possibility of neural-tube defects or other abnormalities.

The American Diabetes Association recommends testing of all pregnant women between the 24th and 26th week of pregnancy for a condition known as gestational diabetes. This testing is accomplished by giving the expectant mother 50 g of glucola, and taking a blood sample 1 hour later. If the glucola level is above 140 mg/dL, gestational diabetes is suspected and the pregnant woman will need further testing. Gestational diabetes will be discussed in depth with other complications of pregnancy.

Group B streptococci infections in the vagina or cervix of the expectant mother have been linked to a high number of neonatal infections and infant deaths. In some areas, antepartum cultures of the birth canal are taken from pregnant women who are at high risk to colonize with Group B streptococci.

There are several rapid (within 10 minutes) screening tests to detect Group B streptococci in pregnant women. This rapid detection can be done in the office or clinic setting. The test allows the physician time to treat the affected woman adequately to avoid exposing the newborn.

RETURN VISITS

The patient under the doctor's care returns every three or four weeks during the first seven months of pregnancy. During the last two months, she is usually seen more frequently. At each visit, careful inquiries are made regarding any unusual signs or symptoms. Blood pressure and weight are noted each time, and the urine specimen is examined for the presence of albumin, sugar, and sometimes nitrites, and leukocytes.

Weight gain or loss is an important detail of prenatal care. A diet to control weight may be prescribed, but an adequate diet is important to maintain daily strength and health. Usually there is little, if any, weight gain during the first three months of pregnancy. A woman gains about ¾ to 1 pound a week during the last six months of pregnancy. The recommended weight gain in pregnancy is 25 to 30 pounds.

At each visit, many doctors examine the abdomen to determine the growth and size of the uterus and the fetus; they also listen to the fetal heartbeat, which usually ranges from 120 to 160 beats per minute. Within a month to six weeks before the fetus is full term, the doctor is able to determine whether the presenting part is engaged by performing a pelvic exam.

PALPATION OF THE ABDOMEN

Palpation of the abdomen, which doctors include in their examination, is a useful skill for the nurse to acquire also. As a diagnostic measure, its value is greatest after the 13th or 14th week, when the uterus has risen from the pelvic cavity. The progress of a pregnancy can be determined by measuring the height of the **fundus** (top of the uterus). Fundal height can be measured in centimeters, using calipers, or by placing the hand over the fundus and estimating the height in relation to anatomical landmarks such as the symphysis pubis or umbilicus.

By 12 weeks, the fundal height is at the top of the symphysis. At 16 weeks, the fundus can be palpated midway between the symphysis and umbilicus. By 20 weeks the fundal height has reached the umbilicus, and by 36 weeks, it is often at the xiphoid, or tip of the chestbone called the sternum. The height of the fundus is measured at each prenatal visit, usually with a caliper or tape measure. The measurement is taken from the pubic bone to the fundus. Between 18 and 30 weeks gestation, the height of the uterus in centimeters approximately equals the age of the baby in weeks. This measurement is a good indicator that the baby is growing appropriately.

Presentation and position of the developing baby can be determined by techniques called **Leopold's maneuvers**. The outline of the fetus is determined by palpation, see Figure 6–5. Sliding warmed hands down the sides of the mother's abdomen and applying gentle but deep pressure, the nurse may feel firmness and resistance on one side (fetal back) and nodularity on the other (feet, elbows, and so on, of the fetus). With thumb and fingers of one hand, the nurse can determine the presenting part (fetal head or breech) by grasping the lower portion of the uterus just above the symphysis pubis. If the presenting part is freely movable above the brim of the pelvis, it is said to be **floating**; if it is firmly fixed in the pelvis, it is said to be **engaged**.

PLANNING FOR THE BABY

The nurse who sees the pregnant woman throughout her pregnancy is in a unique position to help her make decisions about what will happen after she gives birth. These decisions require information gathering, discussion, and introspection on the part of the expectant mother. Questions she might explore include:

- Who will provide health care for the baby — a pediatrician, family practice physician, nurse practitioner, or well-child clinic?
- Will I breast feed or bottle feed my baby?
- If my baby is male, should I have him circumcised?
- What preparations are needed for the baby — car seat, crib, clothes, and so on?
- What do I know about child care, and where can I get information and support if I need it?
- Will I work outside the home after the baby is born? If so, who will provide child care?

The prenatal care nurse can help the expectant mother find answers to her questions and ease the transition to parenthood.

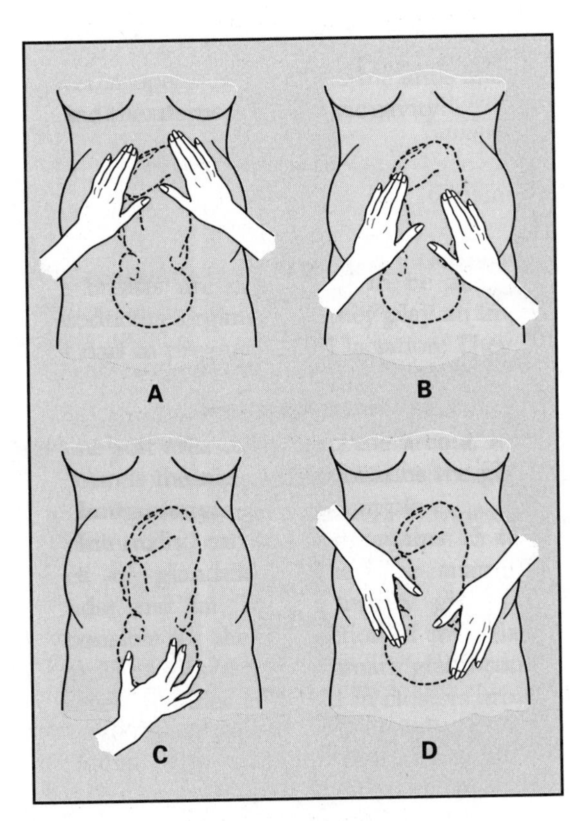

Figure 6–5 Palpating the outline of the fetus to determine its position and presentation

DANGER SIGNALS

The patient should be instructed to immediately report any of the following symptoms to the doctor. They may indicate major complications:

- vaginal bleeding, no matter how slight
- severe, continuous headache
- swelling of the face and hands
- dimness or blurring of vision
- flashes of light; spots before the eyes
- pain in the abdomen and back
- persistent nausea or vomiting
- chills and fever over 100°F (37.8°C)
- sudden escape of fluid from the vagina
- painful, burning sensation on urination
- irritating vaginal discharge
- dizziness

These danger signals and the complication that they may indicate will be dealt with more fully in Chapter 8, Complications of Pregnancy.

OTC DRUGS, ALCOHOL, TOBACCO, AND CAFFEINE

Drugs such as aspirin, acetaminophen, sedatives and tranquilizers, antihistamines, antacids, and antiemetics are frequently used during pregnancy. These drugs do not treat illness; they relieve symptoms. Other medications such as antibiotics, insulin, and steroids cure or control an illness. The benefit of these drugs will outweigh the potential hazards in most cases. The nurse must be sure to instruct the pregnant woman to report all drugs she is taking.

Aspirin. Even one aspirin will affect the body's ability to clot blood and may prolong bleeding time. Two tablets will double the bleeding time. This effect can last from four to seven days after a single dose. Aspirin present in the baby's circulation at birth also prolongs bleeding time for the newborn and increases the likelihood of jaundice.

Acetaminophen. No adverse fetal effects have been reported with moderate use of acetaminophen. If, however, excessive amounts of this drug are used, there may be kidney damage in the fetus.

Alcohol. Until the mid-1970s, alcohol was thought to be harmless to the fetus. We now know that alcohol has a direct toxic effect on the developing fetus. Alcohol quickly passes through the placenta and enters the baby's blood in the same concentration as in the mother's blood. In the first trimester, alcohol may affect the cell membrane and alter the embryonic organization of tissue. Throughout pregnancy, alcohol may interfere with the metabolism of carbohydrates, lipids, and proteins and thus retard cell growth and division. The central nervous system probably is most vulnerable in the third trimester, during which time rapid brain growth occurs.

More than 1½ ounces of absolute alcohol (three to four drinks) per day is likely to produce an adverse effect, and moderate drinking (defined anywhere from daily to monthly) may also have negative effects, see Figure 6–6. Babies born to alcoholic mothers are at risk.

ALCOHOL CONSUMPTION

Heavy drinker	More than 45 drinks per month, or more than 5 drinks per occasion
Moderate drinker	Between 1 and 45 drinks per month, never more than 5 drinks per occasion
Light or rare drinker	Fewer than 1 drink per month

One drink is equal to ½ ounce of alcohol, or:

- One beer
- 4 ounces of wine
- 1.2 ounces of liquor

Figure 6–6 *Medical classification of alcohol consumption*

The most serious adverse effect associated with alcohol is the **fetal alcohol syndrome (FAS)**. FAS is diagnosed when there are abnormalities in each of the following three categories:

- prenatal or postnatal growth retardation
- neurological abnormality, developmental delay, or intellectual impairment
- characteristic facial dysmorphology (abnormal shape) with at least two of the following signs:

  microcephaly (small head)

  microphthalmia (small eyes) or short palpebral (eyelid) fissures

  poorly developed philtrum (groove on upper lip), thin upper lip, or flattening of the maxillary area

While assessment and support for behavioral changes in the expectant mother who consumes alcohol need to begin at the first prenatal visit, continuing such efforts throughout the woman's pregnancy is equally important.

Tobacco. Tobacco smoking should also be discouraged in pregnancy. Cigarette smoke contains tars, nicotine, carbon monoxide, lead, and other substances that are harmful to both a woman and an unborn child. Evidence exists that smoking reduces placental blood flow. On average, pregnant women who smoke give birth to lower birth weight babies. They have a greater chance of premature rupture of the membranes, premature birth, perinatal death, placental abnormalities, and bleeding during pregnancy. These conditions are directly proportional to the amount of smoking. The effects on the woman herself are also destructive. There is a greater risk of lung cancer; cancer of the oropharyngeal cavity, esophagus, and larynx; emphysema; coronary artery disease; cerebrovascular disease; and cardiac arrhythmias.

Caffeine. Caffeine, present in coffee, tea, cocoa, and cola-flavored drinks is probably safe in pregnancy if consumed in moderation, provided there is the absence of peptic ulcer or hypertensive heart disease. Caffeine causes an increased production of epinephrine (adrenalin) and norepinephrine (noradrenalin). These hormones constrict peripheral blood vessels, including those of the uterus. This restriction can result in a temporary decrease of oxygen available to the fetus. According to a National Academy of Sciences report, many pregnant women take in an average of 144 mg of caffeine per day. This is equivalent to about one to two cups of coffee or two to three cups of tea. Caffeine readily enters the fetal bloodstream and can cause some mild tachycardia. The effects of caffeine on pregnancy have not been proved as conclusively and consistently as those of alcohol and tobacco. But a pregnant woman who consumes drinks or foods with caffeine should be advised to do so in moderation, see Figure 6–7.

CAFFEINE CONTENT

Food	Caffeine in Milligrams
Decaffeinated coffee (cup)	2
Instant coffee (cup)	66
Brewed coffee (cup)	110
Dr. Pepper (can)	38
Pepsi-Cola (can)	37
Coca-Cola (can)	34
Cocoa (cup)	10
One ounce milk chocolate	6
One ounce dark chocolate	20
One tea bag brewed 1 minute	21
One tea bag brewed 5 minutes	40
Iced tea (can)	36
Drugs	
NoDoz	200
Anacin	64
Excedrin	130
Dristan	32
Dexatrim	200

Figure 6–7

REVIEW QUESTIONS

A. Multiple choice. Select the best answer.

1. The length of pregnancy varies, but the average duration is
   a. 266 days from the time of conception
   b. 280 days from the time of conception
   c. 320 days from the last normal menstruation
   d. 240 days from the last normal menstruation

2. The woman's urine is routinely checked for the presence of
   a. an infection
   b. albumin, sugar, nitrites, and leukocytes
   c. blood
   d. a sexually transmitted disease

3. Which of the following body signals does not need to be reported to the doctor?
   a. vaginal bleeding
   b. nausea or vomiting
   c. frequency of urination
   d. continuous headaches

4. Naegle's rule is used for calculating the expected date of confinement. This is done by
   a. adding 7 days to the first day of the last menstrual period, subtracting 3 calendar months from the new date, and adding one year
   b. adding 7 days to the last day of the last menstrual period, subtracting 3 calendar months from the new date, and adding one year
   c. subtracting 7 days from the first day of the last menstrual period, adding 3 calendar months and one year to that date
   d. adding 3 days to the first day of the last menstrual period, subtracting 4 calendar months from the new date, and adding one year

5. If the first day of a woman's last menstrual period is August 21, 1992, her expected date of confinement is
   a. May 14, 1993
   b. June 7, 1993
   c. June 1, 1993
   d. May 28, 1993

6. A blood sample is taken during the first visit (within the first 2 months of the pregnancy) to determine
   a. blood type, Rh factor, and syphilis screen
   b. whether the patient has chlamydia or other STDs
   c. whether the patient has an abnormal alphafetoprotein
   d. whether the patient has gestational diabetes

7. Important information to obtain during a patient's first prenatal visit includes
   a. the age at which menstruation began
   b. the duration of her normal menstrual cycle
   c. the first day of her last period
   d. all of the above
   e. none of the above

8. When doing an abdominal examination, the doctor is determining
   a. the growth of the uterus
   b. the growth of the fetus
   c. the size of the fetus
   d. all of the above
   e. none of the above

9. The initial internal examination of the vagina and pelvis is made to
   a. determine signs of pregnancy
   b. take a Pap smear
   c. determine if the true pelvis is large enough to allow an average-size baby to pass through at birth
   d. all of the above
   e. none of the above

10. Medications that can have an effect on the fetus are
    a. vitamin K preparations
    b. thalidomide
    c. salicylate
    d. none of the above
    e. all of the above

B. Match the step of the nursing process in column I to the correct activity in column II.

Column I	Column II
1. assessment	a. identifying and organizing patient needs and problems and documenting them
2. planning	b. giving direct nursing care
3. implementation	c. determining whether goals have been met
4. evaluation	d. gathering information about the patient

C. Complete the following statements.

1. On the basis of knowledge of the patient and the participation of the woman or couple in childbirth preparation, ________ ________ are developed.

2. The nurse can be assured that care has been effective when ________ ________ have been met.

SUGGESTED ACTIVITIES

- Practice writing a nursing care plan for a specific patient problem.
- Practice taking the medical and obstetrical history of a student who role plays a pregnant woman.
- Practice setting up equipment and draping the patient for the obstetrical examination.
- Make a list of community resources that provide classes for the prospective parents.
- Develop a list with pros and cons to consider to help the expectant mother make a decision regarding child care (breast versus bottle; circumcision of the male infant; health-care provider, and so on).

- Make a chart using the SOAP format on a new patient who presents with the following history:
  - currently at 20 weeks gestation
  - smokes one package of cigarettes a day
  - admits to taking aspirin for headaches, which she has frequently
  - drinks wine, beer, or liquor once or twice a week with meals
  - vital signs and lab work within normal range
- Demonstrate the ability to ascertain the fundal height by abdominal palpation and measurement. Correlate the fundal height with gestational age.
- Demonstrate the ability to perform an abdominal exam. Outline the fetal structures, describe the fetal lie, presentation, position, and attitude using Leopold's maneuvers.
- Demonstrate the ability to obtain a health-screening history from a patient with respect to the following:
  - patient identification
  - social history
  - medical history
  - habits
  - family history
  - obstetrical and menstrual history
  - review of systems

BIBLIOGRAPHY

Aaronson, L. S., and C. L. Macnee, "Tobacco, Alcohol and Caffeine Use during Pregnancy," *JOGNN* 18(4):279–286. July-August, 1989.

Berkowitz, R., Coustan, D., and T. Mochizuke. *Handbook for Prescribing Medication during Pregnancy*. 2nd ed. Boston: Little, Brown and Co., 1986.

Brackbill, Y. "Medication in Maternity," *Childbirth Educator* 6(2):28–32, Winter, 1986–1987.

Engstrom, J. "Measurement of Fundal Height." *JOGNN* 17(3):172–177, May-June, 1988.

Fischbach, F. T. *A Manual of Laboratory Diagnostic Tests*, 3rd ed. Philadelphia: J. B. Lippincott, 1988.

Hamilton, P. M. *Basic Maternity Nursing*, 6th ed. St. Louis, MO: C. V. Mosby, 1989.

Hassid, P. *A Textbook for Childbirth Educators*. New York: Harper and Row, 1978.

Hawkins, J. W., and L. Pierfedeici. *Maternity and Gynecological Nursing*, New York: J. B. Lippincott, 1981.

Jenson, M. D., Benson, R., and I. Bobsk. *Maternity Care: The Nurse and the Family*, 3rd ed. St. Louis, MO: C. V. Mosby, 1985.

Lynch, M., and V. A. McKeon. "Cocaine Use during Pregnancy." *JOGNN* 19(4):285–291, July-August, 1990.

McNall, L. K. *Obstetric and Gynecologic Nursing*. St. Louis, MO: C. V. Mosby, 1980.

Niswander, K. R. *Manual of Obstetrics, Diagnosis and Therapy*, 3rd ed. Boston: Little, Brown and Co., 1987.

Oxorn, H. *Oxorn-Foote Human Labor and Birth*, 5th ed. E. Norwalk, CT: Appleton-Century-Crofts, 1986.

Pillitteri, A. *Maternal-Newborn Nursing: Care of the Growing Family*, 2nd ed. Boston: Little, Brown and Co., 1981.

Pletsch, P. "Birth Defect Prevention: Nursing Interventions." *JOGNN* 19(6)482–487, November-December 1990.

Pritchard, J. A., Paul C. MacDonald, and Norman F. Grant. *Williams Obstetrics*, 17th ed. E. Norwalk, CT: Appleton-Century-Crofts, 1985.

Reeder, S., Luigi Mastroianni, Jr., and Leonide Martin. *Maternity Nursing*, 16th ed. New York: J. B. Lippincott, 1987.

Tucker, Susan Martin, et al. *Patient Care Standards: Nursing Process, Diagnosis, and Outcome*, 5th ed. St. Louis, MO: C. V. Mosby, 1992.

Wason, C., and B. Metzger. *Diabetes Management for the Mother-to-Be*. Chicago: Abelson-Taylor-Frizsimmons, 1986.

Worthington-Roberts, B. S., and S. R. Williams. *Nutrition in Pregnancy and Lactation*, 4th ed. St. Louis, MO: Times Mirror-Mosby, 1989.

CHAPTER

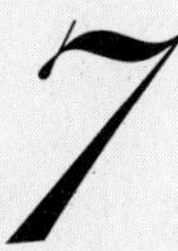

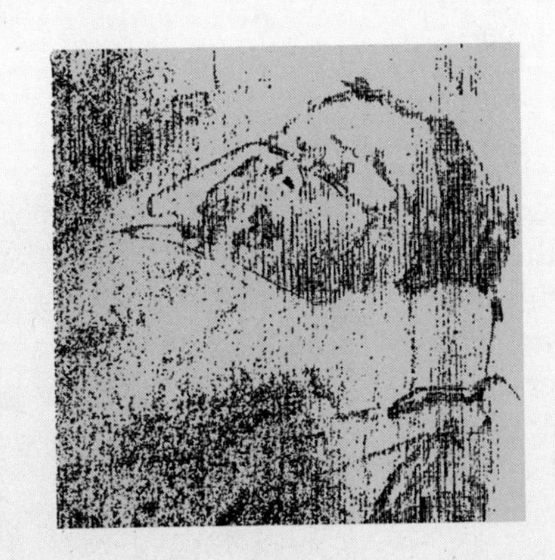

Normal Pregnancy

Objectives

After studying this chapter, the student should be able to:

- Explain what personal care is recommended during pregnancy and why.
- Identify the common discomforts of pregnancy and explain their preventive measures and treatment.
- Using the basic four food groups, state dietary requirements of the pregnant woman.
- State the psychological concerns of the single mother.
- Identify the cultural groups in your area of practice and discuss three or more health beliefs of each of the groups.
- Discuss what impact these beliefs have on the quality of medical care.
- Identify and discuss cultural biases and how they are related to the ability to provide optimum health care.

Key Terms

Colostrum
Perineal squeeze
Kegel exercise
Pica
Prepared childbirth classes
Psychoprophylaxis
Episiotomy
Breech presentation

The value of medical supervision and specific examinations and tests were covered in the preceding chapter. This chapter deals with the physical needs of the pregnant woman, the importance of diet, the benefits of proper exercise, and the discomforts of a normal pregnancy. The nurse must understand these aspects of prenatal care in order to be able to advise and assist the pregnant patient toward a normal, healthy pregnancy.

PHYSIOLOGICAL CARE

The physical care required during pregnancy is not unusual. It generally calls for moderation in normal habits and minor adjustments as pregnancy develops.

CLOTHING

Clothing should be practical, attractive, and nonconstricting. Stockings with elastic tops should be avoided because they interfere with venous return and aggravate varicosities. Low-heeled shoes are more practical than high heels. But if a patient does not develop a backache from the abnormal curving of the spine and is able to maintain good balance, there is no medical reason for not wearing high heels. A well-fitting bra is recommended, and a properly fitted maternity "girdle" or support lingerie may be of some help in combatting excessive backache and pressure due to the change in posture, Figure 7–1.

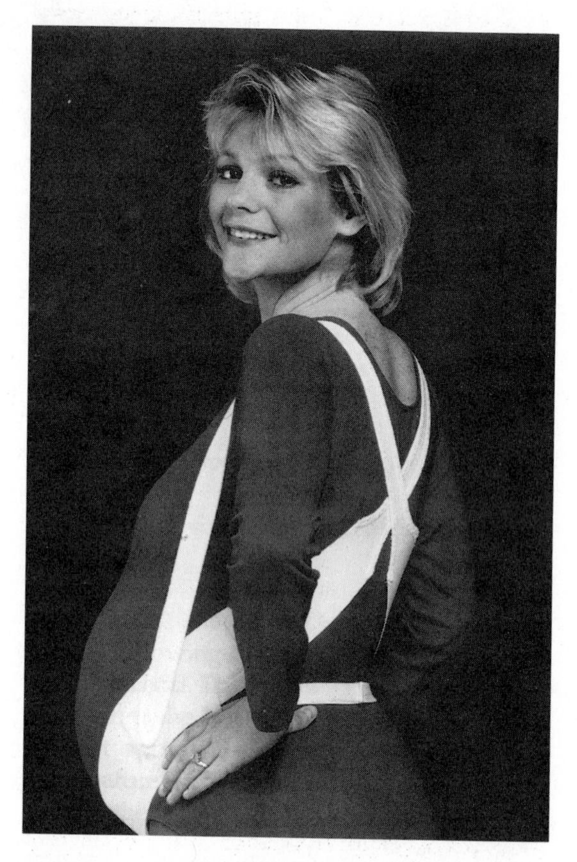

Figure 7–1 *Loving Lift™ maternity support lingerie (Courtesy Moore Products, Redwood City, CA)*

BATHING

Daily bathing is encouraged. If the skin is sensitive, however, the use of soap should be restricted. Tub baths may be taken until labor begins unless the membranes have ruptured. Body balance is not at its best; the patient must be careful not to slip and fall in the tub. The old notion that bath water may enter the vagina and carry infection to the uterus is now believed to have little validity.

DENTAL CARE

Good oral hygiene should be practiced during pregnancy. There is no proven basis for the idea that dental problems are aggravated by pregnancy. The doctor should be consulted, however, if extensive or difficult repairs or extractions are required. X-rays of the teeth should be delayed until after the pregnancy unless absolutely necessary. If x-rays cannot be avoided, a lead apron should by used to shield the mother's abdomen. The pregnant woman should also be encouraged to notify and consult her doctor when any medications have been prescribed by her dentist before she takes them.

BREAST CARE

Special care of the breasts is advised in order to increase the ability to nurse and to lessen discomfort. The breasts should be adequately supported and not bound too tightly by a bra that is too small. The precaution becomes most important during the last trimester and after delivery.

If the nipples are inverted or depressed, they should be massaged gently to draw them out. It is extremely important that the breasts are kept clean in order to prevent infection during nursing. Late in pregnancy a secretion called **colostrum** exudes from the breasts. It is sometimes recommended that a woman who plans to breast feed her baby express a few drops of colostrum from each breast every day during the last six weeks of her pregnancy. This procedure helps to open milk ducts, thereby reducing the engorgement that often occurs when the milk first comes in.

A regular bathing routine is all the washing that nipples will require, now or later. Soap should be used sparingly if at all because it dries the skin; dryness encourages cracked nipples.

ELIMINATION

Constipation may become a problem during pregnancy. A woman who normally has a tendency toward constipation will experience increased discomfort in pregnancy caused by decreased physical exertion, relaxation of the smooth muscle system all over the body, and the obstruction of the lower bowel by the presenting part of the fetus. When constipation remains a problem, the doctor may order a mild laxative. A woman also should be advised to increase the amount of fiber in her diet. An increase in fiber and water can greatly reduce constipation problems.

Fluid requirements are increased. A pregnant woman should drink the equivalent of at least 8 to 10 glasses of water daily for kidney regulation. The condition of the kidneys is extremely important during pregnancy; the kidneys help to filter the waste products of the fetus as well as those of the mother. The urine may have a strong odor during the first period of gestation, but this odor is not a sign of urinary infection. It is an indication of the excessive production of hormones in the body.

SEXUAL INTERCOURSE

Sexual intercourse in moderation usually does no harm. If there is a history of abortion or premature labor, the question of intercourse should be discussed with the physician.

FEMININE HYGIENE

More than 50% of pregnant women complain of increased vaginal secretions. If the flow of secretions is not heavy enough to necessitate wearing a pad, the woman should be informed that is a normal state. If there is an excess, however, the physician may wish to check for infection or irritation and treat appropriately. In most cases, douching in pregnancy is unnecessary and usually is not recommended. (See discussion of vaginal infections and sexually transmitted diseases in Chapter 8.)

POSTURE AND EXERCISE

In order to maintain her balance, the pregnant woman tends to lean backward to offset the heavy weight in front. This posture puts increased strain on the muscles and ligaments of the back and thigh, causing muscular cramps and aches. Certain specific muscle exercises are helpful in maintaining the tone of the abdominal, back, and perineal muscles. The exercises shown in Figure 7–2 may help to maintain good muscle tone and ease some of the discomforts of pregnancy. (*Caution:* These exercises should be performed under the direction of the doctor.)

PELVIC FLOOR CONTRACTIONS (PERINEAL SQUEEZE OR KEGEL EXERCISE)

The pelvic floor, or perineal, muscles are attached to the insides of the pelvic bones and act like a hammock to support the abdominal and pelvic organs, Figure 7–3. During pregnancy, these muscles may sag in response to the increased weight of the uterus and the relaxing effect of pregnancy hormones. During pregnancy and labor, muscle tone of the pelvic

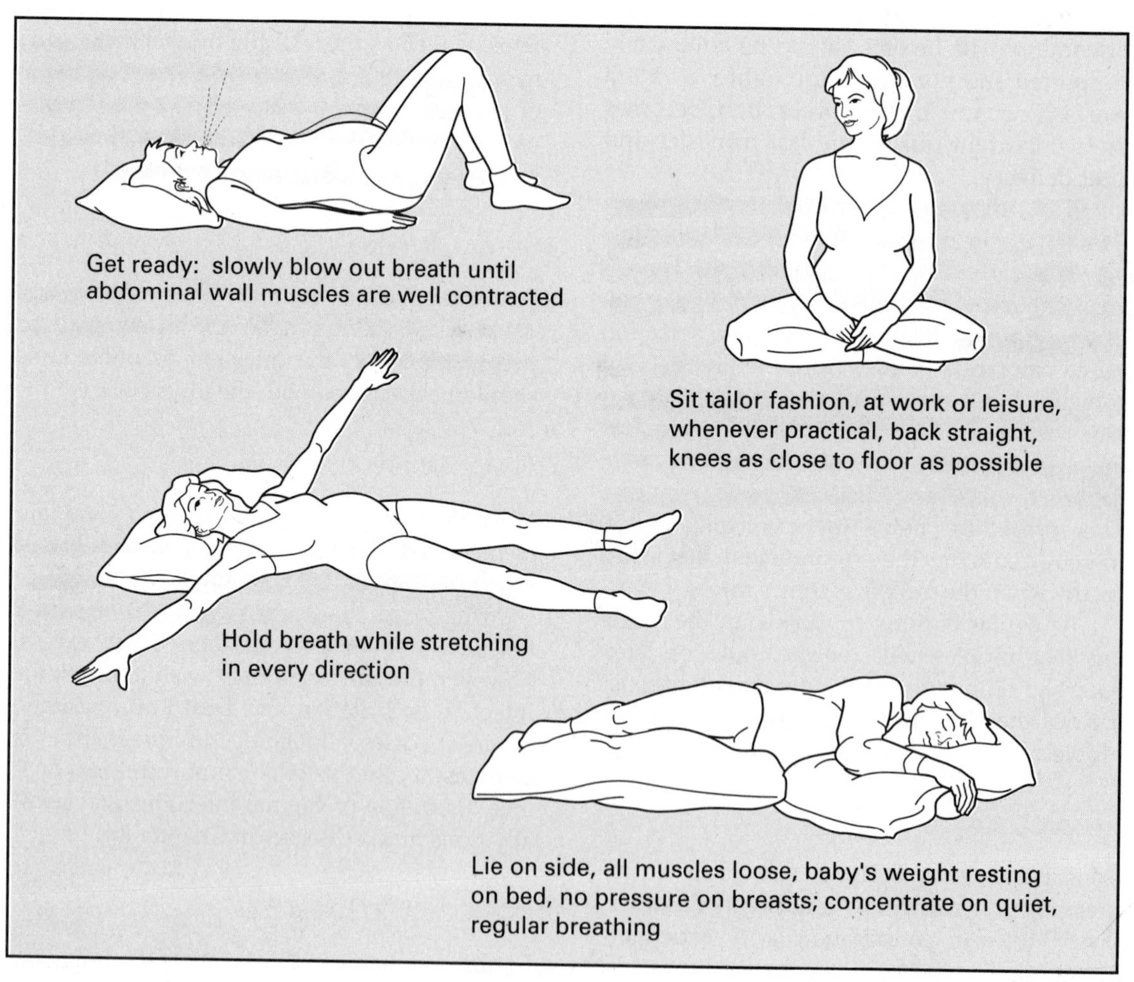

Get ready: slowly blow out breath until abdominal wall muscles are well contracted
Sit tailor fashion, at work or leisure, whenever practical, back straight, knees as close to floor as possible
Hold breath while stretching in every direction
Lie on side, all muscles loose, baby's weight resting on bed, no pressure on breasts; concentrate on quiet, regular breathing

Figure 7–2 *Relaxation exercises*

floor is important. To become aware of how the muscle works, the mother should learn to tighten and relax the muscles surrounding the urethra, vagina, and anus. She can practice in any position. One simple method for exercising the perineal muscle can be done each time the patient urinates. The mother should try to halt the flow of urine midstream, then empty the bladder.

The exercise called the **perineal squeeze** or **Kegel exercise**, can be used to tone the muscle of the pelvic floor: tighten up the pelvic floor muscle and hold to a slow count of five; relax; bulge the muscle downward gently by holding breath and bearing down; relax; tighten again; relax. This exercise should be practiced often each day.

The perineal squeeze (Kegel exercise) helps avoid involuntary loss of urine during the last few weeks of pregnancy. It helps to support the uterus and bladder in their proper position and will aid in pushing out the baby. It is also used

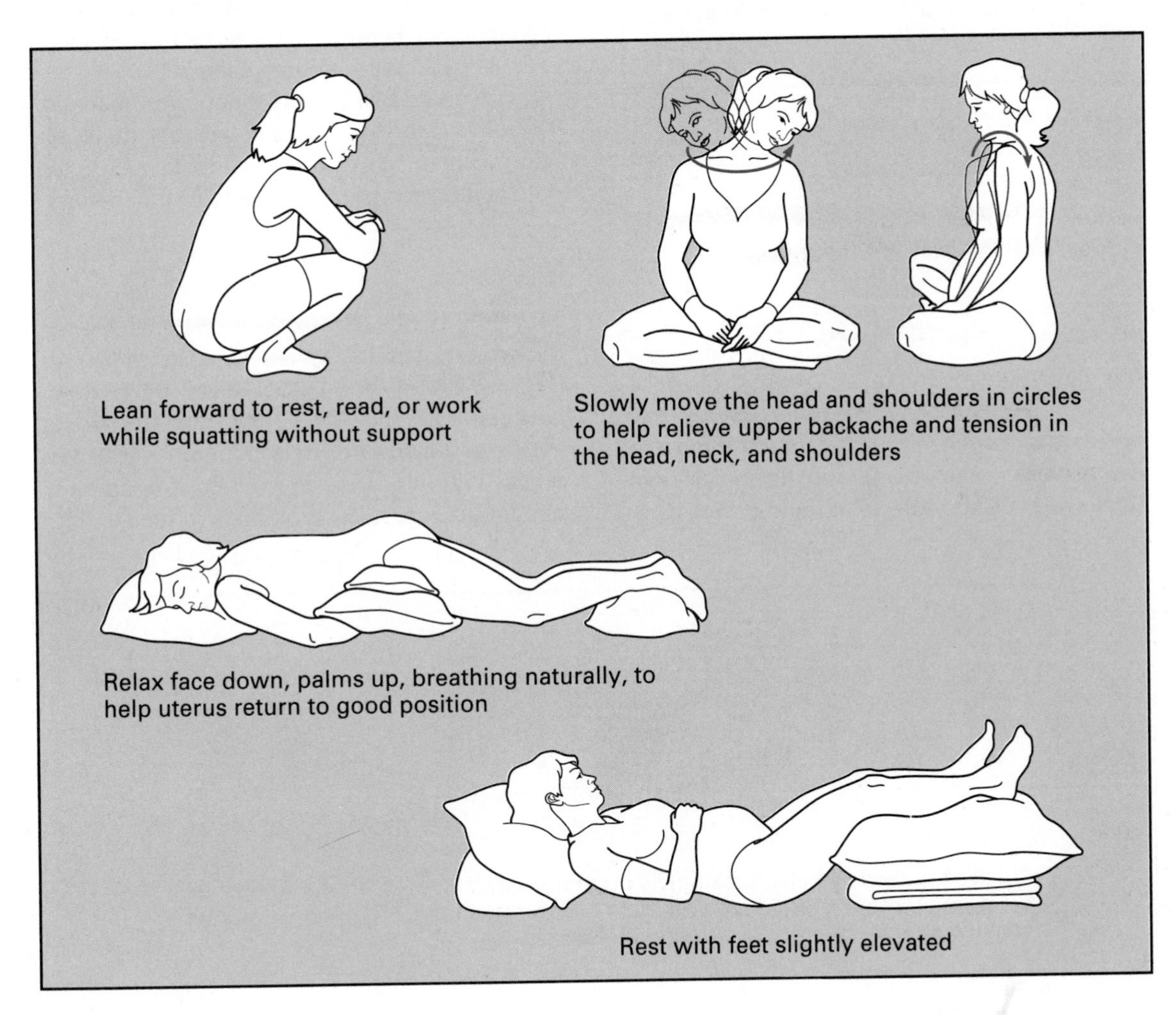

Lean forward to rest, read, or work while squatting without support
Slowly move the head and shoulders in circles to help relieve upper backache and tension in the head, neck, and shoulders
Relax face down, palms up, breathing naturally, to help uterus return to good position
Rest with feet slightly elevated

Figure 7–2 *continued*

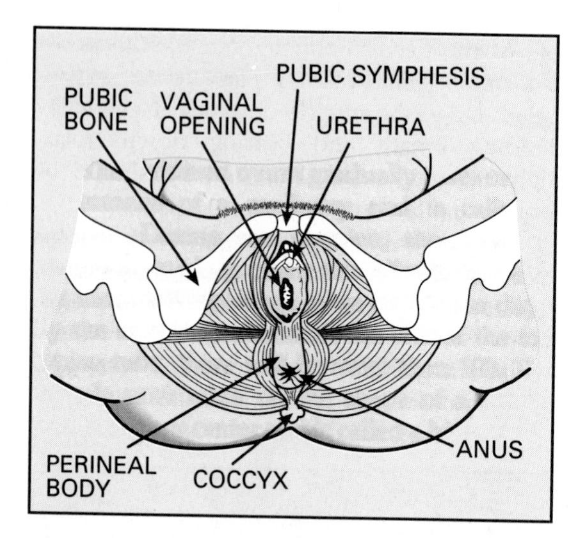

Figure 7–3 *Pelvic floor muscles*

to tighten the perineum (pelvic floor muscle) back to its former state after delivery.

ACTIVITY, REST, AND RECREATION

Pregnant women tire easily. Fatigue must be avoided. Normal activities in recreation and housework may be continued but should not be excessive. A woman who does her own housework needs little or no additional exercise. However, she does need fresh air, sunshine, and diversion. Walking is valuable for the maintenance of correct carriage. Any activity that incurs sudden jolts, changes of momentum, or physical trauma should be avoided. Sports and exercise may be enjoyed at a mild pace, Figure 7–4. The American College of Obstetricians and Gynecologists (ACOG) recommends that a pregnant woman's heart rate should not exceed 140 beats per minute during exercise. Aerobic and low-impact exercise can increase a woman's sense of well-being and can help build endurance that may be helpful during labor. See Figure 7–5 (page 106) for ACOG's exercise guidelines in more detail.

Adequate rest periods should be planned. The physician may recommend that the pregnant woman stop work before the expected date of delivery, but this usually is unnecessary.

TRAVEL

Traveling is fine during pregnancy. However, the woman should be cautioned to avoid sitting still for long periods in a car, boat, plane, or train. She should be encouraged to walk about for a few minutes each hour or hour and a half. Walking helps to prevent slowdown of her circulation. If the woman is in the last four

Don't fly last 2 mths

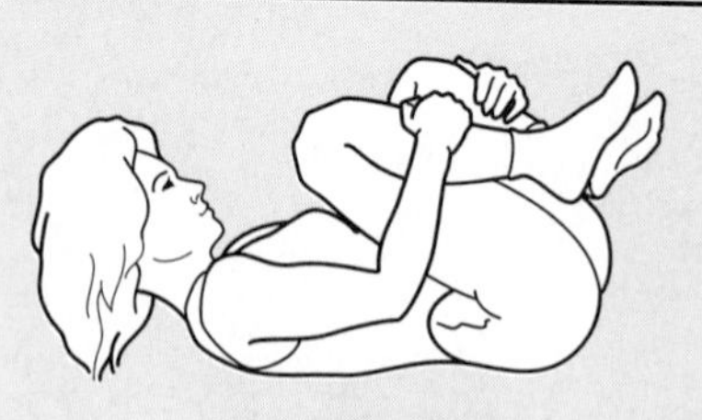

LEG STRETCHES

Pull legs up beside baby; rock pelvis up in front; relax pelvic floor muscles; take quick, deep costal-sternal breaths. Hold as if for pushing, alternating with quick shallow panting breaths, as if to avoid pushing

Figure 7–4 *Stretching exercises*

to six weeks of her pregnancy, she should consult with her doctor and be aware of alternative available care if labor should begin prematurely.

THE IMPORTANCE OF DIET

The pregnant woman who follows a well-balanced diet feels better and is more apt to retain her health than one who chooses her food thoughtlessly. Preeclampsia does not occur as often among pregnant women on excellent diets as among those on poor diets. Studies show a relationship between the mother's diet and the health of the baby at birth. A relationship also has been established between maternal nutrition and the subsequent mental development of the child. It appears that an insufficient quantity of protein in the diet during pregnancy may affect the quantity of brain cells in the developing fetus.

Although it is often said that "a pregnant woman must eat for two," that statement is not entirely true. Quality rather than quantity is the main consideration in planning a diet. During pregnancy a woman's recommended dietary allowances increase considerably. Protein demands increase from 46 g per day to 60 g per day; calcium from 0.8 g per day to 1 or 2 g per day. Thirty milligrams of iron is required daily but is difficult to get in foods. An iron supplement and prenatal vitamin preparation may be prescribed by the obstetrician. During pregnancy a woman will need approximately 300 additional calories a day. Thus, a woman of average weight would need about 2,200 to 2,700 calories per day. The nurse should be familiar with the four basic food groups in order to give adequate dietary counseling.

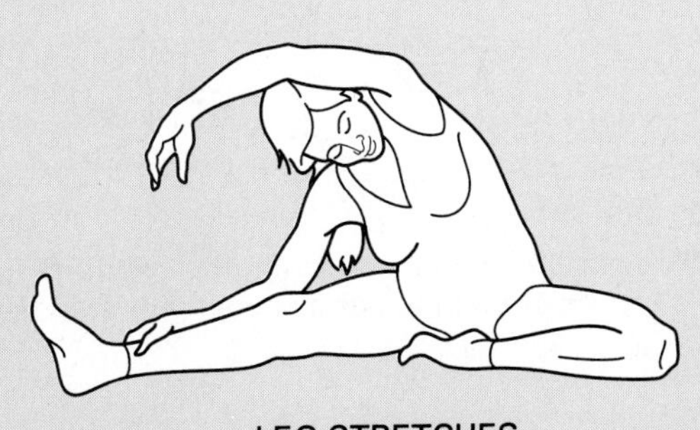

LEG STRETCHES

Stretching legs relieves tension in hips and legs, and helps relieve or prevent leg cramps

- Sit on floor with right leg stretched out toward the side, foot flexed and left leg folded in
- Facing forward, lean upper body to the right side, so right ear is directly over right leg. At same time, lift left hand over your head so it is directly over left ear
- Using right hand, grasp right foot, ankle or calf, whichever is most comfortable
- Hold this position for a count of 10. Relax and release the stretch
- Repeat on the left side. Do three times, holding longer as you become more comfortable with this exercise

Figure 7–4 *continued*

VEGETABLES AND FRUITS

Four or more servings should be included from the vegetable and fruit group, especially leafy green and yellow vegetables. Citrus fruits or tomatoes should also be included daily because vitamin C cannot be stored by the body. Vegetables are rich in iron, calcium, and several vitamins. Vegetables also act as laxative agents. Their fibrous framework increases the bulk of the intestinal content and stimulates action of the intestines. Vegetables should

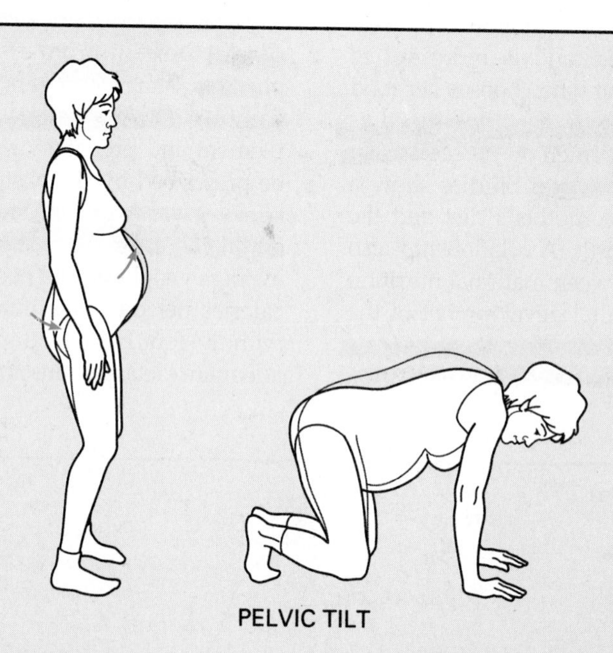

PELVIC TILT

Tilting the pelvis back toward the spine can strengthen abdominal muscles and relieve backache. This can be done in either a kneeling or standing position.

Standing

- Stand in a comfortable position. Inhale and relax
- Exhale as you roll hips and buttocks forward, as if trying to lift the fetus up toward your chest
- Hold for a count of five. Inhale and relax
- Repeat three to five times, several times a day

Kneeling

- Kneel on hands and knees, with back relaxed but not arched
- Inhale and relax a moment
- Exhale and pull buttocks under and forward — you should feel abdomen tighten and back straighten at the waist
- Hold for a count of five. Inhale and relax

Figure 7–4 *continued*

be carefully prepared and cooked to maintain maximum vitamin and mineral content.

Oranges, lemons, and other citrus fruits are the best sources of vitamin C. Most of these fruits also supply vitamins A and B.

DAIRY FOODS

The expectant mother should have at least a quart of milk daily. The high content of calcium and phosphorus make milk indispensable for good growth of bone and teeth in the fetus. Milk is also a good source of protein and a tissue-building material rich in energy-providing values. Milk contains some of the most important vitamins, particularly vitamin A. Vitamin A increases resistance to infection and safeguards the development of the fetus. Other foods that contain milk, such as ice cream, cheese, and yogurt can be substituted for part of the milk requirements. These, how-

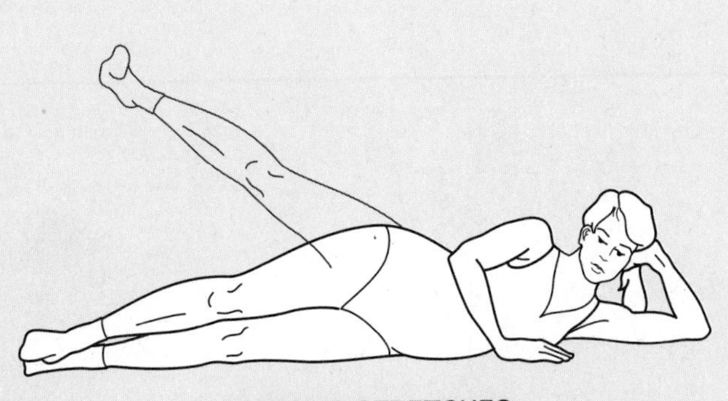

SIDE LEG STRETCHES

Side leg stretches improve circulation and tone muscles of the hips, buttocks, and thighs.

- Lie on left side, with knees, hips, and shoulders in straight line
- Put right hand on floor in front of you and use left hand to support head
- Inhale and relax
- Exhale while slowly raising the right leg as high as possible without bending knee or body. Keep foot flexed, with right outer ankle bone facing up
- Inhale while slowly lowering leg
- Repeat ten times
- Turn to right side and repeat ten times with left leg

You can change this exercise two different ways for more variety:

1. Instead of raising the leg all the way up, raise it only halfway and make small circles with it. Make ten clockwise circles and then ten counterclockwise circles
2. Instead of keeping upper leg straight, bend your knee so upper thigh is at right angle to body. Keeping knee bent, do the side raises, making sure knee faces forward and outer ankle bone faces upward

Figure 7–4 *continued*

ever, contain extra calories, which the expectant mother may not need.

BREADS AND CEREALS

At least four servings of bread or cereal should be included in the diet daily. Whole wheat bread, enriched flour products, brown rice, oatmeal, and noodles are included in this group. The bread and cereal group provides carbohydrates, thiamine, riboflavin, niacin, phosphorus, and magnesium.

MEATS

Meat is a rich source of the essential nutrient protein. The main value of the meat group is the amino acids it provides. Amino acids are needed by the mother as well as by the fetus for the development of all the delicate and intricate systems of the body. Three or more servings of beef, pork, lamb, veal, organ meats, fish, poultry, eggs, or cheese are recommended daily. Dried beans and peas or nuts may be used as alternates. Two eggs can also substi-

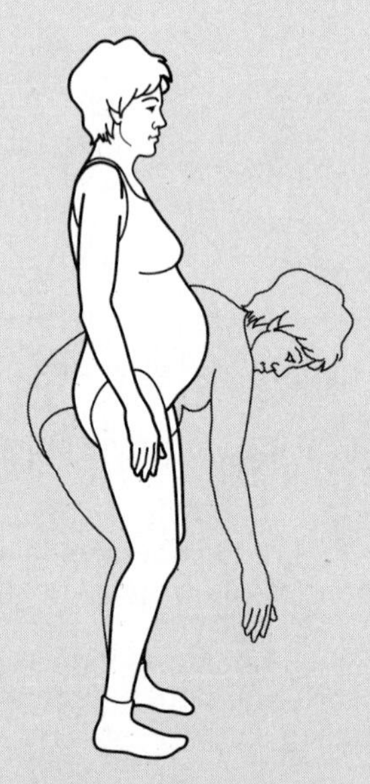

FORWARD BEND

This exercise stretches and relaxes the muscles in your back to help relieve tension and fatigue

- Stand with feet about 12–18 inches apart and knees slightly bent. As this exercise is done, spread legs, bend knees, or do both, as needed for comfort. Do not try to keep knees straight
- Exhale and bend forward from the waist, letting upper body slowly sag toward the floor, uncurling slowly
- Inhale and slowly uncurl the back, one vertebra at a time, until standing

Figure 7–4 *continued*

tute as a serving of meat. Figure 7–6 summarizes the normal daily nutritional requirements for the nonpregnant woman, pregnant woman, and nursing mother. A pregnant adolescent would require more of the essential nutrients. Because she has not yet attained full maturity her own body needs are higher than an adult's. She must meet those higher needs as well as those of the fetus.

The unusual craving for certain foods during pregnancy does no harm unless eating the foods interferes with the normal diet and causes excessive weight gain. **Pica**, cravings for nonfood substances such as starch or clay, can interfere with the normal diet and can irritate the salivary glands.

WEIGHT GAIN

Usually there is little, if any, weight gain during the first three months of pregnancy. A woman gains about ¾ to 1 pound a week during the last six months of her pregnancy. Excessive weight gain should be avoided because it may predispose a woman to preeclampsia or cause complications during delivery. The recommended weight gain in pregnancy is 25 to 30 pounds.

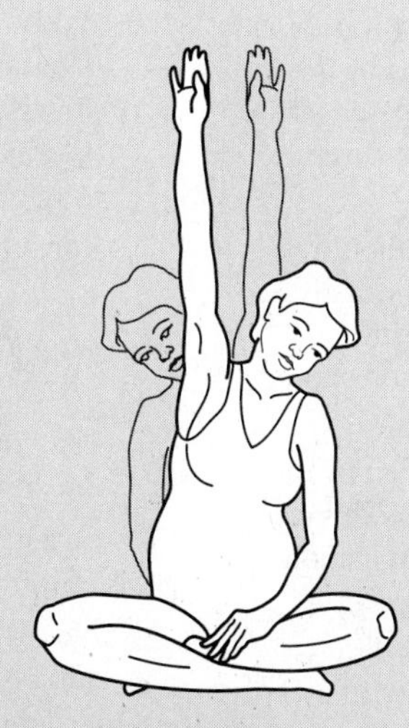

ARM REACHES

Stretching sides and upper body helps relieve upper backache. It also is helpful when feeling out of breath

- Stand or sit comfortably
- Inhale while raising right arm above head, reaching as high as possible. Stretch from the waist without letting hip or foot rest
- Exhale, bending elbow and pulling arm down to side
- Repeat on left side. Do three to five repetitions

Figure 7–4 continued

COMMON DISCOMFORTS

Pregnancy sometimes brings discomforts that, when recognized as normal, should cause the patient no undue alarm. Two of the most common discomforts are morning sickness, or nausea, and frequent urination. Additional discomforts include heartburn, distress after eating, flatulence, swelling of feet, varicose veins, hemorrhoids, leg cramps, constipation,

ACOG EXERCISE GUIDELINES

During Pregnancy and Post Partum

1. Regular exercise (at least three times a week) is preferable to intermittent activity. Competitive activities should be discouraged.
2. Vigorous exercise should not be performed in hot, humid weather or during a period of febrile illness.
3. Ballistic movements (jerky, bouncy motions) should be avoided. Exercise should be done on a wooden floor or a tightly carpeted surface to reduce shock and provide a sure footing.
4. Deep flexion or extension of joints should be avoided because of connective tissue laxity. Activities that require jumping, jarring motions, or rapid changes in direction should be avoided because of joint instability.
5. Vigorous exercise should be preceded by a 5-minute period of muscle warmup. This can be accomplished by slow walking or stationary cycling with low resistance.
6. Vigorous exercise should be followed by a period of gradually declining activity that includes gentle stationary stretching. Because connective tissue laxity increase the risk of joint injury, stretches should not be taken to the point of maximum resistance.
7. Heart rate should be measured at times of peak activity. Target heart rates and limits established in consultation with the physician should not be exceeded.
8. Care should be taken to gradually rise from the floor to avoid orthostatic hypotension. Some form of activity involving the legs should be continued for a brief period.
9. Liquids should be taken liberally before and after exercise to prevent dehydration. If necessary, activity should be interrupted to replenish fluids.
10. Women who have had sedentary lifestyles should begin with physical activity of very low intensity and advance activity levels very gradually.
11. Activity should be stopped and the physician consulted if any unusual symptoms appear.

Pregnancy Only

1. Maternal heart rate should not exceed 140 beats per minute.
2. Strenuous activities should not exceed 15 minutes in duration.
3. No exercise should be performed in the supine position after the fourth month of gestation is completed.
4. Exercises that employ the Valsalva maneuver should be avoided.
5. Caloric intake should be adequate to meet not only the extra energy needs of pregnancy, but also of the exercise performed.
6. Maternal core temperature should not exceed 38°C (100.4°F).

Figure 7–5 *(Adapted from* Exercise during Pregnancy and the Postnatal Period, *The American College of Obstetricians and Gynecologists, ACOG Home Exercise Programs, Washington, D.C. © 1984)* shortness of breath, dizziness and fainting, fatigue and drowsiness, bleeding gums and nose bleeds, backache, vaginal discharge, itchy skin (urticaria), and salivation (mouth watering), and mood swings. Figure 7–7 summarizes these common patient problems and outlines the appropriate nursing actions and the rationales for those actions. It should be studied carefully.

NUTRIENTS AND VITAMINS

Key nutrient & RDA*	Important functions	Important sources	Comments
Calories N—2,200 P—2,200 (1st trimester) P—2,500 (2nd & 3rd trimesters) L—2,700	• Provide energy for tissue building and increased metabolic requirements	Carbohydrates, fats, and proteins	Calorie requirements vary according to the stage of pregnancy, size, activity level, prepregnant weight, and how well nourished the patient is.
Water or liquids N—4 cups P—8+ cups L—8+ cups	• Carries nutrients to cells • Carries waste products away • Provides fluid for increased blood, tissue, and amniotic fluid volume • Helps regulate body temperature • Aids digestion	Water, juices, and milk	Liquid is often neglected, but it is an important nutrient.
Protein N—46 g P—60 g L—65 g	• Builds and repairs tissues • Helps build blood, amniotic fluid, and placenta • Helps form antibodies • Supplies energy	Meat, fish, poultry, eggs, milk, cheese, dried beans and peas, peanut butter, nuts, whole gains, and cereals	Fetal requirements increase by about one-third in late pregnancy as the baby grows.

*N—nonpregnant P—pregnant L—lactating (first 6 months)

continues

Figure 7–6 *(Reprinted from* Becoming Parents *with permission by the Childbirth Education Association of Seattle, 1443 N.W. 54th, Seattle, WA)*

Key nutrient & RDA*	Important functions	Important sources	Comments
MINERALS			
Calcium N—800 mg P—1,200 mg L—1,200 mg	• Helps build bones and teeth • Important in blood clotting • Helps regulate use of other minerals in the body	Milk, cheese, whole grains, vegetables, egg yolk, whole canned fish, and ice cream	Fetal requirements increase in late pregnancy. Caffeine can decrease the amount of calcium available to the fetus.
Phosphorus N—800 mg P—1,200 mg L—1,200 mg	• Helps build bones and teeth	Milk, cheese, and lean meats	Calcium and phosphorus exist in a constant ratio in the blood. An excess of either limits
Iron N—15 mg P—30 mg L—15 mg	• Combines with protein to make hemoglobin • Provides iron for fetal storage	Liver, red meats, egg yolk, whole grains, leafy vegetables, nuts, legumes, dried fruits, prunes, and prune and apple juice	Fetal requirements increase tenfold in last 6 weeks of pregnancy. Supplement of 30 to 60 mg of iron daily is recommended by the National Research Council.
Zinc N—12 mg P—15 mg L—19 mg	• Component of insulin • Important in growth of skeleton and nervous system	Meat, liver, eggs, and seafood — especially oysters	Deficiency can cause malformations of fetal skeleton and nervous system.
Iodine N—150 mcg P—175 mcg L—200 mcg	• Helps control the rate of body's energy use • Important in thyroxine production	Seafoods, iodized salt	Deficiency may cause goiter in infant.
Magnesium N—280 mg P—320 mg L—355 mg	• Helps energy, protein, and cell metabolism • Enzyme activator • Helps tissue growth and muscle action	Nuts, cocoa, green vegetables, whole grains, and dried beans and peas	Most is stored in bones. Deficiency may cause neuromuscular dysfunction.

*N—nonpregnant P—pregnant L—lactating (first 6 months)

continues

Key nutrient & RDA*	Important functions	Important sources	Comments
FAT-SOLUBLE VITAMINS			
Vitamin A N—800 mcg RE (Retinol equivalent) P—800 mcg RE L—1,300 mcg RE	• Helps bone and tissue growth and development • Essential in development of enamel-forming cells in gum tissue • Helps maintain health of skin and mucous membranes	Butter, fortified margarine, green and yellow vegetables, and liver	In excessive amounts, it is toxic to the fetus. It loses its potency when exposed to light.
Vitamin D N—5 mcg P—10 mcg L—10 mcg	• Needed for absorption of calcium and phosphorus and mineralization of bones and teeth	Fortified milk, fortified margarine, fish liver oils, and sunlight on skin	Toxic to the fetus in excessive amounts.
Vitamin E N—8 mg ∝-TE (Alpha Tocopherol) P—10 mg ∝-TE L—12 mg ∝-TE	• Needed for tissue growth, cell wall integrity, and red blood cell integrity	Vegetable oils, cereals, meat, eggs, milk, nuts, and seeds	Enhances absorption of vitamin A.
Vitamin K N—65 mcg P—65 mcg L—65 mcg	• Essential for the synthesis of blood-clotting factors		Produced in the body by the intestinal flora.
WATER-SOLUBLE VITAMINS			
Folic acid N—180 mcg P—400 mcg L—280 mcg	• Essential in hemoglobin synthesis • Involved in DNA and RNA synthesis • Needed for synthesis of amino acids	Liver, leafy green vegetables, and yeast	Deficiency leads to anemia. Can be destroyed in cooking and storage. Supplement of 400 mcg per day is recommended by the National Research Council. Oral contraceptives may reduce blood level of folic acid.

*N—nonpregnant P—pregnant L—lactating (first 6 months)

continues

Key nutrient & RDA*	Important functions	Important sources	Comments
Niacin N—15 mg P—17 mg L—20 mg	• Needed for energy and protein metabolism	Pork, organ meats, peanuts, beans, peas, and enriched grains	Stable; only small amounts are lost in food preparation.
Riboflavin N—1.3 mg P—1.6 mg L—1.8 mg	• Essential for energy and protein metabolism	Milk, lean meat, enriched grains, cheese, and leafy greens	Oral contraceptives may reduce serum concentration of riboflavin.
Thiamin (B_1) N—1.1 mg P—1.5 mg L—1.6 mg	• Important for energy metabolism	Pork, beef, liver, whole grains, and legumes	Essential for conversion of the carbohydrates into energy in the muscular and nervous systems.
Pyridoxine (B_6) N—1.6 mg P—2.2 mg L—2.1 mg	• Important in amino acid metabolism and protein synthesis • Required for fetal growth	Unprocessed cereals, grains, wheat germ, nuts, seeds, legumes, and corn	Excessive amounts may reduce milk supply in lactating women. May help reduce nausea in early pregnancy.
Cobalamin (B_{12}) N—2.0 mcg P—2.2 mcg L—2.6 mcg	• Essential in protein metabolism • Important in formation of red blood cells	Milk, eggs, meat, liver, and cheese	Deficiency leads to anemia and central nervous system damage. Is manufactured by microorganisms in the intestinal tract. Oral contraceptives may reduce serum concentration.
Vitamin C N—60 mg P—70 mg L—95 mg	• Helps tissue formation and integrity • Is the "cement" substance in connective and vascular tissue • Increases iron absorption	Citrus fruits, berries, melons, tomatoes, chili peppers, green vegetables, and potatoes	Large supplemental doses in pregnancy may create a larger-than-normal need in infant. Benefits of large doses in preventing colds have not been confirmed.

*N—nonpregnant P—pregnant L—lactating (first 6 months)

CHILDBIRTH PREPARATION

Many physicians today recommend that an expectant mother and father attend **prepared childbirth classes** in the last 9 to 12 weeks of pregnancy. If a woman understands what is happening within her body, she will be less fearful and less tense. She will be able to relax more with her labor and help effectively with delivery. A supportive person acting as a labor coach enhances the experience. Many hospitals allow the father to follow the course of labor and delivery along with the mother. He may give emotional support and help to relax the mother-to-be so that she can take advantage of body muscle control reflexes. His presence may help reduce fear and tension in both the labor room and delivery room.

There are three basic components of prepared childbirth education: (1) factual information about pregnancy, labor, and delivery; (2) physical conditioning, relaxation techniques, and breathing patterns; and (3) information about breast feeding, postpartum experiences, and infant care.

Childbirth education is available from a variety of sources:

- nonprofit groups such as the Childbirth Education Association
- private instructors trained to teach expectant parents
- public-service groups such as the Red Cross
- hospitals
- doctors
- books, films, and tapes

DICK-READ METHOD OF NATURAL CHILDBIRTH

Dr. Grantly Dick-Read, an English obstetrician, was a pioneer in the movement for natural childbirth. The Dick-Read method of childbirth is based on (1) a thorough understanding of the anatomy and physiology of pregnancy and labor by the patient and (2) the use of exercises designed to strengthen useful muscles and mentally condition the patient to painless labor. It also teaches a woman to visualize the internal process of birth. In this respect this method resembles techniques of meditation and differs from the Lamaze and Bradley methods.The breathing required also is different in that is uses abdominal breathing rather than chest breathing, and light panting is used during the expulsion stage. The method is instituted early in pregnancy, when the woman takes a training course that prepares her for labor.

LAMAZE METHOD OF NATURAL CHILDBIRTH

Another natural childbirth method, called **psychoprophylaxis**, has become very popular. Dr. Fernand Lamaze of Paris brought this technique to Western Europe in 1952. Psychoprophylaxis (commonly called the Lamaze method) depends on educating the mother-to-be about childbirth and training her through exercise and various breathing techniques to control her activity during labor. It is an intellectual, physical, and emotional preparation for childbirth. This preparation can be helped by good nursing support and acceptance of the laboring woman's desire to experience her own childbirth with a degree of control. A coach, usually the expectant father, also serves a vital role in helping the mother stay in control with breathing techniques and relaxation. The nurse must recognize this coach as an important team member and keep him informed of the laboring woman's progress, Figure 7–8.

Childbirth, no matter how normal, is accompanied by some degree of discomfort. Exercises using the psychoprophylactic method

NURSING CARE PLAN: Common Discomforts

PATIENT PROBLEM	GOAL(S)
Nausea and vomiting often caused by hormonal changes during pregnancy (occurs in approximately 50% of patients) Causes: • decreased gastric emptying time (increased progesterone) • nutritional deficiency • iron supplementation or other drugs • emotional ambivalence about pregnancy • increased hCG • acute infection or other illness • fatigue	Patient accepts a certain amount of nausea as a normal discomfort of pregnancy. She attempts intervention explained to her by the nurse in attempts to control symptoms. She reports excessive vomiting so medication can be ordered as needed.

Figure 7–7 Nursing care plan for common problems associated with pregnancy

are based on what is known as the theory of conditioned reflexes. It takes advantage of the fact that the brain can accept only one set of signals at a time. If the stronger signals are of conditioned responses to exercise and control of the muscles to expel the baby instead of signals of pain, then the muscle control takes precedence over the signal from the uterine contractions. Fear must be reduced to a minimum, and tension must be defeated during labor.

NURSING INTERVENTION	RATIONALE
Instruct the patient in general principles of prevention: • rest • relaxation • happy frame of mind • exercise • fresh air	A lowered state of anxiety and a healthy environment decrease the chance of nausea and vomiting.
Advise the patient of specific measures that may prevent or lessen nausea and vomiting: • limiting liquid intake upon waking or with meals • eating two or three crackers or a piece of toast immediately upon waking • lying quietly for 20–30 minutes after waking • dressing slowly • eating a regular breakfast in due time; may be advantageous to eat frequent, small meals • eating primarily carbohydrates, taking liquids and solid foods separately, and avoiding foods with strong odors and extremes of temperature • resting after meals • taking sedatives, as ordered by physician • taking medication to control nausea and vomiting, as ordered by physician	Dry, carbohydrate food is easily digestible. Limiting the amount of food in the stomach helps to improve the usually slowed gastric motility in pregnant patients. Decreasing agitation by moving slowly and avoiding unnecessary stimuli is often helpful.

BRADLEY METHOD OF PREPARED CHILDBIRTH

The Bradley method of prepared childbirth was introduced in the 1940s by an American obstetrician, Robert A. Bradley. It differs from the other methods in that it emphasizes the use of a trained, prepared husband to coach his wife in achieving a spontaneous delivery without med-

Text continues on page 126

PATIENT PROBLEM	GOAL(S)
Heartburn Causes: • gastric reflux–relaxation of the cardiac sphincter (progesterone) • decreased hydrochloric acid and pepsin secretion in the stomach (estrogen) • displacement of stomach and duodenum by enlarging uterus • emotional problems	Patient understands the cause of heartburn and the interventions explained to her by the nurse. Heartburn is minimized by these actions. Patient reports any other associated symptoms.
Distress after eating Causes: • decreased gastric emptying time (increased progesterone) • nutritional deficiency • iron supplementation or other drugs • emotional ambivalence about pregnancy • increased hCG • acute infection or other illness • fatigue	Distress is minimized or eliminated and food is digested well. Decrease in gas and constipation.
Flatulence Causes: • ingestion of gas-forming foods • decreased exercise • decreased motility of the gut • compression of the uterus on the gut • constipation • fecal impaction	Symptoms are minimized by the prescribed intervention. Bowels function normally.

Figure 7–7 *continued*

NURSING INTERVENTION	RATIONALE
Discuss with the patient ways to prevent heartburn: • eating frequent, small amounts of food • avoiding greasy foods • taking an antacid preparation, as ordered by physician	Eating small amounts and avoiding greasy foods decreases gastric acidity.
Advise patient to avoid sodium bicarbonate.	Sodium bicarbonate may cause fluid retention because of its sodium content.
Instruct the patient to: • eat slowly • chew food thoroughly • eat small amounts • rest after meals	Improves digestive process
Be available to offer support and listen to patient's feelings.	
Identify for the patient some common gas-forming foods and discuss the importance of regular bowel movements with her. Advise the patient of the importance of exercise and rest.	Regular bowel movements, avoidance of gas-forming foods, and adequate rest and exercise all contribute to the normal functioning of the digestive system.
Advise the patient that a suppository may be ordered by the physician.	Constipation may be the cause of flatulence; a stool softener or laxative suppository may be prescribed for the constipation.

PATIENT PROBLEM	GOAL(S)
Constipation Causes: • decreased GI tract motility • increased absorption of water from the bowel • pressure of the uterus on the bowel • decreased physical exercise • decreased fluid intake • inadequate food roughage in diet • dry stool due to iron therapy • fecal impaction	Bowels function normally. Stools are soft-formed.
Hemorrhoids Causes: • all the causes under varicosities apply • straining at stool due to predisposition to hemorrhoid formation	Patient understands the cause or aggravation of hemorrhoidal development and minimizes these factors. Patient is comfortable with intervention techniques to alleviate discomfort. Patient understands the need to report any excessive rectal bleeding so further evaluation can be made as necessary.
Mouth watering	Patient is reassured there is nothing abnormal about this symptom in pregnancy. Patient is willing to attempt techniques to control symptoms if bothersome.

Figure 7–7 continued

NURSING INTERVENTION	RATIONALE
Review the patient's diet for adequate amounts of fluids, fresh fruits, vegetables, and fiber; discuss the importance of these foods with the patient.	Fluids, fresh fruits, vegetables, and fiber foods aid in digestion.
Discuss the importance of regular bowel movements with the patient.	A relaxed, regular routine for bowel movements decreases the incidence of constipation.
Advise the patient that a stool softener, mild laxative, or suppository may be ordered by her physician.	A laxative or stool softener (suppository) will aid in bowel evacuation.
Discuss with the patient ways to prevent constipation.	Constipation increases the need for straining, placing additional pressure on the hemorrhoid.
If hemorrhoids are present, instruct the patient to: • gently push hemorrhoids back into rectum • elevate hips on a pillow • apply cold witch hazel compresses • take sitz baths	Pushing hemorrhoids back into the rectum decreases irritation. Elevating the hips relieves pressure. Cold witch hazel compresses and sitz baths help decrease discomfort and promote healing.
Reassure the patient that this is a normal occurrence in pregnancy and that it usually disappears on its own.	During pregnancy, the salivary glands increase production. In a few women, this increase may be excessive. Knowledge of the condition and its usual disappearance over time will decrease patient anxiety.
Advise patient to eat several small meals per day, rather than large ones.	Eating several small feedings a day will help prevent excessive salivation, which is the first step in the digestive process.

PATIENT PROBLEM	GOAL(S)
Swelling of the feet Causes: • sodium and water retention from hormonal influences • increased venous pressure • varicose veins with congestion • dietary protein deficiency • increased capillary permeability	Patient understands the physiology of edematous ankles and feet. Patient also aware of importance of reporting any persistence of the problem along with other symptoms that may indicate preeclampsia.
Varicose veins (aching, pain) Causes: • increased blood volume adds additional pressure on the venous circulation • increased stasis of blood in the lower limbs due to pressure of the enlarged uterus on the venous circulation • congential predisposition to weakness in the vascular walls • inactivity and poor muscle tone decrease optimum blood circulation • prolonged standing causes venous pooling in lower limbs and pelvis • obesity places increased pressure on blood circulation	Patient is willing to elevate legs frequently and wear elastic support stockings as directed by the physician. Patient understands that this condition is aggravated by pregnancy and will improve after delivery.
Leg cramps (numbness and tingling) Causes: • a diet, containing large amounts of milk and milk products, can disturb the body's calcium and phosphorus balance. Increased phosphorus causes a predisposition to leg cramps. • fatigue or muscle strain on extremities • blood vessel occlusion in the legs • sudden stretching of the leg and foot or pointing the toes	Patient understands this can be a normal discomfort of pregnancy and can demonstrate techniques to decrease muscle spasm.

Figure 7–7 continued

NURSING INTERVENTION	RATIONALE
Advise the patient that restricting sodium intake will help prevent swelling. Advise the patient to elevate her feet and legs whenever possible. Warn the patient that persistent swelling should be reported to her physician.	Sodium can cause fluid retention. Foot and leg elevation helps promote blood return from the legs. Persistent swelling is a sign of preeclampsia and should be investigated promptly.
Instruct the patient to: • avoid constrictions of any type (e.g., tight clothing) • rest with feet and legs elevated • move about while standing rather than remaining stationary • use elastic stockings, if indicated, and elevate legs for aching pain	Constrictions impair blood circulation. Elevation of the legs helps promote blood return from the legs. Movement and exercise promote blood circulation. Elastic stockings provide support to weak-walled veins.
Monitor the patient for adequate intake of vitamin B complex and calcium; if determined to be inadequate, instruct the patient to drink milk regularly in order to increase calcium intake. Discuss with the patient measures to prevent or alleviate leg cramps: • rest to avoid fatigue • place a hot water bottle on affected area • extend affected leg and flex ankle, pointing toes to knees • adequate exercise • elevate the legs	A lack of calcium and vitamin B complex is thought to be a cause of leg cramps. Muscle fatigue may cause leg cramps. Warmth helps to relax a cramped muscle. Stretching the calf muscle by flexing the ankle and extending the leg will decrease muscle spasm. Adequate exercise promotes circulation. Elevation of the legs helps promote blood return from legs.

PATIENT PROBLEM	GOAL(S)
Backache Causes: • relaxation of body joints from the hormonal influence of estrogen and relaxin • muscle strain from increased weight of the growing uterus • excessive weight causes added strain on back muscles • exaggerated lordosis can cause aching and numbness of the upper extremities • wearing high-heeled shoes causes postural change • fatigue and muscle tension will cause back pain	Backache is minimized with proper body alignment and stretching exercises.
Shortness of breath Causes: • supine hypotensive syndrome • increased awareness of breathing • pressure from uterus on lung expansion (This is questionable.)	Patient understands and accepts explanation of shortness of breath. This knowledge alleviates anxiety that can compound problem.
Dizziness and fainting Causes: • sudden standing from a supine or sitting position will cause pooling of blood in the lower extremities • supine hypotension caused by compression of the uterus on the vena cava, resulting in decreased blood flow to the heart and brain • hypoglycemia • hyperventilation • anemia decreases the oxygen-carrying capacity of the red blood cell	Patient reports any symptoms for evaluation. Patient understands the effects of diet and rest on symptoms.

Figure 7–7 *continued*

Nursing Intervention	Rationale
Discuss with the patient measures to alleviate or prevent back pain: • adequate rest to avoid fatigue • good posture and body alignment • proper shoes • exercise to strengthen muscles	As the patient's body weight, shape, and balance change, posture may be altered, causing muscle strain. Exercises designed to strengthen abdominal and back muscles will help maintain good posture and will prevent backache.
Explain to the patient the usual cause of shortness of breath during pregnancy. Instruct the patient to sleep in semi-Fowler's position, supported by two or three pillows.	Knowledge of the cause of the breathlessness (usually, pressure exerted on the diaphragm by the growing uterus) will alleviate patient's anxiety about the condition. Anxiety may exacerbate the problem. A semi-upright position reduces the pressure on the diaphragm.
Instruct the patient to avoid: • rapid changes in position • standing for long periods of time • fatigue • extreme excitement and nervousness Advise the patient to: • rest on her left side • report any dizziness to her physician	Low blood pressure, which can occur in a pregnant woman if she stands for a long time or changes position rapidly, may cause dizziness or faintness. Excitement or anxiety may affect respiratory function, leading to hyperventilation and dizziness. Faintness or dizziness may also result from low blood sugar or too little iron in the blood. Resting on the left side rather than in a supine position reduces the risk of hypotension, as it promotes blood return by shifting the baby's weight off the mother's inferior vena cava.

PATIENT PROBLEM	GOAL(S)
Fatigue and drowsiness Causes: • influence of increased hormone production • lack of exercise • malnutrition • anemia • psychogenic causes • excessive weight gain • infection	Patient understands the reason for fatigue and complies with the advice for additional rest as her body dictates.
Bleeding gums and nose bleeds Causes: • diet with lack of vitamin C • increased blood volume applies additional strain to mucous membranes • increased hormones	Bleeding gums and nose bleeds are kept to a minimum by preventive measures. Patient reports any persistent or prolonged bleeding to her physician.
Vaginal discharge Causes: • increased estrogen secretion during pregnancy causes increased production of cervical mucus — more vaginal discharge becomes evident	Patient accepts increased vaginal discharge as normal but reports any significant change that causes tissue irritation, itching, or odor. Patient keeps vulva as clean and dry as possible to minimize irritation.

Figure 7–7 *continued*

NURSING INTERVENTION	RATIONALE
Explain to the patient the importance of adequate rest, particularly in the very early and late weeks of pregnancy. Advise the patient to: • experiment with pillow props to make the lying position more comfortable • practice relaxation techniques taught in childbirth education classes • interpret body signals and respond to them; if she feels tired, she should rest	Fatigue is a natural effect of hormones of pregnancy. Extra energy is needed to carry and care for the developing baby, and thus, additional rest is necessary.
Evaluate the patient's diet to ensure adequate intake of vitamin C. Advise the patient to: • have a dental checkup • apply pressure or ice or both to lower soft part of nose for nose bleeds • keep nasal passages lubricated	A lack of vitamin C in the diet may contribute to these conditions. Membranes become overloaded in pregnancy because volume of circulation is increased. Nose bleeds may result. An increased supply of hormones as well as the increase in volume of circulation may cause tenderness, swelling, and bleeding of gums. Applying ice or pressure or both to the soft part of the nose will decrease the blood flow. Dryness of the nasal passages increases the risk of nose bleeds.
Explain the cause of vaginal discharges in pregnancy. Discuss cleanliness.	Increased blood supply and hormones cause the vagina to increase its normal secretions. The normal acidic atmosphere changes, too, creating a more fertile setting for common vaginal infections, including monilia.

PATIENT PROBLEM	GOAL(S)
Itchy skin Causes: • infection or allergy • stretching tissue due to an enlarging uterus • soap can contribute to dry skin, which will increase itching • dehydration	Patient understands influence of certain drying agents used on the skin and avoids these products. Patient is comfortable with the knowledge that itchy skin may be caused by stretching during pregnancy. Patient drinks an adequate amount of fluids.
Frequent urination Causes: • enlarging uterus stretches the base of the bladder, producing a sensation of fullness • bladder capacity is diminished by the enlarging uterus • excessive fluid intake • increased urine output by the kidney occurs in the supine position • urinary tract infection	Patient reports any dysuria or other symptoms of a bladder infection and accepts the changes in her urinary frequency as part of a normal pregnancy.
Mood swings Causes: • hormonal changes can affect mood • inadequate rest • inadequate diet • ambivalent feelings regarding the pregnancy and responsibility of parenting	Patient verbalizes her fears, concerns, and anxieties openly. She seeks supportive people to talk with about these feelings.

Figure 7–7 continued

NURSING INTERVENTION	RATIONALE
Evaluate patient's hygiene practices and the type of soap used. Advise the patient to: • take starch baths • increase fluid intake somewhat	A lack of good hygiene or the use of a drying soap may cause skin irritation. Itching may also be caused by stretching of the skin of the abdomen. An increased fluid intake may improve the elasticity of the skin.
Reassure the patient that this is a normal condition during pregnancy and that fluids should *not* be restricted in an attempt to alleviate the problem. Advise the patient to empty her bladder whenever necessary.	A frequent urge to urinate is usually caused by the growing uterus exerting pressure on the bladder; this symptom increases in the latter weeks of pregnancy, when the baby drops lower into the pelvis. Fluid restriction may lead to dehydration.
Explain that mood swings are common during pregnancy. Encourage patient to communicate fears and feelings. Explain the importance of proper nutrition and rest.	Hormonal changes may affect some women emotionally. Fear of changes in lifestyle and adaptation to a new role may also contribute to mood alterations; expression of these feelings and fears will help allay them. Adequate rest and good nutrition will promote a state of general good health and will allow the woman to cope with emotional changes more easily.

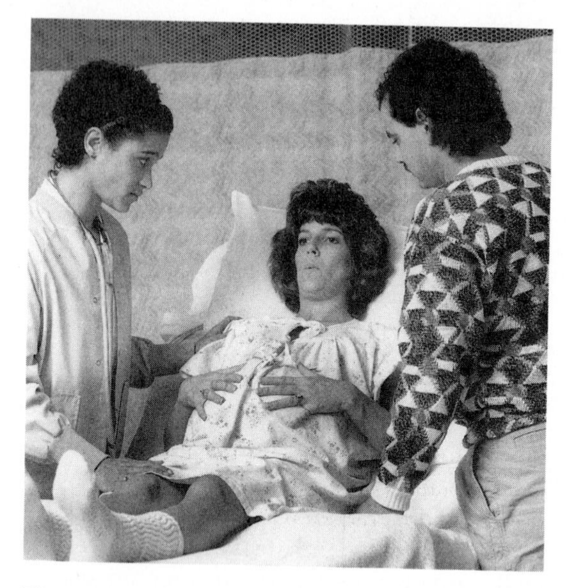

Figure 7–8 *Husband-coached childbirth*

ication. It has been called the "husband-coached childbirth" method. Techniques include relaxation of all muscle groups, normal diaphragmatic breathing, use of different positions during labor, and various pushing techniques.

In most areas where childbirth classes are taught, there is little distinction between the various methods. Many instructors incorporate principles from several methods and refer to their classes as prepared childbirth education.

PREGNANCY AND BIRTH IN DIFFERENT CULTURES

In all cultures, since before recorded history, birth has been a special, magical event. Birth is linked to the basic spiritual concepts of creation, life, and death. It is at the center of many religious rituals. Each culture has evolved rituals and techniques symbolizing that culture's world view. To a great extent, the mother's perception of her birth experience is set by her society's practices and attitudes toward birth. Our culture, for example, attempts to solve its problems scientifically and views childbirth as a medical event that can sometimes be perilous for the baby or the mother.

Almost all cultures have views on when the life force or "spirit" enters the baby. Canadian Eskimos believe that the spirit enters the baby in early pregnancy. Africans believe the father's clan spirit enters the baby in early pregnancy. The mother's clan spirit does not enter until the naming ceremony after the baby's birth. In Western cultures, views on when the spirit enters the baby vary. The Roman Catholic Church, for example, believes that the spirit enters upon conception. English common law deems that it enters at the time that the mother first feels the baby move. The question of when the spirit enters the baby is at the heart of the abortion issue.

Cultures vary widely in terms of whether they view pregnancy and childbirth as an illness or as a healthy, natural event. Brigitte Jordan, a medical anthropologist, notes a wide variation even in Western countries. In the United States, birth is viewed as a medical procedure; in Holland, as a natural process; in Sweden, as a fulfilling personal achievement; and among the Indians of the Yucatan, as a stressful but normal part of family life. The French view the birth process with reverence, an attitude that may explain in part why France has an official policy encouraging women to have as many babies as possible. In contrast to the United States, where having more than two children is seen as an assault on the environment, in France motherhood is seen as a significant national service. Because of this attitude, in France the mother-to-be benefits from several social services, including free perinatal (the first weeks after birth) care and physical therapy sessions to get her body back into shape after delivery and monthly stipends for each child regardless of the family's income. French women are not forced to bear children they do not want. Although France is a

Catholic country, abortion and the abortion pill (RU-486) are legal there, but everything possible is done to enable a woman to have as many children as she wants.

Cultural patterns dealing with childbearing encompass all aspects of the experience, including behavior during pregnancy, labor, delivery, and the postpartum period. Childbearing is taken seriously in all cultures, with an emphasis on responsibility about the parenting role. In almost every culture, there are dietary guidelines for the expectant mother. Depriving the mother of certain foods, rather than adding foods, is the most common pattern. For example, one Philippine community believes that eating a bird can keep the baby small and eating octopus can make the fetus stick inside the mother.

Guidelines related to activity during pregnancy also vary and are very much culture-related. The most common advice is to be active so that the baby does not grow too big. The Hopi and the Sanpoil Indians have a whole exercise regimen for expectant mothers. ACOG's exercise guidelines, listed in Figure 7–5, are typical in mainstream obstetrical practice in the United States.

It was recommended at a conference sponsored by the National Institutes of Health, in Bethesda, Maryland, that ultrasound examinations in a normal pregnancy not be used routinely. In England, the official recommendation is for one sonogram during pregnancy. French health insurance covers two sonograms for every pregnancy, and some French obstetricians routinely ask for four or more.

Yale anthropologist Clellan Ford charted 60 cultures regarding their practices of discouraging sexual intercourse during pregnancy. It was found that 70% permitted intercourse in the second month; only 30% permitted it by the ninth month.

Practices in labor and delivery also vary among cultures. How can medicine, which purports to be a science, differ so radically among people who are so genetically similar? Few procedures in medicine have been well evaluated, with only about 15% of all contemporary clinical interventions having scientific evidence to do more good than harm. In the face of uncertainty, doctors tend to do what makes sense to them, but their decisions are highly susceptible to cultural influences. As early as 1922, for example, a well-performed study showed that women whose pubic hair was shaved before they gave birth had more infections than women who weren't shaved. The same conclusions were reached in a 1965 study. Yet many hospitals in England and the United States continued to give pubic shaves. In France, the practice was never widespread.

In 58 out of 60 cultures that anthropologist Ford studied, older women assisted the mother during childbirth. Often the women were related in some way to the laboring woman. Usually, men were not allowed in the room with the mother. In another study, Marshall Klaus, an American pediatrician and bonding expert, also found that the majority of helpers were women. In addition, at least one helper remained with the woman continuously throughout labor and delivery. In the United States today, fathers are not only allowed but are encouraged to "coach" the expectant mother through her labor and delivery and to take an active part in bonding with their baby.

Birthing positions also vary among cultures. Out of the 76 cultures in the Yale human relations area file, 63 had the mother give birth in a vertical rather than horizontal position. Of those, 22 had mothers upright on their knees, 19 sitting, 15 squatting, and 7 standing. Many cultures also provide pulling devices to help the laboring woman increase the force of her efforts to expel the baby.

The routine use of **episiotomy** (a perineal incision) in childbirth in the United States can be traced to Joseph DeLee, an obstetrician who in 1920 recommended the routine use of forceps, episiotomy, and early removal of the placenta. An artificial cut, argued DeLee, was much cleaner and more controlled than a jagged, natural tear. While DeLee eventually had second thoughts about prophylactic obstetrics when such practices were shown to be a major cause of birth-related accidents, the practices concurred too much with the American view of medicine to be abandoned. Consideration of other countries whose infant and maternal mortality and life expectancy are as good or better than our own shows that such aggressive practices are not the inevitable result of medical progress but of choices that arise from cultural biases.

Cutting the umbilical cord is another issue that has cultural variances. In the Philippines, the cord is traditionally cut with a piece of sharp bamboo and then dusted with powder. In another Philippine community, the cord is left long enough to touch the baby's forehead so the child will be wise.

Postpartum methods of caring for a new mother also vary greatly from one people to another. Many cultures isolate the mother and her newborn, sometimes for an extended period of time. Among the Goajiro Indians of Colombia, a well-to-do mother may remain in bed for a month after delivery. In other cultures, the woman returns to her normal activities and work less than a day after she has given birth.

Another major difference among cultures is the pattern of closeness between the baby and the mother after birth. Among the cultures that Ford studied, 1 baby was weaned at 6 months, 13 at 18 months, 16 at 2 years, 15 at 3 years, and 19 were unclear. In a few cultures, breast feeding continued up to 6 years of age.

Tribal cultures had a fairly long period in which the baby was nursed and carried about by the mother. As societies became industrialized, there was a tendency to shorten this period and wean the child earlier.

There are also many contrasting beliefs regarding **breech presentation**, where either buttocks or feet are presented first. Mexican-American midwives *(parteras)* are reluctant to deliver a baby in breech position and many believe it is a curse to do so. If they are unable to manually rotate the child to a cephalic position, they will send the laboring mother to the hospital. Some cultures believe that if a baby is born in breech position the mother is sure to die; other cultures believe that the child will die and perceive breech births as bad luck. Conversely, other cultures see breech babies as lucky and wise, to have magical gifts, and to be ambitious.

Innumerable cultures have traditional ways of protecting a baby and young child from illness and harm believed to be caused by the "evil eye" or "evil spirits." Figure 7–9 lists some practices derived from an ethnocultural background.

Studying various cultures helps the nurse to view all systems with an open mind. The nurse must recognize different cultural practices and respect the individual's right of choice. A mother-to-be's choices might include (1) which people she wants to have support her during labor, (2) how she will cope with the discomforts of labor, (3) her position for delivery, and (4) how she responds to her newborn. The nurse should remember that there is no one right way to have a baby. Knowledge of the pregnancy and birth practices of the various cultures within the nurse's community is vital for the nurse to be an effective health-care provider.

THE SINGLE MOTHER

The emotional needs of the single pregnant woman are many, complex, and often incompatible. Unfortunately, all too little is being done to meet those needs. In their attempts to gain privacy and to hide their pregnancy, these women may cut themselves off from all communication. In addition, when they come

ETHNOCULTURAL PRACTICES

Origin	Practices
Eastern European Jews	Weave red ribbon into clothes or attach it to crib
Sephardic Jews	Put a blue ribbon or blue bead on baby
Italians	Put a red ribbon (*corno*) on baby
Greek	Put blue "eye" bead, crucifix, charms on baby
	Put *phylact* (a baptismal charm) on baby
	Pin cloves of garlic to baby's shirt
Tunisia	Pin amulets consisting of tiny figures or writings from the Koran on baby's clothing
	Use charms of the fish symbol to ward off evil
Iran	Cover child with amulets — agate, blue beads
	May leave children unwashed to protect them from the evil eye
India /Pakistan	Hindus: give baby copper plates with magic drawings rolled in them
	Muslims: give baby slips of paper with verses from the Koran
	Tie black or red string around baby's wrist
Guatemala	Place small red bag containing herbs on baby or crib
Mexico	Put amulet with red yarn on baby
Philippines	Put charms, amulets, medals on baby
Scotland	Knot red thread into baby's clothing
	Put fragment of Bible on baby's body
South Asia	Put knotted hair or fragment of Koran on baby's body

Figure 7–9

to the hospital to deliver their babies, the staff, with the kindest of intentions, may avoid mentioning the fact that they are single mothers. Every mother about to give birth should have the opportunity to talk about it if she wishes to do so. She may need to express her feelings about her pregnancy and to discuss her baby with someone who cares about her as a person. If a mother has greater needs because she is a single woman, then she must be afforded greater opportunities to meet those needs. The health-care team must deal with the numerous medical, psychological, educational, and social concerns of the single mother.

It is highly probable that the unmarried woman about to deliver did not consciously choose to be in this position. However, this should not be assumed by the nurse. A caring, nonjudgmental attitude and good communication skills assist the nurse in giving supportive care. This mother-to-be is fulfilling her unique function as a woman. To rob her of a sense of dignity and accomplishment at this time is inexcusable.

Pregnancy outside of marriage for the adolescent is especially stressful. The young unmarried mother-to-be is particularly vulnerable since she has neither the emotional nor financial security needed to manage an unplanned, or even a planned, pregnancy. She may lose not only the emotional support of her parents but also the approval of her peer group. Such losses make it very difficult to accept the pregnancy. For individuals in cultures where pregnancy is viewed favorably, the psychological adjustment is not as severe.

To work with the single mother is a challenge. The nurse must be sensitive to changing emotions, have knowledge of the mother's family background, be honest, and create a trust necessary for interaction and effective communication.

The pregnant single woman must decide whether she will keep her baby or give the baby up for adoption. This task would be difficult for any woman. Culture, the financial and family situation, emotional maturity, and reliable support systems are factors that directly or indirectly affect her feelings and judgment. The nurse must not project personal values; rather, the nurse can reduce the patient's mental anguish through effective communication in the difficult decision-making process. If the baby is given up for adoption, the nurse can then support the mother through the grieving process. If the woman decides to keep the baby, many decisions need to be made; education is necessary to the well-being of baby and mother. The father also should be encouraged to participate in all discussions.

REVIEW QUESTIONS

A. Multiple choice. Select the best answer.

1. Morning sickness may be relieved by all the following except
   a. eating dry toast on awakening
   b. eating frequent small meals
   c. increasing liquid intake
   d. resting after meals

2. Swelling (edema) of the feet
   a. calls for restricted sodium intake
   b. is relieved by elevating the feet
   c. should be reported to the doctor
   d. all of the above
   e. none of the above

3. Itchy skin, or urticaria, may be relieved by
   a. increasing calcium intake
   b. increasing fluid intake
   c. taking starch baths
   d. using milder soap
   e. b, c, and d

4. During the early months of pregnancy, a woman should be sure that her diet includes
   a. an extra portion of carbohydrates daily
   b. foods rich in iron
   c. at least one quart of milk daily
   d. 55 to 76 g of protein daily
   e. b, c, and d
   f. b and c only

5. Milk is important to a pregnant woman's diet because it is an excellent source of
   a. body-building protein and calcium, which aids the development of the fetal skeleton
   b. vitamin A, which increases resistance to infection
   c. iron, which is necessary for a rich blood supply
   d. a and b only
   e. all of the above

6. Which of the following statements are true about management of the diet during pregnancy?
   a. Excessive weight gain should be avoided because it can complicate delivery.
   b. A weight gain of 25 to 30 pounds is normal during pregnancy.
   c. Preeclampsia does not occur as often among women on excellent diets as among women on poor diets.
   d. A pregnant woman must increase her calories because now she is eating for two.
   e. b and c only
   f. a, b, and c

7. Psychological concerns of the single adolescent mother include
   a. possible loss of emotional support from her parents
   b. possible loss of financial support from her parents
   c. possible loss of peer group approval
   d. deciding to keep the baby or give it up for adoption
   e. all of the above

8. The main causes of constipation during pregnancy are
   a. decreased physical exertion
   b. changes in the diet
   c. relaxation of the smooth muscle system
   d. obstruction to the lower bowel by the presenting part of the fetus
   e. a, c, and d
   f. a, b, and d

9. Some common discomforts of pregnancy that usually are not medically serious include all the following except
   a. heartburn and flatulence
   b. shortness of breath
   c. headaches and dizziness with blurred vision
   d. vaginal discharge

10. Special care of the breasts during pregnancy that helps to increase the ability to nurse include
    a. having adequate support that is not too tight
    b. massaging nipples if inverted or depressed
    c. expressing a few drops of colostrum from the breasts each day during the last six weeks
    d. washing the breasts daily, using soap sparingly
    e. all of the above

11. The basic components of childbirth classes are
    a. factual information about pregnancy, labor, and delivery
    b. physical conditioning, relaxation, and breathing techniques
    c. information about breast feeding, postpartum experiences, and infant care
    d. a and b
    e. a, b, and c

12. Fetal requirements of iron increase tenfold in the last six weeks of pregnancy. Foods high in iron include
    a. liver and red meats
    b. egg whites
    c. dried fruits and prunes
    d. nuts and legumes
    e. a, c, and d
    f. a, b, c, and d

13. A pregnant woman can decrease the possibility of varicose veins by
    a. avoiding any type of constriction and resting with her feet and legs elevated
    b. eating foods high in calcium
    c. sleeping 12 or more hours a day
    d. exercising regularly
    e. wearing low-heeled shoes

SUGGESTED ACTIVITIES

- Discuss the adjustment in body care required as pregnancy progresses.
- Practice the exercises shown in this chapter so that you will be able to show a pregnant patient how to perform them.
- Review the important nutrients and the four basic food groups. Which nutrients does the pregnant woman need? Explain. Which nutrients can she limit? Explain.
- Plan a diet for the normal pregnant woman.
- Plan a diet for the normal pregnant woman who dislikes milk.
- Discuss the common discomforts of pregnancy and their prevention and nursing care.
- Discuss the fetal physiological response to maternal exercise.
- Discuss the current controversy about vigorous exercise during pregnancy.
- Demonstrate the ability to take a thorough and useful diet history for a patient.
- Identify at least four good sources for the following:
  - low sodium content
  - vitamins D, A, C, and B
  - high iron content
  - folic acid
  - high protein content
  - calcium (other than milk)

BIBLIOGRAPHY

Greif-Fishbein, E. "How Safe Is Exercise during Pregnancy." *JOGNN* 19(1):45–49, January-February, 1990.

Hamilton, P. M. *Basic Maternity Nursing*, 6th ed. St. Louis, MO: C. V. Mosby, 1989.

Hassid, P. *A Textbook for Childbirth Educators*. New York: Harper and Row, 1978.

Hawkins, J. W., and Loretta Pierfedeici. *Maternity and Gynecological Nursing*. New York: J. B. Lippincott, 1981.

Jenson, M. D., Benson, R., and I. Bobsk. *Maternity Care: The Nurse and the Family*, 3rd ed. St. Louis, MO: C. V. Mosby, 1985.

Kay, M. A. *Anthropology of Human Birth*. Philadelphia: F. A. Davis, 1982.

Lowenstein, V. "Who's in Control: Personal Behaviors and Pregnancy." *Childbirth Educator* 8(4):20–25, 1989.

Mattson, S., and L. Lew. "Culturally Sensitive Prenatal Care for Southeast Asians." *JOGNN* 21(1):48–54, January-February, 1992.

McNall, L. K. *Obstetric and Gynecologic Nursing*. St. Louis, MO: C. V. Mosby, 1980.

Moore, M. L., and Ora Strickland. *Realities in Childbearing*, 2nd ed. Philadelphia: W. B. Saunders, 1983.

Oxorn, H. *Oxorn-Foote Human Labor and Birth*, 5th ed. E. Norwalk, CT: Appleton-Century-Crofts, 1986.

Payer, L. "Medicine and Culture." *Childbirth Educator* 9(2):28–31, Winter 1989–1990.

Pillitteri, A. *Maternal-Newborn Nursing: Care of the Growing Family*, 2nd ed. Boston: Little, Brown and Co., 1981.

Porter-Lewallen, L. "Health Beliefs and Health Practices of Pregnant Women." *JOGNN* 18(3):245–246, May-June 1989.

Pritchard, J. A., Macdonald, P. C., and N. F. Grant. *Williams Obstetrics*, 17th ed. E. Norwalk, CT: Appleton-Century-Crofts, 1985.

Reeder, S., Mastroianni, L., Jr., and L. Martin. *Maternity Nursing*, 16th ed. New York: J. B. Lippincott, 1987.

Scott, J. R., et al. *Danforth's Obstetrics and Gynecology*, 6th ed. Philadelphia: J. B. Lippincott, 1990.

Simkin, P., Whalley, J., and A. Keppler. *Pregnancy, Childbirth and the Newborn*. Deephaven, MN: Meadowbrook Books, 1991.

Worthington-Roberts, B. S., and S. R. Williams. *Nutrition in Pregnancy and Lactation*, 4th ed. St. Louis, MO: Times Mirror-Mosby, 1989.

CHAPTER

8

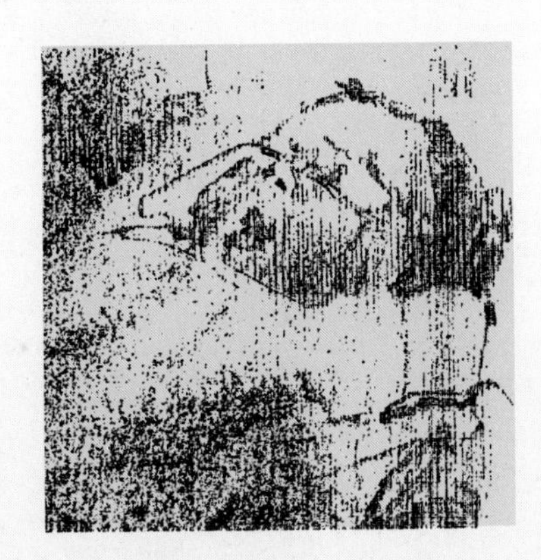

Complications of Pregnancy

Objectives

After studying this chapter, the student should be able to:

- List the danger signals that may indicate complications in pregnancy.
- Describe the symptoms, prevention, and treatment of the more common complications.
- Describe the procedure for an intrauterine transfusion.
- Describe the risks of gestational diabetes.
- List common sexually transmitted diseases and their effect on pregnancy.
- Explain the Rh factor and how it affects the mother and the fetus.

Key Terms

- ECTOPIC PREGNANCY
- TUBAL PREGNANCY
- HYDATIDIFORM MOLE
- ABORTION
  - SPONTANEOUS
  - INDUCED
  - COMPLETE
  - INCOMPLETE
  - MISSED
  - HABITUAL
- D&E
- MULTIPLE PREGNANCY
- HYPEREMESIS GRAVIDARUM
- PIH
- HYPERTENSION
- PREECLAMPSIA
- ECLAMPSIA
- HELLP SYNDROME
- PLACENTA PREVIA
- PLACENTA ABRUPTIO
- GESTATIONAL DIABETES
- HYDRAMNIOS
- LEUKORRHEA
- CANDIDIASIS
- TRICHOMONIASIS
- BACTERIAL VAGINOSIS
- HERPES GENITALIS
- CONDYLOMATA ACUMINATO
- GONORRHEA
- SYPHILIS
- CHLAMYDIA
- PID
- AIDS (ACQUIRED IMMUNE DEFICIENCY SYNDROME)
- FIFTH DISEASE
- TOXOPLASMOSIS
- RH FACTOR
- RHOGAM
- ERYTHROBLASTOSIS FETALIS
- AMNIOCENTESIS
- INTRAUTERINE TRANSFUSION

This unit discusses complications of pregnancy and symptoms that must be called to the doctor's attention immediately.

Danger Signals

It is always desirable to be able to assure the patient that the findings on examination are normal and that she may anticipate an uneventful pregnancy. At the same time, however, the patient should be instructed tactfully regarding danger signals.

DANGER SIGNALS

Symptom	Possible problem
• Any vaginal bleeding	Miscarriage, placenta previa, placenta abruptio, preterm labor
• Severe, continuous headache	Preeclampsia
• Swelling of the face, fingers, or feet	Preeclampsia
• Dimness or blurring of vision or spots before the eyes	Preeclampsia
• Pain in the abdomen or back	Ectopic pregnancy, miscarriage, placenta abruptio, preterm labor contractions
• Persistent nausea and/or vomiting	Infection, hyperemesis gravidarum
• Chills and fever (oral over 100°F or 38°C)	Infection
• Sudden escape of fluid from the vagina	Rupture of the membranes
• Decrease in urine output	Dehydration
• Noticeable reduction in fetal movement	Fetal distress
• Constant, painful firmness of the abdomen, with or without vaginal bleeding	Placenta abruptio

Treatment is prescribed according to the severity of the situation; therapy should be individualized.

ECTOPIC PREGNANCY

An **ectopic pregnancy** is an extrauterine pregnancy; that is, the fertilized ovum begins to develop outside the uterus. Ninety-five percent of ectopic pregnancies occur in the fallopian tubes. Occasionally, the fertilized egg starts to develop in the ovary, or in rare cases, within the abdominal cavity. When the fertilized ovum becomes implanted within the wall of the fallopian tube, it is called a **tubal pregnancy**. The wall of the tube is not elastic enough for the fertilized ovum to grow and develop in it, so inevitably it ruptures. Symptoms before rupture include abdominal pain and some vaginal bleeding. A diagnosis is usually be made with ultrasound. When the tube ruptures, the abdomen becomes tender and rigid and the pain increases. The patient may go into shock if the internal hemorrhage is massive. Upon diagnosis, surgery is indicated; usually an ectopic pregnancy becomes apparent between the second and fourth months. Early diagnosis is imperative because a ruptured ectopic pregnancy can be life-threatening to the mother.

HYDATIDIFORM MOLE

Hydatidiform mole, or molar pregnancy, is an abnormal condition in which the fertilized ovum degenerates and dies; the chorionic villi convert into a mass of transparent cysts resembling a cluster of grapes that fill the uterus, Figure 8–1.

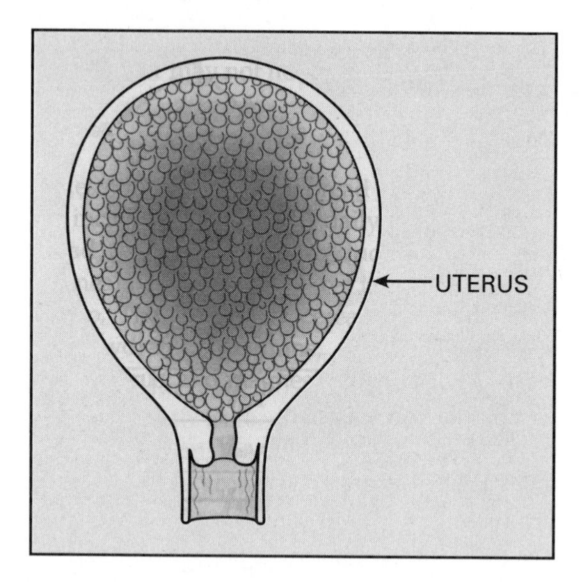

Figure 8–1 *Hydatidiform mole. The chorionic villi convert to a mass of cysts that fill the uterus.*

Molar pregnancy occurs about once in every 2,000 pregnancies. Signs and symptoms that can suggest hydatidiform mole include (1) dark red or brown bleeding, (2) severe nausea and vomiting, (3) an absence of fetal heart tones, (4) a larger uterus than expected for the dates, and (5) pregnancy-induced hypertension before the 24th week of pregnancy. Diagnosis is readily made with ultrasound.

Treatment consists of emptying the uterus. A spontaneous abortion may occur, or induced abortion may be necessary. In some cases a hysterectomy may be performed. Follow-up care is very important. Although hydatidiform mole usually is benign, malignant chorion carcinoma can sometimes add further complications. The most common site of metastasis is the lungs (more than 75%); the second most common is the vagina. The vulva, kidneys, liver, ovaries, and brain can also contain metastases. Close follow-up is needed for up to a year after hydatidiform mole. Human chorionic gonadotropin (hCG) hormone is measured frequently to be sure it is decreasing to a normal range. Pregnancy should be avoided for at least a year after a hydatidiform mole.

EVALUATION OF POSSIBLE HYDATIDIFORM MOLE

Hydatidiform mole is a developmental placental abnormality in which some or all the chorionic villi become edematous and degenerate into grapelike vesicles. Etiology is unknown, but it is more common in women over 40 who have had more than three births plus a history of prior hydatidiform moles. There is a higher incidence of this problem in women residing in Asia and the South Pacific than in the United States and Europe.

Subjective Observations (patient's description)

- vaginal bleeding, minimal, at end of first and beginning of second trimester
- severe nausea and vomiting due to high hCG levels associated with hydatidiform mole
- absence of fetal movement
- passage of grapelike vesicles

Objective Observations (nurse's comments)

- uterus can be larger or smaller than expected by the due date
- anemia is out of proportion to blood loss
- signs of pregnancy-induced hypertension developing before 24 weeks of pregnancy
- absence of fetal heart tones and inability to feel fetal parts when palpating the abdomen
- adnexal mass due to ovarian lutein cysts
- visualization of passed grapelike vesicles

Assessment

Presumptive diagnosis of hydatidiform mole is made on the basis of subjective symptoms and objective findings. This condition is confirmed with the visualization of grapelike vesicles. It is associated with elevated blood pressure and proteinuria before the 24th week of gestation.

Plan

- diagnostic tests
  1. sonogram
- treatment
  1. refer immediately to physician
- education
  1. Women with molar pregnancies and their families must be helped to understand and deal with
     a. what a molar pregnancy is
     b. the favorable statistics for benign resolution
     c. what symptoms might indicate malignancy
     d. possible serious complications
     e. need to delay the next pregnancy
     f. importance of follow-up testing and close supervision by physician
  2. assist in resolution of feelings of grief, anger, and fear.

ABORTION AND BLEEDING

Abortion is the termination of pregnancy at any time before the fetus has obtained a stage of viability. Abortion may be subdivided into two main forms: spontaneous and induced. **Spontaneous abortion** (or miscarriage) is the termination of pregnancy through natural causes. **Induced abortion** is the termination of pregnancy with the aid of mechanical or medical agents. A **complete abortion** is one in which the entire product of conception is expelled. An **incomplete abortion** is one in which part of the product of conception is passed, but part remains in the uterus. A **missed abortion** is one in which the fetus dies in utero, but the product of conception is retained. **Habitual abortion** is the condition in which three or more successive pregnancies are terminated by spontaneous abortion. Abortion, in any form, has a tremendous psychological impact on a woman and should be understood by the nurse in order for her to be supportive.

Before 1803, in the United States and Great Britain, induced abortion was either lawful or widely tolerated if performed before quickening occurred. In 1803, a general reform of British criminal law made it illegal to perform abortions before quickening. Canon law, established by Pope Pius IX in 1869, stated that under no circumstances is abortion justifiable. Since the 1960s, people increasingly have favored liberalization of abortion laws. In 1969, 11 states had amended their laws by extending the indications for therapeutic termination of pregnancy. In 1973 the U.S. Supreme Court ruled that a state may not prevent a woman from having an abortion during the first six months of pregnancy. By 1977, all states had reevaluated their abortion laws; each state now abides by its own standards and regulations. Canon law remains unchanged.

One of the most essential issues that a woman must face is her own moral view of induced abortion. The U.S. Supreme Court decision of 1973 gives each woman the right to freedom of conscience in this matter. Martin Ekblad interviewed 479 Swedish women in a follow-up study concerning the psychological consequences of elective abortion. He said, "Sixty-five percent of the women stated that they were satisfied with their abortion and had no self-reproaches; 10 percent had no self-reproaches but felt the operation itself was unpleasant; 14 percent had mild degrees of self-reproach or regretted having had the operation." The women who felt the most guilt were those who had allowed their decision to be influenced by others; those who felt the least guilt were those who were confident that they wanted the abortion themselves.

Although abortion continues to be one solution for unwanted pregnancy, many women prefer other alternatives. A woman may choose to make room for a new addition to her existing family, she may decide to keep the child and become a single parent, or she may bring her pregnancy to term and then give the child up for adoption. Supportive counseling and listening are essential from the nurse regardless of her personal views. If the nurse feels incapable of being supportive without bias from her own strong personal beliefs, she should refer the woman to someone who can give unconditional support.

Spontaneous abortion when a child is desperately wanted is another emotional issue the nurse may need to help a family deal with. When a woman who has had a positive pregnancy test presents with bleeding and cramping, the nurse must evaluate the medical implications. An ectopic pregnancy must first be ruled out. An ultrasound usually is effective in determining the status of an early pregnancy. If the woman is in fact "miscarrying," she has some choices to make. The products of conception can be evacuated for her medically with a **D&E** (dilation and evacuation) or she may choose to wait and allow her body to pass the products of conception on its own. There are risks and benefits to both alternatives; they must be discussed with her physician. The nurse also must be familiar with abortion aftercare and future fertility or birth control issues and discuss them with her patient.

MULTIPLE PREGNANCIES

When two or more embryos develop in the uterus at the same time, the condition is known as **multiple pregnancy**. Twins are relatively common, occurring in about 1 of 80 pregnancies. Fraternal twins are produced by the fertilization of two eggs and two sperm. Identical twins occur when one sperm fertilizes one egg, which later divides into two developing babies. Triplets occur in approximately 1 of 6,400 pregnancies, and quadruplets or quintuplets less frequently. A multiple birth may be suspected if two or more fetal heartbeats are heard, if there is a family history of twins, if weight gain is rapid, or if uterine growth exceeds the normal rate. Ultrasound can easily confirm a multiple gestation.

The mother-to-be usually experiences greater discomforts and higher risks than the woman with a single pregnancy. The requirements for calories, protein, minerals, and vitamins are higher in the woman with multiple fetuses. Pregnancy-induced and pregnancy-aggravated hypertension are much more likely to develop in pregnancies with more than one fetus. Prematurity is also more likely to occur, placing the babies at much greater risk. Bed rest has been thought to help prolong such pregnancies to term, but this has been difficult to prove. Medications to decrease premature contractions also may be indicated in some cases. In any event, both the psychological and physical adjustments made by a woman carrying more than one baby need to be recognized and addressed by the nurse. Mothers of Twins is a nationwide community information and support group for families expecting more than one baby and is a good resource for the nurse.

HYPEREMESIS GRAVIDARUM

Hyperemesis gravidarum (excessive vomiting) is a serious complication that is rarely encountered today because of improved prenatal care. Symptoms include constant nausea and vomiting, loss of sleep, restlessness, and exhaustion. Weight loss is rapid, and dehydration of all the body tissues is a marked sign. Hyperemesis gravidarum occurs in the first three months of pregnancy. If excessive vomiting continues, it usually indicates that a condition other than the pregnancy is the immediate cause.

The treatment of hyperemesis gravidarum generally consists of (1) stopping the dehydration and starvation that is a result of the patient's inability to ingest food, (2) improving the general psychological condition of the patient, and (3) administering medication, as ordered by the doctor.

PIH, Preeclampsia, and Eclampsia

Pregnancy-induced hypertension **(PIH)** affects 6% to 8% of pregnant women in the United States. This condition can be divided into three categories: hypertension, preeclampsia, and eclampsia.

Hypertension, or high blood pressure, is defined as blood pressure that exceeds 140/90 for at least two recordings, or as a sustained rise in systolic pressure of more than 30 mmHg or a sustained rise in diastolic pressure of more than 15 mmHg above the first trimester pressures.

Preeclampsia can be dangerous for a pregnant woman and her baby. It is a toxemia shown by swelling of the body tissues (edema) with rapid weight gain, an elevated blood pressure, and the presence of protein in the urine (albuminuria). The woman's urine output may be decreased. She may experience epigastric pain, vision changes, and headache and her reflexes may be hyperactive. Preeclampsia occurs in the last two or three months of gestation; it rarely occurs before the 24th week. The patient often is not aware of anything unusual until she becomes ill. She must be under the strict supervision of a physician, with regular office visits and sometimes hospitalization. If the condition does not progress to eclampsia, the majority of patients return to normalcy within 10 days or so after delivery.

Women younger than 18 or over 35 have a higher chance of developing preeclampsia in pregnancy than women between those ages. Also, women who have a multiple gestation are at greater risk. Preeclampsia is one of the most dangerous conditions of pregnancy. Decreased blood flow through the placenta causes the baby to suffer. Babies of preeclamptic mothers tend to be small in relation to the length of time they are carried; they also have a greater chance of being stillborn than babies of nonpreeclamptic mothers. The prognosis is always serious for both the mother and child.

Eclampsia is an acute toxemia of pregnancy. It is characterized by the same symptoms as preeclampsia plus spasmodic and sustained convulsions and loss of consciousness, followed by coma. It sometimes results in fetal or maternal death. Since eclampsia can be prevented by good prenatal care, it is becoming increasingly rare (1 in 1,000 or 1,500 deliveries) as more women receive adequate medical supervision during pregnancy. It occurs more often in primigravidas than in multiparas. It also occurs in women who are nutritionally deficient or who are diabetic.

The treatment for PIH includes bed rest and close medical supervision to monitor blood pressure and signs of preeclampsia. A blood test for signs of the **HELLP syndrome** (*h*emolysis, *e*levated *l*iver enzymes, and *l*ow *p*latelets) can indicate liver and blood complications. Sometimes medication is ordered to lower blood pressure. If preeclampsia develops, drugs to decrease the risk of seizures may be given. If preeclampsia persists despite efforts to control the symptoms, a cesarean birth may be planned.

Placenta Previa

While spontaneous abortion is the most frequent cause of bleeding early in pregnancy, the most common cause during the later months is placenta previa. **Placenta previa** occurs when the placenta has implanted in the lower segment of the uterus and either wholly or partially covers the cervix, Figures 8–2 and 8–3.

Cesarean section is the treatment of choice in severe forms of placenta previa. Bleeding, shock, and infection are the main dangers. Blood transfusion is important in the management of these cases, as is meticulous attention to antiseptic techniques.

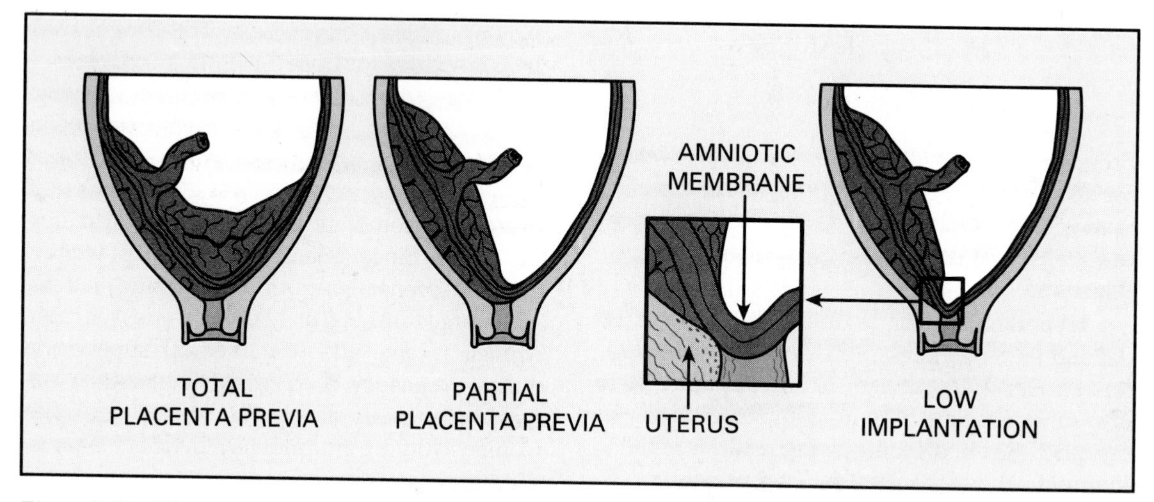

Figure 8–2 *Placenta previa: abnormal implantation (Adapted from Clinical Education Aid, No. 12, Ross Laboratories)*

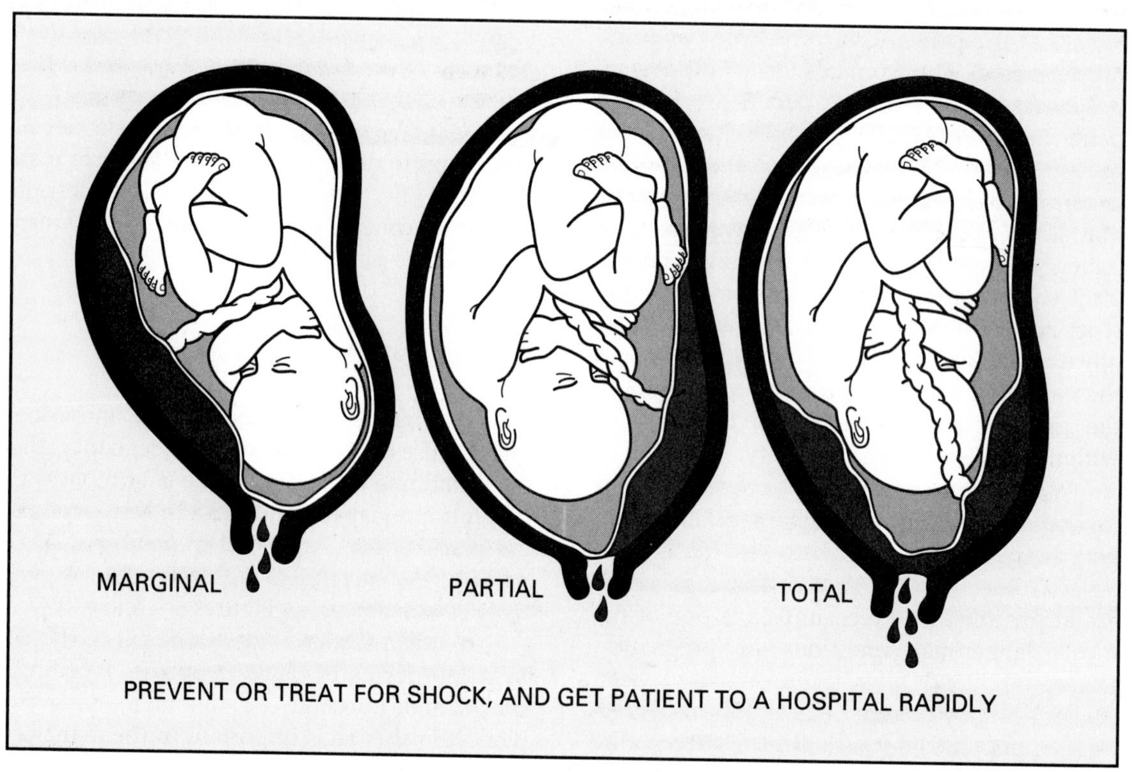

Figure 8–3 *Placenta previa and the fetus*

PLACENTA ABRUPTIO

Placenta abruptio is the premature separation of the normally implanted placenta. It occurs either in the later months of pregnancy or at the beginning of labor and is usually characterized by bleeding and pain, Figures 8–4 and 8–5. Bleeding behind the placenta causes pressure to build up. This pressure causes the uterus to become rigid and painful. Placenta abruptio may be partial or complete, depending on whether all or part of the placenta becomes detached.

Treatment consists of performing a cesarean section, or, in cases when the abruptio is only minor, rupturing the membranes so that the woman delivers vaginally before the detachment increases and bleeding becomes more severe. Shock secondary to blood loss is almost always present and must be dealt with first. The prognosis for the infant depends on the severity of the condition, refer to Figure 8–6.

GESTATIONAL DIABETES

Gestational diabetes is diabetes brought on by pregnancy. In many obstetrical practices, it is routine to screen women for gestational diabetes by giving the expectant mother 50 g of glucola at 24 to 26 weeks of her pregnancy. A blood sample is taken one hour later and evaluated. If the glucola level is above 140 mg/dL, gestational diabetes is suspected, and the pregnant woman needs further testing. A three-hour glucose tolerance test is then taken and evaluated. Many gestational diabetic women can be managed by diet alone; some women may need insulin. But in either case, close management throughout the pregnancy is important.

Gestational diabetes differs from insulin-dependent (type I) and noninsulin-dependent (type II) diabetes in that it is not usually permanent. Once the baby is delivered, the diabetes disappears; the reason for the increased

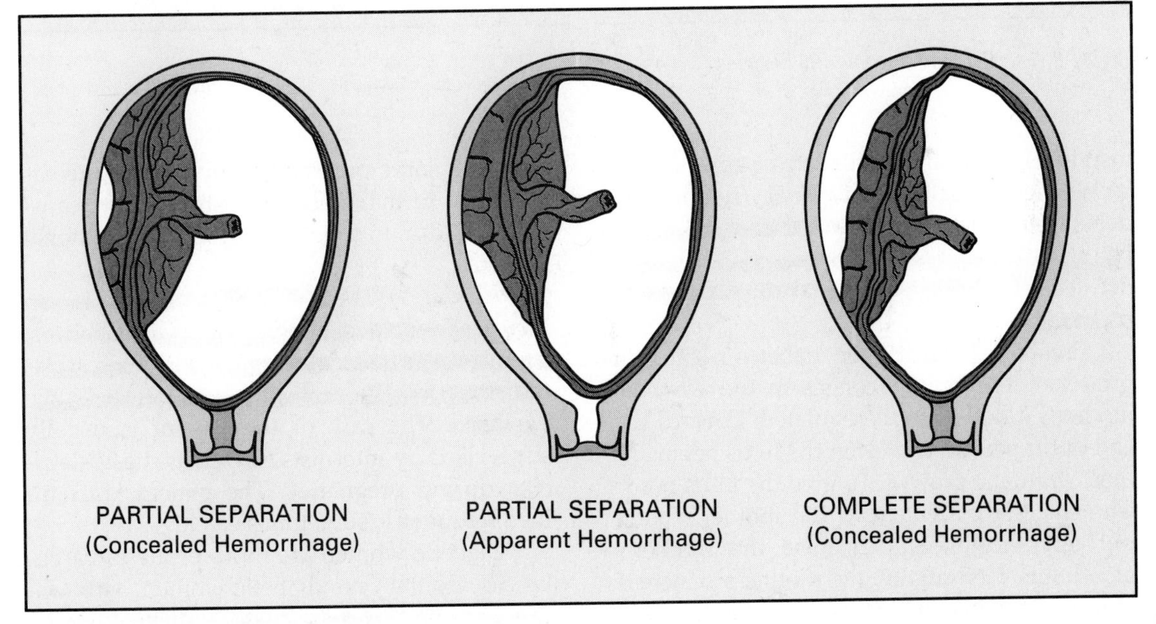

Figure 8–4 *Placenta abruptio: premature separation (Adapted from Clinical Education Aid, No. 12, Ross Laboratories)*

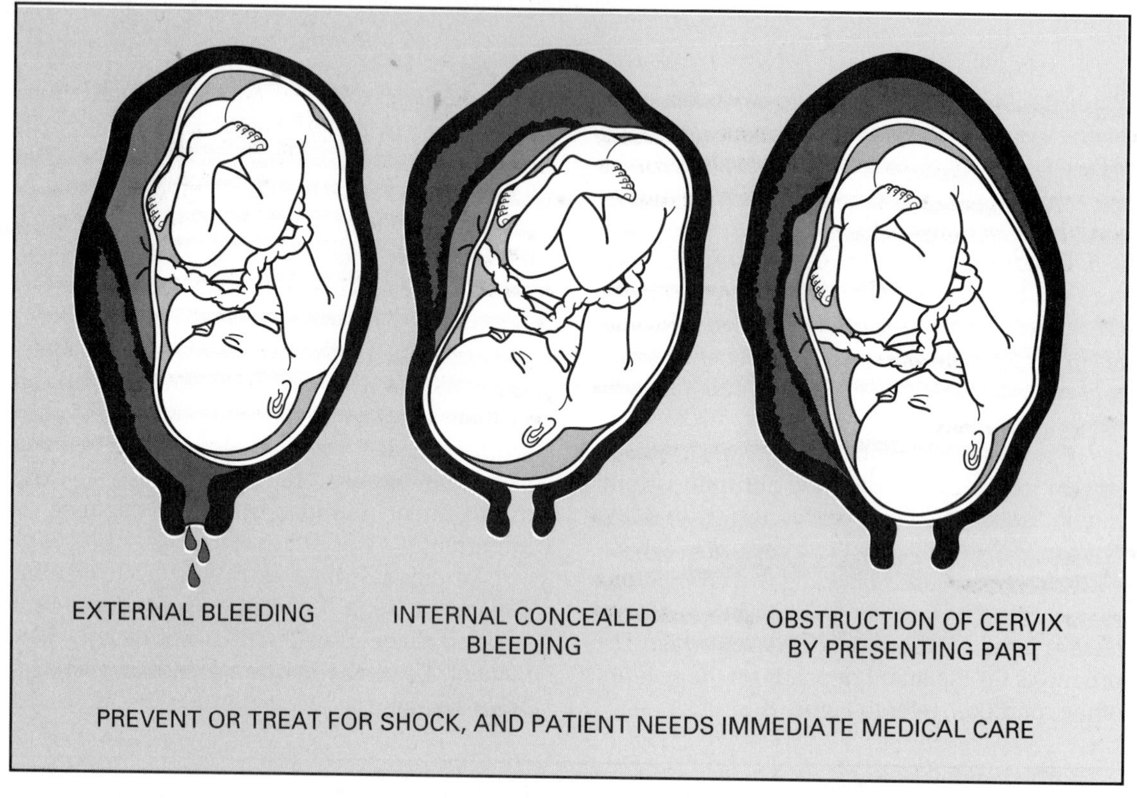

Figure 8–5 *Placenta abruptio and the fetus*

insulin is gone. If the diabetes persists, it is reclassified usually as type II (noninsulin-dependent) diabetes. Women who have diabetes before becoming pregnant are not defined as having gestational diabetes when pregnant.

Pregnancy can trigger diabetes because it produces temporary changes in the way the mother's blood sugar is regulated. Toward the end of the second trimester, the fetus begins its most dramatic growth. To give the fetus nourishment, the placenta and the mother's body put out substances that raise the mother's blood sugar. Normally, the mother's pancreas makes extra insulin in response to the extra sugar in her blood. Insulin allows cells to use sugar for energy and helps to keep the mother's blood sugar level within a normal range. In some pregnant women, the pancreas is unable to make enough extra insulin, causing a buildup in sugar. The result is gestational diabetes.

Among diabetic patients there is an increased incidence of abortion, stillbirths, preeclampsia, premature labor, large-for-gestational-age infants, and congenital defects in the newborn. The care of the patient is usually supervised by internists as well as the obstetrician during pregnancy. The patient is examined frequently, sometimes weekly.

Diabetic women are more prone to vascular disease than nondiabetic women. This tendency may partially explain why diabetic women are more likely to develop pregnancy-induced hypertension (PIH). Urinary tract infections occur more frequently in pregnant

COMPLICATIONS OF PREGNANCY

Complication	Cause	Symptoms	Prevention or Care
Hyperemesis gravidarum	1. Faulty nutrition 2. Vitamin deficiency 3. Hormones 4. Emotional disturbances	1. Vomiting	1. Eight hours sleep and midday rest 2. Avoid sexual relations 3. Avoid odors that precipitate attacks 4. Fresh air and sunshine 5. Proper ventilation 6. Sedation 7. Small amounts of food with high-carbohydrate diet 8. Vitamin B_6 and complex 9. For more severe cases: a. Complete bed rest b. Extreme quiet c. IV fluids d. Sedation: phenobarbital and dramamine e. Vitamin B complex f. Nothing by mouth at first and later small feedings or liquids until tolerated

Figure 8–6 *(Courtesy* Maternal and Child Health, *Littlefield, Adams & Co.)*

women who are diabetic than in those who are not, because the presence of sugar in the urine favors the growth of bacteria.

Another complication that frequently accompanies pregnancy in a diabetic woman is **hydramnios**, an excessive accumulation of amniotic fluid surrounding the fetus in utero. It is not a serious threat to the mother, but it can lead to complications as the mother approaches the time of delivery. If this complication devel-

COMPLICATIONS OF PREGNANCY

Complication	Cause	Symptoms	Prevention or Care
Toxemias 1. Acute a. Preeclampsia b. Eclampsia	1. True cause unknown 2. Probable causes a. Dietary deficiencies b. Infection c. Pressure d. Endocrine imbalance of mother e. Infarct of placenta f. Endocrine imbalance of fetus g. Rh factor of fetus	In preeclampsia: 1. Edema 2. Weight gain 3. Albuminuria 4. Elevated blood pressure 5. Headaches 6. Drowsiness 7. Dizziness 8. Decrease in urine 9. Casts in urine 10. Disturbance of vision 11. Nausea and vomiting 12. Slight jaundice 13. Hyperactive reflexes 14. Epigastric pain	1. Proper prenatal care to prevent 2. Complete bed rest 3. Dark room 4. Isolation 5. Check blood pressure 6. Give antihypertensive drugs 7. Hypertonic solutions 8. Inhalation of oxygen 9. Intake and output
Placenta previa	1. Placenta partially or completely over cervix a. Coitus b. Lifting c. Falls	1. Painless bleeding	1. Same as for bleeding 2. Cesarean section
Placenta abruptio	1. Lifting 2. Falls 3. Without reason	1. Painful bleeding 2. Shock 3. May have no external bleeding	1. Same as for bleeding 2. Cesarean section immediately

Figure 8–6 *continued*

ops, the doctor may wish to deliver the baby earlier than scheduled.

Infants delivered at term to diabetic patients have a higher mortality rate than those delivered earlier because the vascular changes in the placenta compromise the fetus. The larger size of the fetus at term may also complicate delivery. For these reasons, the obstetrician may decide to schedule an early delivery, at about the 36th to 38th week of gestation.

The baby of a mother who has high blood sugar can actually develop low blood sugar

COMPLICATIONS OF PREGNANCY

Complication	Cause	Symptoms	Prevention or Care
Bleeding	1. First and second trimesters a. Abortions b. Chronic epithelium c. Carcinoma of cervix d. Varicose veins e. Erosion of cervix	1. Bleeding 2. Low blood pressure 3. Shock	1. Complete bed rest 2. Elevate feet 3. Check blood pressure 4. Sedation
	2. Second and third trimesters a. Placenta previa b. Premature separation of placenta c. Ruptured uterus d. Carcinoma of cervix e. Varicose veins f. Erosion of cervix		1. Cesarean section if necessary
Abortion	1. Size and shape of uterus 2. Accidental 3. Radiation 4. Electrical shock 5. Alcohol and tobacco 6. Drugs 7. Surgical procedures 8. Coitus	1. Bleeding 2. Expulsion of fetus and placenta	1. Same as for bleeding 2. D&E if incomplete

Figure 8–6 *continued*

after delivery. During pregnancy, the mother's insulin does not reach the baby; the baby produces and uses its own insulin. When a mother has diabetes, the baby gets an overload of sugar, which causes the baby's pancreas to produce a greater amount of insulin. After birth, when the baby is no longer receiving sugar from the mother's system, the child takes a

COMPLICATIONS OF PREGNANCY

Complication	Cause	Symptoms	Prevention or Care
Ectopic pregnancy	1. Growth of fetus outside of uterus 2. Obstruction of uterine tubes 3. Infection	1. Miss one period 2. Nausea and vomiting 3. Stabbing, tearing pain on side 4. Bleeding with pains 5. Cervix tender and painful 6. Rupture brings dizziness, faintness, drop in blood pressure	1. Surgery 2. Antibiotics 3. Bed rest 4. Sedatives 5. Reassurance 6. Cul de sac puncture

Figure 8–6 *continued*

while to adjust the amount of insulin produced. As a result, the baby's blood sugar level can fall too low. Prolonged low blood sugar (below 30 mg/dL) can cause brain damage.

Malformations, which are often a worry for women with uncontrolled type I and type II diabetes, are not a particular problem in babies of women who have gestational diabetes. The baby's organs are formed by the 10th to the 12th week after conception. Gestational diabetes does not usually occur until after the 20th week.

Some women are at greater risk for developing gestational diabetes than others. Obesity increases the odds because excess fat causes cells to resist insulin. Therefore the cells have difficulty using blood sugar for energy. A family history of diabetes can add to the risk because the tendency to diabetes is inherited. Severe emotional or physical stress can trigger diabetes in someone who is prone to the disease. Stress causes a rise in hormones that raise blood sugar and cause sugar that has been stored in the liver to be released into the blood.

Some women have classic symptoms of diabetes, including increased thirst, hunger, urination, and weakness. Often, however, women have no obvious symptoms and feel normal. Therefore the American Diabetes Association recommends testing all pregnant women between the 24th and 26th week of pregnancy, as discussed earlier.

Anyone diagnosed with diabetes during pregnancy should see a diabetic specialist if her obstetrician does not specialize in diabetes. Some doctors believe that a controlled meal plan alone can achieve ideal blood sugar levels. Others believe that insulin is required. Treatment depends on the woman's individual situation.

Insulin dosage and dietary management require adjustment. The woman should be alert for signs of hyperglycemia, hypoglycemia, and acidosis, see Figure 8–7. She should test her urine and blood four times a day, usually upon rising in the morning and two hours after each meal. Tests that measure sugar levels in urine are not accurate enough for use during pregnancy and may be misleading. However, women need to test the urine for ketones. High levels of ketone in the urine is a sign that the body has switched to burning fat for energy and can be harmful to the fetus. It is also a sign that diabetes is out of control. Blood tests for sugar levels are easy to perform and relatively painless. Individual instruction must be given to each woman to learn to interpret her own results. Management of the diet is also on an individual basis. The diet is usually developed from what a woman normally likes to eat. It should include the same balance of nutrients that are considered best for pregnancy. Meals should be scheduled at regular times, keeping the same balance of protein, fat, and carbohydrates each day. A low-sodium diet may be ordered to prevent preeclampsia.

VAGINAL INFECTIONS AND SEXUALLY TRANSMITTED DISEASES

Vaginal infections are more common among pregnant women than among nonpregnant women. Two common vaginal infections are leukorrhea and candidiasis. These vaginal infections are usually mild. Their presence is noted during the internal examination, and the patient is treated accordingly.

The nurse also should be aware of vaginal infections that might be sexually transmitted. They are more serious than leukorrhea and candidiasis, and many sexually transmitted infections can have an adverse effect on the baby if present at the time of birth, refer to Figure 8–8.

LEUKORRHEA

Leukorrhea is a white mucous discharge originating in the cervical canal. Normally there is an increased amount of discharge during pregnancy. Leukorrhea becomes abnormal when the discharge becomes yellow and the odor and consistency change. Hormones change the vaginal pH and sometimes destroy the normal, helpful vaginal bacteria.

CANDIDIASIS

Candidiasis is caused by a yeast organism and results in an irritating, cheesy discharge. Edema (swelling) of the external genitals is sometimes present. Most women who have candidiasis will complain of intense vaginal itching. If the condition is left untreated during pregnancy, the baby may be contaminated while passing through the birth canal. This is how a newborn develops thrush, a fungal infection of the mouth.

TRICHOMONIASIS

Trichomoniasis is caused by the microorganism *Trichomonas vaginalis* (known as a trichomonad) that lives in the vagina and urethra. It produces a profuse irritating discharge and causes itching of the vulva and vaginal opening. This condition is treated with an antibiotic.

BACTERIAL VAGINOSIS (*Gardnerella vaginalis*)

Bacterial vaginosis (also called hemophilus, *Gardnerella vaginalis*, and nonspecific vaginitis) is caused by bacteria that live in the vagina. These organisms cause a chalky white or gray-green vaginal discharge, which can be thick or watery. It usually produces a fishy odor and can be accompanied by itching, dyspareunia (painful intercourse), and dysuria (painful urination). This condition also can be treated with an antibiotic.

NURSING CARE PLAN: Insulin Reaction

PATIENT PROBLEM	GOAL(S)
Insulin reaction (possible overdose) • rapid development of symptoms • cold, clammy skin • trembling, twitching of lips, mental confusion • double vision • shallow breathing • loss of consciousness • NPH insulin overdose has a slow reaction occurring late in day	Patient will be stabilized; blood levels will return to normal; patient will understand symptoms and report any further problems.
Deficiency of insulin, diabetic coma (acidosis) • slow development of symptoms • skin hot and dry • fruity odor to breath • extreme thirst, nausea, vomiting • dull vision • deep, heavy breathing • loss of consciousness	Patient will be stabilized; blood levels will return to normal; patient will understand symptoms and report any further problems.

Figure 8–7

HERPES GENITALIS

Herpes genitalis (genital herpes) is an acute primary or recurrent herpes virus infection of the cervix, vagina, or genitals. Herpes has been called the fastest growing sexually transmitted disease in the United States. It is a lifelong disease that tends to recur again and again. The patient may have itching and a burning sensation at the infection site. Painful blisterlike lesions can be observed. There is often vulvovaginal edema, leukorrhea, and dyspareunia. If a lesion is present at the time of labor, a cesarean section should be performed. If tests show that the infection is not active, the mother may be able to deliver vaginally without infecting the infant. The herpes virus is potentially fatal for a newborn if infected.

CONDYLOMATA ACUMINATO

Condylomata acuminato (genital warts) are pedunculated, elongated, fleshy raised lesions. Large lesions may appear in cauliflower-like masses or clusters. Usually women do not

NURSING INTERVENTION	RATIONALE
Check blood; it will probably be low in glucose. Give orange juice with or without sugar. Call physician for further direction.	Verifies condition and degree of imbalance. Glucose level in orange juice is high and is quickly absorbed in the bloodstream to counteract the insulin.
Check blood; it will have a high sugar content. Call the physician for order of regular insulin and further direction.	Documented levels will help in developing a further care plan.

have any symptoms other than gradual appearance of the warts over the affected area. Occasionally, they can be accompanied with itching and a vaginal discharge. Condylomata acuminato are estrogen-dependent lesions. Therefore, they can enlarge or become more abundant during pregnancy.

GONORRHEA

Gonorrhea is a sexually transmitted disease caused by *Neisseria gonorrheae*, a species of bacteria. Some infected women remain asymptomatic. However, many will complain of a purulent vaginal discharge, urinary frequency and urgency, dysuria, and pelvic pain. If a baby passes through a birth canal infected with gonorrhea, eye infection and blindness can result unless the eyes are treated with an antibiotic or 1% silver nitrate at the time of delivery. Gonorrhea in the mother is generally treated with penicillin. If the mother is sensitive to penicillin, another antibiotic may be used.

SEXUALLY TRANSMITTED DISEASES

	No. Cases in U.S.	Infecting Agent	Female Symptoms
Trichomoniasis	Exact number of cases unknown — millions	*Trichomonas vaginalis* protozoa	None or yellow discharge, irritation, unpleasant odor, painful urination
Genital Herpes	200,000 to 500,000 new cases per year; 30 to 40 million cases total	Herpes simplex virus II	Often none; blisters in or around vagina; sometimes fever or headache
Genital Warts	1 million new cases per year	Human papilloma virus	Single warts or clusters of soft growths in and around vagina or anus; may be microscopic as well as visible
Gonorrhea	1.8 million new cases per year	*Neisseria gonorrhea* bacteria	Often none; sometimes burning at urination, vaginal discharge, fever, abdominal pain
Syphilis	85,000 new cases per year	*Treponema pallidum* bacteria	Sore (chancre) shortly after infection; fever, sore throat, or rashes
Chlamydia	4 million new cases per year	*Chlamydia trachomatis* bacteria	Usually none; sometimes burning at urination, vaginal discharge
AIDS	As of July 1987, 38,808 cases reported; 22,328 deaths	HIV (human immunodeficiency virus)	Headache, fever, night sweats, swollen lymph glands, diarrhea, weight loss, fatigue, infections

Figure 8–8

SYPHILIS

Syphilis is another infectious condition that may affect the development of the embryo. It is caused by the bacteria *Treponema pallidum*. Premarital serological testing, mandatory in some states, has reduced the incidence of deformities due to syphilis. However, if the fetus should be infected before the fifth month, it will probably die. If syphilis is contracted by the mother in the later months of pregnancy

Male Symptoms	Consequences to Women	Treatment Agent	Cure
None or prostitis	Urinary tract infections	Metronidazole	Yes
Often none; sores or clusters of blisters on penis; sometimes fever or headaches	Miscarriage, birth defects, serious infection of newborn; sometimes death of baby	Acyclovir	None
Warts or clusters on or around penis	Increased risk of cervical cancer	Podophyllin, 5–Fluorouracil, surgical removal	Several treatments may be needed
White discharge from penis, itching or painful urination	PID, sterility, arthritis	Penicillin, ampicillin, amoxicillin	Yes
Same as female	Heart disease, brain damage, arthritis, death, damage to babies	Penicillin, erythromycin	Yes
Usually none; itching or burning at urination; white discharge	Pelvic inflammatory disease (PID), sterility, ectopic pregnancies	Tetracycline, erythromycin	Yes
Same as female	Opportunistic infections, some cancers, death	Azidothymidine, Ribavirin	None

and inadequately treated, it may cause congenital syphilis affecting the heart, long bones, skin, and respiratory system of the fetus. It may also cause premature delivery or a stillborn infant. Syphilis is treated with antibiotics.

CHLAMYDIA

The bacteria *Chlamydia trachomatis* is the causative agent for the sexually transmitted disease **chlamydia**. Sixty to eighty percent of infected women will not have symptoms.

Some will have a vaginal discharge and pain when urinating. Others may exhibit symptoms of a **PID** (pelvic inflammatory disease), which include an elevated temperature and pelvic pain. Chlamydia can cause both eye damage and respiratory problems in an infant born through an infected birth canal. This disease has also been linked to prematurity and stillbirths.

AIDS

AIDS (acquired immune deficiency syndrome) is a serious disease caused by a virus that damages the body's immune system. People with AIDS are open to infections and cancers that would not be a threat to someone with a healthy immune system. More than half of all people who are diagnosed with AIDS die within two years after diagnosis. The first cases of AIDS were reported in 1981.

A virus called human T-cell lymphotropic virus, Type III (HTLV-III) causes AIDS. The virus was renamed human immunodeficiency virus (HIV). Symptoms include fever, fatigue, loss of appetite and weight, night sweats, unexplained diarrhea, swollen glands in the neck, axilla, and groin, a dry cough, unexplained skin lesions, and persistent yeast infections. Individuals exposed to AIDS can generally be divided into three categories. Among the population are those who are HIV-antibody reactive but who develop no symptoms; those with AIDS-related complex (ARC), who develop certain physical symptoms but who do not have AIDS; and those with AIDS. A large percentage of people exposed to HIV may never develop the physical symptoms of immune suppression. Many people infected with HIV have no symptoms and feel well. In fact, more than 90% of the people infected with this virus have not developed AIDS. However, people with a positive HIV test are infectious and can pass the virus to others through sexual contact or direct contact with infected blood.

AIDS is spread only by direct contact with infected blood or semen. There are four ways to contract AIDS:

1. Engaging in sexual contact with an infected person (who can look and feel well).
2. Sharing contaminated hypodermic needles.
3. Being given blood transfusions with infected blood.
4. An infected mother can transmit AIDS to her baby during or immediately after pregnancy. A woman who has been exposed to the HIV virus has a 50% chance of producing a child infected with the virus.

There is a concern about transmission of AIDS to medical personnel caring for AIDS patients. Risks encountered during routine nursing care appear to be minimal. The evidence seems clear that transmission by inadvertent needle sticks is much less likely to occur than with patients with hepatitis B virus. Clearly, precautions in handling needles and blood should be followed in patients with AIDS or HIV antibodies. It would be helpful to know the antibody status of all patients, but there is no mandatory or routine screening to date.

The newborn with AIDS poses a potential problem in the delivery suite, for medical staff inevitably encounter blood and secretions that might be contaminated with HIV. Therefore, when there is a possibility of coming into direct contact with blood from either the mother or the newborn, use gloves during any direct care.

The risk to health care workers from occupational exposure to persons infected with AIDS has been evaluated in several medical centers in the United States and is known to be extremely low. However, the Centers for Disease Control, with advice from health-care professionals, has made recommendations to protect workers from AIDS and HIV infections. These precautions are prudent practices that help prevent the transmission of blood-borne infections. They should be followed routinely.

1. Use gloves where blood, blood products, or body fluids will be handled.
2. Use gowns, masks, and eye protectors for procedures that involve more extensive splashing of blood or body fluids.
3. Use pocket masks, resuscitation bags, or other ventilation devices to resuscitate a patient, in order to minimize exposure.
4. Wash hands thoroughly after removing gloves and immediately after contact with blood or body fluids.
5. Use disposable needles and syringes. Do not recap, bend, or cut needles. Place sharp instruments in a specially designated puncture-resistant container located as close as practical to the area where they are used. Handle and dispose of them with extraordinary care to prevent accidental injury.
6. Follow general guidelines for sterilization, disinfection, housekeeping, and waste disposal. Place potentially infected waste in impervious bags and dispose of them as local waste regulations require.
7. Clean up blood spills immediately with detergent and water. Use a solution of 5.25% sodium hypochloride (household bleach) diluted between 1:10 and 1:100 parts water for disinfection.
8. Know the modes of transmission and prevention of these infections.

ACUTE INFECTIOUS DISEASES

Pregnant women who contract German measles (rubella) in the first trimester of pregnancy frequently give birth to infants afflicted with certain malformations such as cataracts, heart lesions, deaf-mutism, and microcephaly (abnormally small head). Opinions differ concerning the medical justification for therapeutic abortion in these cases. In 1969 a vaccine became available to protect against rubella. Routinely, women are tested for rubella antibodies when they become pregnant. If the woman has no immunity, she may be given the vaccine just after delivery. It is best to wait three months after receiving the vaccine before trying to become pregnant again.

The pregnant woman appears to be slightly more susceptible to acute upper respiratory infections than the nonpregnant woman. Therefore, the common cold, sinusitis, laryngitis, and bronchitis should never be regarded lightly.

Influenza is better controlled today with medication and is less serious than the influenza that caused the epidemic of 1918. Although the prognosis is good, complications must be suspected when fever persists. Antibiotic drugs have decreased the danger of pneumonia in pregnancy, and influenza is no longer considered a serious condition.

Measles and scarlet fever tend to cause premature labor or abortion. They do not cause congenital defects. However, women known to be pregnant should not be subjected to routine immunization against mumps, measles, German measles, or yellow fever. Live virus vaccines in these immunizations can infect the fetus.

Immunizations in which killed or inactivated vaccines are used are considered safe. Such vaccines are used against influenza, epidemic typhus and typhoid, tetanus, and diphtheria. Rabies anti-serum vaccine, killed cholera vaccine, and attenuated live oral polio vaccine or killed injectable polio vaccine may also be given to pregnant women when protection is required.

Fifth disease is so called because it was the fifth to be discovered among a group of diseases that cause fever and skin rash in children. It is caused by human parvovirus B19. Fifth disease usually results in a mild flu-like illness with a rash. If a woman is exposed to fifth disease in the first trimester or early second trimester, she is at an increased risk for miscarriage. If infection occurs later in pregnancy, it can cause anemia in the fetus and may require treatment.

Toxoplasmosis is a condition caused by the parasite *Toxoplasma*, which lives in some mammals, such as cats. Humans can become infected by eating raw or undercooked meats, especially lamb or mutton, or by coming into contact with feces from a cat who harbors the parasite. Toxoplasmosis causes only mild illness in adults, and often those exposed have no symptoms. This illness can create a problem in pregnancy only when the mother has a primary (first-time exposure) infection. When the infection first occurs in pregnancy, the fetus is also infected in about one-third of the cases. Because the risk to the fetus occurs only when a woman becomes ill during pregnancy, routine blood testing of pregnant women is not recommended. Infection during pregnancy can cause the baby to be born prematurely or to be too small. It can also cause fever, jaundice, eye problems, or other long-term problems.

RH FACTOR

The **Rh factor** is an antigen found on the surface of the red blood cells. About 85% of the white population in the United States have this antigen present; they are called Rh positive. About 15% lack the antigen and are called Rh negative. This percentage differs with various racial groups. The factor is of consequence only if the mother is Rh negative and the father is Rh positive.

An Rh-negative woman may carry an Rh-positive baby as a result of mating with an Rh-positive male. In rare instances, fetal red blood cells enter the mother's circulation by passing through the placental barrier. When this happens, her body may become sensitized and develop antibodies to fend off the "foreign" invaders. These antibodies cross the placental barrier and enter the circulation of the fetus, destroying the fetal red blood cells. This destruction begins during gestation and continues after the baby is born. Usually antibodies do not develop in quantities large enough to harm the fetus until the woman has had at least one Rh-positive baby. Treatment involves transfusing the infant with Rh-negative erythrocytes.

Constant revisions in the methods of dealing with Rh are made as new antigens are discovered. It is now possible to prevent Rh sensitization by administering an anti-Rh globulin that causes passive immunity in the woman so that she does not produce anti-Rh antibodies if she becomes pregnant with an Rh-positive fetus. **RhoGAM** (solution of gamma globulin that contains a concentration of Rh antibodies) is given to the Rh-negative woman shortly after the delivery of an Rh-positive baby or after a midtrimester abortion or miscarriage, Figure 8–9. RhoGAM may be given during pregnancy at about 28 weeks to prevent sensitization that may occur during fetal-maternal transfusion. Fetal-maternal transfusion occurs in less than 2% of cases.

Knowledge of the Rh factor is important in order to prevent hemolytic disease of the fetus and newborn. The physician determines whether or not an intrauterine transfusion (see below) or an exchange transfusion and phototherapy for the newborn will be required, and plans accordingly.

ERYTHROBLASTOSIS FETALIS

Erythroblastosis fetalis is a hemolytic disease of the newborn. It is characterized by anemia, jaundice, enlargement of the liver and spleen, and generalized edema of the newborn. It is caused by the development of antibodies from an Rh-negative mother that react against an Rh-positive fetus. The infant's red blood cells are hemolyzed (broken down) and destroyed, producing severe anemia. If anemia is severe enough, heart failure, brain damage, or death of the fetus can occur.

In the early 1950s, a British doctor named D. C. A. Bevis, ignoring a centuries-old taboo, injected a long sterile needle through the abdomen of a pregnant woman and drew out a few drops of amber-colored amniotic fluid. Analysis of the bilirubin (pigment of red blood cells) in the syringe enabled Dr. Bevis to determine just how sick the fetus was. Doctors began using this technique **(amniocentesis)** to tell them when to induce labor prematurely so that the fetus could undergo immediate postnatal transfusion. This procedure cut the death rate from erythroblastosis fetalis in many hospitals by more than 50%.

INTRAUTERINE TRANSFUSION

An **intrauterine transfusion** is the injection of Rh-negative erythrocytes into the peritoneal cavity of the fetus while it is still in the uterus. The fetus absorbs these erythrocytes in order to combat anemia, Figure 8–10.

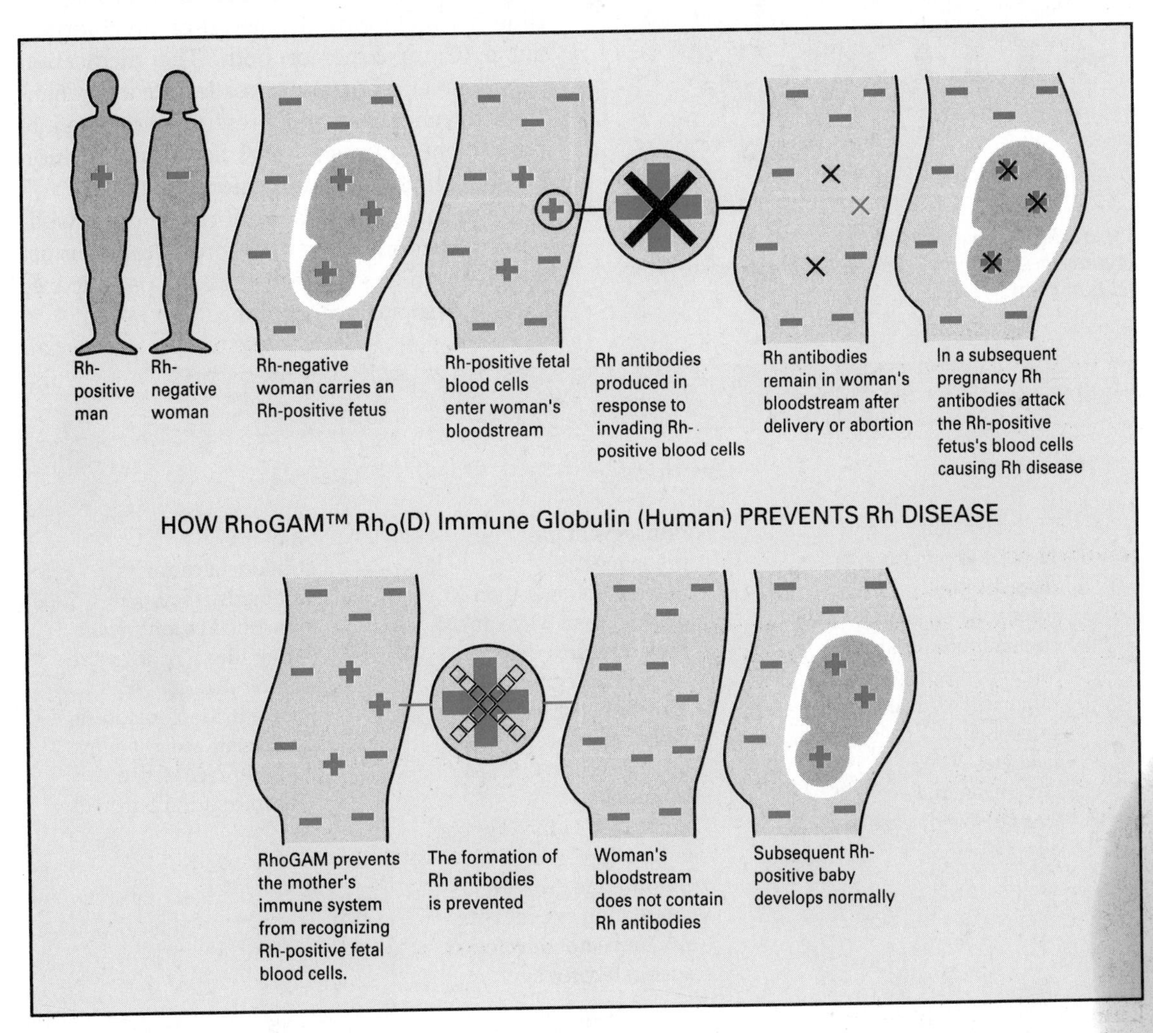

Figure 8–9 *How Rh disease develops (Adapted from* A Discussion about the Rh Factor and RhoGAM™ *by Ortho Diagnostic Systems, Inc., and Johnson & Johnson Company, Raritan, NJ)*

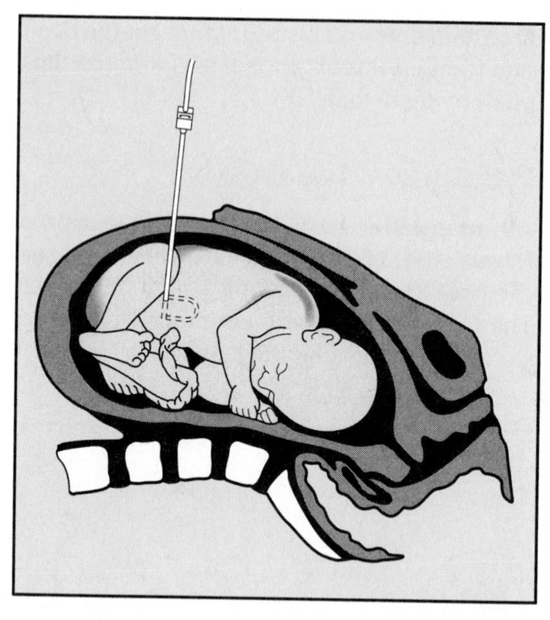

Figure 8–10 Intrauterine transfusion. Rh-negative erythrocytes are injected into the peritoneal cavity of the fetus in utero.

This transfusion was developed in 1963, in Auckland, New Zealand, when Dr. A. W. Liley performed the first intrauterine transfusion for the treatment and, it was hoped, correction of erythroblastosis fetalis. Since then, skilled workers around the world have been performing the procedure with promising results. The fetal survival rate from this procedure is approximately 50%.

The morning of the transfusion, the patient is allowed to have a regular breakfast. She may then be given a medication, such as meperidine hydrochloride (Demerol) or prochlorperazine (Compazine) or both. The medication serves several purposes: to alleviate apprehension; to relieve pain, if present; and to sedate the patient, since she must lie in one position for some time on an uncomfortable table.

The procedure is performed in a well-equipped room. Care and consideration must be given to the patient, and all participants should wear surgical clothing.

FACTORS THAT CAN COMPLICATE PREGNANCY

Medical

- Hypertension
- Heart, kidney, lung, or liver diseases
- Infections — sexually transmitted diseases, vaginal infections, or other viral or bacterial infections
- Diabetes
- Severe anemia
- Convulsive disease, such as epilepsy

Obstetrical

- Problems in past pregnancies
- Mother younger than 15 or older than 35 years old
- Previous birth defects
- Multiple pregnancy (e.g., twins or triplets)
- Bleeding, especially during the second or third trimester
- Pregnancy-induced hypertension (preeclampsia)
- Intrauterine growth retardation or prematurity (fetus not developed adequately for age)

Lifestyle

- Smoking
- Drinking alcohol
- Taking drugs not prescribed by physician (either illegal or over-the-counter drugs)
- Poor nutrition, including inadequate weight gain
- Lack of prenatal care
- Multiple sexual partners

Figure 8–11

After the transfusion has been completed, the patient is returned to her room and is carefully observed for fetal activity, premature labor, peritonitis, and hemorrhage. Fetal heart tones are checked every four hours. The patient may have a liquid diet for lunch and a general diet toward evening. If necessary, Compazine may be ordered to relieve nausea and distress. Fetal complications are difficult to detect, but liver injuries, hemothorax, and sepsis have occurred as a direct result of this transfusion.

If the transfusions are successful, labor is induced with oxytocin (Pitocin) about the 35th week of gestation. The mother may receive an anesthetic to help her during delivery. After the child is born, the pediatrician carefully observes the child. Cord studies are done, and bilirubin levels are measured to determine when and how frequently exchange transfusions are necessary. It is not unusual for a transfusion to be performed within the first hour of life and repeated as necessary.

A summary of factors that can complicate pregnancy is shown in Figure 8–11.

REVIEW QUESTIONS

A. Multiple choice. Select the best answer.

1. An acute infectious disease that often results in malformation of the infant is
   a. pneumonia
   b. polio
   c. influenza
   d. rubella

2. Severe anemia of the fetus that could cause its death in utero is
   a. respiratory disease syndrome
   b. erythroblastosis fetalis
   c. hydatidiform mole
   d. creatinemia

3. Scarlet fever or measles contracted during pregnancy may cause
   a. premature labor
   b. congenital defects
   c. acidosis
   d. all of the above

4. The termination of pregnancy through natural causes is
   a. therapeutic abortion
   b. complete abortion
   c. spontaneous abortion
   d. incomplete abortion

5. Injection of Rh-negative erythrocytes into the peritoneal cavity of the fetus is
   a. amniocentesis
   b. intrauterine transfusion
   c. bilirubin sampling
   d. none of these

B. Match the symptom in column II to the correct complication in column I.

Column I	Column II
1. placenta previa	a. painful bleeding and shock
2. ectopic pregnancy	b. stabbing pain in side
3. placenta abruptio	c. painless bleeding
4. eclampsia	d. disturbance of vision
5. preeclampsia	e. excessive vomiting
6. hyperemesis gravidarum	f. convulsions

C. Briefly answer the following questions.

1. List the danger signals that may indicate a complication in pregnancy.
2. Why is labor induced for the pregnant diabetic patient?
3. List the four observations to be made about a patient who has had an intrauterine transfusion.
4. What is a tubal pregnancy?

SUGGESTED ACTIVITIES

- Discuss bleeding in pregnancy and the possible causes.
- Define molar pregnancy. List the signs suggesting molar pregnancy and the precautions necessary after a molar pregnancy is terminated.
- Define ectopic pregnancy. List the factors that increase a woman's risk of an ectopic pregnancy.
- Define preeclampsia and eclampsia. Discuss the present theories regarding their causes.
- Identify the signs and symptoms of preeclampsia and the patients at risk.
- List the danger signals of pregnancy.
- Review Figure 8–6 which summarizes the complications of pregnancy. Note especially the symptoms that characterize each condition.

BIBLIOGRAPHY

Benson, R. C. *Current Obstetric and Gynecologic Diagnosis and Treatment*, 5th ed. Los Altos, CA: Lange Medical Publications, 1984.

Buckingham, S., and S. Rehm. "AIDS and Women at Risk." *Health and Social Work* 0360–7283/87, Winter, 1987.

Burrow, G. N., and T. F. Ferris. *Medical Complications during Pregnancy*, 3rd ed. Philadelphia: W.B. Saunders, 1988.

Coughlin, S. "STD/HIV Risk Assessment and Counseling by Primary Care Providers." *Nurse Practitioner Forum* 2(2):84–86, June, 1991.

Hawkins, J. W., and L. Pierfedeici. *Maternity and Gynecological Nursing*. New York: J. B. Lippincott, 1981.

Hill-Blakley, L. "Gestational Diabetes." *Childbirth Educator* 8(2):24–29, 1989.

Jornsay, D., Duckles, A., and L. Javanovic. *Gestational Diabetes*. Indianapolis, IN: Boehringer Mannheim, 1986.

Long, K., and R. Long. "Treatment Modalities for HPV Infection." *Nurse Practioner Forum* 1(1):8–9, 1990.

Loveman, A., Colburn, V., and A. Dobin. "AIDS in Pregnancy." *JOGNN* 15(2):91–96, March-April, 1986.

Niswander, K. R. *Manual of Obstetrics, Diagnosis and Therapy*, 3rd ed. Boston: Little, Brown and Co., 1987.

Oxorn, H. *Oxorn-Foote Human Labor and Birth*, 5th ed. E. Norwalk, CT: Appleton-Century-Crofts, 1986.

Pletsch, P. "Birth Defect Prevention: Nursing Interventions." *JOGNN* 19(6)482–487, November-December, 1990.

Pritchard, J. A., Macdonald, P. C., and N. F. Grant. *Williams Obstetrics*, 17th ed. E. Norwalk, CT: Appleton-Century-Crofts, 1985.

Reeder, S., Mastroianni, L., Jr., and L. Martin. *Maternity Nursing*, 16th ed. New York: J. B Lippincott, 1987.

Scott, J. R., et al. *Danforth's Obstetrics and Gynecology*, 6th ed. Philadelphia: J. B. Lippincott, 1990.

Shannon, D. M. "HELLP Syndrome: A Severe Consequence of Pregnancy-Induced Hypertension." *JOGNN* 16(6):395–402, November-December, 1987.

Smith, P. C. "Diabetes in Pregnancy." *Childbirth Educator* 1(2):8–12, 1982.

Wason, C., and B. Metzger. *Diabetes Management for the Mother-to-Be*. Chicago: Abelson-Taylor-Frizsimmons, 1986.

Wiley, K., and J. Grohar. "Human Immunodeficiency Virus and Precautions for Obstetric, Gynecologic and Neonatal Nurses." *JOGNN* 17(3)165–168, May-June 1988.

Zigrossi, S., and S. Riga-Ziegler. "The Stress of Medical Management on Pregnant Diabetics." *MCN* 11:320–323, September-October, 1986.

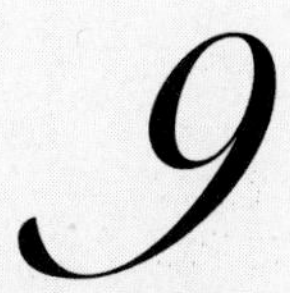

CHAPTER 9

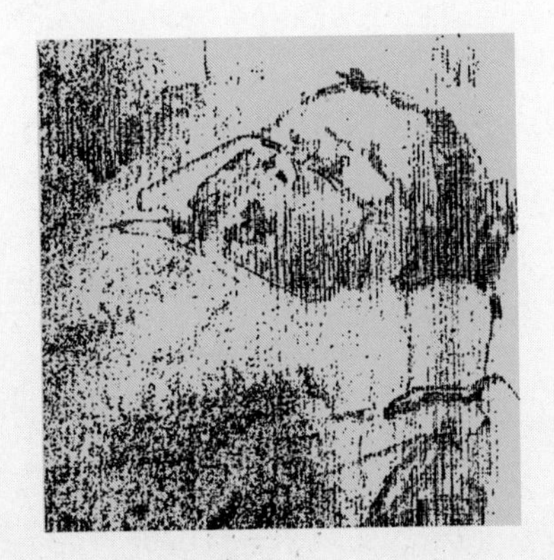

Assessing Fetal Well-Being

Objectives

After studying this chapter, the student should be able to:

- Explain the procedure and value of amniocentesis.
- Explain the purpose of chorionic villi sampling.
- List the uses of ultrasound.
- Name the tests that may be made on amniotic fluid.
- Explain the significance of the alpha fetoprotein test.
- Compare the differences between a biophysical profile and a nonstress test.

Key Terms

alpha fetoprotein (AFP)
neural tube defects
amniocentesis
genetic abnormalities
meconium
lecithin-sphingomyelin (L-S) ratio
respiratory distress syndrome (RDS)
shake test

AMNIOTIC FLUID CREATININE

AMNIOTIC FLUID BILIRUBIN

NILE BLUE SULFATE

CHORIONIC VILLI SAMPLING (CVS)

ULTRASONOGRAPHY

URINARY ESTROGENS

FETAL BLOOD SAMPLING

BIOPHYSICAL PROFILE

NONSTRESS TEST

Fetal well-being can be assessed by performing various tests. Amniotic fluid obtained by amniocentesis can be used to assess for meconium, lecithin-sphingomyelin ratio, creatinine, bilirubin, sex of fetus, and for the Nile blue sulfate and the shake tests. Chorionic villi sampling is also a way to evaluate cells directly from the fetus. Ultrasound (looking directly at the fetus with the use of sound waves), urine studies, blood studies, and nonstress tests also give hints at fetal well-being. Asking the expectant mother to monitor her baby's movements is one of the simplest ways to evaluate fetal well-being.

ALPHA FETOPROTEIN (AFP) TEST

As stated in Chapter 6, a measure of **alpha-fetoprotein (AFP)** may be used for prenatal detection of **neural tube defects** such as spina bifida (open spine) and anencephaly (abnormal brain development). The alphafetoprotein test is performed between the 15th and 20th week of pregnancy by taking a sample of the mother's blood. AFP is made by the baby's liver and concentrates in the spinal fluid. Some of this protein passes into the amniotic fluid and crosses the placenta into the mother's blood. When the fetus has an open neural tube defect (open spine), large amounts of AFP leak into the amniotic fluid and then into the mother's blood. If the test is abnormal, it may be repeated. Abnormal results are common if the dates are incorrect for gestational age or if there is a multiple gestation. Ultrasound will confirm those causes and also show abnormalities in the baby. Amniocentesis is sometimes necessary to confirm a problem. An abnormally low AFP may suggest Down syndrome. A "triple screen for trisomy 21" (Down syndrome) may then be ordered. This test looks at the maternal serum alpha fetoprotein (MSAFP), the level of hCG (human chorionic gonadotropin), and estriol level. This triple screen can predict Down syndrome accurately approximately 60% of the time. The alpha fetoprotein test needs to be adjusted for weight of the mother, race, and weeks gestation to be accurate. Also, if the mother is an insulin-dependent diabetic, an adjustment in the value will be made by the laboratory to reflect a more accurate value.

AMNIOCENTESIS

Amniocentesis is the method of obtaining fluid and cells from the amniotic sac (bag of waters) as shown in Figure 9–1. When fluid and fetal cells from a sample of amniotic fluid are analyzed, specific abnormalities can be identified and appropriate treatment can be initiated.

With any pregnancy there is a small chance that some birth defect will occur. The likelihood becomes greater when the woman is over age 35 or when one or both parents have a family history of genetic disorders.

Often, a family history or studies performed on a couple suggest the possibility of an abnormality in the fetus. In cases where there is an increased risk of a specific disorder, amniocentesis may determine whether the fetus is affected. When an abnormality is detected, however, the severity of the disorder cannot always de determined; it is left to the couple to decide whether they want to terminate or continue the pregnancy. Amniocentesis is generally performed for any one of three reasons: genetic testing, testing for enzymes and proteins, and in a problem pregnancy.

Genetic testing (chromosomal analysis for **genetic abnormalities**, such as Down syndrome, in the fetus) is the most common reason for an amniocentesis. Although only certain defects can be detected by amniocentesis, the benefits can be significant to the couple at risk of producing a child with one of them. For the purpose of genetic testing, amniocentesis should be performed relatively early in the pregnancy. The usual reasons for genetic testing are: the mother is over 35; one or both parents have a family history of specific genetic abnormalities; or the parents already have had a child with a genetic abnormality.

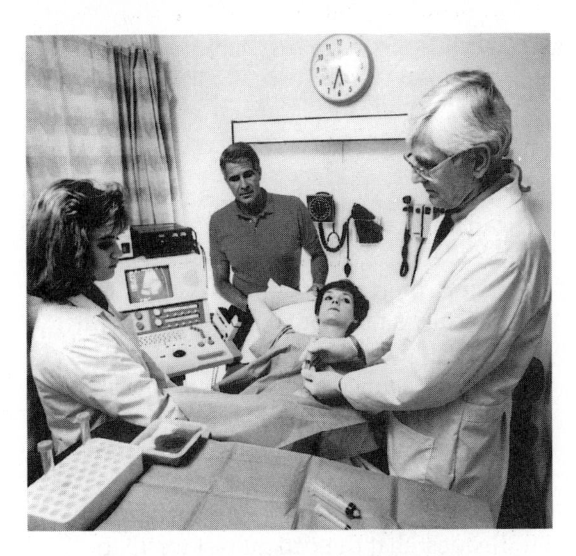

Figure 9–1 *A small amount of amniotic fluid is withdrawn for study through amniocentesis. (Courtesy Evergreen Hospital Medical Center, Kirkland, WA)*

Testing for enzymes and proteins is another application of amniocentesis. The fluid is tested for the presence of abnormal levels of certain enzymes that may indicate that the child is affected by some rare congenital defect (e.g., muscular dystrophy), which usually is familial. The fluid is also tested for alpha fetoprotein. Abnormal levels may indicate that the child is affected by a neurological abnormality such as meningocele or anencephalus.

A problem pregnancy might also indicate amniocentesis. If there is any known or suspected condition that might jeopardize the pregnancy, amniocentesis could help to detect the problem and might provide the doctor with information needed to plan for the last few months of pregnancy and for the delivery. For this purpose, amniocentesis is usually performed rather late in the pregnancy. Amniocentesis can also help determine the maturity of the fetus when size and menstrual dates are uncertain.

Amniocentesis can provide a wide range of information, including the sex of the unborn baby. However, it should not be used for casual screening or simply to learn the sex of the child. If there is no history of genetic abnormalities, or if no specific situation exists that requires closer investigation, there is usually no reason to perform amniocentesis. Amniocentesis carries a very slight risk of injury to the fetus and a very slight risk of causing an abortion. The physician discusses these risks with the mother in some detail if amniocentesis is to be considered.

Amniocentesis for genetic testing usually is done sometime between the 15th and 18th weeks of pregnancy. At this time, the procedure is relatively simple and safe because the uterus is large enough and there is an adequate amount of amniotic fluid. In the case of a problem pregnancy, amniocentesis usually is done later in pregnancy, depending on the doctor's recommendation. Amniocentesis is usually performed in a hospital as an outpatient procedure.

Although amniocentesis is done by the physician, the nurse must be familiar with the procedure.

The amniotic fluid obtained by amniocentesis is sent to the laboratory for analysis. The following tests can be conducted on the fluid.

MECONIUM

Meconium (dark green tarlike substance in fetal intestine) obtained by amniocentesis indicates that the fetus is not getting enough oxygen. Meconium is, therefore, a sign of fetal distress. Lack of oxygen, which may have been acute or continuing, has caused the rectal sphincter muscle of the fetus to relax. Meconium also interferes with other tests, making them either unreliable or reliable only after difficult extraction methods.

LECITHIN-SPHINGOMYELIN RATIO

The **lecithin-sphingomyelin (L-S) ratio** measures fetal lung surfactant phospholipids. It approaches 100% reliability in determining fetal pulmonary maturity; it requires several hours for results. An L-S ratio of greater than 2 to 1 indicates lung maturity. This test indicates the possibility of **respiratory distress syndrome (RDS)**, also known as hyaline membrane disease.

SHAKE TEST

The **shake test** (or rapid surfactant test) is also used to determine RDS. However, it requires only 10 minutes to obtain results. It is reliable

PROCEDURE

Amniocentesis

1. Explain the procedure to the patient and obtain an informed consent.
2. Check and record all vital signs.
3. Have the patient empty her bladder just before the doctor begins the procedure.
4. After the doctor palpates the abdomen, prep the abdomen with soap and sterile water.
5. Open the amniocentesis tray on patient's bedside table and add the spinal needle and syringes.
6. Pour betadine into the medicine glass.
7. Hold the Xylocaine bottle so the doctor can draw solution with the syringe and needle.
8. Using direct ultrasound to determine the baby's position, the physician withdraws fluid from the amniotic sac.
9. Label specimen and send it to the laboratory with a request form.
10. After completion of procedure, recheck vital signs and record in nurse's notes. Attach nurse's notes to prenatal record.
11. Request that the patient rest for 15 to 20 minutes after the procedure.

when interpreted as "mature, low-risk RDS." There are very few false positive tests; however, there are many false negative tests. If the test is negative, an L-S ratio test must be done to obtain an accurate assessment.

AMNIOTIC FLUID CREATININE

The **amniotic fluid creatinine** test is also reliable to a high degree. It assesses fetal muscle mass and renal function. Large amounts of creatinine indicate a large fetus. Large fetuses, however, such as those of diabetic mothers, may have pulmonary immaturity, and growth-retarded fetuses may be mature. Therefore, false high and false low values are sometimes obtained.

AMNIOTIC FLUID BILIRUBIN

Spectrophotometric measurement of **amniotic fluid bilirubin** assesses fetal liver maturation. The optical density of amniotic fluid bilirubin is 450 μm (O.D.450μm). This test is not as reliable as the L-S or creatinine tests for determining fetal maturity. But it is highly important in managing Rh-sensitized pregnancies, because the levels of amniotic fluid bilirubin are correlated with the degree of anemia in the fetus.

NILE BLUE SULFATE TEST

Nile blue sulfate stains the cutaneous lipid-containing cells of the fetus, which increase in number near term. The number of these cells indicates whether the fetus is mature. Because L-S ratios and creatinine are more reliable, this test is rarely used at present.

SEX DETERMINATION TEST

A procedure introduced in 1968 can tell the prospective parents the sex of the fetus. Examination of the genes in the amniotic fluid that has been extracted can identify the sex of the fetus with 100% accuracy.

CHORIONIC VILLI SAMPLING

Chorionic villi sampling (CVS) is a procedure where samples of placental tissue are obtained and assessed for fetal well-being. It is conducted under direct ultrasound. The patient is in a lithotomy position. A speculum is inserted into the vagina, and a tenaculum is affixed to the anterior wall of the cervix. The depth of the uterus is determined by a uterine sound. Then a catheter is directed through the cervical os into the chorionic villi site, Figure 9–2. Chorionic villi are then aspirated through the catheter into a syringe. A few selected institutions are performing CVS through the abdomen rather than through the cervix. That procedure is illustrated in Figure 9–3.

The biggest advantage of chorionic villi sampling is that the procedure is performed early in the first trimester of pregnancy (9 to 12 weeks gestation). Since the cells do not have to be grown in the lab, laboratory results are obtained earlier than with amniocentesis. First-trimester cells divide rapidly, and karotyping is performed during the metaphase of mitosis.

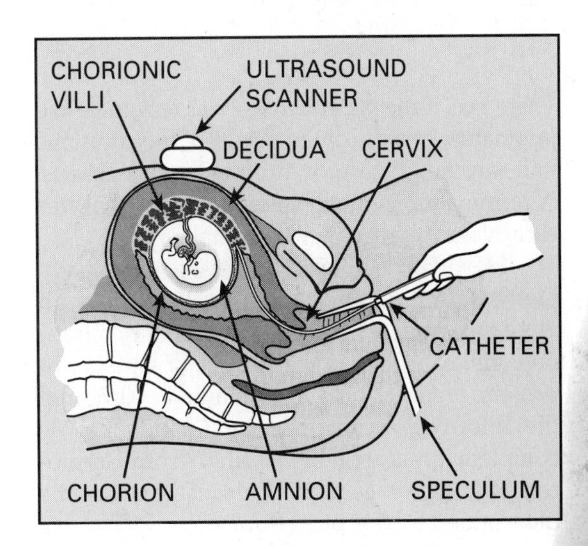

Figure 9–2 *Chorionic villi sampling at 12 weeks*

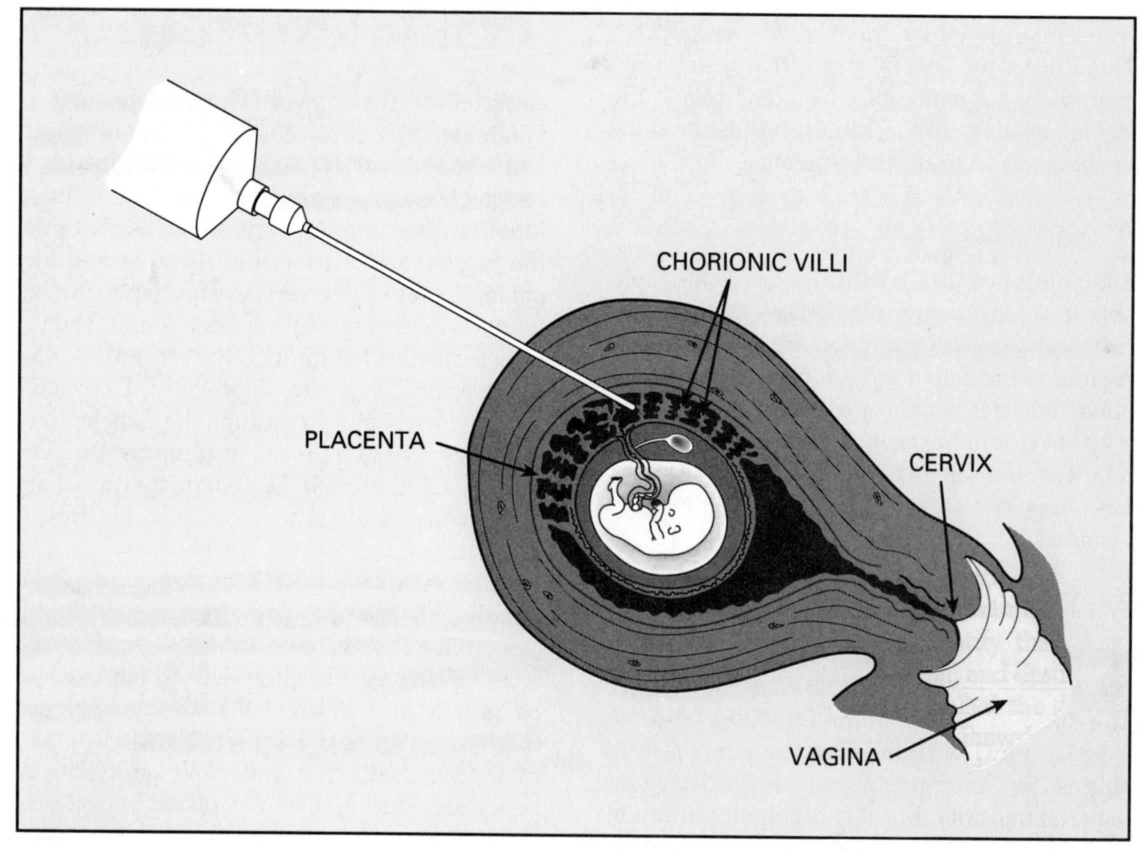

Figure 9–3 *Transabdominal chorionic villi sampling*

Therefore, if the patient chooses to terminate the pregnancy because of the results of the chorionic villi sampling, the procedure is less hazardous. A termination is much easier to perform at this early stage of pregnancy than later.

The disadvantages include a slightly higher rate of spontaneous abortion than with amniocentesis. Also, one limitation of chorionic villi sampling is that values of alpha fetoprotein levels cannot be obtained. Although the information obtained by CVS is not as complete or as reliable as that from amniocentesis, many genetic abnormalities can be determined by this procedure.

ULTRASONOGRAPHY

Ultrasonography (ultrasound) is a fast-developing technology that allows the physician to see into the uterus of the pregnant woman without exposing her and her baby to the known dangers of x-rays and without pain or intrusions. See Figure 9–4. The technique uses high-frequency, inaudible sound waves, which are directed into the abdomen of the pregnant woman and then reflected back to a receiver. The reflected waves give a visual "echo" of what is inside the uterus. This echo is transformed electronically into an image on a

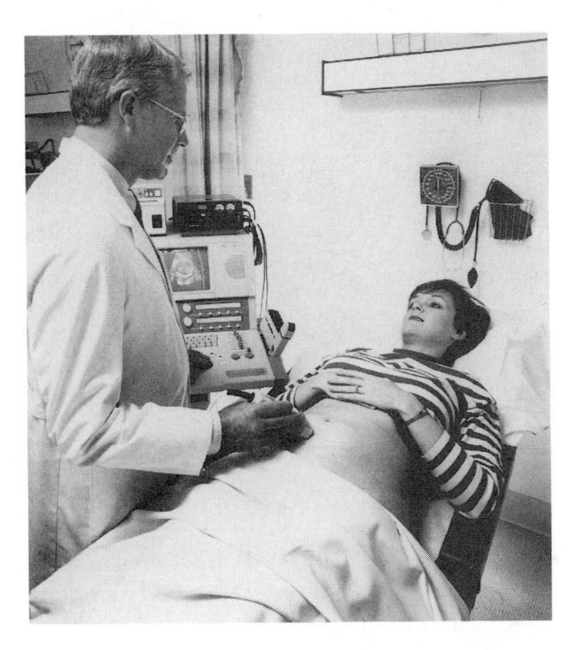

Figure 9–4 An ultrasound exam creates a picture of the baby, called a sonogram, from sound waves. (Courtesy Evergreen Hospital Medical Center, Kirkland, WA)

screen. Bone, the densest tissue, appears as white areas in the ultrasound picture. Muscles and less dense tissue appear in shades of gray. Fluid-filled areas give no reflection at all and appear black as shown in Figures 9–5 and 9–6. From the image, the physician can learn an enormous amount about the conditions in the uterus and the health of the fetus.

By far the most common use of diagnostic ultrasound is to determine true fetal age when the date of conception is unknown or mistaken by the mother. By allowing measurement of the fetal head and femur and assessment of the fetus's physical development, ultrasound can pinpoint the length of pregnancy to within a week or so. Certain abnormalities within the heart, the abdomen, or in the spinal column can also be seen and evaluated. In a mother who has diabetes or high blood pressure, a series of sonograms taken every two weeks can show if

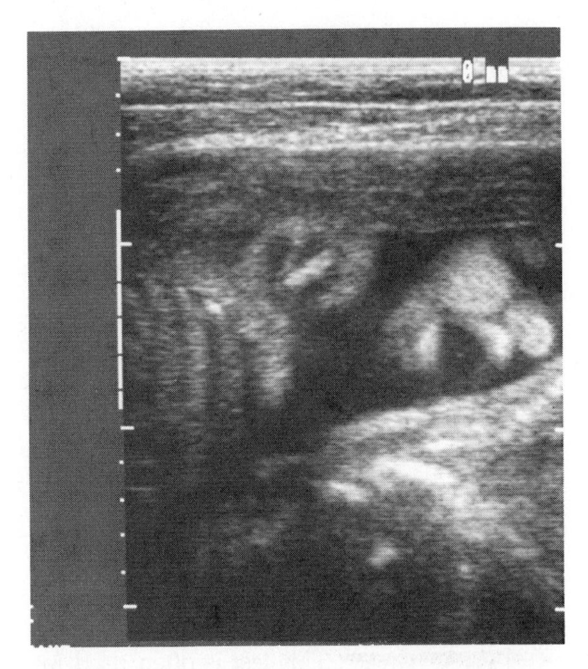

Figure 9–5 Current ultrasound technology allows highly detailed fetal imaging.

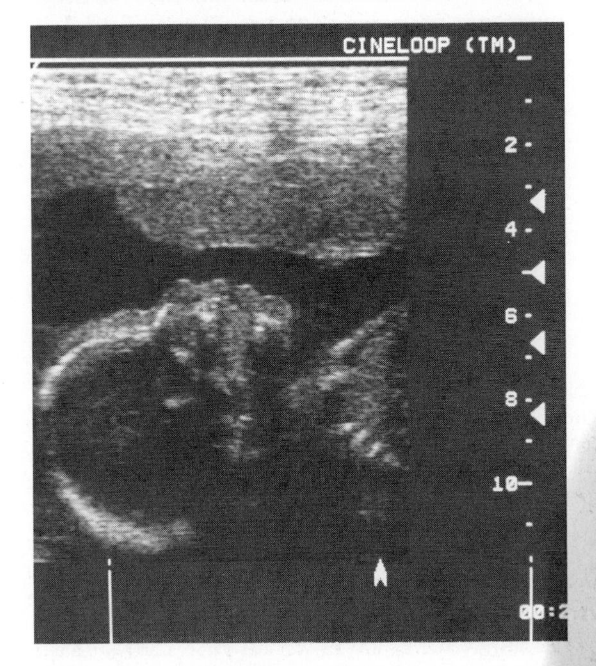

Figure 9–6 Fetal skull

the baby is growing properly. If it is not, the doctor can perform a cesarean to save the child. Dangerous uterine conditions such as placenta previa can be detected early. Structural abnormalities of the fetus or the presence of more than one fetus can also be diagnosed with the help of ultrasonography, see Figure 9–7. There are numerous other obstetrical and gynecological indications for ultrasound.

Ultrasound is being used before amniocentesis. Sonography lets the doctor see where to insert the needle safely by locating the position of the fetus and placenta.

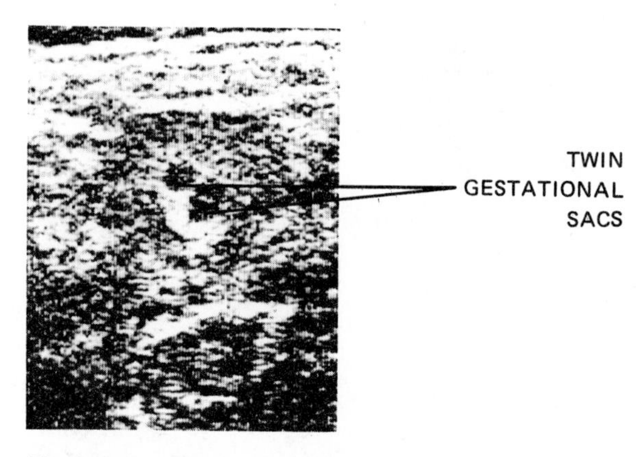

Figure 9–7 *Twin gestational sacs at five weeks*

24-Hour Urinary Estrogens

The 24-hour **urinary estrogens** collected in a 24-hour urine specimen are a measure of the fetal-placental unit. This test is often used for fetal assessment. Estriol is an estrogen produced by the fetal-placental unit in increasing amounts as pregnancy progresses. Estriol is excreted in the mother's urine, where it can be measured as necessary. Testing the level of estriol in the urine and blood can provide important information about how well the placenta is functioning. Estriol tests may be ordered for a mother with diabetes, preeclampsia, or severe hypertension, or if a baby is thought to be too small or considerably overdue. A significant drop in estriol levels from one test to another may indicate the need to induce labor. The estriol level can also be tested by drawing the necessary blood sample.

Fetal Blood Sampling

The purpose of **fetal blood sampling** is to determine the status of the fetus during labor. A sample of blood is withdrawn from a small skin puncture in the presenting part of the fetus. The blood sample is then analyzed to determine fetal distress. Fetal blood sampling is discussed in Chapter 11.

Biophysical Profile

Biochemical assessment of the fetus has largely been replaced by biophysical and biometric evaluation **(biophysical profile)**. The fetal central nervous system (CNS) is very sensitive. Hypoxia and its resultant metabolic acidosis will produce pathological CNS depression with changes in biophysical activity. The demonstration of several biophysical activities, showing a normal pattern collectively, assures fetal well-being. A score of eight or more demonstrates probable fetal well-being, see Figure 9–8.

Nonstress Test

A **nonstress** test can be performed on the patient who is not in labor. It is based on the observation that acceleration of the fetal heart rate in response to fetal movement or uterine

BIOPHYSICAL PROFILE

	Score 2	Score 0
Fluid Assessment	One or more pockets of amnionic fluid 1 cm × 1 cm or more	No pocket greater than 1 cm
Fetal Breathing	Sustained for 30 seconds	Not sustained for 30 seconds or not present
Fetal Movement	Two gross body movements in 20 minutes	Fewer than two gross body movements in 20 minutes or no movement
Fetal Tone	One episode of flexion/ extension	No flexion/extension
Fetal Reaction	At least two FHT reactions greater than 15 beats per minute lasting 15 seconds in a 40-minute period	Less than two FHT reactions in 40 minutes

Figure 9–8 *Biophysical profile (use of ultrasound)*

contractions is a reliable indicator of immediate fetal well-being. Fetal heart rate is obtained by using an external ultrasound monitor. It is considered reactive if two or more fetal heart accelerations occur in a 10- to 20-minute period of observation. These accelerations should be greater than an increase of 15 beats per minute and should persist for 15 seconds or more. This evaluation is useful in determining fetal well-being in situations where patients are at risk for uteroplacental insufficiency (post-term pregnancy, maternal diabetes, oligohydramnios, and maternal hypertension). It is also indicated if there is a decrease or absence of normal fetal movements as perceived by the mother. In most cases, testing is instituted at 32 to 34 weeks of gestation. For more detail, see Chapter 11.

FETAL MOVEMENTS

One of the best ways to monitor a healthy fetus is to notice its movements. Healthy fetuses are active, particularly in the evening after supper. However, some perfectly normal fetuses may go for as long as 60 minutes without moving. Fetuses who are experiencing stress are sluggish and move less. Asking the expectant mother to count her fetus's movements in a given period of time can warn the physician of developing problems. "Kick counts" should begin in the seventh month (28 weeks). The mother should feel at least 10 movements (kick, turn, flip, or a combination of movements) in a two-hour period, counted at some time during her day. In the evening, after dinner, when the mother can lie down and concentrate on the fetus's movements is often the best time. Ten movements may be felt within less than two hours. The mother should be instructed to inform her physician if:

1. Ten movements are not felt within a two-hour period. If two hours pass with fewer than 10 movements during the day, repeat the counting routine in the evening.
2. No movement is felt all day.
3. It takes longer and longer each evening to get to the tenth movement.

REVIEW QUESTIONS

A. Multiple choice. Select the best answer.

1. Fetal assessment is made by
   a. directly looking at chromosomes
   b. ultrasound
   c. fetal blood sampling
   d. all of the above
2. Amniocentesis is usually performed
   a. before 8 weeks gestation
   b. between the 8th and the 13th week of gestation
   c. between the 15th and 18th week of gestation
   d. after 20 weeks
3. Alphafetoprotein tests for all the following except
   a. neural tube defects
   b. fetal maturity
   c. Down syndrome
   d. spina bifida
4. The biggest advantage to chorionic villi sampling is
   a. it is less risky than amniocentesis
   b. it can be performed early in the pregnancy and the results are obtained faster
   c. it can be obtained through the cervix as well as through the abdomen
   d. it is less likely than amniocentesis to injure the fetus
5. Fetal blood sampling is done to determine
   a. the age of the fetus
   b. the lung maturity of the fetus
   c. fetal distress
   d. all of the above

B. Briefly answer the following questions.

1. Name five tests that are made on amniotic fluid.
2. What is the alpha fetoprotein screen and when is it used?
3. Describe the difference between a biochemical assessment and a biophysical profile.

SUGGESTED ACTIVITIES

- Describe the most common techniques of prenatal diagnosis including: (a) ultrasound (b) amniocentesis (c) CVS.
  - Discuss their risks and limitations.

BIBLIOGRAPHY

Benson, R. C. *Current Obstetric and Gynecologic Diagnosis and Treatment*, 5th ed. Los Altos, CA: Lange Medical Publications, 1984.

Fischbach, F. T. *A Manual of Laboratory Diagnostic Tests*, 3rd ed. Philadelphia: J. B. Lippincott, 1988.

Flood-Chez, B., Skurnick, J., Chez, R., Verklan, T., Biggs, S., and M. Hage. "Interpretations of Nonstress Tests by Obstetric Nurses." *JOGNN* 19(3)227–231, May-June, 1990.

Lavery, J. P. "Nonstress Fetal Heart Rate Testing." *Clinical Obstetrics and Gynecology* 25(4):689, December, 1982.

Niswander, K. R. *Manual of Obstetrics, Diagnosis and Therapy*, 3rd ed. Boston: Little, Brown and Co., 1987.

Oxorn, H. *Oxorn-Foote Human Labor and Birth*, 5th ed. E. Norwalk, CT: Appleton-Century-Crofts, 1986.

Pletsch, P. "Birth Defect Prevention: Nursing Interventions." *JOGNN* 19(6)482–487, November-December, 1990.

Pritchard, J. A., MacDonald, P. C., and N. F. Grant. *Williams Obstetrics*, 17th ed. E. Norwalk, CT: Appleton-Century-Crofts, 1985.

Sabbagha, R. E. *Diagnostic Ultrasound Applied to Obstetrics and Gynecology*, 2nd ed. Philadelphia: J.B. Lippincott, 1987.

Stringer, M. "Chorionic Villi Sampling: A Nursing Perspective." *JOGNN* 17(1):19–22, January-February, 1988.

Tucker, S. M., and S. L. Bryant. *Fetal Monitoring and Fetal Assessment in High-Risk Pregnancy*. St. Louis: C. V. Mosby, 1978.

UNIT

iii

Labor and Delivery

CHAPTER

10

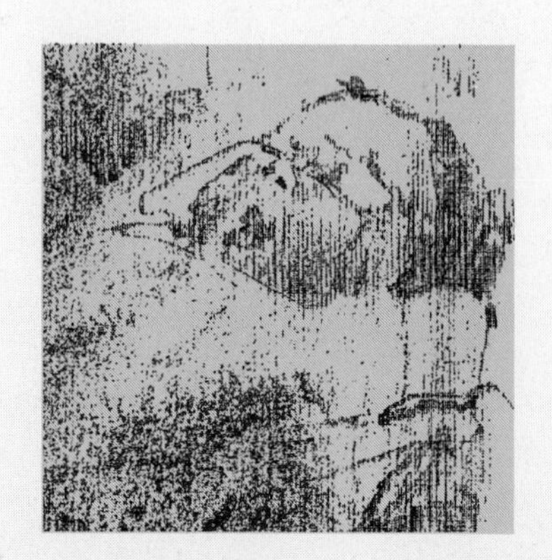

The Stages and Mechanism of Labor and Delivery

Objectives

After studying this chapter, the student should be able to:

- Define the four stages of labor.
- List the signs and symptoms of each stage of labor.
- Explain the birth process in terms of presentation, position, and station.
- List the abbreviations for categories of presentations.
- Describe the seven movements in the mechanism of labor.

Key Terms

Engagement	Increment
Lightening	Acme
Show	Decrement

FREQUENCY

DURATION

FALSE LABOR

TRUE LABOR

EFFACEMENT

DILATATION

ATTITUDE

LIE

LONGITUDINAL LIE

TRANSVERSE LIE

PRESENTATION

CEPHALIC PRESENTATION

BREECH PRESENTATION

POSITION

OCCIPUT

SACRUM

MENTUM

STATION

CORD PROLAPSE

LATENT PHASE

ACCELERATED PHASE

TRANSITION PHASE

MECHANISM OF LABOR

RESTITUTION

EXPULSION

EPISIOTOMY

AFTERBIRTH

LOCHIA

AFTERBIRTH PAIN

In the final two to four weeks of gestation, the fetal head sinks into the pelvis. The passing of the widest diameter of the presenting part of the fetus through the pelvic inlet is known as **engagement**. Its effect on the mother is called lightening. In **lightening**, the fundus of the uterus lowers, making the upper part of the abdomen flatter and lowering the waistline, see Figure 10–1. Breathing becomes easier, but walking and moving are more difficult. As in early pregnancy, the pressure of the uterus causes frequency of urination.

The actual onset of labor is marked by one or more of the following signs:

- the "show"
- rupture of the membranes (bag of waters)
- regular contractions of the uterus

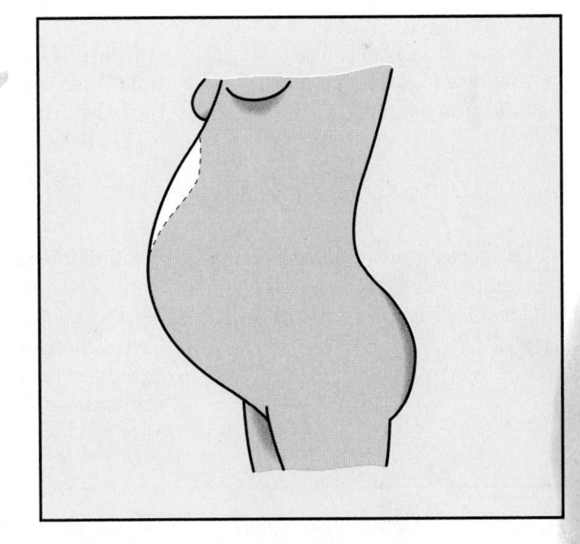

Figure 10–1 Lightening

The **show** is a pink vaginal discharge consisting of thick, stringy mucus streaked with blood (called the mucous plug); the blood is due to the rupture of capillary vessels in the cervix and lower segment of the uterus. Actual bleeding at any time during labor is abnormal, and the doctor should be notified. Rupture of the membranes (bag of waters) is the tearing of the membranes that contain the amniotic fluid, which supported the baby during the term of pregnancy. The amniotic fluid may gush or trickle out of the vagina, depending on the degree of tear in the amniotic sac. Rupture of the membranes may or may not occur with the onset of contractions. Refer to Figure 10–2 for signs of approaching labor.

LABOR SIGNS

Sign	What it is	When it happens
Feeling as if the baby has dropped lower	**Lightening** is commonly referred to as the "baby dropping." The baby's head has settled deep into pelvis.	From a few weeks to a few hours before labor begins
Discharging a thick plug of mucus or having an increase in vaginal discharge (clear, pink, or slightly bloody)	**Show:** a thick mucus plug has accumulated at the cervix during pregnancy. When the cervix begins to open wider, the plug is pushed into the vagina.	Several days before labor begins or at the onset of labor
Discharging a continuous trickle or a gush of watery fluid from vagina	**Rupture of membranes:** the fluid-filled sac that surrounded the baby during pregnancy breaks ("water breaks").	From several hours before labor begins to any time during labor
Feeling a regular pattern of cramps or what may feel like a bad backache or menstrual cramps	**Contractions:** uterus tightens (contracts) and relaxes; feels hard when it's tightening. Contractions may cause pain, as the cervix opens and the baby moves through the birth canal.	Usually at the onset of labor

Figure 10–2 *Signs of approaching labor (The American College of Obstetricians and Gynecologists.* How to Tell when Labor Begins. *ACOG Patient Education Pamphlet AP004. Washington, D.C. © 1984)*

The contractions of the uterus are an involuntary tightening of the uterine muscle. These contractions are often referred to as "labor pains." Each contraction lasts from 45 to 90 seconds (less than 1½ minutes). The average contraction is about one minute long. Each contraction has three phases:

- **increment:** the intensity of the contractions increases
- **acme:** the contraction is at its height
- **decrement:** the intensity of the contraction diminishes

The contractions of the uterus are intermittent, with periods of relaxation between them. Contractions are timed from the beginning of one to the beginning of the next contraction; the **frequency** is measured in minutes. The **duration** is timed from the beginning to the end of one contraction and is measured in seconds; the intensity can be measured with a uterine monitor and is in direct relation to the progress of labor.

FALSE LABOR

It is often difficult to determine whether a patient is in labor, see Figure 10–3. Abdominal discomfort may occur a few days to three weeks before labor actually begins. This discomfort may be due to gas in the bowels or

TRUE versus FALSE LABOR

Type of Change	True Labor	False Labor
Timing of contractions	Come at regular intervals and, as time goes on, get closer together	Often are irregular and do not consistently get closer together (called Braxton-Hicks contractions)
Change with movement	Contractions continue, despite movement	Contractions may stop when patient walks or rests or may even stop with a change of position
Location of contractions	Usually felt in the back coming around to the front	Often felt in the abdomen
Strength of contractions	Increase in strength steadily	Usually weak and do not get much stronger

Figure 10–3

irregular uterine contractions. These contractions are annoying and closely resemble true labor. **False labor** contractions, however, are irregular, and the intensity does not increase with time. Also, they are usually confined to the lower abdomen. If examined, there is no marked change in the cervix. A warm bath or light activity, such as walking, will often relieve the symptoms. False labor may occur for a period of a few minutes to hours and then disappear, only to return in a similar manner or develop into true contractions.

TRUE LABOR

True labor is characterized by a rhythmic, increasingly intense uterine contraction that occurs at intervals of 5 to 15 minutes; each contraction lasts 30 seconds or more and is accompanied by typical changes in the lower portion of the body of the uterus and the cervix. The cervix, normally long and narrow, shortens and widens. The shortening is called **effacement**; the widening, **dilatation**, Figure 10–4. Effacement is measured in percentages. The higher the percentage, the thinner and shorter the cervix. Dilation is measured in centimeters (2½ cm = 1 in.). These changes are accomplished by the uterine contractions and hormonal influence.

Dilatation and effacement of the cervix distinguish true labor from false labor. The internal os of the cervix enlarges from a few millimeters to a diameter of about 10 cm, as shown in Figure 10–5. At this stage, cervical dilatation is commonly said to be "complete" or "full." The amount of dilation and effacement of the cervix may be determined by vaginal or rectal examination.

When labor first begins, the patient usually feels an uncomfortable tenseness in her lower abdomen, back, or rectum, followed by another contraction in 20 to 30 minutes. These contractions gradually become more frequent and regular.

FOUR STAGES OF LABOR

Labor progresses in four stages. The first stage, called the *period of dilatation and effacement*, extends from the time cervical dilatation and effacement begin until they are complete. The second stage, the *period of expulsion*, is the period between complete dilatation of the cervix to the delivery of the fetus. The third stage begins with the birth of the baby and lasts until the placenta and membranes are expelled. This stage is known as the *placental stage*. The fourth stage of labor, *recovery*, begins after the birth of the placenta and lasts for the first few hours after delivery.

Before you can fully understand the stages of labor, you must know the relationships of the baby and birth canal. The terms *attitude*, *lie*, *presentation*, and *position* are used to describe these relationships. **Attitude** is the relationship of the

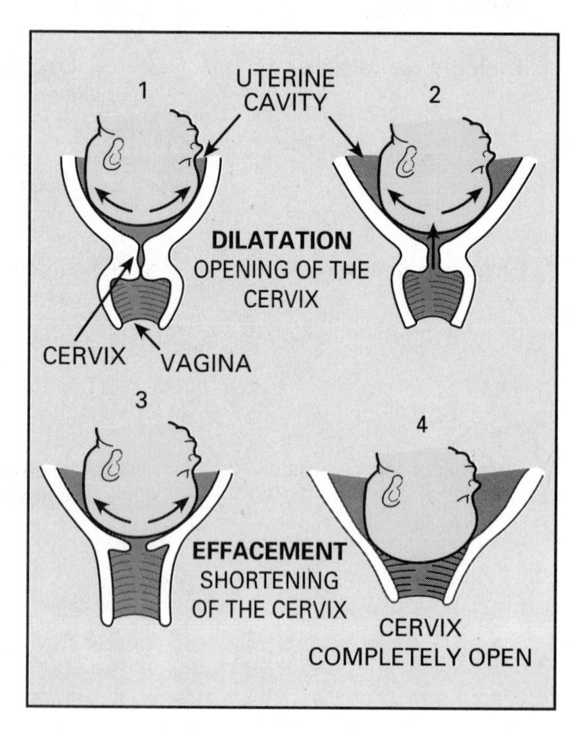

Figure 10–4 *Dilatation and effacement of the cervix during labor*

fetus's body to itself. The most common attitude is flexion, and it needs the least amount of space. The head is flexed on the chest, arms are folded, legs are flexed and drawn up on the abdomen. When the head is extended, the chin will present.

Lie refers to the relation of the long axis of the baby to that of the mother. In most cases,

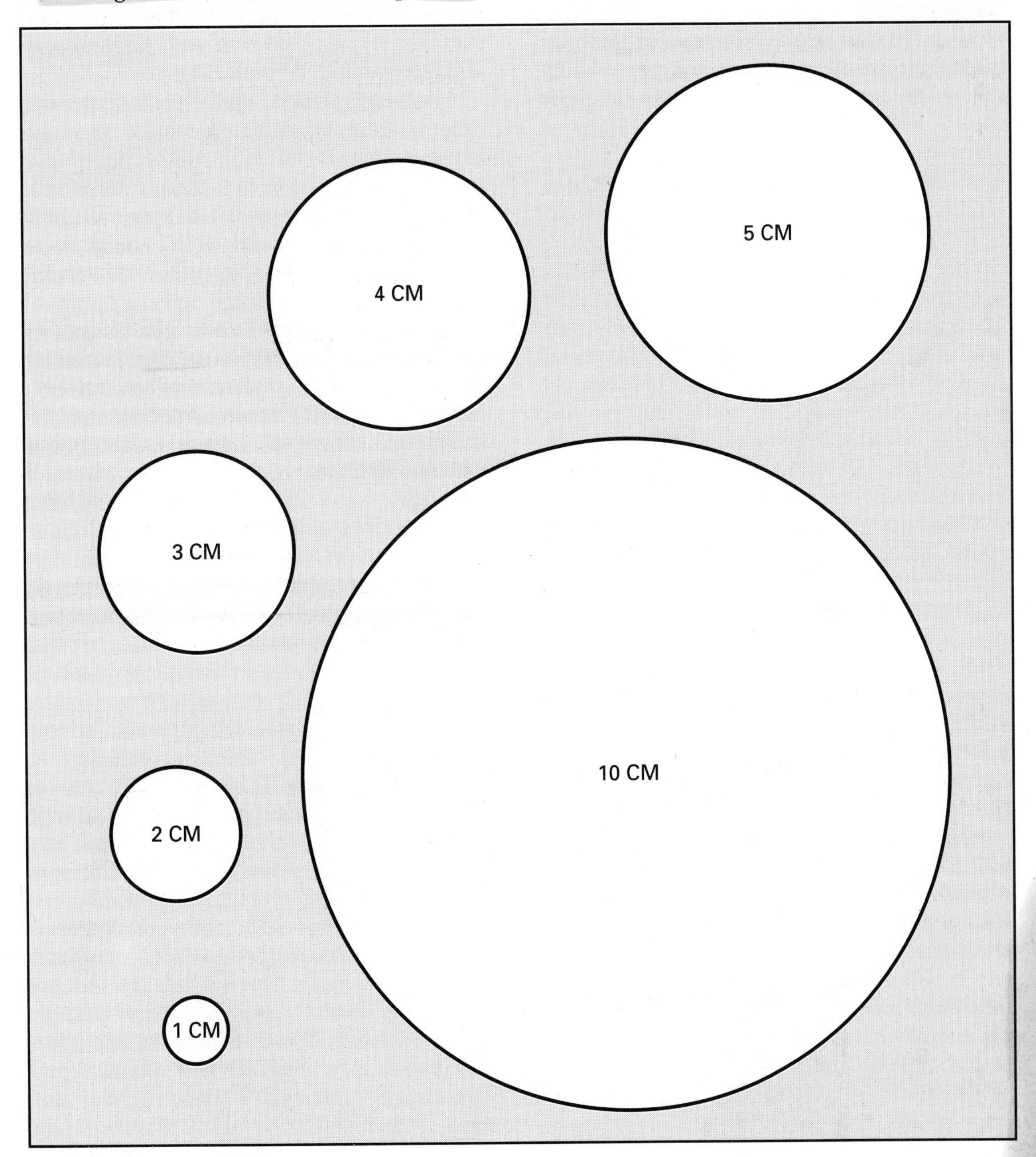

Figure 10–5 *Cervical dilatation*

this axis is parallel to or in the same plane as the mother's and is called a **longitudinal lie**, Figure 10–6. A much rarer occurrence is a **transverse lie**, in which the baby lies across the mother's pelvis, Figure 10–7.

Presentation refers to the part of the baby that enters the internal os for delivery. In longitudinal lie, the presenting part may be either the head **(cephalic presentation)** or the buttocks **(breech presentation)**. Cephalic presentation may be either vertex, brow, or face, depending on whether the occipital area, frontal area, or chin is presenting. In transverse lie, the shoulder is the presenting part. Cephalic presentation occurs 96% of the time.

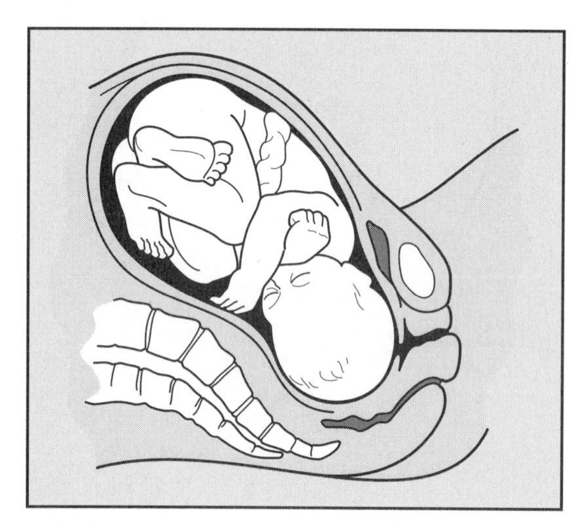

Figure 10–6 *Longitudinal lie*

Position refers to the relation of the presenting part of the child to the right or left side of the mother, Figure 10–8. The relationship of the presenting part to the anterior, transverse, or posterior portion of the mother's pelvis is also considered in determining the position. There are six positions for each presentation, Figure 10–9.

When the **occiput** (head) is the presenting part, it is identified by the letter *O*. Its position in relation to the quadrants of the mother's pelvis may be: left occiput anterior (L.O.A.), left occiput transverse (L.O.T.), or left occiput posterior (L.O.P.), Figure 10–10. Similarly, if on the right, it may be right occiput anterior (R.O.A.), right occiput transverse (R.O.T.), or right occiput posterior (R.O.P.).

The **sacrum** (buttocks) is designated by the letter *S*, **mentum** (face) by the letter *M*, and

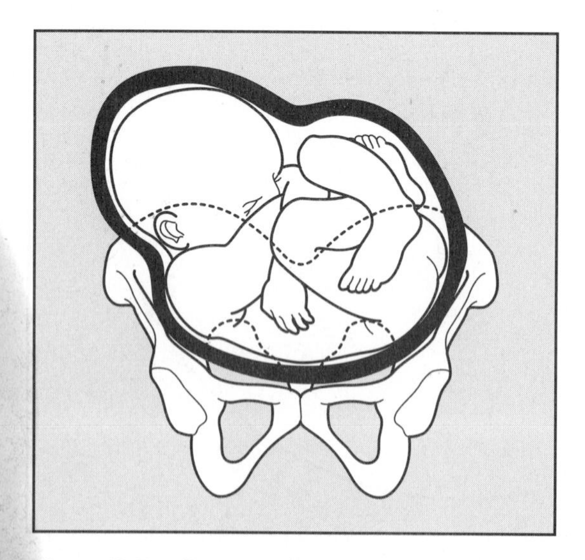

Figure 10–7 *Transverse lie*

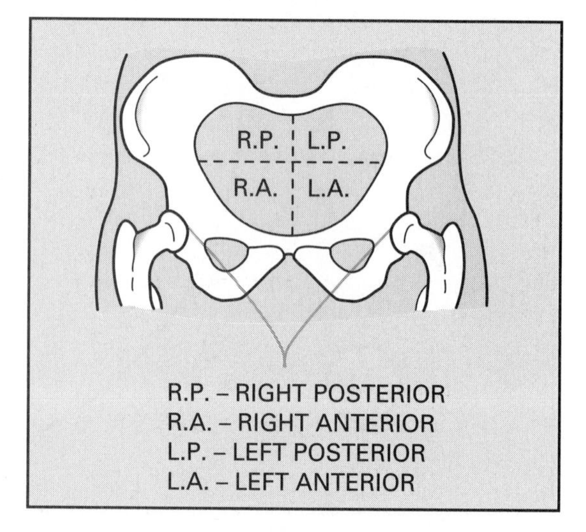

Figure 10–8 *Pelvic quadrants*

POSITIONS OF PRESENTATION

A. Cephalic Presentations
1. L.O.A. — Left occiput anterior
2. L.O.T. — Left occiput transverse
3. L.O.P. — Left occiput posterior
4. R.O.A. — Right occiput anterior
5. R.O.T. — Right occiput transverse
6. R.O.P. — Right occiput posterior

B. Breech Presentations
1. L.S.A. — Left sacrum anterior
2. L.S.T. — Left sacrum transverse
3. L.S.P. — Left sacrum posterior
4. R.S.A. — Right sacrum anterior
5. R.S.T. — Right sacrum transverse
6. R.S.P. — Right sacrum posterior

C. Face Presentations
1. L.M.A. — Left mentum anterior
2. L.M.T. — Left mentum transverse
3. L.M.P. — Left mentum posterior
4. R.M.A. — Right mentum anterior
5. R.M.T. — Right mentum transverse
6. R.M.P. — Right mentum posterior

D. Transverse Presentations
1. L.Sc.A. — Left scapula anterior
2. L.Sc.T. — Left scapula transverse
3. L.Sc.P. — Left scapula posterior
4. R.Sc.A. — Right scapula anterior
5. R.Sc.T. — Right scapula transverse
6. R.Sc.P. — Right scapula posterior

Figure 10–9

scapula (shoulder) by the letters *Sc*. The presentation and position can be determined by abdominal palpation, vaginal examination, and auscultation. The left occiput anterior (L.O.A.) position is the most common position and the most favorable for the welfare of the mother and baby.

ENGAGEMENT AND STATION

When the presenting part descends and fully enters the true pelvis, it is said to be engaged. The degree of engagement is called **station**, Figure 10–11. There are five stations:

1. floating: presenting part high above inlet; –4, –5 cm
2. fixed: presenting part in the inlet; –3, –2, –1 cm
3. engaged: the largest diameter of the presenting part has reached the level of the ischial spines; 0 cm
4. midplane: presenting part is between the inlet plane and maximum depth of pelvis; +1, +2, +3 cm
5. on the perineum: presenting part is deep in the pelvis; +4, +5 cm

The degree of engagement is determined by rectal and vaginal examination.

FIRST STAGE: DILATATION AND EFFACEMENT

Although labor varies in length, the first stage of labor in the average primipara lasts about 16 hours. It may be difficult to determine exactly when true labor begins since contractions may occur before dilatation starts. Dilatation and effacement may be slow or rapid depending upon the age of the patient, her general physical condition, and the number of previous pregnancies. The membranes may

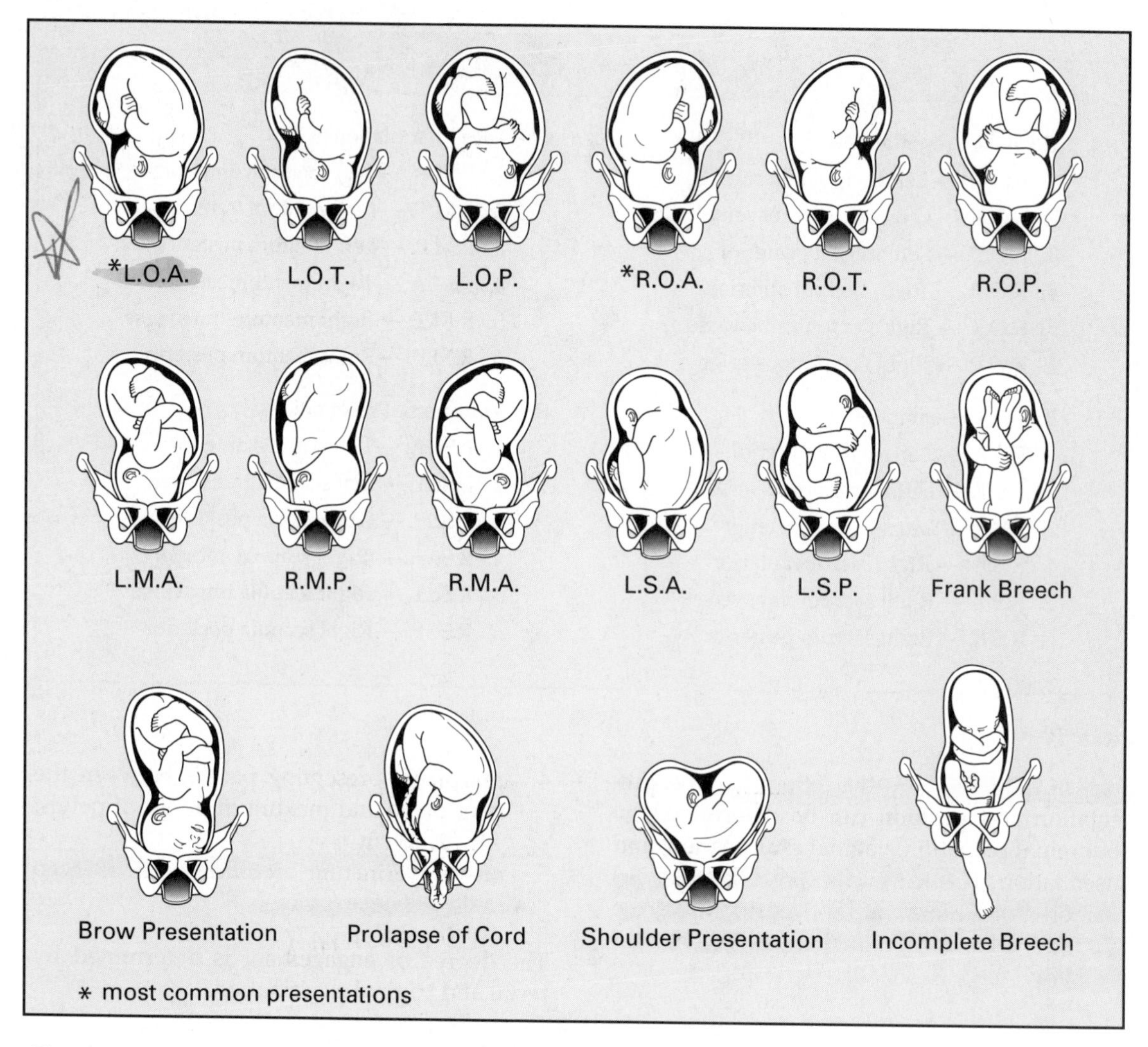

Figure 10–10 *Categories of presentations (Courtesy Ross Laboratories)*

rupture before the beginning of labor, or they may remain and assist in the dilatation of the cervix. If the membranes rupture at home, the patient should be brought to the hospital immediately. It is important to note the exact time that the membranes rupture because there is now an entry for infection. Also **cord prolapse** (premature expulsion of the cord) could occur, causing more complications. The entire first stage is an involuntary act; the only assistance that the patient can give is to relax.

As the contractions continue through the first stage of labor, a pull is exerted on the cervix and supporting ligaments. This pulling, combined with a reduction in oxygen supply to the contracted muscle and tissue, can cause discomfort. The more intense the contraction, the more pull is exerted on the cervix; the more

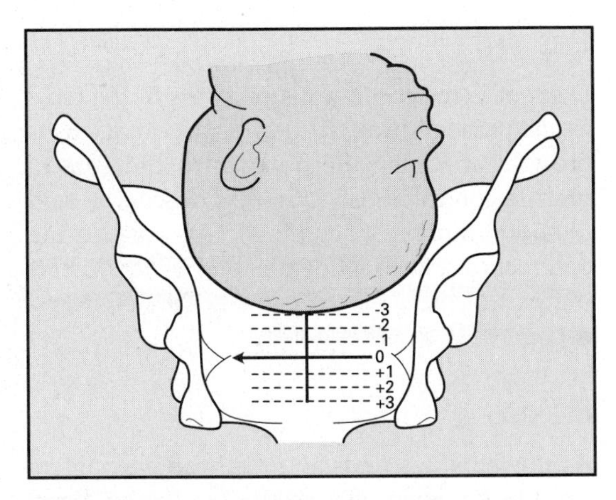

Figure 10–11 *Station is the relationship of the baby's head to a bony landmark in the pelvis; measured in centimeters. (Adapted from Ross Laboratories)*

often the contractions occur, the more frequently that pull is exerted. As the upper portion of the uterus contracts, the lower portion relaxes, allowing the baby to descend farther toward the vagina. The pressure of the baby's head against the cervix stimulates the release of the hormone oxytocin, which in turn stimulates further contractions.

In a typical pattern of labor contractions, the period from 1 to 4 cm is called the **latent phase** of labor; from 5 to 7 cm, the **accelerated phase**; and from 8 to 10 cm, the **transition phase**. Each of these periods is shorter and more intense than the one before it, with the transition period being shortest and most difficult, see Figure 10–12.

SECOND STAGE: EXPULSION

The position of the fetus must change as it passes through the pelvis and birth canal. Note in Figure 10–13 that the long diameter of the inlet of the pelvis is side to side. The long diameter at the outlet is from front to back. Therefore, the baby's head must turn 90 degrees to emerge from the outlet. A series of movements, called the **mechanism of labor**, or cardinal movements, Figure 10–14, adjusts the position

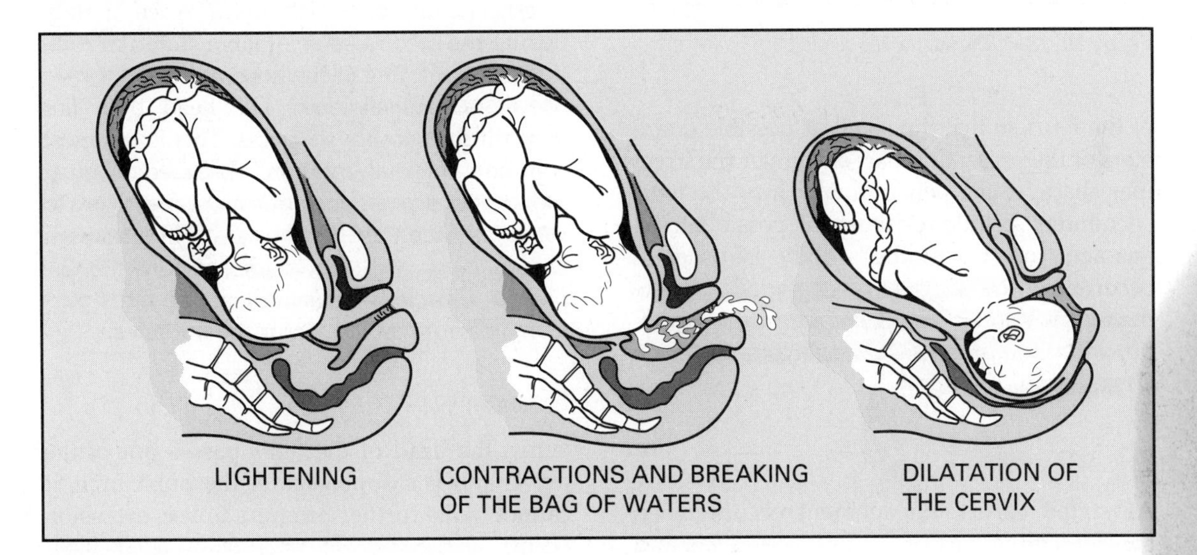

Figure 10–12 *The first stage of labor (Courtesy Carnation Company)*

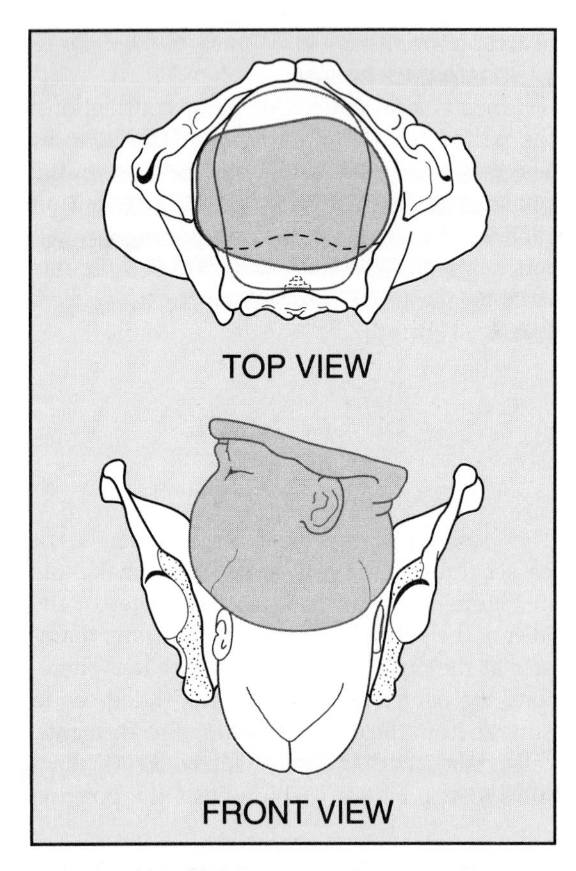

Figure 10–13 *The inlet of the pelvis*

of the fetus so that the smallest possible diameters of the presenting part encounter the irregular shape of the pelvic canal. Thus, the fetus encounters as little resistance as possible to its passage from the mother's body. In order of occurrence, these movements are: (1) engagement, (2) descent, (3) flexion, (4) internal rotation, (5) extension, (6) external rotation, and (7) expulsion.

ENGAGEMENT

As stated earlier, engagement occurs when the presenting part of the fetus descends and fully enters the pelvis. In multiparas, engagement sometimes does not occur until dilatation begins.

DESCENT

Descent is the continuous progress of the fetus as it passes through the birth canal. It is brought about by the downward pressure of uterine contractions. Although descent is said to be continuous, it actually occurs only during contractions. Descent begins when the presenting part of the fetus fully enters the pelvis and engagement is accomplished.

FLEXION

As the fetus descends and the head encounters resistance, flexion (condition of being bent) occurs. During flexion, the head of the fetus is bent forward, causing its chin to rest on its sternum (breastbone). Flexion is important because the narrowest part of the head must enter the pelvic outlet. Flexion can occur either at the edge of the pelvis or when the head reaches the pelvic floor.

INTERNAL ROTATION

The next step in the mechanism of labor is internal rotation, which takes place mainly during the second stage of labor. Internal rotation is the rotating of the head of the fetus 45 to 90 degrees to the left. The head then lies beneath the symphysis pubis. This is the most common internal rotation. If the fetus must move from a posterior position, it may have to rotate as much as 135 degrees. This means a longer labor with more discomfort for the patient, especially back pain, as the fetus puts extra pressure on the sacrum as it rotates.

EXTENSION

When the head of the fetus passes out of the pelvis and is stopped under the pubic arch, it cannot make further progress unless extension occurs. Extension is when the fetal head becomes unflexed and pushes upward out of the vaginal canal. The head of the fetus is actually delivered during extension.

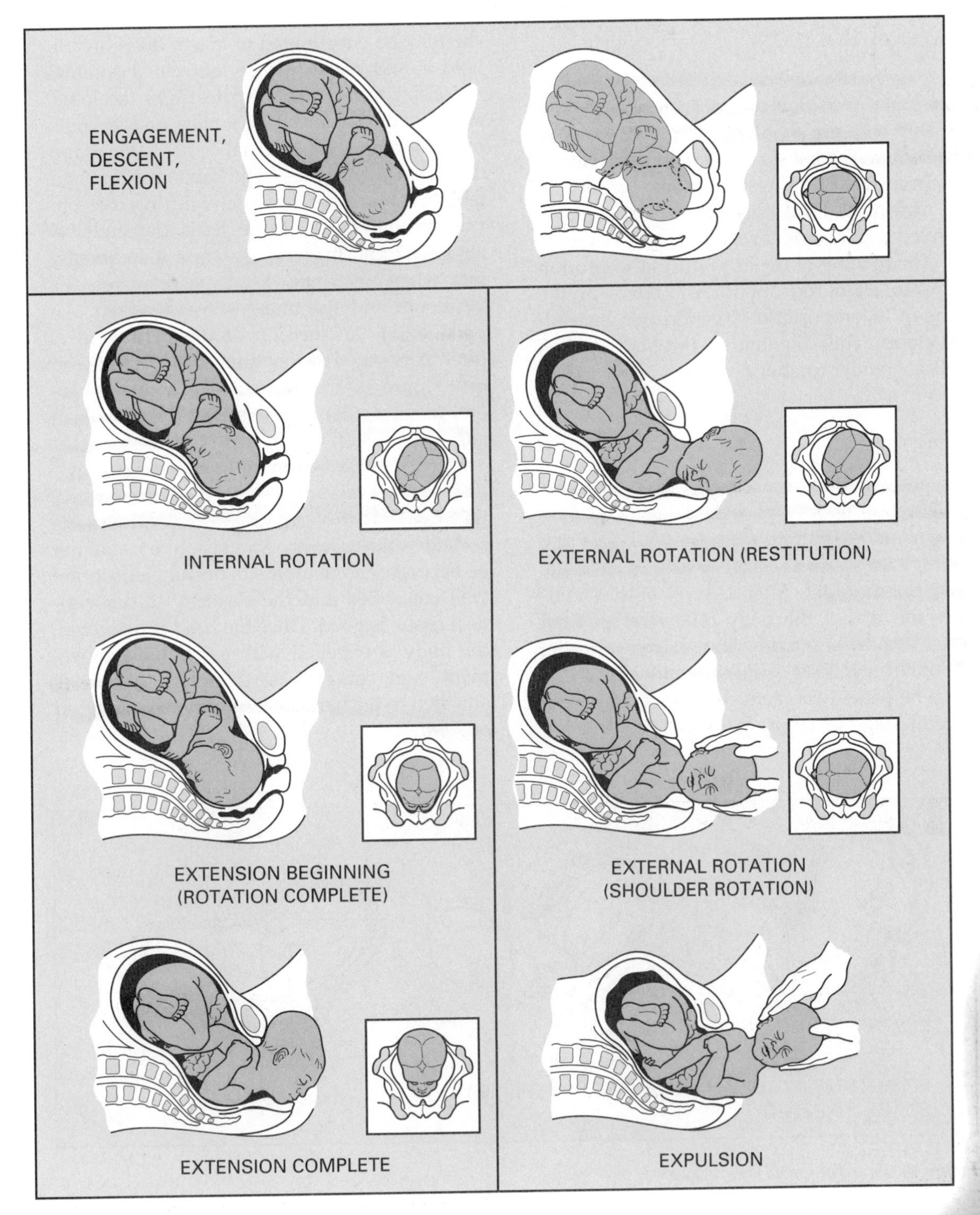

Figure 10–14 *Mechanism of normal labor, the process by which the baby traverses the birth canal*

EXTERNAL ROTATION

After the head is delivered, it rotates back 45 to 90 degrees or until it resumes its normal relationship with the shoulders. This step is called **restitution.** The baby's position in utero can be determined during restitution by observing the turn of its head. Restitution is sometimes coupled with shoulder rotation.

The rotating of the head during restitution helps to align the unborn shoulders of the fetus in anteroposterior position just beneath the pubis. This aligning of the shoulders is called shoulder rotation.

EXPULSION

The anterior shoulder emerges first, aided by the doctor, who applies a gentle but firm downward pressure on the baby's head. The doctor then raises the head gently to clear the posterior shoulder. After delivery of the shoulders the rest of the body follows. This final step, which is actually the delivery of the shoulders and body, is called **expulsion**.

The patient can actively participate in the second stage of labor. With each contraction she may be encouraged to take a deep breath, hold it, and bear down so that the abdominal muscles contract and help to expel the fetus. As the contractions last longer and become more frequent, the vaginal tissue bulges and the rectum stretches. The labia majora and labia minora separate widely; during the contraction the head of the fetus descends. A stretching and burning sensation is frequently felt when the fetal head passes over the perineum and the muscles are stretched. An **episiotomy** (an incision of the perineum) is often performed at this time to facilitate delivery, Figure 10–15. The episiotomy serves several purposes: (1) it substitutes a straight, clean surgical incision for a ragged laceration that otherwise could occur; (2) it spares the baby's head from pressure against perineal obstruction; and (3) it shortens the duration of the second stage of labor. An episiotomy may not be necessary if the mother's pushing efforts are well controlled and the elasticity of her perineal tissue is good. Once the head is delivered, the body is expelled with a rotational movement, and complete birth occurs. The cord attached to the newborn infant is then clamped and cut.

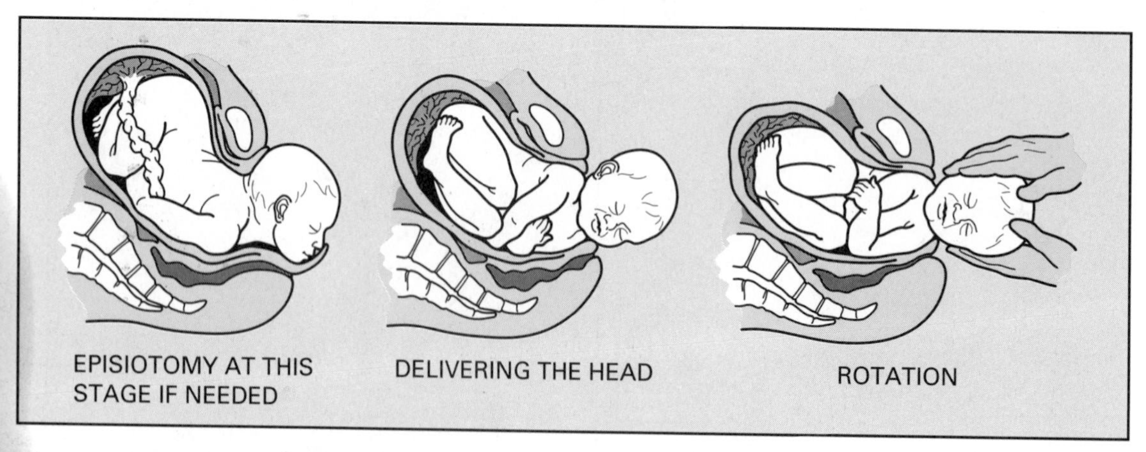

Figure 10–15 *The second stage of labor*

THIRD STAGE: PLACENTAL STAGE

The third stage of labor, the placental stage, usually begins with a gush of blood. The placenta and its membranes are still attached to the wall of the uterus; contractions of the uterus continue for a time before the placenta separates. These contractions are not severe at first; they become stronger to expel the **afterbirth** (placenta, membranes, and umbilical cord). Bleeding from the vagina occurs at the time of separation of the placenta.

With the contractions of the uterus, the placenta is expelled into the vagina, bringing the membranes after it, Figure 10–16. With moderate pressure on the fundus, the placenta leaves the vagina. The fundus usually lies in the vicinity of the umbilicus (the navel). The uterus then becomes hard and firm and once more lies in the pelvis. Occasionally, the uterus may soften, rise up, and relax. This condition could be a symptom of hemorrhage. (*Caution:* It is most important that the uterus be massaged carefully until it remains firm.) Oxytocin may be given to aid in contracting the uterus and controlling bloody discharge.

FOURTH STAGE: RECOVERY

The fourth stage consists of the first few hours after birth. The first hours after birth are a very special time for a family, Figure 10–17. The baby is usually more alert and receptive to the parents at this time than during the ensuing 24 hours.

When the mother's condition is considered stable, she is moved to a bed, where she continues to recover. Some hospitals are equipped with birthing rooms, where the mother will labor, deliver her baby, and stay during her recovery period without changing location. The first hours after birth are a time when the mother must be watched closely. Her uterus is checked for firmness and location. Her normal flow of blood, excess tissue and fluids from the uterus, called **lochia**, are checked for amount and consistency. Her blood pressure, temperature, and pulse are checked for stabilization and normalcy. She is asked to urinate, and her bladder is checked for complete emptying.

The mother may experience some trembling of her legs, which may be relieved by covering them with a warmed blanket. She may also experience a burning discomfort in

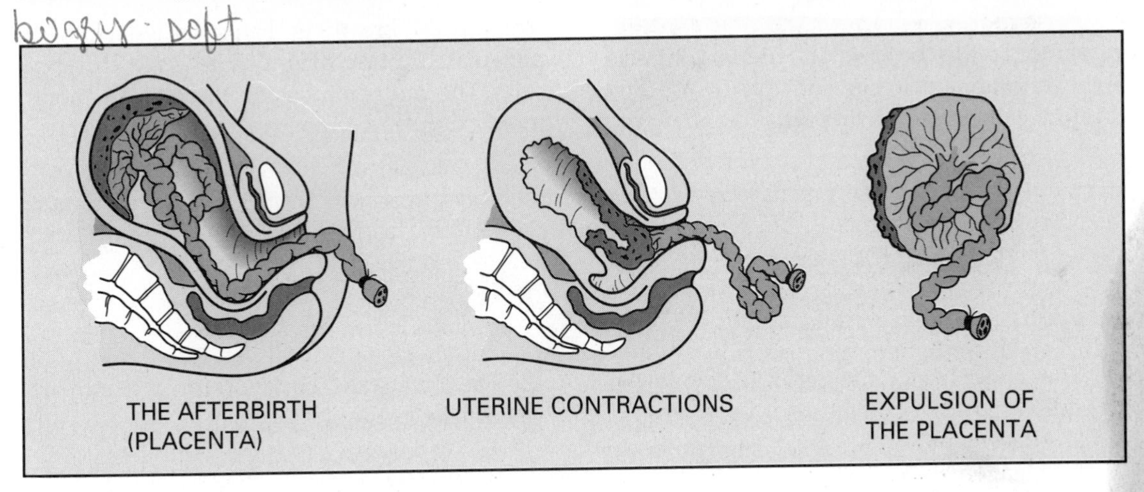

Figure 10–16 *The third stage of labor*

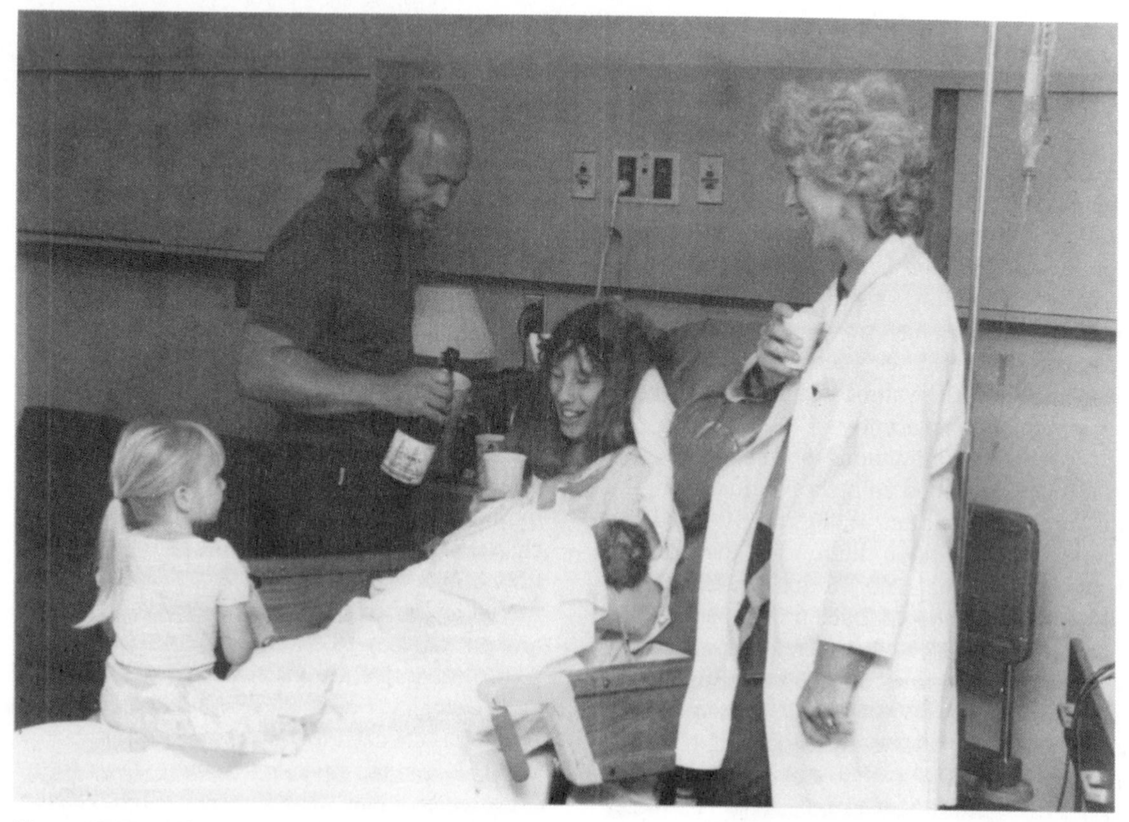

Figure 10–17 *The expanding family gets acquainted.*

her perineum, which may be eased by applying an ice bag to the area. The uterus contracts for a time after delivery and may cause discomfort called **afterbirth pains**, or afterpain. Slow, deep breathing helps to lessen these pains. Medication may also be given if necessary. The mother must continue to be monitored carefully during her entire hospital stay.

REVIEW QUESTIONS

A. Multiple choice. Select the best answer.

1. The widening of the cervical opening is called
   a. effacement
   b. engagement
   c. dilatation
   d. prolapse

2. The first stage of labor for a primipara usually lasts
   a. 3 to 6 hours
   b. 6 to 10 hours
   c. 10 to 16 hours
   d. 24 hours

3. Descent of the fetal head into the pelvis is called
   a. lightening
   b. effacement
   c. labor
   d. presentation

4. Duration of the contractions of the uterus (labor pains) ranges from
   a. 10 to 45 seconds
   b. 20 to 40 seconds
   c. 45 to 90 seconds
   d. 60 to 120 seconds

5. The patient has an active role to play during the
   a. first stage of labor
   b. second stage of labor
   c. third stage of labor
   d. all of the above

6. True labor is characterized by
   a. increasingly intense uterine contractions
   b. contractions that occur at regular 5- to 15-minute intervals
   c. dilatation of the cervix
   d. all of the above

7. The four stages of labor are
   a. dilatation and effacement, expulsion, placental, recovery
   b. dilatation, presentation, engagement, expulsion
   c. early, latent, transition, expulsion
   d. none of the above

8. *Lie* refers to
   a. how deep the baby's head has dropped into the pelvis
   b. the relation of the long axis of the baby to that of the mother
   c. the baby's head being on the right or left side of the mother
   d. how long it takes for the baby to move down the birth canal

9. When the presenting part descends fully into the true pelvis, it is said to be
   a. floating
   b. fixed
   c. engaged
   d. midplane

10. If the baby is in a head-down position, with back facing out toward the mother's abdomen and the occiput on the left side, the position is termed
    a. L.O.A.
    b. L.O.P.
    c. L.S.A.
    d. L.O.T.

11. An episiotomy is performed
    a. when the laboring woman has the urge to push
    b. when the fetal head is stretching the perineum and muscles
    c. when the vaginal tissue bulges and the rectum stretches
    d. when it appears that the perineum has torn

12. The process by which the baby traverses the birth canal is called
    a. presentation
    b. station
    c. position
    d. mechanism of labor

13. The percentage of births that occur with a cephalic presentation is
    a. 50%
    b. 4%
    c. 96%
    d. 75%

14. The physician can determine the presentation and position of the baby by
    a. vaginal examination
    b. abdominal palpation
    c. auscultation
    d. all of the above

15. The presenting part is usually engaged when it reaches the level of the
    a. ischial tuberosities
    b. ischial spines
    c. iliac crests
    d. perineum

16. Provisional determination of fetal lie, position, and presentation may be made by
    a. abdominal palpation after the 6th month
    b. the fetal heart rate
    c. vaginal exam
    d. all of the above

SUGGESTED ACTIVITIES

- Submit a written, documented report on one of the following:
  - Cervix in primigravida
  - Four stages of labor: Nursing care according to the nursing process
- Identify each category of presentation (see Figure 10–10).
- Define labor. Describe the changes in each stage.
- Identify the signs of approaching labor.
- Define station, engagement, and crowning.
- Differentiate between true labor and false labor.
- List the cardinal movements in birth.

BIBLIOGRAPHY

Hamilton, P. M. *Basic Maternity Nursing*, 6th ed. St. Louis, MO: C. V. Mosby, 1989.

Hawkins, J. W., and L. Pierfedeici. *Maternity and Gynecological Nursing*, New York: J. B. Lippincott, 1981.

Jenson, M. D., Benson, R., and I. Bobsk. *Maternity Care: The Nurse and the Family*, 3rd ed. St. Louis, MO: C. V. Mosby, 1985.

McNall, L. K. *Obstetric and Gynecologic Nursing*. St. Louis, MO: C. V. Mosby, 1980.

Oxorn, H. *Oxorn-Foote Human Labor and Birth*, 5th ed. E. Norwalk, CT: Appleton-Century-Crofts, 1986.

Pillitteri, A. *Maternal-Newborn Nursing: Care of the Growing Family*, 2nd ed. Boston: Little, Brown and Co., 1981.

Pritchard, J. A., MacDonald, P. C., and N. F. Grant. *Williams Obstetrics*, 17th ed. E. Norwalk, CT: Appleton-Century-Crofts, 1985.

Reeder, S., Mastroianni, L. Jr., and L. Martin. *Maternity Nursing*, 16th ed. New York: J. B Lippincott, 1987.

Simkin, P., Whalley, J., and A. Keppler. *Pregnancy, Childbirth and the Newborn*. Deephaven, MN: Meadowbrook Books, 1991.

CHAPTER

11

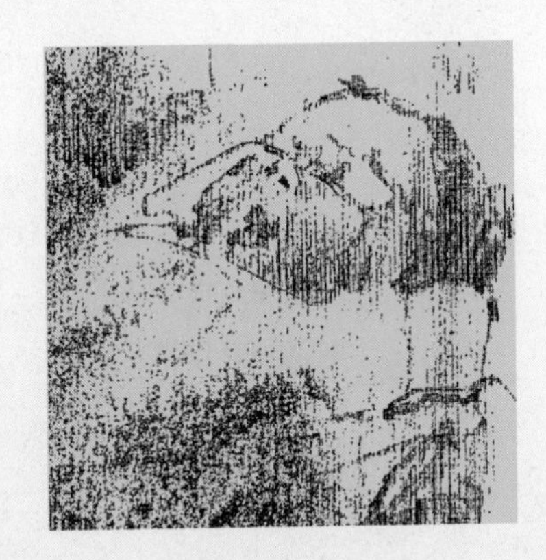

Management of the Patient in Labor

Objectives

After studying this chapter, the student should be able to:

- Describe the nursing care given during the first stage of labor.
- State the purpose and describe the procedure for a rectal examination, vaginal examination, enema, and catheterization.
- Name four factors that affect the rapidity of labor.
- List six signs of abnormal labor.

Key Terms

- TPAL
- vital signs
- abdominal palpation
- fetal heart tones (FHT)
- fetoscope
- Doppler

AUGMENTATION

CONTRACTION RING

AMNIOTOMY

PERINEAL PREPARATION

MINIPREP

AMNIHOOK

MECONIUM-STAINED FLUID

PROLAPSED CORD

INDUCED LABOR

PROSTAGLANDIN

OXYTOCICS

When the first hospitals were built in the Middle Ages, only the very poor were confined in them for childbearing. There was a 30% mortality rate due to infection and lack of knowledge in nursing techniques and isolation care. Progress in the fields of science and education greatly improved conditions. In 1847, the cause and prevention of childbed fever were discovered. In the late 1800s, Pasteur's and Lister's theories on the spread of infection were accepted, and obstetricians introduced aseptic techniques into maternity wards. With the advance of science and improved patient care, an obstetrical patient is given the same consideration as surgical patients.

Admission Procedures

Admission procedures vary among hospitals. But the patient in labor undergoes basically the same examinations and care upon admission that are given to other patients.

Greeting and Welcoming the Patient

Nurses should greet the expectant parents in a warm, friendly manner and introduce themselves. If the nurse has studied the prenatal record, the background information will help personalize and individualize the greeting, Figure 11–1.

Helping the Patient Undress

The nurse provides the patient with a hospital gown and helps her undress. The clothing that she intends to keep with her is tagged to make sure it is properly identified. Generally, the patient will have been told to leave valuables at home.

Obtaining the Patient's History

When the mother-to-be in labor is admitted to the hospital, the obstetrics nurse should determine how much sleep she has been getting, her last sleep period before admission — how long and how well — and her physical activity before coming to the hospital. The nurse reviews the prenatal record for the background of the patient and ascertains the following:

- time contractions began; their frequency and duration
- presence of show or vaginal bleeding
- state of bag of waters

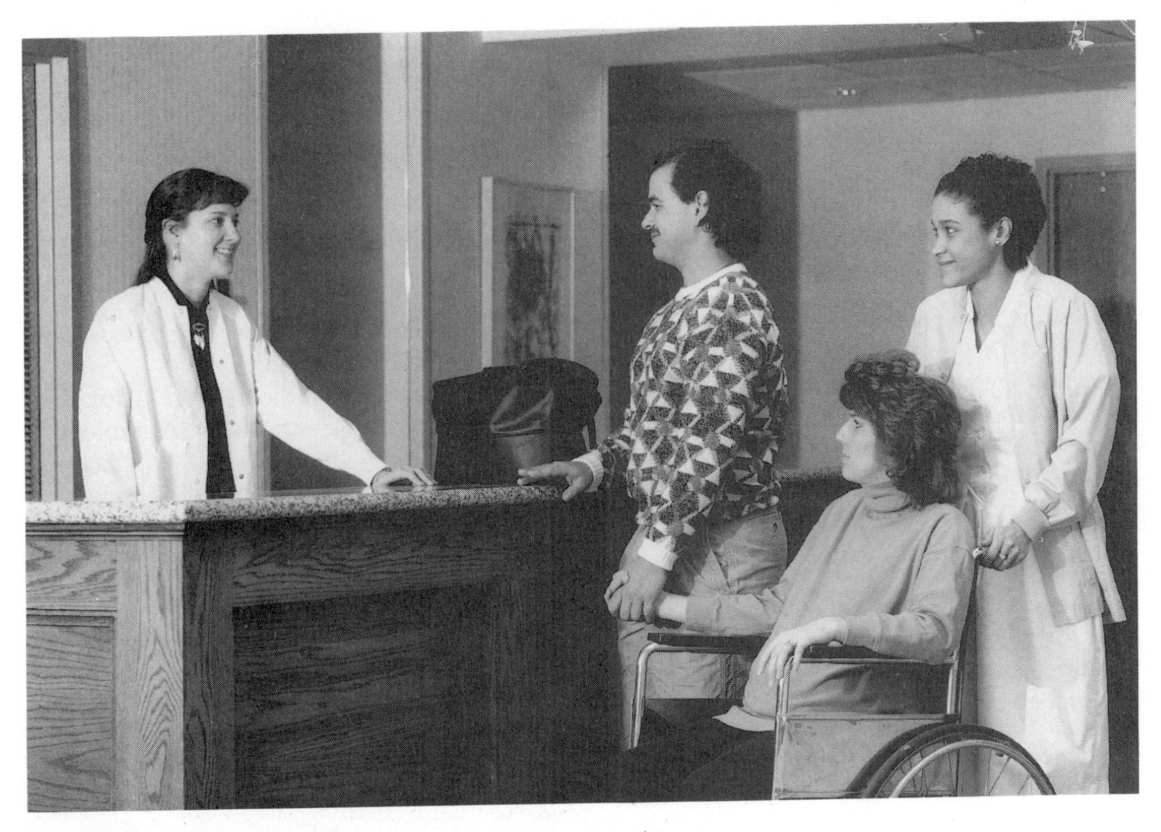

Figure 11–1 *Welcoming the laboring couple to the maternity unit*

- expected date of delivery or "confinement" (EDC); last menstrual period (LMP)
- when patient last ate and what she ate, including fluids
- number of pregnancies patient has had (gravida/para)
- any complications during the pregnancy

The nurse includes miscarriages in recording the number of pregnancies and the number of children the patient has borne. *Gravida* refers to the total number of pregnancies including the present one. *Para* refers to the number of pregnancies that have continued through the period of viability (20 weeks of gestation), including any stillborn babies.

A term that may be frequently seen in hospital charting is **TPAL**. This term refers to the number of term or completed gestational pregnancies (T); premature deliveries (P); abortions, including miscarriages (A); and number of living children (L). It is charted simply as numbers. For example 3-1-0-4 indicates three term pregnancies, one premature birth, no abortions, and four living children.

EXAMINATIONS AND PROCEDURES

The first stage of labor (the dilatation and effacement stage) begins with the first symptoms of true labor and ends with the complete dilatation of the cervix. Usually, the doctor examines the patient early in labor. But, for the welfare of the mother and child, the nurse must constantly be aware of all changes in the patient's condition and vital signs. This information must be recorded accurately and promptly reported to the attending physician.

TEMPERATURE, PULSE, AND RESPIRATIONS

Vital signs (temperature, pulse, respirations, and blood pressure) are taken and recorded every four hours while the patient is in labor. A rise in temperature may indicate an infection; an increased pulse rate may be a sign of dehydration. Report any abnormalities immediately.

URINE SPECIMEN

A urine specimen may be analyzed immediately for blood, sugar, albumin, and amniotic fluid. If it contains blood or amniotic fluid, the doctor may order a catheterized specimen.

BLOOD PRESSURE

Blood pressure is generally taken every two hours. If preeclampsia or pregnancy-induced hypertension (PIH) is present or suspected, the blood pressure is taken more often. Report any abnormalities immediately.

UTERINE CONTRACTIONS

At first, as labor begins, contractions are mild. They last about 30 seconds and occur at about 20-minute intervals. As labor progresses, they increase in intensity, last longer, and occur more frequently.

Uterine contractions of labor and the dilatation of the cervix occur in an intense, wavelike pattern. The duration of muscular contractions ranges from 30 seconds to over one minute. Each contraction is made up of three phases: a period of increasing intensity, known as *increment;* a period when the contraction is at its height, called *acme;* and a period of diminishing intensity, or *decrement*. The increment is longer than the other two periods combined. The nurse can actually feel the muscular action by placing one hand on the abdomen at the level of the fundus, see Figure 11–2. The nurse can see the action as the abdominal wall rises and relaxes again. The frequency of contractions is timed from the beginning of one contraction to the beginning of the next contraction. The duration of each contraction (number of seconds each lasts) should also be noted.

Record and report the frequency, duration, and intensity of contractions. A prolonged contraction lasting more than 90 seconds could lead to fetal hypoxia and should be brought to the physician's attention.

ABDOMINAL PALPATION

Abdominal palpation is used to check the

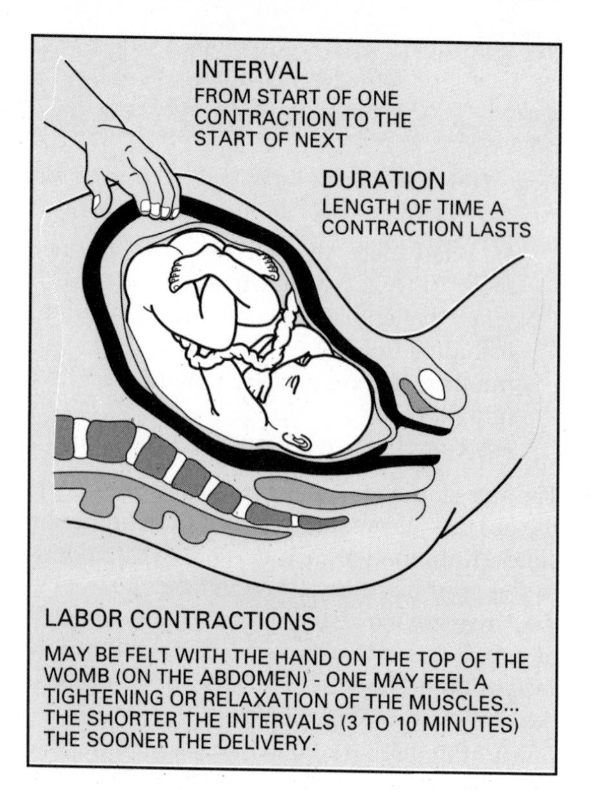

INTERVAL
FROM START OF ONE CONTRACTION TO THE START OF NEXT
DURATION
LENGTH OF TIME A CONTRACTION LASTS
LABOR CONTRACTIONS
MAY BE FELT WITH THE HAND ON THE TOP OF THE WOMB (ON THE ABDOMEN) - ONE MAY FEEL A TIGHTENING OR RELAXATION OF THE MUSCLES... THE SHORTER THE INTERVALS (3 TO 10 MINUTES) THE SOONER THE DELIVERY.

Figure 11–2 *Contractions of the uterus*

position and presentation of the baby. The size of the baby can also be estimated.

FETAL HEART TONES

Fetal heart tones are heard with a **fetoscope** (obstetrical stethoscope), which is worn on the examiner's head (see Figure 11a, b), or with a **Doppler** instrument or electron fetal monitor (Figure 11c, d). The heart tones are checked between contractions and during a contraction. They normally slow down during a contrac-

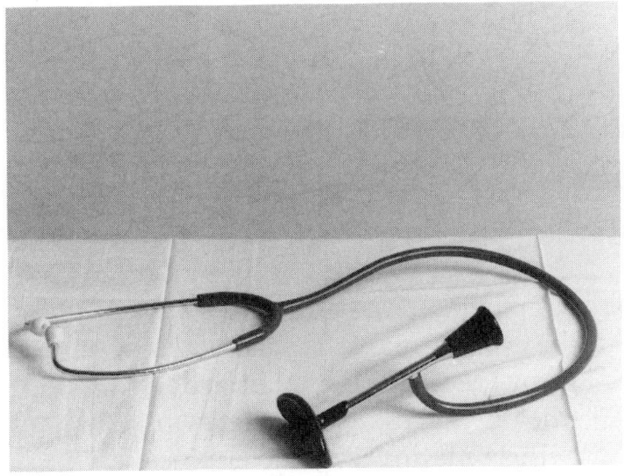

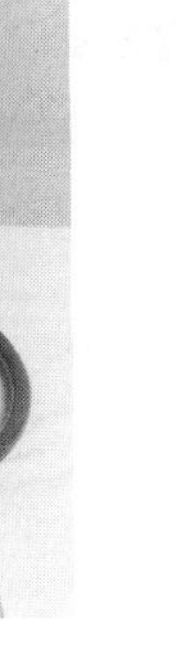

a.

b.

c.

d.

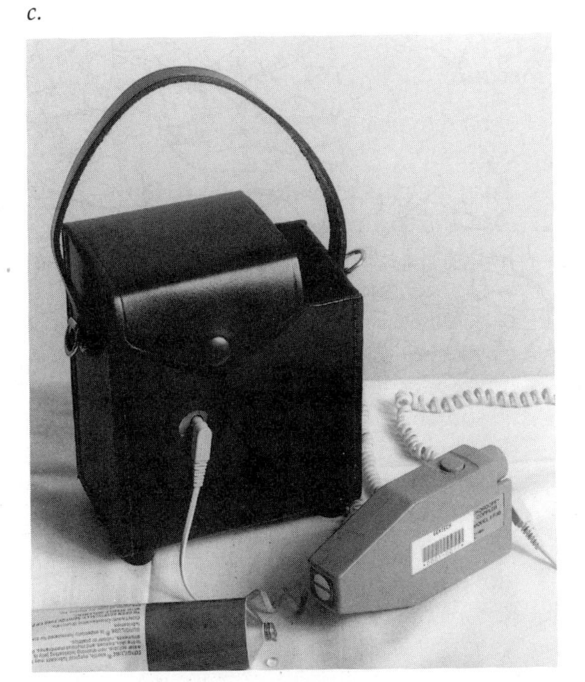

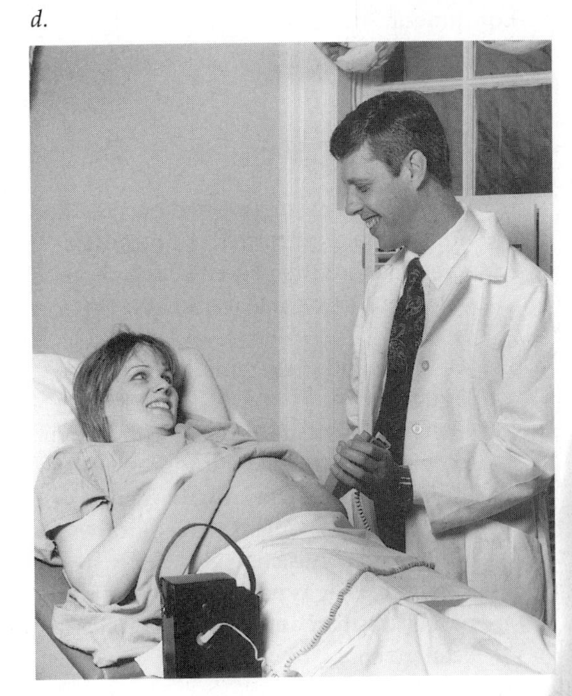

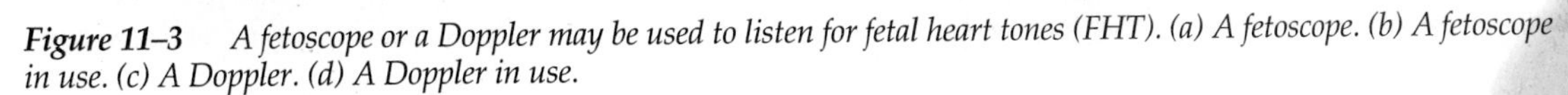

Figure 11–3 *A fetoscope or a Doppler may be used to listen for fetal heart tones (FHT). (a) A fetoscope. (b) A fetoscope in use. (c) A Doppler. (d) A Doppler in use.*

tion, but return to the normal rate as the contraction ends. The normal fetal heart rate ranges from 120 to 160 beats per minute. Fetal heart tones must be checked frequently during the first stage of labor. Any slowing down or speeding up of the heart tones beyond the normal limits should be reported immediately to the doctor. These changes may indicate fetal distress, and the doctor may wish to **augment** (increase) labor or perform a cesarean section if the heart rate indicates that the baby is in jeopardy.

PROCEDURE

Rectal Examination

Purpose: The rectal examination is done to determine the progress of labor: dilatation, effacement, and presentation. Usually vaginal examinations are performed, but there may be times when a rectal exam is preferred.

Equipment:

- 1 disposable glove
- lubricant

Precautions

1. Only the doctor or an experienced nurse should perform this procedure.
2. Keep in mind the patient's history, and determine a possible termination of labor.
3. Keep in mind the size of the cervix (see Figure 10–5).
4. Check the patient during a contraction to determine the rate of progress. Note the descent of the head with each contraction and whether the membranes bulge with contraction.
5. Remember the type of medication the patient has had and how often it has been given.
6. Keep in mind the difference between the external and internal os and always go by the size of the **"contraction ring"** (the internal os). Note other symptoms at this time and try to determine the delivery time.
7. Prevent contamination of the vaginal area.

Procedure:

1. Screen the patient and explain the procedure.
2. Turn the patient on her back or left side, knees flexed, and tell her to relax.
3. Put on the glove; lubricate index finger well and insert it into the rectum slowly and carefully, both for the comfort of the patient and to prevent reflex resistance. Press on the upper abdomen (uterus); locate the cervical opening and ascertain the dilatation, station, effacement, and presenting part of the fetus.
4. After the examination, discard the glove. Clean the anus.
5. Record the findings in the chart.

RECTAL EXAMINATION

The rectal examination may be done to determine the progress of the patient. The cervical opening can be felt to ascertain dilatation; the level of descent of the presenting part can also be determined as shown in Figure 11–4.

VAGINAL EXAMINATION

More commonly, the vaginal examination is performed to evaluate (1) the dilatation of the cervix, (2) the effacement of the cervix, (3) the station of the presenting part, and (4) the identification of the presenting part, see Figure 11–5.

PROCEDURE

Vaginal Examination

Purpose: A vaginal examination is done to ascertain the amount of cervical dilatation, presenting part, station, and effacement of the cervix, or to rupture the membranes.

Equipment:

- Sterile glove
- Bacteriostatic agent
- Membrane hook for rupturing membranes
- Adequate lighting

Precautions:

1. This procedure is usually done by the patient's physician or an experienced labor nurse.
2. Stay with the doctor during the procedure.

Procedure:

1. Explain the procedure if the patient seems tense.
2. Pull the curtain around the patient to ensure privacy.
3. Open glove packet for the doctor.
4. Pull covers to bottom of bed and drape the patient.
5. Have the patient lie on her back, knees up, soles of feet together, and legs flexed apart. Help her to relax.
6. Cleanse the vulva with a bacteriostatic agent.
7. The doctor, nurse, or midwife puts on a glove and inserts the examining fingers into the vagina and ascertains the dilatation, station, effacement, and presenting part.
8. If the doctor wishes to rupture the membranes, open up the **amnihook** (membrane hook). Put a protective pad under the patient's hips to absorb the fluid.
9. Check the fetal heart tones after the examination.
10. Cleanse the external genitals of the patient with a bacteriostatic agent after the examination.
11. If the doctor has ruptured the membranes, tell the patient that she must now remain in bed.
12. Inform the patient that she will have leakage from time to time. Slip a protective pad under her hips and have others available for use.

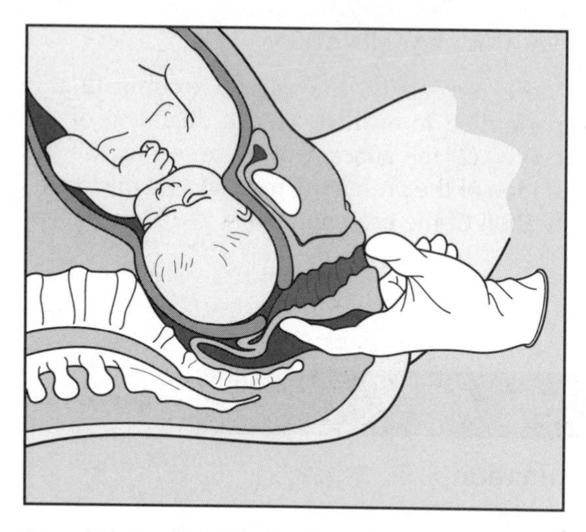

Figure 11–4 *Rectal examination of patient in labor*

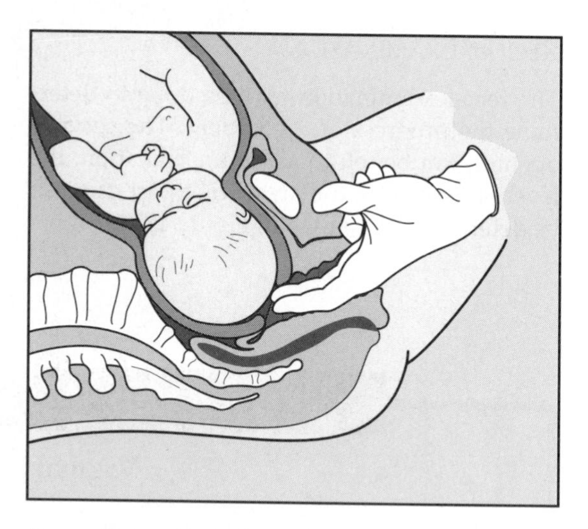

Figure 11–5 *Vaginal examination of patient in labor*

It is also performed when **amniotomy** (physical rupture of the bag of waters) is required.

PERINEAL PREPARATION

Perineal preparation used to involve perineal shaving and cleansing to remove the pubic, perineal, and anal hair in preparation for delivery of the infant. Recent studies, however, have demonstrated that the infection rate is lower among women who have not been shaved; shaving can nick or irritate the skin, leaving openings for bacteria. A complete perineal shave is rarely performed in today's obstetrical practice. Many physicians require no perineal preparation other than cleansing before an episiotomy. Some require only a **miniprep** (shaving anal and perineal area only). Perineal preparation serves to (1) make repair of the episiotomy easier, (2) ensure quicker healing and cleanliness of the area after delivery, (3) help prevent infection of the episiotomy, and (4) allow a better view during labor. For women with very long perineal hair, a scissor clip can be used as an alternative to shaving.

ENEMA

If the membranes have not ruptured, an enema may be ordered by the physician to empty the rectum and prevent contamination during delivery or to stimulate uterine contractions. With a multipara, the enema usually is not given if the first stage of labor is well advanced because it hastens labor.

CATHETERIZATION

It is essential that the patient void during labor. If other measures to encourage voiding fail, catheterization may be necessary. A distended bladder may hinder labor and cause a slight abrasion, which favors bacterial growth and cystitis.

POSITIONS FOR THE FIRST STAGE OF LABOR

A change of position during the first stage of labor can not only make a woman more comfortable, but can also enhance the progress of

PROCEDURE

Catheterization

Purpose: Catheterization is done to empty the bladder if the patient is unable to void. A distended bladder may hinder labor by preventing the head from descending and contributes to the patient's discomfort. Overdistention may cause stretching of the bladder so that a slight abrasion occurs, which favors bacterial growth and cystitis.

Equipment:

- Disposable catheterization set
- Disposable sterile gloves
- Adequate lighting
- Sterile sheet
- Sterile towels
- Zephiran or Betadine solution
- Cotton balls
- Lubricant

Procedure:

1. Explain the procedure to the patient.
2. Have the patient lie on her back with her legs up, apart, and flexed.
3. Screen the patient, and cover her with a bath blanket, exposing only the perineal area.
4. Arrange for a bedside light (a relaxed patient and good light are important to a successful catheterization).
5. Wash hands and open the tray.
6. Pour Zephiran or Betadine solution over the cotton balls.
7. Put on the sterile gloves.
8. Place a sterile sheet under the patient's buttocks.
9. Drape the patient with sterile towels.
10. Squeeze lubricant on clean area of tray.
11. Gently expose the meatus by holding the labia open with left hand, Figure 11–6.
12. Cleanse the perineal area, using a cotton ball for one downward stroke, and discard into box. Use last cotton ball for cleaning the urinary meatus. (Squeeze excess solution out of cotton ball.)
13. Pick up catheter with right hand about 3 to 4 inches from tip; lubricate tip of catheter.
14. Gently insert the catheter into the urinary meatus until urine flows through the tubing. Ask the patient to take deep breaths through her mouth. If there is any difficulty in locating the meatus, ask for assistance.
15. Hold catheter in place with left hand and place specimen bottle at end of catheter to obtain a sterile specimen. Allow excess urinary flow to collect in the large portion of the catheterization tray.

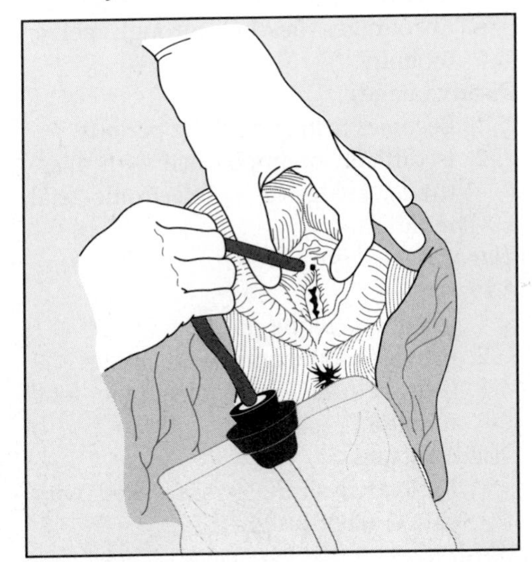

Figure 11–6 *Meatus made visible by separating the labia in order to insert catheter*

labor. Some standard positions and their advantages and disadvantages follow.

Standing or standing and leaning forward, Figure 11–7

Advantages

1. Takes advantage of gravity during and between contractions.
2. Contractions are less painful and more productive.
3. Fetus is well-aligned with angle of pelvis.
4. May speed labor.

Disadvantages

1. Becomes tiring after long periods.
2. May not be possible with anesthesia.

Walking

Advantages

1. Takes advantage of gravity.
2. Contractions are often less painful and more productive.
3. Fetus is well-aligned with angle of pelvis.
4. May speed labor.
5. May relieve backache.
6. Encourages descent through pelvic mobility.

Disadvantages

1. Becomes tiring after long periods.
2. Is difficult or impossible with anesthesia, analgesia, or electronic fetal monitoring.

Sitting upright, Figure 11–8

Advantages

1. Is a good resting position.
2. Provides some gravity advantage.
3. Can be used with electronic fetal monitor.

Disadvantages

1. Prolonged sitting is associated with slower labor progress.

Semisitting

Advantages

1. Is a good resting position.
2. Provides some gravity advantage.
3. Can be used with fetal monitor.

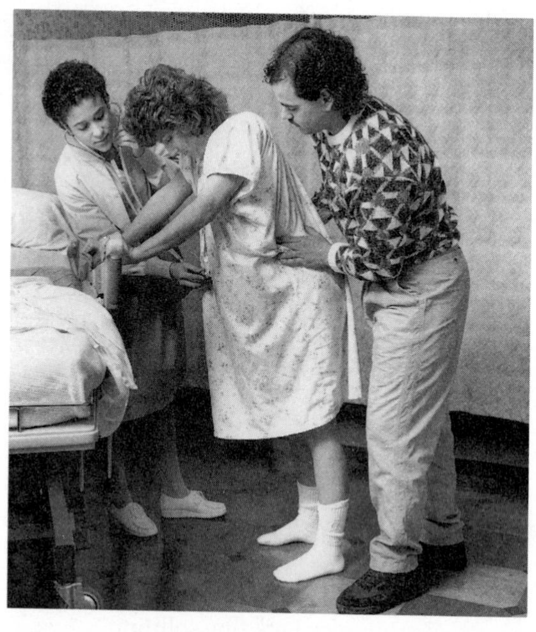

Figure 11–7 *Standing during labor takes advantage of gravity to help effacement and dilatation progress.*

4. Makes vaginal exam possible.

Disadvantages

1. Increases back pain.
2. May slow labor progress if used for long periods.

Hands and knees, Figure 11–9

Advantages

1. Helps relieve backache.
2. Helps baby in O.P. position rotate.
3. Allows pelvic rocking.

Disadvantages

1. Is uncomfortable and tiring for long periods.
2. May interfere with external monitoring.

Side-lying

Advantages

1. Is a good resting position.
2. Is convenient for intervention.
3. Helps lower elevated blood pressure.
4. Is safe if pain medications have been used.
5. Increases blood flow to placenta.

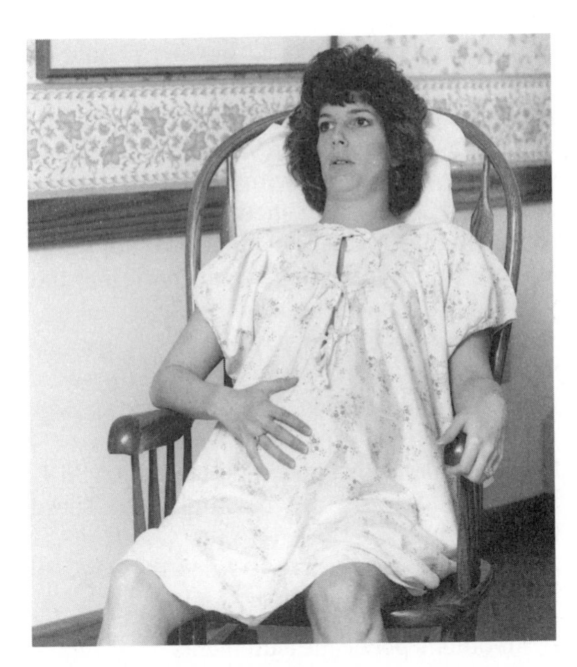

Figure 11–8 Sitting during labor aids in focusing and reflexing through each contraction.

Disadvantages
1. Contractions may be less effective and longer.
2. Is inconvenient for vaginal exams.

Squatting

Advantages
1. Takes advantage of gravity.
2. Relieves backache.

Disadvantages
1. Becomes tiring after long periods.

Back-lying

Advantages
1. Is convenient for caregiver, for procedures, and for vaginal exams.
2. Is restful.

Disadvantages
1. May cause supine hypotension.
2. Increases backache.
3. Labor contractions found to be longest, most painful, and least productive in this position.

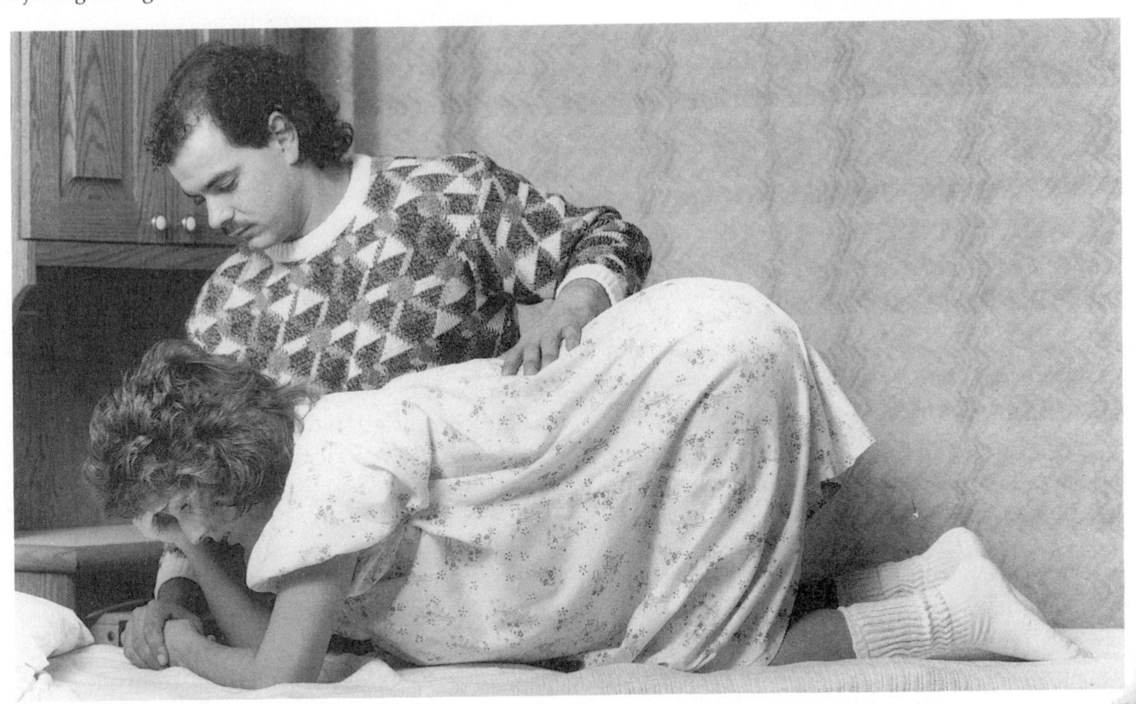

Figure 11–9 The hands-and-knees position may reduce backache and help an occiput posterior baby rotate.

ABNORMAL SIGNS

While observing the patient in labor, the nurse must constantly be alert to indications that labor is not progressing normally. The nurse must report the following signs immediately to the physician:

- abnormal vaginal bleeding with pain
- irregular, too fast, too slow, or absent fetal heart tones
- cessation of contractions after labor has begun
- a rise in blood pressure
- rigid uterus after contractions
- severe headaches and dizziness
- passage of **meconium-stained fluid**
- prolapse of the umbilical cord

PROLAPSED CORD

When the umbilical cord lies beside or below the presenting part, it is called a **prolapsed cord**. Although an infrequent complication, it is significant because of the high fetal mortality rate. It occurs more frequently with breech presentations than with cephalic presentations. Compression of the umbilical cord between the presenting part and the maternal pelvis reduces or cuts off the blood supply to the fetus, and the baby may die.

Immediate diagnosis is most important. The only ways to diagnose a prolapsed cord are by seeing the cord outside the vulva or by feeling the cord during a vaginal examination. It may be diagnosed whenever the presenting part does not fit closely in the inlet of the pelvis and fails to fill it. The cord may occupy one of three positions: it may lie beside the presenting part at the pelvic inlet; it may descend into the vagina; or it may pass out of the vagina.

The longer the cord, the more apt it is to prolapse. If the cord is seen at the vaginal entrance during labor, the nurse should place the patient in the knee-chest position and notify the physician at once. No time should be wasted. If this position is not possible, help the patient to turn onto her side, and place pillows under her hips. If the cord is visible, the nurse should keep it moist with sterile wet saline dressings. Special care should be taken not to compress the cord. The nurse should never attempt to put a prolapsed cord back into the vagina.

RAPIDITY OF LABOR

Many factors affect the rapidity with which labor and delivery are accomplished. These factors include:

- size of the baby
- position of the baby
- mother's pelvic measurements
- rupture of the membranes
- muscle tone of mother's cervix
- quality of the contractions
- relaxation of the patient
- effect of medication on the patient
- whether the patient is primipara or multipara (the multipara generally completes labor faster)

STIMULATION OF LABOR

The physician may **induce** (cause) labor if complications of pregnancy have occurred. Such complications include preeclampsia or PIH, a marginal placenta previa, a mild placenta abruptio, diabetes, and hydramnios. Other indications that the physician considers are: fetal distress, the Rh factor, a multipara with a history of short labors, and a past-due (42 plus weeks gestation) baby. The simplest method of inducing labor is to rupture the membranes (amniotomy). In some cases, it may be necessary to administer medication to induce labor. If complications jeopardize the health and safety of the mother and baby, a cesarean section may be necessary.

One of the main problems in inducing labor is an unripe cervix. **Prostaglandin** (a substance that causes contraction of smooth muscles) placed close to the cervix has been shown to be effective in ripening the cervix, and sometimes as an initiator of active labor. Prostaglandin brings about biochemical changes in the cervix that result in softening, and it stimulates the uterus to contract gently. This action leads to retraction and partial dilatation of the cervix.

If the cervix is soft but the uterus is not contracting sufficiently to cause labor to progress, an **oxytocic** drug may be given, usually Pitocin or Syntocinon. This medication increases the strength and frequency of contractions. It is usually administered through intravenous drip but can be given by an intramuscular injection or in tablet form. Induction is necessary to cause the onset of labor when the membranes have ruptured and contractions have not begun. Augmentation (increasing) is necessary if contractions are not strong enough to cause the cervix to dilate and efface once labor has actively begun.

NURSING CARE DURING THE FIRST STAGE OF LABOR

During the early part of labor the patient may be out of bed if the membranes have not ruptured. Food may or may not be given, depending on the progress of labor and the doctor's orders. Ice chips or a clean, wet washcloth to suck on can be substituted for water to relieve a dry mouth, but a record of fluid intake and output should be kept. The father or labor coach may wish to participate in some of these comforting activities. If a couple has attended prepared childbirth classes, they may wish to proceed through labor using their learned techniques of relaxation and breathing exercises. The nurse's role remains one of support, close observation, and informing the couple of how the labor is progressing. Refer to Figure 11–10.

Bed linen is replaced as necessary. Emotional support to keep the mother-to-be as relaxed and comfortable as possible is important for labor to progress actively through this stage. If the father is not with the patient, the nurse's role becomes even more important.

The nurse should explain the examinations and procedures required during the first stage of labor. The patient will be more relaxed and more willing to accept these treatments and procedures when she knows what to expect. See Figure 11–11 (page 205). Specific nursing care includes the following:

- Encourage the patient with comfort, cheerfulness, and empathy. Give assurance of the progress she is making.
- Observe the character of the patient's contractions: frequency, duration, intensity.
- Observe the presence of show. In good amounts, show denotes rapid progress. The color of show usually changes from pink to red as progress is made.
- Check the pulse. If the pulse is over 100 beats per minute, the patient may be dehydrated.
- Check the blood pressure. Elevation may suggest PIH or preeclampsia. Report any abnormalities, and recheck frequently.
- Observe the fetal heart tones. The normal rate is 120–160 beats per minute. The rate decreases slightly during each contraction. Slowing or speeding of the fetal heart tones suggests distress if the rate does not return to the normal range between contractions.
    a. Report all abnormal signs immediately.
    b. Maintain accurate records.
- Urge the patient to void frequently. A distended bladder can be palpated above the symphysis pubis. Labor may be slowed by a distended bladder.

NURSING CARE PLAN: First Stage of Labor

PATIENT PROBLEM	GOAL(S)	NURSING INTERVENTION	RATIONALE
Slight contractions	The woman remains calm and relaxed with an understanding of what is happening to her body.	Mother usually feels elated at this time; help prolong this feeling through encouragement.	A woman's psychological attitude and ability to remain calm and relaxed have a great effect on her ability to cooperate during labor.
		Allow her to engage in quiet activities such as reading, playing cards, watching TV, or listening to the radio.	Pursuing familiar activities will help promote relaxation.
		Avoid bustling preparations, noises, whispering, and rattling of utensils.	
		If the membranes are intact, permit the patient to walk about and to shower if she wishes.	
Thirst	Thirst is satisfied without compromising health.	Permit fluid intake until contraindicated.	Adequate intake of fluids prevents dehydration.

Figure 11–10 *Nursing care plan for discomfort during the first stage of labor (Adapted from* Maternal and Child Health, *Littlefield, Adams & Co.)*

PATIENT PROBLEM	GOAL(S)	NURSING INTERVENTION	RATIONALE
Backache	Back pain is reduced or alleviated.	Put pressure on the small of mother's back, or try rubbing her lower back briskly. Advise the patient that pelvic rocking or arching of her back may help alleviate the backache.	These maneuvers offer counterpressure to the force that the baby is exerting on the back as it descends into the pelvis.
Profuse perspiration	Woman feels comforted and comfortable.	Wash patient's hands and face with cool water.	Offers comfort through "therapeutic touch" and may help relax her.
Fear and anxiety	Information helps to reduce woman's concerns.	Reassure the parents; encourage the father to provide mother with emotional support and keep him informed of the progression of labor.	Such emotional support will help prevent the fear-tension-pain syndrome. Father can help to reassure the mother if he is informed.
Fear of anesthesia	Fear is reduced with explanation and understanding.	Explain the effect of the agent to be used prior to administration. Use a quiet, reassuring voice.	Prior knowledge will help allay anxiety.

Figure 11–10 *continued*

PATIENT PROBLEM	GOAL(S)	NURSING INTERVENTION	RATIONALE
Full bladder	The bladder is emptied routinely and monitored for distention.	Encourage the patient to void every 3 or 4 hours. If catheterization is necessary, insert the catheter between contractions.	A full bladder could interfere with the normal progress of labor.
Irritability	Symptom is accepted as a normal part of labor.	Accept any expression of irritability cheerfully. Explain to the mother and father that an irritable reaction is normal during labor.	The mother needs to feel supported and "accepted" during labor. Increased irritability often indicates that the first stage of labor is nearly ended.

Figure 11–10 continued

- Record the fluid and food intake.
  a. Liquids may be given up to about four to six hours before delivery, depending on the type of anesthesia to be administered.
  b. Good fluid balance forestalls dehydration and exhaustion. The physician may order an IV in case of long labors.
- Help the mother to remain as relaxed as possible.
- Watch for signs of the second stage of labor. Maintain close observation so that the physician can be notified in sufficient time before delivery.
- When delivery seems imminent or when the perineum begins to bulge and the head of the fetus can be seen, take the patient to the delivery room and prepare her for delivery. Hospitals with birthing rooms may simply need to have the equipment for the delivery ready and available for the doctor.

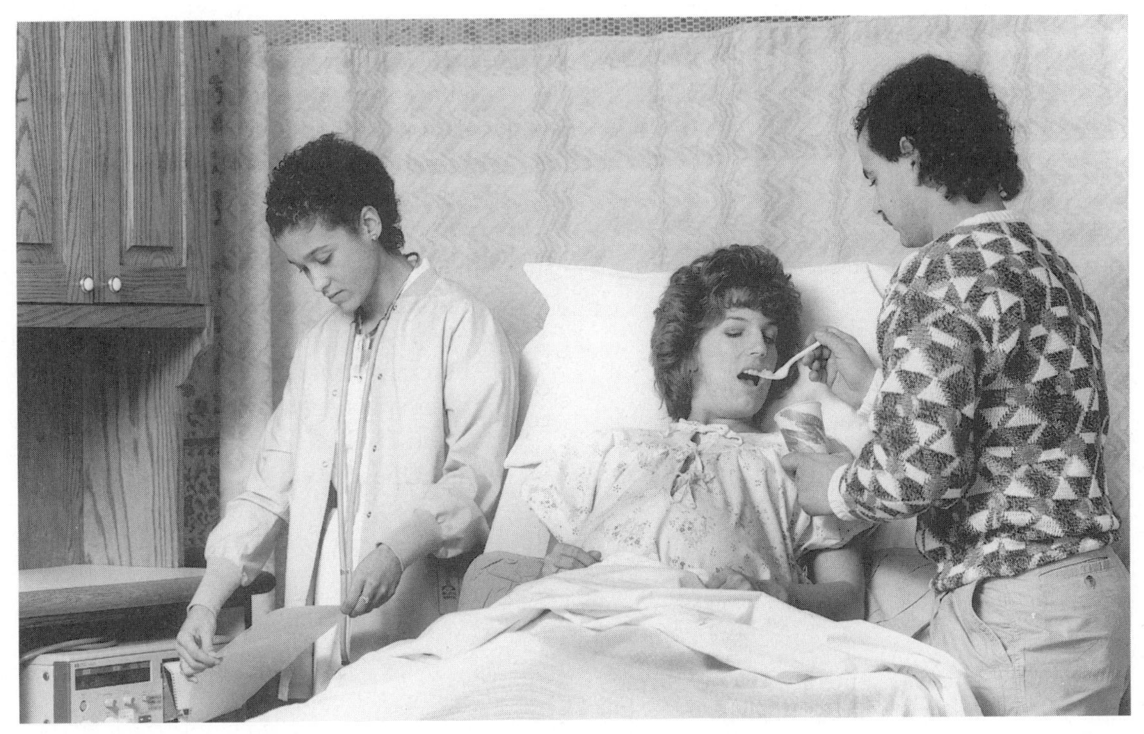

Figure 11–11 *The nurse keeps the couple informed regarding their labor process.*

REVIEW QUESTIONS

A. Multiple choice. Select the best answer.

1. Surgical rupture of the membranes is called
   a. amniotomy
   b. amniocentesis
   c. fetation
   d. augmentation

2. The normal rate of the fetal heart tone is
   a. 90–100 beats per minute
   b. 180 beats per minute
   c. 90–140 beats per minute
   d. 120–160 beats per minute

3. The blood pressure of a patient in uncomplicated labor is taken every
   a. 15 minutes
   b. half hour
   c. hour
   d. two hours

4. Temperature, pulse, and respirations of a patient in labor are taken every
   a. hour
   b. two hours
   c. four hours
   d. six hours

5. The term used to refer to the number of pregnancies that have continued through 20 weeks of gestation is
   a. gravida
   b. para
   c. prima
   d. parturient

6. The three phases of uterine contractions are termed
   a. increment, acme, decrement
   b. increment, intensity, duration
   c. frequency, duration, intensity
   d. onset, intensity, decrement

7. An increased pulse rate for the mother during labor may indicate
   a. fetal distress
   b. fatigue
   c. infection
   d. dehydration

8. Catheterization is sometimes done during labor if the patient is unable to void because
   a. a distended bladder may hinder labor by preventing the fetal head from descending and could lead to cystitis
   b. the laboring mother has no control over her bladder
   c. an overdistended bladder may rupture if not drained for the laboring mother
   d. overdistention of the bladder may cause severe backache

9. A vaginal examination is done to determine
   a. effacement and dilatation of the cervix
   b. station of the presenting part
   c. identification of the presenting part
   d. all of the above

10. Nursing care during labor includes
    a. recording fluid and food intake
    b. observing character of patient's contractions and checking vital signs
    c. observing fetal heart tones
    d. b and c only
    e. all of the above

B. Briefly answer the following questions.

1. List six signs that labor is not progressing normally.

2. Name four factors that may affect the rapidity of labor.

SUGGESTED ACTIVITIES

- State how you would determine whether the membranes are ruptured.
- List the major signs of fetal distress. Briefly describe diagnosis and management.
- Describe ways in which the father may be encouraged to participate in the labor and birth experience.
- Describe techniques that nurses and other support people can use to enhance the comfort of the laboring woman.
- With the assistance of the instructor and the permission of the patient, listen for fetal heart tones.

BIBLIOGRAPHY

Hamilton, P. M. *Basic Maternity Nursing*, 6th ed. St Louis, MO: C. V. Mosby, 1989.

Hawkins, J. W., and L. Pierfedeici. *Maternity and Gynecological Nursing*. New York: J. B. Lippincott, 1981.

Jenson, M. D., Benson, R., and I. Bobsk. *Maternity Care: The Nurse and the Family*, 3rd ed. St. Louis, MO: C. V. Mosby, 1985.

McNall, L. K. *Obstetric and Gynecologic Nursing*. St. Louis, MO: C. V. Mosby, 1980.

Oxorn, H. *Oxorn-Foote Human Labor and Birth*, 5th ed. E. Norwalk, CT: Appleton-Century-Crofts, 1986.

Pillitteri, A. *Maternal-Newborn Nursing: Care of the Growing Family*, 2nd ed. Boston: Little, Brown and Co., 1981.

Pritchard, J. A., MacDonald, P. C., and N. F. Grant. *Williams Obstetrics*, 17th ed. E. Norwalk, CT: Appleton-Century-Crofts, 1985.

Reeder, S., Mastroianni, L., Jr., and L. Martin. *Maternity Nursing*, 16th ed. New York: J. B. Lippincott, 1987.

Tucker, S. M., et al. *Patient Care Standards: Nursing Process, Diagnosis, and Outcome*, 5th ed. St. Louis, MO: C. V. Mosby, 1992.

CHAPTER

12

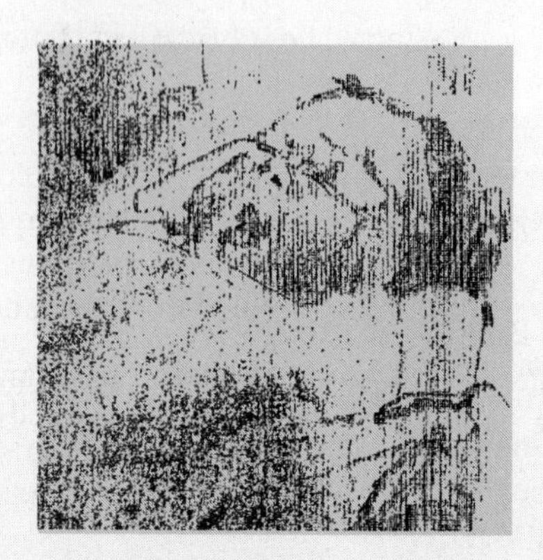

Fetal Monitoring

Objectives

After studying this chapter, the student should be able to:

- Define transducer.
- Explain the process of indirect fetal monitoring.
- Name three types of external transducers used for fetal monitoring.
- Explain the process of direct fetal monitoring.
- Describe the procedure for obtaining a fetal blood sample.
- Name the conditions that would indicate the need for fetal monitoring.
- Name the conditions that would indicate the need for a fetal blood sample.
- Read a fetal monitor chart.

Key Terms

- FETAL HEART RATE (FHR)
- TRANSDUCER
- INDIRECT METHOD
- PARTURITION
- TOCOTRANSDUCER
- UTERINE ACTIVITY TRANSDUCER
- PHONOTRANSDUCER
- DOPPLER TRANSDUCER
- DIRECT METHOD
- FETAL SCALP ELECTRODE
- ATRIAL CONTRACTION
- AV VALVE CLOSURE
- SEMILUNAR VALVE OPENINGS
- BASELINE
- VARIABILITY
- BRADYCARDIA
- TACHYCARDIA
- EARLY DECELERATION
- LATE DECELERATION
- VARIABLE DECELERATION
- OXYTOCIN CHALLENGE TEST (OCT)
- NONSTRESS TEST (NST)
- FETAL BLOOD SAMPLING

References to fetal observation for distress can be found in print as far back as the 1600s. In 1821, obstetrical auscultation was described as a potentially important diagnostic tool to detect fetal life and distress during labor. Attempts to record fetal heart tones were made by Pestolozza in 1891, Seitz in 1903, and Hofbauer and Weiss in 1908. Cremer used a vaginal electrode to obtain a fetal ECG tracing in 1906. During the late 1930s and 1940s, research into fetal heart rate monitoring increased. By 1964, the Doppler device was available. The first successful recording of a fetal ECG (electrocardiogram) through the abdomen was reported by Hon in 1957. The idea was then conceived to pass an electrode through the cervix and clip it to the fetal scalp in order to record the fetal ECG. Major improvements were made in 1972. Today, monitoring is done either externally or internally.

A major goal in obstetrics is to be able to assess the condition of the fetus during labor and delivery. Fetal monitoring is one method used for diagnosing fetal condition. In some hospitals, the only practical method for evaluating fetal status in the normal, uncomplicated pregnancy is regular listening with a fetal stethoscope or a Doppler. Accuracy of the count, however, depends upon the person counting. A **fetal heart rate (FHR)** greater than 160 or less than 120 beats per minute may indicate fetal distress.

If the fetal heart is listened to with a fetal stethoscope every 15 minutes for a duration of 30 seconds, only 3% of the available information is obtained. Modern technology permits monitoring of the FHR with a precision and endurance far exceeding the capabilities of the human ear. Newer methods of continuous auscultation (listening for sound within body cavities) are provided by ultrasonic devices that amplify the fetal heart sound. By using these newer approaches to evaluate the relationship of the FHR to uterine contractions, medical personnel can obtain reliable and predictive information about the fetus from the FHR. Even during contractions, when the possibility of FHR changes and fetal stress are greatest, the fetal monitor allows doctors to follow the FHR and thereby maintain fetal surveillance. Fetal monitoring has proven to be valuable in the management of high-risk pregnancies, where fetal tolerance of the stress of labor is low and the risk of fetal damage is high. Monitoring makes possible early detection of fetal distress due to umbilical cord compression, which is the most common cause of fetal distress during labor. It also helps in the early detection of abnormal uterine activity.

The following is a list of patient categories for which fetal monitoring is desirable when feasible. It is meant to be a guide in selecting patients for monitoring and represents a suggested order of preference by category. It should not be construed as a list of those who are the only patients to be monitored.

Category I

1. Abruptio placenta
2. Prolonged rupture of membranes
   a. with fever
   b. without fever
3. Amnionitis
4. Preeclampsia/PIH
5. Uterine inertia or dystocia problems
6. Fetal jeopardy or fetal distress (meconium staining alone included, unless associated with breech presentation)
7. 42 weeks or more gestation
8. Prolonged labor

Category II

1. Rh incompatibility
2. Breech position
3. Cardiovascular or renal disease (especially hypertension)
4. Diabetes
5. Other medical problems including suspected postmaturity without other complications
6. Prematurity without other complications
7. Multiparity

Category III

1. History of unexplainable death in utero
2. Hydramnios
3. Induction of labor for patient or physician convenience

Fetal monitoring is accomplished by either indirect methods using external transducers or direct methods using fetal scalp electrodes or an internal catheter. A **transducer** is a piece of equipment used to convert one form of energy into another form of energy. In medical terminology, a transducer receives energy produced by pressure or sound and relays it to another transducer as an electrical impulse. The second transducer can either convert the energy back to its original form or make a record of it on a recording instrument, as shown in Figure 12–1.

The sequence of electrical impulses that reproduce the fetal heartbeat makes it possible to detect the motion of fetal heart valves and the actual sound made by fetal blood. Fetal heart function can be monitored either indirectly or directly.

INDIRECT METHOD

The **indirect method** monitors the fetus without directly contacting it. During **parturition** (childbirth) the uterus contracts periodically. These contractions can be detected by changes in the body or by the forces exerted by the uterine muscle tissue. External geometrical changes may be detected by a transducer strapped to the patient's abdomen. Such a transducer is often called a tocotransducer, or uterine activity transducer. External transducers used in indirect fetal monitoring include the uterine activity transducer, the phonotransducer, and the Doppler transducer. Indirect monitoring usually takes place early in labor but can be used throughout labor.

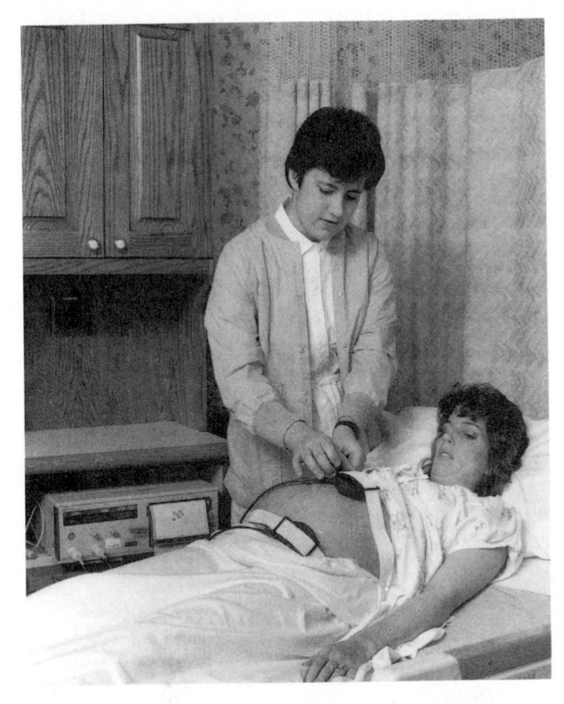

Figure 12–1 *A fetal monitor such as this records information received from some types of transducers. The transducer picks up a signal and transmits it as an electrical impulse that is recorded by the monitor.*

THE UTERINE ACTIVITY TRANSDUCER

The **tocotransducer (uterine activity transducer)** monitors uterine activity during labor and delivery by responding to the muscle tone in the abdominal wall, Figure 12–2. The transducer is placed on the abdomen in an area where the uterine contour changes the most during a contraction — usually a little to either side of midline. The transducer is strapped securely to the skin surface of the patient's abdomen; the strap must not be too tight for comfort. A record of the intrauterine pressure is transmitted by the transducer onto a chart.

PHONOTRANSDUCER

The **phonotransducer** (microphone amplification) technique offers the doctor a means of screening for possible complications early in labor, Figure 12–3. The phonotransducer is a combination of mechanical and electrical filtering of fetal heart activity. It is an effective means of obtaining reliable information in more than 80% of early labor cases.

The phonotransducer is the easiest transducer to apply. The area of maximum fetal heart sound is located by using a fetal stethoscope. The best FHR signal is usually heard through the back and shoulder of the fetus.

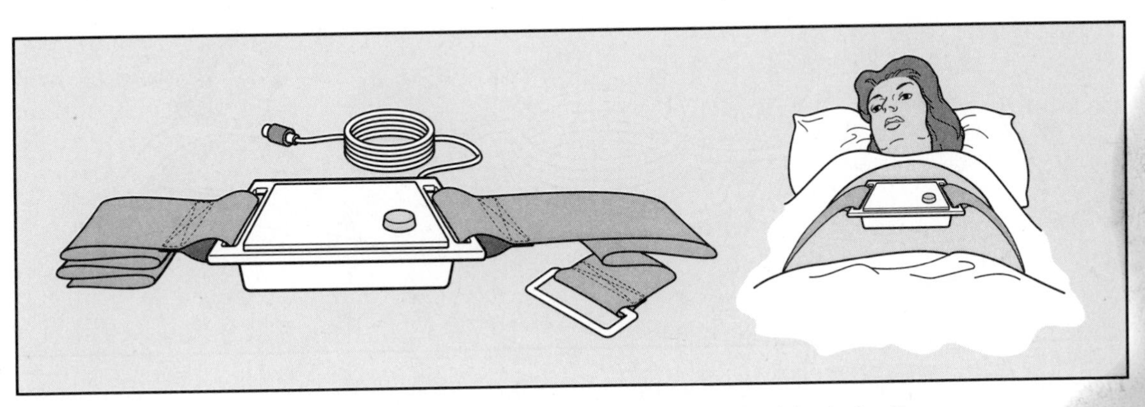

Figure 12–2 *The uterine activity transducer responds to the muscle tone in the abdominal wall.*

The phonotransducer is placed over the area and secured with tape or an elastic belt that comes with the unit.

THE DOPPLER TRANSDUCER

The **Doppler transducer** is an ultrasonic device that monitors the fetal heart rate by detecting the fetal heart movements, Figure 12–4. Its primary advantage over the phonotransducer is its relative insensitivity to talking, abdominal noises, and maternal heart sound. It provides excellent information on fetal heart activity. It can be used to localize the placenta.

The Doppler transducer is placed on the abdomen. After a waiting period of 10 to 20 seconds, which is needed for the amplifier to stabilize, it is manually moved along the contour of the abdomen until the spot is found where the fetal heartbeat is strongest. The transducer is then secured to this spot by tape or by the elastic strap supplied with the unit. The transducer must be repositioned if the patient or fetus changes positions.

Movement of the fetal body or of an extremity produces an abrupt, short, large-amplitude signal. Other detectable movement includes fetal hiccups and breathing and maternal bowel peristalsis.

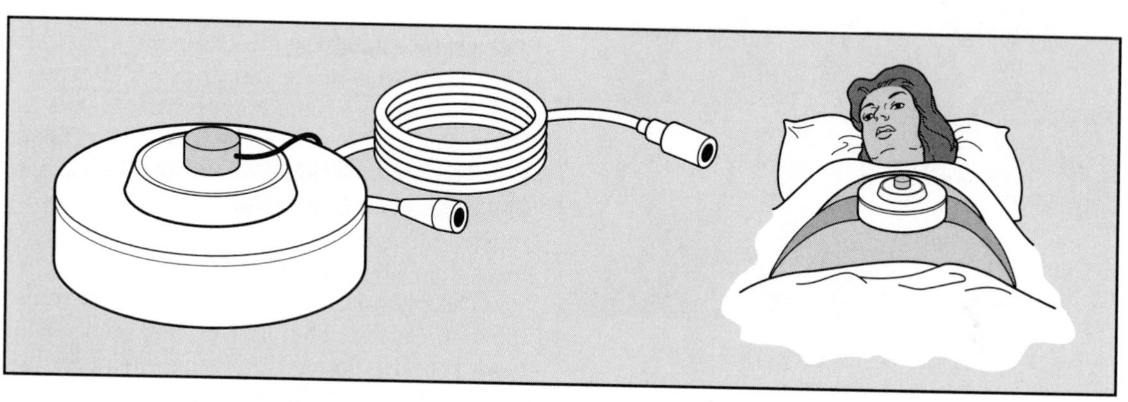

Figure 12–3 *The phonotransducer is placed on the abdomen over the spot of maximum fetal heart sound.*

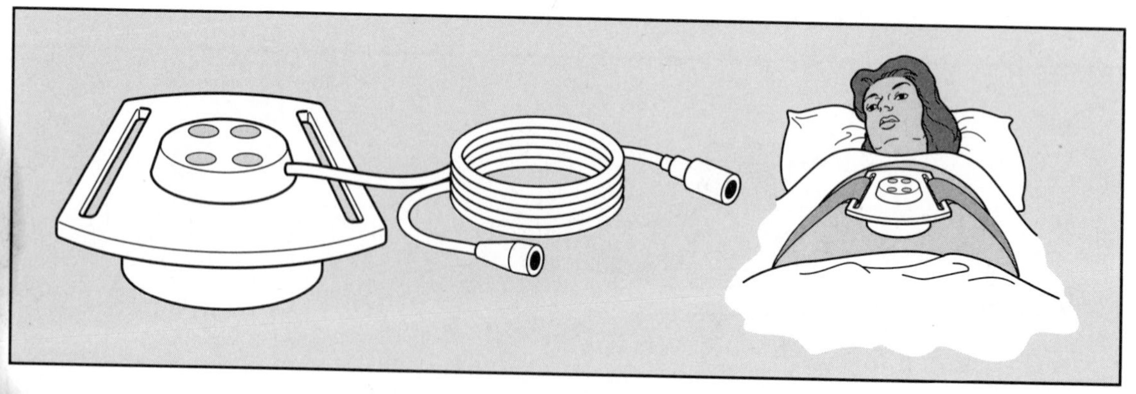

Figure 12–4 *The Doppler transducer uses ultrasound to detect fetal heart movements.*

Clinical situations in which the Doppler instrument has been found to be useful include early detection of pregnancy, diagnosis of fetal death in utero, detection of a remote fetal heartbeat, intermittent observation of the rate and rhythm of the fetal pulse, placental localization, diagnosis of multiple pregnancy, the differential diagnosis of vaginal bleeding during pregnancy, and fetal monitoring in the third trimester and during labor.

An incidental discovery attributable to use of the Doppler instrument is that the average fetal pulse rate is 170 to 179 in the 8th to 11th week of pregnancy and slows to an average of 149 by the 16th week.

DIRECT METHOD

The **direct method** of fetal monitoring involves the use of various types of ECG electrodes with or without an intrauterine catheter. The direct method is more reliable and exact than the indirect method. It permits monitoring of the fetal ECG both during and between contractions. However, it is limited because it requires skilled personnel to attach the electrode and place the catheter, see Figure 12–5. Also, the patient must have ruptured membranes, and the presenting part must be low enough to allow for the correct placement of the electrode. Direct fetal monitoring cannot be used with such complications as placenta previa and premature labor, nor can it be used for monitoring the second twin.

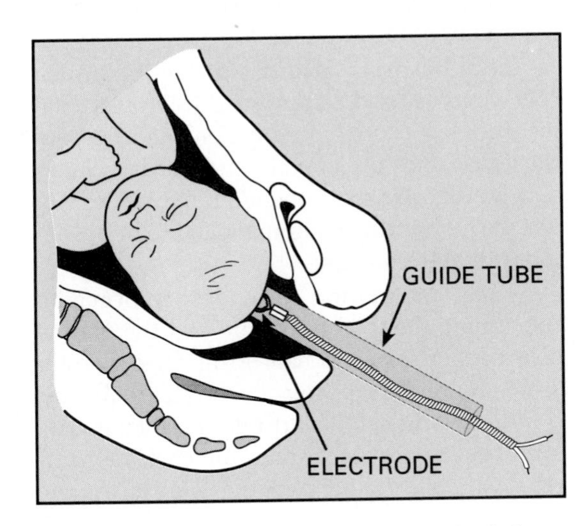

Figure 12–5 Attaching an electrode to the head of a fetus

INTRAUTERINE CATHETER

Within the uterus, uterine contractions cause pressure changes in the trapped fluid. A thin, flexible polyethylene catheter filled with distilled water may be used as a fluid trap to bring these pressure changes out to a transducer, which in turn translates the fluid pres-

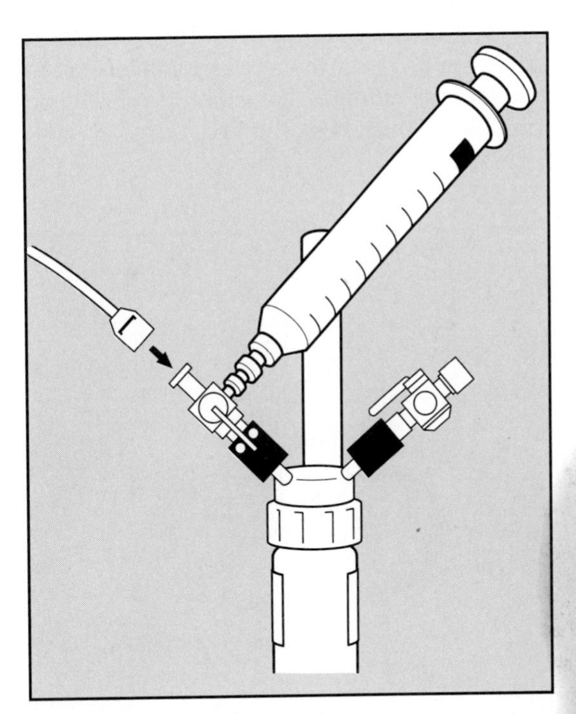

Figure 12–6 A syringe of distilled water is connected to the catheter.

sure into an electrical signal, Figure 12–6. This signal gives simple, reliable information on the beginning of the uterine contraction, its duration, and absolute strength.

Sterile technique is used when inserting the catheter. If a **fetal scalp electrode** is to be used with the catheter, the catheter is inserted before the electrode is attached, to minimize the possibility of dislodging the electrode during insertion of the catheter.

ECG ELECTRODE

The ECG electrode is attached to the presenting part of the fetus in order to directly monitor the fetal heart rate. Sterile technique is used when attaching the electrode to the fetus. The presenting part of the fetus must be clearly identified and must be far enough into the birth canal to allow for correct placement of the electrode, see Figure 12–7. The electrode is never applied over the face or fontanels of the fetus. If membranes have not ruptured, an amniotomy must be performed.

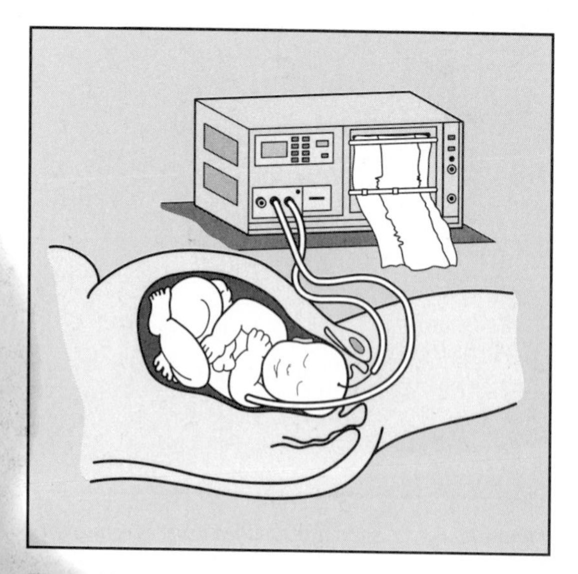

Figure 12–7 Insertion of the intrauterine catheter and the ECG electrode

INTERPRETATIONS

There are many companies that manufacture monitoring systems. Each system is accompanied by specific instructions for its use. Most companies send a representative to give operating instructions to the obstetrical staff.

Every obstetrical nurse should pursue the study of fetal monitoring and the interpretations of fetal heart rate patterns. The fetal heart signal has a two-phase, galloping rhythm with a rate of 120 to 160 beats per minute (b.p.m.). The first phase represents **atrial contraction**; the second reflects **AV valve closure** and **semilunar valve opening**. Pulsatile blood flow in the umbilical and other fetal vessels produces single-phase sounds that are higher pitched than the fetal heart signal. The umbilical sound is characterized also by frequent changes in location. The placental sound is complex, combining a windlike sound at the maternal pulse rate (70–90 b.p.m.) and the umbilical signal at the fetal rate (120–160 b.p.m.). The placental sound is generated only in the area of the umbilical cord insertion and cannot be detected over the remainder of the placenta.

Fetal heart rate patterns can indicate such conditions as head compression, uteroplacental insufficiency, cord compression, uterine contractions, and prolonged bradycardia. Study and practice are recommended to learn how to use the monitoring equipment and to be able to interpret the readings.

Fetal monitoring provides information concerning the fetal heart rate and the uterine contractions. The top half of the fetal monitor screen represents the fetal heart rate frequency. It indicates the fetal heart rate instantaneously with beat-to-beat recording, the baseline heart rate, variability, and periodic fetal heart rate changes.

The fetal heart rate **baseline** is usually 120 to 160 b.p.m. The degree of deviation from the baseline (called **variability**) reflects autonomic control. Good variability is 3% to 10% of the baseline. Excessive variability (15%) may be an early sign of distress or stress. Minimal variability is 3% of the baseline. Loss of beat-to-beat variability must be checked, as it is a sign of nervous system hypoxia. Minimal variability could also be an indication of prematurity or the presence of drugs in the fetal circulation. Minimal variability is especially likely to occur if tranquilizers, narcotics, and phenothiazines are given during labor.

A heart rate of less than 120 b.p.m. is fetal **bradycardia**. Moderate bradycardia in the fetus is 100 to 119 b.p.m.; marked bradycardia is 99 b.p.m. or less. Bradycardia usually clears up at the time of delivery, but it could be an indication of a congenital heart lesion.

Fetal **tachycardia** is a rapid heart rate, usually 160 or more beats per minute. It may be associated with maternal fever, dehydration and acidosis, fetal immaturity or prematurity, or mild fetal hypoxia. It is a serious sign when associated with any uteroplacental insufficiency pattern, severe cord compression, thick meconium stain, or loss of beat-to-beat variability of the baseline. Transient rises in fetal heart rate are referred to as accelerations; transient falls are decelerations.

The bottom half of the fetal monitor screen represents the uterine contractions. The increment, acme, and decrement of the contraction are shown as well as the baseline tone, frequency, duration, and intensity of the contraction.

DECELERATIONS OF FETAL HEART RATE

	Early Decelerations	Late Decelerations	Variable Decelerations
1. Shape	Uniform	Uniform	Variable
2. Association with baseline	None	Tachycardia; normal (120–160)	No change unless severe, then bradycardia
3. Timing	Early	Late	Variable
4. Physiology	Head compression	Uteroplacental insufficiency	Cord compression
5. Clinical input	Innocuous	Ominous	Variable
6. Duration	Usually <60 seconds almost never >90 seconds	Usually under 90 seconds	Usually <60 seconds; if longer, of clinical importance
7. Lower level of FHR	Not usually below 110; almost never below 100	Usually not under 110; if under 110, of grave importance and particularly if associated with loss of variability	Not unusual to go below
8. Effect of O_2	None	Positive (?)	None
9. Effect of position change	Little or none	Possible	Possible
10. Effect of atropine	Positive	None	Positive

Figure 12–8 *(Courtesy Jack M. Schneider, M.D.)*

ACUTE FETAL DISTRESS

Fetal heart rate patterns indicating acute fetal distress are: (1) late decelerations of any severity and (2) variable decelerations that last more than one minute, where the fetal heart rate has dropped to 60 b.p.m. or less, see Figure 12–8. Acute fetal distress during labor may be defined as fetal compromise related to the recurring stress of the uterine contractions or umbilical cord compression. Diagnosis of fetal distress and appropriate nursing actions are shown in Figure 12–9.

FETAL HEART RATE PATTERNS

Fetal heart rate patterns are a visible means of determining the condition of the fetus throughout labor. Although the majority of uterine contractions occur without fetal heart rate changes, the contractions do affect the fetus, umbilical cord, and intervillous (between villi) blood flow, Figures 12–10 and 12–11.

An irregularity of the baseline fetal heart rate appears to be an important indication of the maturity of the autonomic nervous system. An increased baseline change between uterine

NURSING CARE FOR FETAL DISTRESS

Diagnosis of Fetal Distress

Warning signs

Mild cord compression (variable deceleration)
Tachycardia of 160 b.p.m. or greater
Smooth baseline FHR (i.e., absence of the normal baseline FHR variability)

Ominous signs

Cord compression (variable deceleration) that lasts longer than one aminute and drops to less than 60 b.p.m. or less, progressively worsening

Uteroplacental insufficiency (late deceleration) of any magnitude, with or without tachycardia. If it is associated with a very smooth baseline FHR, the situation is serious. It is less serious if it is associated with normal baseline FHR variability.

Nursing Intervention for Fetal Distress

1. Change mother's position in order to relieve pressure on the umbilical cord and to correct maternal supine hypotension by taking the weight of the uterus off the vena cava.
2. Monitor FHR frequently to detect changes in pattern.
3. Decrease uterine activity by discontinuing administration of Pitocin. Abnormally strong contractions, or those that last for a long time, may impair placental circulation.
4. Administer oxygen to the mother at a rate of 6–7 L/min by a tightly fitted face mask.
5. Monitor mother's blood pressure.
6. Prepare for operative delivery. (If ominous FHR patterns persist for 30 minutes after the institution of the above measures, immediate termination of labor may be considered.)

Figure 12–9

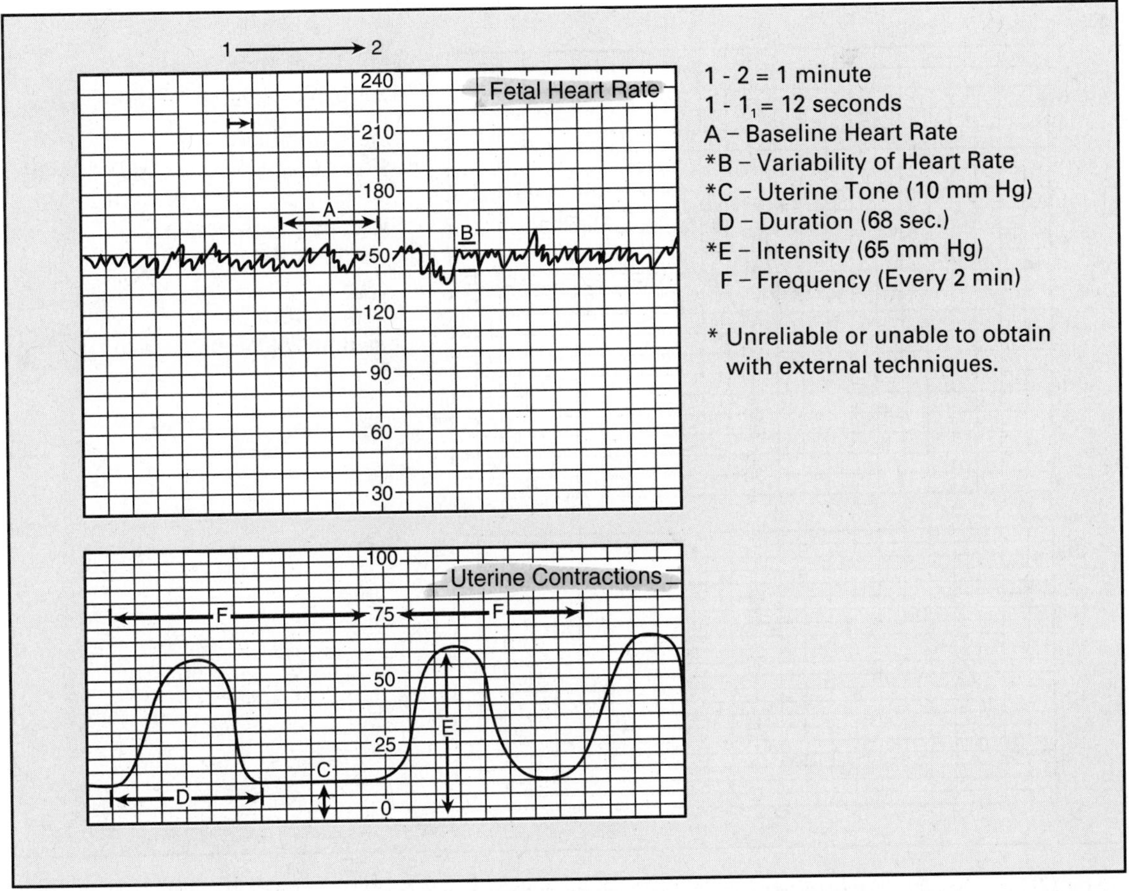

Figure 12–10 *The top half of the monitor tracing indicates beat-to-beat recording of the FHR, baseline heart rate, variability, and periodic FHR changes. The bottom half indicates the increment, acme, and decrement of uterine contractions as well as the baseline tone, frequency, duration, and intensity of the contractions.*

contractions may indicate fetal tachycardia. Fetal tachycardia is frequently associated with immaturity, maternal fever, or minimal fetal hypoxia. Tachycardia shown late in the contracting phase of the uterus may be an early sign of fetal distress. When it is associated with late or prolonged variable deceleration and especially if minimal irregularity is present, fetal distress is occurring. Persistent pure bradycardia of the baseline, not associated with other periodic fetal heart rate changes, has not been associated with depressed newborns, but pure bradycardia may be associated with congenital heart lesions. Sympathetic drugs such as adrenalin increase heart rate, while parasympathetic drugs decrease heart rate.

Acceleration occurs in about 30% of all labors. If the drug atropine is given, the occurrence is 80%. The accelerations are due to intermittent bursts of sympathetic activity and do not reflect any fetal jeopardy.

Decelerations tend to mirror the uterine contraction curve. As shown in Figure 12–12, there are three types of decelerations: **Early**

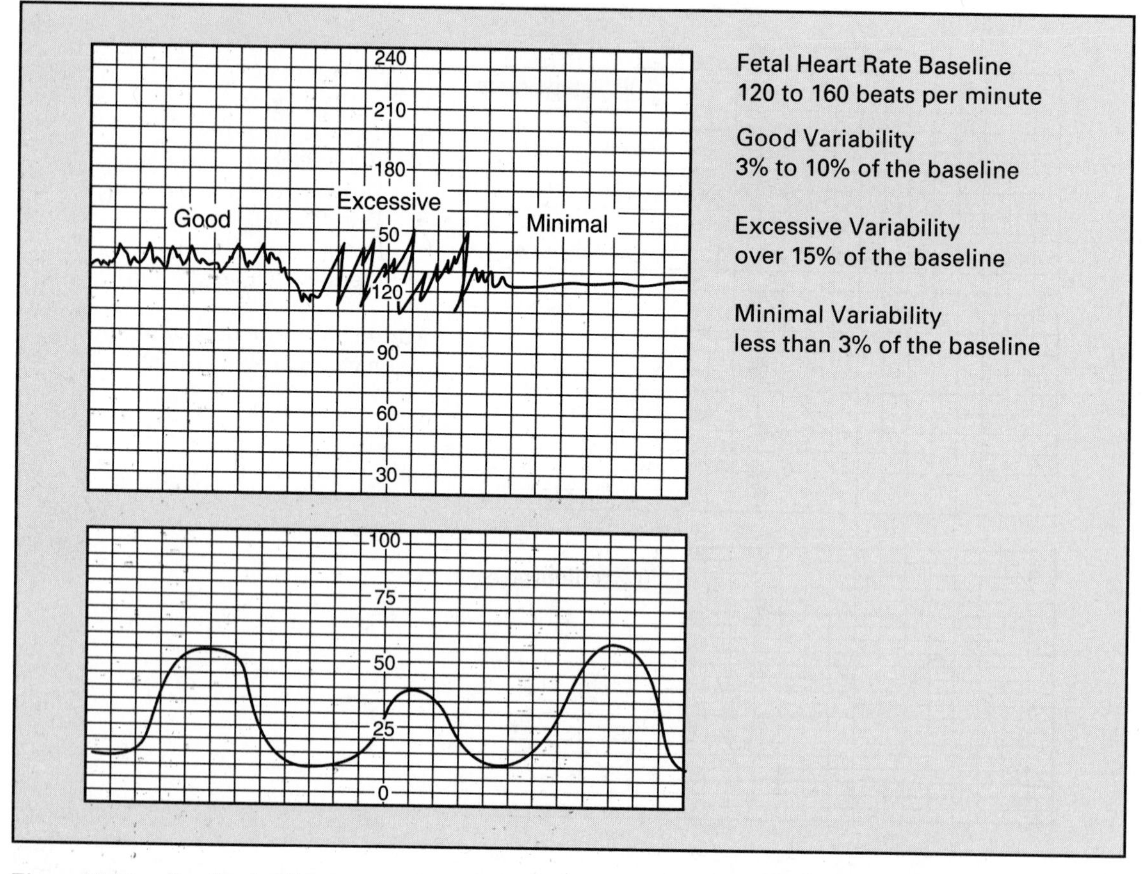

Figure 12–11 *Baseline fetal heart rate variability. Excessive variability or loss of beat-to-beat (minimal) variability may be a sign of fetal distress. The bottom portion of the chart indicates uterine contractions.*

deceleration from head compression; **late deceleration**, which denotes uteroplacental insufficiency and is always sinister; and **variable deceleration**, which is the most common pattern and denotes umbilical cord compression. There is no treatment for early deceleration and none is necessary. But late deceleration is always harmful. Late decelerations are characterized by:

- late onset in the contracting phase of the uterus
- consistent specific fetal heart rate pattern, uniform in shape
- fetal heart rate that usually does not fall below 120 b.p.m., but may fall to 60 b.p.m.
- duration that is usually less than 90 seconds
- baseline rate within normal or upper-normal range

Late decelerations are a probable indication of uteroplacental insufficiency. Administration of high concentrations of oxygen may modify the decelerations; or they may be partially modified by administration of atropine. Other causes are hypertension and too-frequent contractions.

A variable deceleration changes both in its shape and in the timing of its onset. Its shape does not reflect the smooth rise and fall of

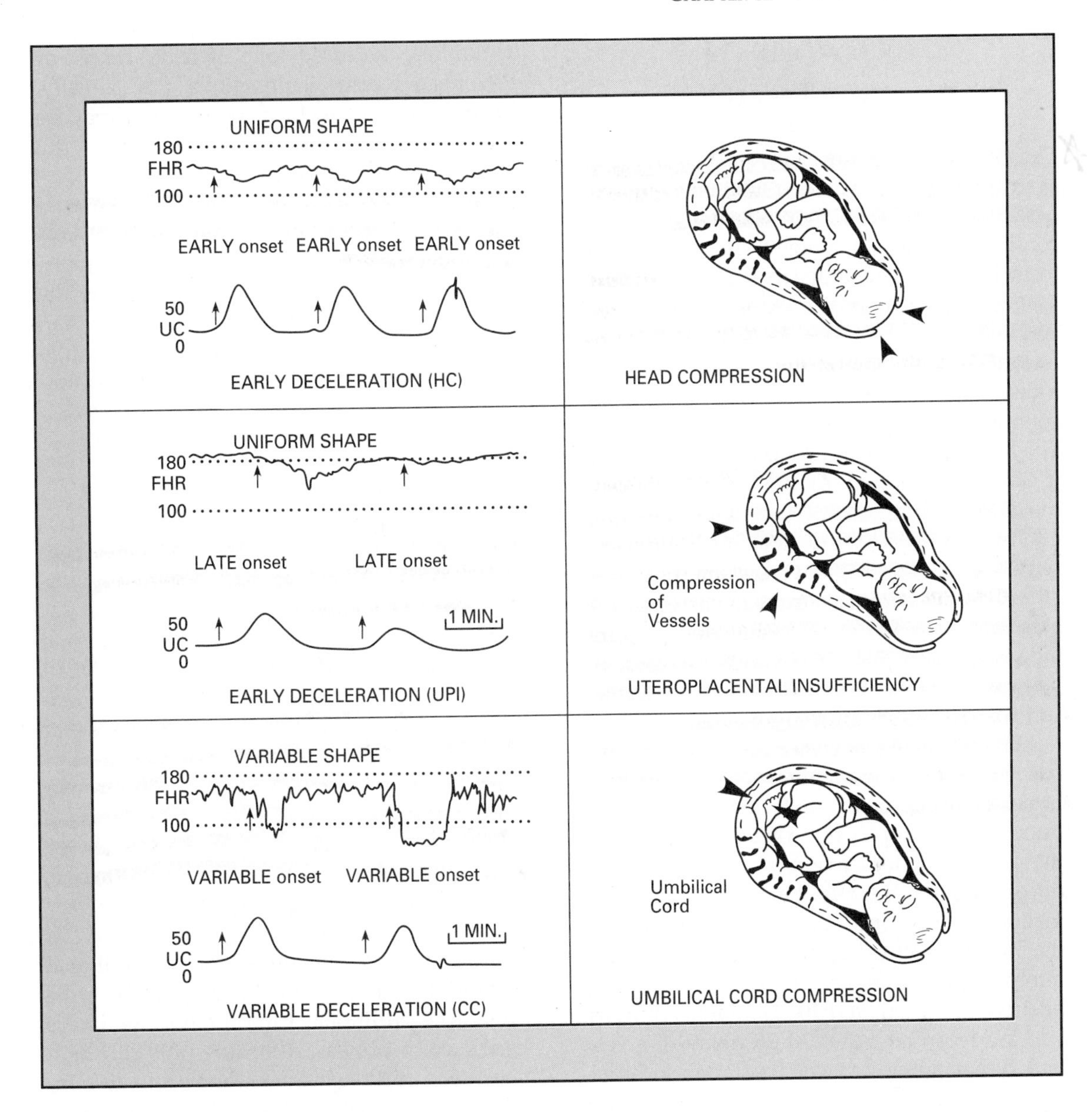

Figure 12–12 *Fetal heart rate patterns*

intrauterine pressure, and its onset shows no consistent relationship to the contraction. It is probably due to a compressed umbilical cord, and usually it is alleviated by the mother changing position. Fetal pH falls slightly in response to transitory variable deceleration but recovers within one to two minutes if there is no added injury.

OXYTOCIN CHALLENGE TEST (OCT)

The **oxytocin challenge test (OCT)** is a means of evaluating how well the placenta is nourishing and supplying oxygen to the fetus. The test consists of giving the patient intravenous oxytocin by controlled infusion sufficient to produce three contractions in a 10-minute period and simultaneously recording the fetal heart rate and uterine contractions with an external transducer. The reaction of the fetal heart to the contractions supplies the needed information. The test may be performed as early as 28 weeks if clinically indicated. Indications are: diabetes mellitus, PIH or chronic hypertension, preeclampsia, intrauterine growth retardation, Rh-sensitized pregnancy with meconium-stained amniotic fluid, maternal cyanotic heart disease, and history of previous stillborn. Contraindications are: prematurely ruptured membranes, placenta previa, previous cesarean section, or history of premature labors.

The oxytocin challenge test is not dangerous for either the mother or the baby, but labor could begin as a result. A uterine activity transducer and a Doppler transducer are placed on the patient's abdomen and secured. The transducers pick up the fetal heart rate and information on the contractions. They then transmit the information to a monitor, which records the information on a paper strip. A slow-drip IV of dextrose is started, and 10–20 minutes of heart rate are recorded. After 10–20 minutes, a second IV containing oxytocin is started in order to make the uterus contract. The rate of infusion is controlled by a pump, increasing the rate until three contractions occur in a 10-minute period. There is no way to predict how long this will take. When three contractions within a 10-minute period have been recorded, the intravenous is stopped and the test results are read.

(*Caution:* Avoid hyperstimulation; signs are uterine contractions closer than every 2 minutes, increased tone of contractions, or prolonged uterine contractions. Occasionally, 10 milliunits of oxytocin per minute may be necessary. Generally, the dosage does not exceed 2.5 milliunits per minute.)

If late decelerations develop, the test is called positive and suggests diminished uteroplacental reserve. If no late decelerations develop, the test is negative. If negative, the test may be repeated weekly. Tests other than negative (positive, suspicious, hyperstimulation, or unsatisfactory) can be repeated as clinically indicated.

NONSTRESS TEST (NST)

The **nonstress test** evaluates the fetal heart rate in response to natural uterine activity or to increased fetal activity. The significant correlation between the presence of fetal heart rate accelerations and the negative oxytocin challenge test led to the development of the nonstress test. In this test, a 10-minute period of fetal heart rate is evaluated. If the fetal heart rate reacts to fetal movements with two or more accelerations of at least 15 b.p.m. above the baseline and lasts at least 15 seconds, an oxytocin challenge test need not be performed, Figure 12–13. The length of the test may vary in different hospitals. If the nonstress test is nonreactive and remains so for an additional 20 minutes, an oxytocin challenge test may be done. The additional time for nonreaction is necessary to prevent recording only during a fetal sleep cycle, which can last up to 20 minutes. If the nonstress test is suspicious, it is repeated in 24 hours, see Figure 12–14.

The value of the nonstress test is twofold. First, it is a simpler test than the oxytocin challenge test and requires less time. Thus, it represents an economic saving to the hospital. Second, when administration of oxytocin is inadvisable, the nonstress test provides a noninvasive means of evaluating the fetus. If the woman is experiencing sufficient spontaneous

PROCEDURE

Oxytocin Challenge Test

Purpose: The oxytocin challenge test is done to determine how well the placenta is performing its function of feeding and supplying oxygen to the fetus.

Equipment:

- Fetal monitor
- Uterine activity transducer and a Doppler transducer or abdominal ECG or phonotransducer
- Blood pressure equipment
- Slow-drip IV of dextrose
- IV solution containing oxytocin
- IV pump

Procedure:

1. Place patient in semi-Fowler's position to prevent supine hypotension.
2. Check blood pressure every 10 minutes to avoid supine hypotension.
3. Strap transducer to the patient's abdomen.
4. Obtain a baseline FHR (noting rate, variability, and so on) and uterine contraction pattern, if any, for 10 minutes prior to oxytocin infusion. If three contractions are obtained within this 10-minute period with interpretable FHR, it is not necessary to give oxytocin.
5. Start oxytocin, via IV pump, at rate ordered by the doctor.
6. Increase oxytocin every 20 minutes until contractions are three in 10 minutes. If late decelerations are repetitive, regardless of uterine contraction frequency, it is not necessary to increase the oxytocin.
7. Discontinue oxytocin and record until uterine contractions diminish and become farther apart or until they stop completely.

Interpretation of Test:

1. Negative:
   a. No late periodic FHR changes.
   b. Usually shows FHR acceleration with fetal movement.
   c. Implies no placental insufficiency and fetus in good environment for at least one week.
2. Positive: Consistent and persistent late decelerations of FHR occurring repeatedly with most contractions even if frequency is less than three in 10 minutes.
   a. Usually shows absence of FHR acceleration with fetal movement.
   b. Implies placental insufficiency may be present and suggests need for intervention depending on fetal maturity.
3. Suspicious:
   a. Lack of FHR acceleration with movement is suspicious.
   b. Inconsistent but definite late deceleration that does not persist with continued contractions.
   c. Consider repeating the test in 24 hours or intervening if fetus is mature.
4. Hyperstimulation: Late deceleration with hyperstimulation suggests a need to repeat the test in 24 hours with lower doses of oxytocin. However, if no decelerations occur with hyperstimulation, the test is interpreted as negative.

A good recording of the FHR and uterine contraction is needed to ensure an interpretable test. If fetal distress is indicated by a positive test or prolonged bradycardia, take the following steps.

1. Stop oxytocin.
2. Increase plain IV fluids.
3. Turn patient to left side.
4. Give oxygen at 6–7 L/min.
5. Place in Trendelenburg position.
6. Check blood pressure frequently.

PROCEDURE

Nonstress Test

Purpose: The nonstress test is used to evaluate fetal heart rate in response to fetal or uterine activity when the oxytocin challenge test is contraindicated.

Equipment:

- External monitor
- Blood pressure equipment

Procedure:

1. Place the woman in semi-Fowler's position with a pillow under her right hip.
2. Take the woman's blood pressure and pulse every 10 minutes.
3. Strap the monitor to the woman's abdomen at a site where the FHR can best be heard.
4. Instruct the woman to press a button on the monitor each time she feels movement. The movement is then recorded on a tape as a dot or line.
5. If there is no movement within 20 minutes, stimulate the fetus by abdominal or vaginal examination.
6. Record fetal heart rate for an additional 20 minutes.
7. Note the date, time, gestational age of fetus and reason for the test on the tape; sign the tape.

Interpretation of the NST:

1. Reactive in 10 minutes: At least 2 accelerations of at least 15 b.p.m. and lasting 15 seconds or more with fetal movement.
2. Nonreactive: Any of the reactive conditions not met.
3. Suspicious: Fewer than two accelerations, 15 b.p.m., lasting 15 seconds with movement; or accelerations, but unassociated with movement.
4. Unsatisfactory: Recording inadequate for interpretation.

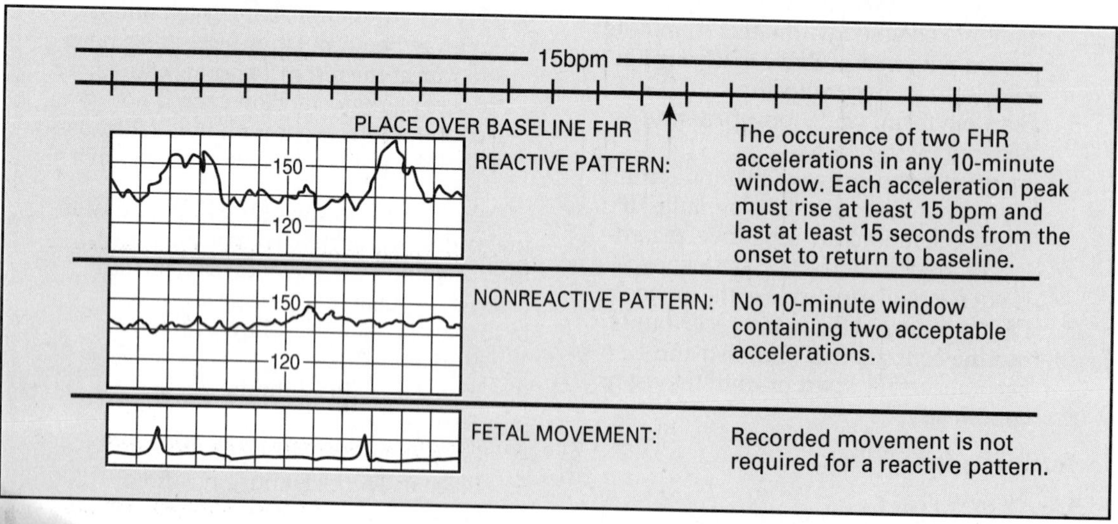

Figure 12–13 *Nonstress test for fetal heart rate patterns (Adapted from materials supplied by Corometrics Medical Systems, Inc.)*

PROCEDURE

Insertion of Intrauterine Catheter

The intrauterine catheter is inserted by the physician, but the nurse should be familiar with the procedure.

Purpose: An intrauterine catheter is inserted to determine pressure changes within the uterus by monitoring uterine contractions in order to assess fetal distress.

Equipment:

- Sterile gloves and drape
- Cleansing solution
- Catheter insertion guide
- Catheter
- Catheter adapter
- Syringe containing 5–10 mL of distilled H_2O
- Micropore tape

Procedure:

1. Perform a vaginal exam.
2. Place the middle and index fingers between the posterior cervix and the presenting part of the fetus.
3. Place the catheter insertion guide between the fingers.
4. Insert the catheter following the curvature of the pelvis. It must pass the presenting part of the fetus and enter the amniotic cavity.
5. Lower the catheter insertion guide so that its front end moves behind the presenting part of the fetus. Amniotic fluid will flow out if it is positioned correctly.
6. Insert the perforated end of the catheter into the catheter insertion guide to the mark indicated on the catheter. The catheter may be lowered to check for amniotic fluid, if necessary.
7. Remove the insertion guide when the catheter is properly positioned.
8. Connect the catheter to the stopcock using the catheter adapter.
9. A syringe containing 4–5 mL of distilled water is connected to the catheter by way of the stopcock. (*Caution:* Never use normal saline in the catheter.)
10. Flush the catheter with the distilled water to ensure there is no air in the catheter.
11. Turn off the stopcock.
12. Tape the catheter to the patient's thigh to avoid accidental displacements.
13. Place the transducer at a level even with the maternal xiphoid.

uterine activity (as often happens after an amniocentesis), the nonstress test might also be used as a contraction stress test without the use of oxytocin, Figure 12–15.

FETAL BLOOD SAMPLING

Fetal blood sampling is a method of determining fetal distress by analyzing a small sample of blood taken from the presenting part of the fetus. This procedure can be done during the course of labor if the cervix is dilated enough to allow withdrawal of fetal blood into a capillary tube from a small puncture in the skin of the presenting part of the fetus. The fetal pH blood values normally decline during the intrapartum period from 7.30–7.35 to 7.20–7.25. It is recommended that delivery be accomplished immediately if two successive determinations are below 7.20.

PROCEDURE

Internal Fetal Heart Monitor

Purpose: The purpose of the internal fetal heart monitor is to assess fetal distress by monitoring the fetal heart rate with the use of an electrode attached to the presenting part of the fetus. The procedure is performed by a physician with nursing assistance.

Equipment:

- Sterile gloves
- Leg plate coated with conductive gel
- Velcro strap
- Appropriate ECG electrode
- Drive tube
- Guide tube

Precautions:

1. Clearly identify the fetal presenting part. Do not apply the electrode over the face or fontanels of the fetus.
2. When removing the electrode, do not pull it from the fetal skin.
3. Use sterile technique.

Preparation:

1. Apply conductive gel to the metal surface on the back of the leg plate.
2. Place the leg plate on the inner upper aspect of the thigh.
3. Fasten leg plate with a Velcro strap.

Procedure:

1. Unpack and remove ends of electrode wires from between the drive and guide tubes.
2. Retract the drive tube and electrode one inch inside the guide tube.
3. Do a vaginal examination, and advance the guide tube between the examining fingers until it reaches the presenting part.
4. Hold the guide tube so that it is at a right angle to, and pressing firmly against, the presenting part.
5. Grasp the guide tube grip. Advance the drive tube and the electrode through the guide tube until the electrode reaches the fetus.
6. Maintain pressure against the presenting part and rotate the drive tube clockwise until slight resistance is met.
7. Attachment is indicated by resistance to further rotation and recoil of the drive tube, which usually occurs after one or two turns.
8. Release the locking device on the drive tube by slipping wires out of the slotted drive tube handle. Carefully slide the guide and drive tubes off the electrode wires.
9. Attach the other end of the electrode to the leg plate on the mother's thigh.

The strip chart and the rate meter on the monitor should show the instantaneous fetal heart rate. The patient's name, hospital number, position (of the presenting part), dilatation, date, onset time of monitoring, and reason for monitoring should be written on the recorded information. To remove the electrode, simply rotate the body or wires of the electrode counterclockwise. (*Caution:* Do not pull the electrode from the fetal skin.)

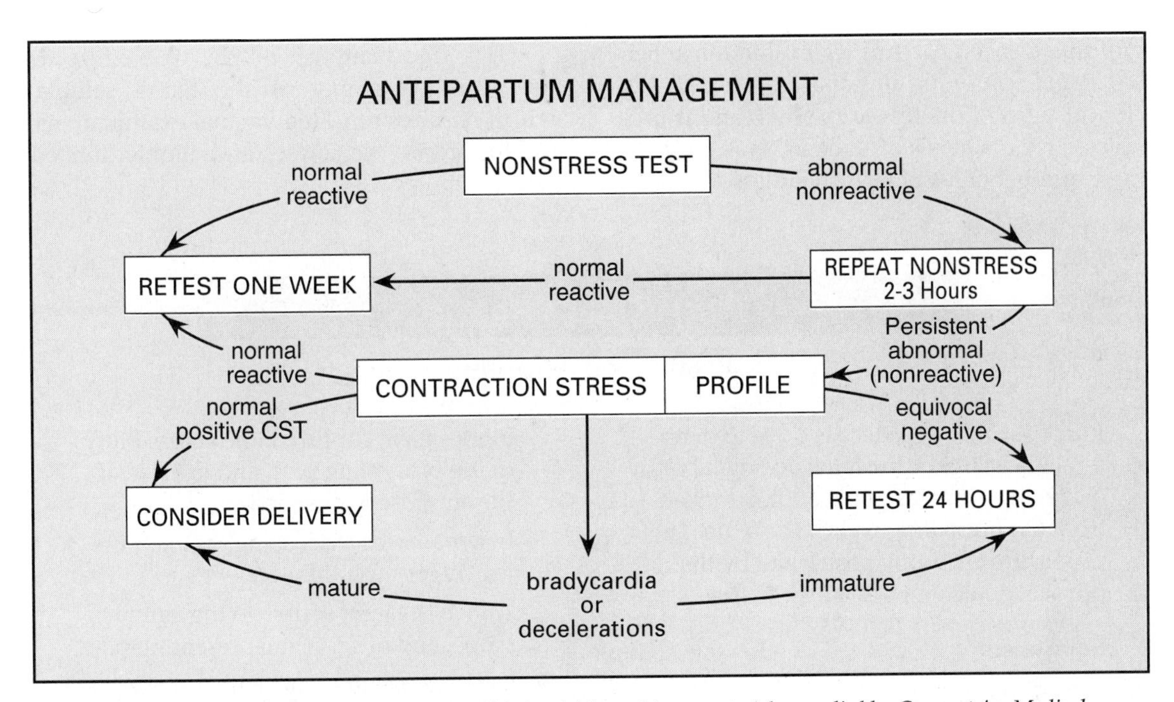

Figure 12–14 *Nonstress test to assess fetal well-being (Adapted from materials supplied by Corometrics Medical Systems, Inc.)*

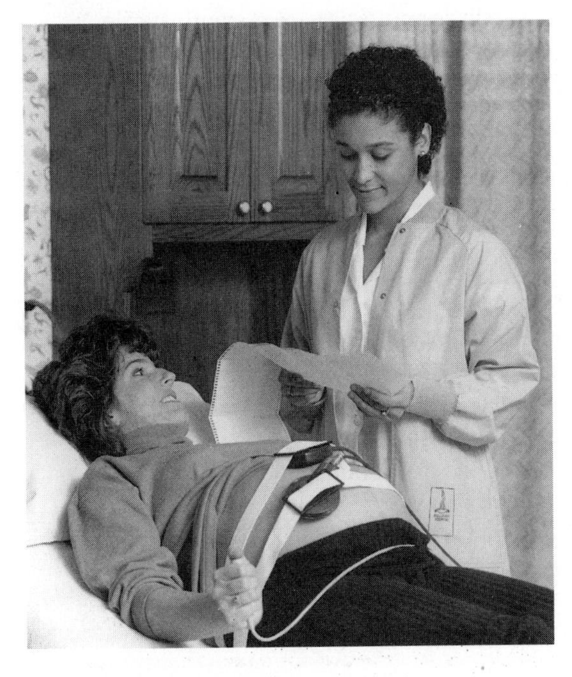

Figure 12–15 *Nonstress test*

Indications that a sample of fetal blood should be obtained for analysis include: (1) abnormal baseline fetal heart rate (under 120 or over 160 b.p.m.); (2) presence of late deceleration periodic heart rate pattern; (3) presence of severe variable deceleration periodic heart rate pattern; (4) loss of beat-to-beat heart rate variability; (5) inability to define type of deceleration pattern; (6) assessment of fetal glucose level, gases, and other values.

Before the procedure for obtaining the blood sample is performed, informed consent of the mother, and ideally the father, must be obtained. The position and station of the fetus must be determined. The presenting part of the fetus must be at least to the –2 station; dilatation of the cervix must be at least 2 cm. If the procedure is done transvaginally the membranes must be ruptured.

Fetal blood sampling has several advantages. It prevents unnecessary intervention; it indicates a need for further evaluation when blood pH values are unsatisfactory and other clinical signs of distress are absent; and it provides early diagnosis of acidosis, thus preventing a number of neonatal difficulties.

The disadvantage of the procedure is the actual obtaining of the blood sample, which requires repeated vaginal examinations, careful sterile technique, and highly refined skills.

PROCEDURE

Fetal Blood Sampling

Purpose: The procedure is done to determine the status of the fetus during labor by analyzing a small sample of blood taken from the presenting part of the fetus. The procedure is usually performed by the physician, who is assisted by a nurse.

Equipment:

- Sterile gloves
- Sterile tray with cover
- Amnioscope (device for looking inside the amniotic cavity)
- Light source for amnioscope
- Long-handled forceps for cotton balls
- Cotton balls or large, long swab
- Ethyl chloride and silicone ointment
- Handle for puncture blade
- Appropriate shallow, squared puncture blade (do *not* substitute)
- Long, heparinized capillary tube
- Transport tubing for capillary tube
- Magnetic stirring rod and magnet; sealing wax
- Ice tray

Procedure:

1. Place the patient in stirrups in lithotomy position or on her side.
2. Perform a vaginal examination. This is done to determine whether the membranes have ruptured, the accessibility of the presenting part, and the size of the amnioscope needed.
3. Insert amnioscope, using the examining finger for guidance.
4. Attach the light source to the amnioscope, and observe the presenting part.
5. Clean presenting part with a sterile cotton swab.
6. Apply ethyl chloride to the presenting part; remove any excess with sterile swab.
7. Apply silicone ointment to the area.
8. Puncture appropriate area with the fetal scalp blade.
9. Withdraw a sample of fetal blood from the puncture site with a heparinized capillary tube.
10. Mix the blood sample with a magnetic stirring rod in the capillary tube. Place the transport tubing in the ice tray.
11. Clean the puncture site with sterile cotton swabs. Apply gentle pressure for at least 90 seconds in order to stop the bleeding.
12. Observe the puncture site to determine if bleeding has stopped.
13. Analyze the blood sample immediately.

REVIEW QUESTIONS

A. Multiple choice. Select the best answer.

1. Slow heart rate of less than 120 b.p.m. is fetal
   a. tachycardia
   b. acceleration
   c. bradycardia
   d. cardiac arrest

2. Information on how well the placenta is nourishing and supplying oxygen to the fetus is obtained by the
   a. phonotransducer
   b. uterine activity monitor
   c. intrauterine catheter
   d. oxytocin challenge test

3. Direct fetal monitoring can take place
   a. any time after 28 weeks gestation
   b. early in labor
   c. only after the membranes have ruptured
   d. a and b

4. For a fetal blood sample to be obtained, the presenting part must be at least to the
   a. –2 station
   b. ischial spine
   c. +2 station
   d. ischial tuberosity

5. The phonotransducer is able to supply information on fetal heat rate by using
   a. recorded electrical impulses
   b. ultrasonic sound
   c. microphone amplification
   d. a gauge to record intrauterine pressure

6. Nervous system hypoxia may be indicated on the fetal monitor as
   a. excessive variability of heart rate
   b. minimal variability of heart rate
   c. heart rate of over 160 b.p.m.
   d. heart rate of less than 120 b.p.m.

7. The top half of the fetal monitor indicates
   a. fetal heart rate
   b. uterine contractions
   c. pH of fetal blood
   d. all of the above

8. The purpose of the intrauterine catheter is to determine
   a. whether meconium is present
   b. muscle tone in the abdominal wall
   c. fetal heart rate
   d. pressure changes within the uterus

B. Match the description in column I to the correct term in column II.

Column I	Column II
1. uterine contractions closer than every 2 minutes or prolonged contractions	a. acceleration
2. rapid heart rate or more than 160 b.p.m.	b. amnioscope
3. transient rise in fetal heart rate	c. deceleration
4. transient fall in fetal heart rate	d. hyperstimulation
5. device for looking inside the amniotic cavity	e. loss of beat-to-beat variability
6. minimal variability of fetal heart rate baseline	f. fetal tachycardia

C. Briefly answer the following questions.

1. What is a transducer?
2. Name three types of external transducers used for fetal monitoring.
3. Explain the direct method of fetal monitoring. What are its limitations?
4. List five of the most important reasons for performing fetal monitoring.
5. Name three indications for fetal blood sampling.
6. Define acute fetal distress.

SUGGESTED ACTIVITIES

- Arrange to have a representative of a company that sells fetal monitors visit the class and demonstrate the use of fetal monitors.
- With the aid of the instructor, practice reading fetal monitor strips.
- Under the supervision of the instructor, arrange with the obstetrical unit of a local hospital to observe the attachment of a fetal electrode or obtaining of a fetal blood sample.
- Make a chart indicating one type of fetal monitor, how it is applied, the condition that indicates its use, and the contraindications, if any.
- Define and indicate the significance of the following:
  - early deceleration
  - variable decelerations
  - late decelerations
  - prolonged decelerations

BIBLIOGRAPHY

Egansouse, D. "Electronic Fetal Monitoring." *JOGNN* 20(1):16–22, January-February, 1991.

Pritchard, J. A., MacDonald, P. C., and N. F. Grant. *Williams Obstetrics*, 17th ed. E. Norwalk, CT: Appleton-Century-Crofts, 1985.

Tucker, S. M., and S. L. Bryant. *Fetal Monitoring and Fetal Assessment in High-Risk Pregnancy*. St. Louis, MO: C. V. Mosby, 1978.

CHAPTER

13

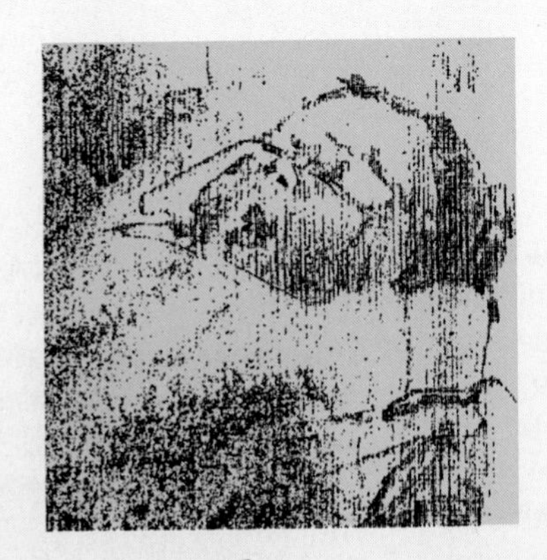

Pain Relief for Labor and Delivery

OBJECTIVES

AFTER STUDYING THIS CHAPTER, THE STUDENT SHOULD BE ABLE TO:

- STATE THE PURPOSE OF ANESTHESIA.
- DISTINGUISH BETWEEN THE ANESTHESIA GIVEN DURING CHILDBIRTH IN TERMS OF ADMINISTRATION, DESIRED EFFECT, AND UNTOWARD EFFECTS.
- NAME THE ADVANTAGES OF USING REGIONAL RATHER THAN GENERAL ANESTHESIA.

KEY TERMS

ANALGESIA
ANESTHESIA
TRANQUILIZERS
BARBITURATES
AMNESIAC
NARCOTICS
INHALATION AGENT
GENERAL ANESTHESIA
REGIONAL ANESTHESIA
PARACERVICAL BLOCK
CAUDAL ANESTHESIA
LUMBAR EPIDURAL BLOCK
SPINAL ANESTHESIA
SPINAL HEADACHE
SADDLE BLOCK
PUDENDAL BLOCK
LOCAL ANESTHESIA
FEAR-TENSION-PAIN SYNDROME

Although the modern philosophy of childbirth stresses the fact that it is a completely normal and natural process, there are occasions when medication to relieve pain is needed. It must be understood that any drugs taken by the mother before delivery also affect the baby. Some drugs produce a sleepy and lethargic baby; other drugs have little effect on the baby. Since the chief objective is to deliver a healthy baby with as little discomfort as possible for the mother, the choice of medication is left to the obstetrician.

The labeling of drugs used in labor and delivery must include a list of the known short-term and long-term effects that the drug can have on the mother and the child. This information must describe the effect the drug has on the duration of labor or delivery. The label also indicates whether forceps or other interventions or resuscitation of the newborn are likely to be needed. The effect the drug has on the later growth, development, and maturation of the child must be indicated. Labeling must include the effect the drug has on the mother's milk and how it can affect the nursing infant.

There is no drug that overcomes the discomfort of labor completely and yet is perfectly safe for both mother and baby. There are many drugs, however, that permit the patient to relax between contractions, thus conserving the patient's strength. Pain-relieving medications fall into two general categories. **Analgesia** is the relief of pain without total loss of sensation. A woman receiving an analgesic medication remains conscious. Although analgesics don't always completely stop pain, they do lessen it. **Anesthesia** refers to the total loss of sensation. Some forms of anesthesia cause a loss of consciousness, whereas others remove the sensation of pain from specific areas of the body while the woman remains conscious.

ANALGESIA

Analgesic drugs reduce the sensation of pain and are generally used in the first stage of labor. These include tranquilizers, barbiturates, amnesiacs, narcotic analgesics, and inhalation agents.

TRANQUILIZERS

Tranquilizers such as hydroxyzine hydrochloride (Vistaril), promethazine (Phenergan), and promazine (Sparine) are often used to relieve anxiety and to relax the patient. These drugs help to relieve tension without confusing the brain. They have little effect on the labor or the fetus, but should not be given when the baby is premature. Hypotension (lowered blood pressure) may be seen in the mother. They are particularly helpful for long labors if tension is building.

BARBITURATES

Barbiturates such as secobarbital (Seconal) and pentobarbital (Nembutal) are given to sedate the mother and produce sleep. Barbiturates do not relieve pain. If it is suspected that the mother is in false labor, she may be given a barbiturate so that she can go to sleep. Barbiturates, however, cross the placental barrier rapidly and are not handled well by the newborn. They are not used near the time of delivery.

AMNESIACS

Amnesiac drugs may be used throughout labor to induce loss of memory of pain. Scopolamine is an amnesiac that was used quite commonly in the past but is rarely used today. Scopolamine does not stop the pain sensation but it does alter thought processes.

Women who receive this drug feel all the pain sensation of labor but do not remember the pain later.

NARCOTIC ANALGESICS

Narcotic analgesics such as meperidine (Demerol) act to relieve pain. They also produce sedation and decrease anxiety. Narcotics have a depressant effect on neonatal respiration and so are not given close to the time of delivery. They also can have adverse effects on the mother. Side effects include respiratory depression, hypotension, nausea, and vomiting. They may also decrease the rate of cervical dilatation if given in excessive quantity early in labor.

INHALATION AGENTS

Inhalation agents such as nitrous oxide can be used during the first stage of labor to produce an analgesic effect. The gas is inhaled during the contraction and makes the mother feel lightheaded. It does not cause any significant respiratory depression or other side effects on the mother and baby and does not interfere with the uterine contractions or labor progress, unless used to excess. It can be administered by the patient herself after an explanation of its purpose and use. Although an effective analgesic during contractions, it is inadequate for delivery if difficult maneuvers such as forceps are planned.

ANESTHESIA

Anesthesia relieves pain at specific sources. It may be used in both the first and second stages of labor and during the episiotomy procedure and repair. Anesthesia can be administered as general anesthesia or regional anesthesia.

GENERAL ANESTHESIA

If used, **general**, or inhalation, **anesthesia** is usually administered in the second stage of labor. It affects the entire system of the patient and may be passed to the fetus through the placenta. Because it may cause toxic effects in the fetus, interfere with the normal establishment of the baby's respiration, and cause postpartum hemorrhage in the mother, it must be administered only by a skilled anesthetist. This technique is generally reserved for situations in which rapid delivery is important, for example, fetal distress, or when intrauterine manipulation is required. Intravenous anesthesia agents are administered for rapid induction of general anesthesia. They are usually followed by inhalational agents for maintenance of the anesthetic state. General anesthesia is seldom used in a normal birth situation.

REGIONAL ANESTHESIA

Regional anesthesia interrupts the pain pathway at a specific source. It is the safest method of anesthetizing a patient because it involves only a localized area. Regional anesthesia has little direct effect on the baby. It also is desirable for the mother as it causes no nausea or vomiting and it lets her be awake to help during the delivery. Examples of regional anesthesia procedures are paracervical block, caudal, lumbar epidural block, spinal, saddle block, pudendal block, and local.

Paracervical Block Anesthesia. **Paracervical block** anesthesia can be administered to the patient in labor when only partial dilatation of the cervix has occurred, see Figure 13–1. An anesthetic solution is injected into the region around the cervix to reduce the pain caused by cervical dilatations. Some obstetricians believe that this kind of anesthesia could have a depressing effect on the infant and may slow

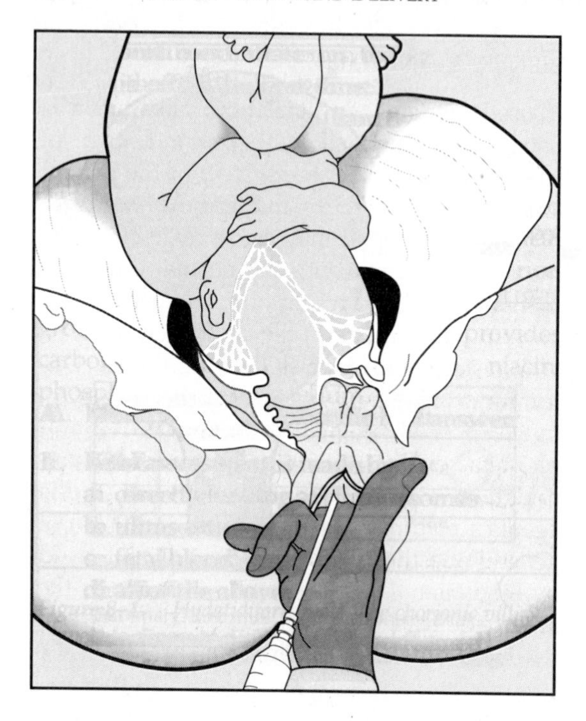

Figure 13–1 *Paracervical block*

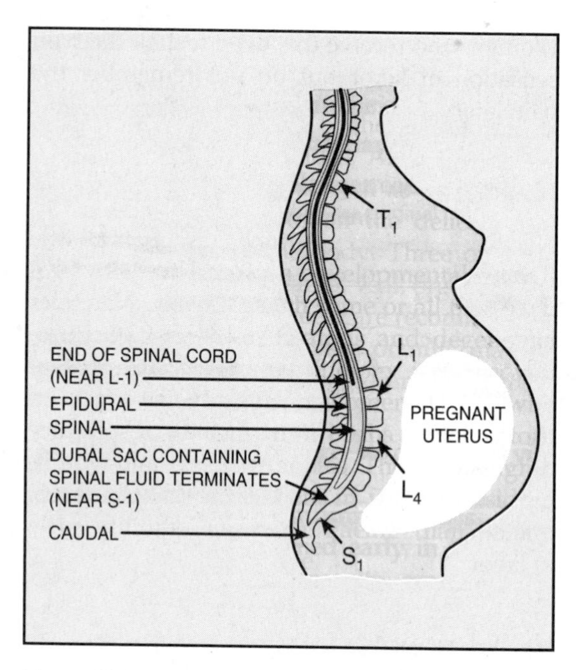

Figure 13–2 *Injection sites for regional anesthesia in obstetrics*

the rate of cervical dilatation. Also, the high incidence of complications has reduced the popularity of this technique.

Caudal Anesthesia. In **caudal anesthesia**, a local anesthetic is injected into the caudal space in the sacrum, see Figure 13–2. The advantage of this form of anesthesia is that the mother is not able to feel the labor contractions. She must have careful nursing care. The nurse must time and evaluate the contractions by placing her hand on the patient's abdomen or by using a fetal monitor. The bladder must be kept empty, by catheterization if necessary, since the patient is not able to void spontaneously. The patient's blood pressure must be taken frequently. Caudal anesthesia sometimes causes a drop in the mother's blood pressure, which can have an adverse effect on the fetus.

The technique of caudal anesthesia, discovered in 1901, was first applied to childbirth in 1909. Use of the continuous technique was limited because of its reputed high rate of failure. With increased clinical experience, however, the failure rate has been considerably reduced. If properly administered, continuous caudal anesthesia (caudal block) is one of the safest techniques for both mother and fetus.

Anesthesia is begun when the patient is in active labor; that is, contractions are 45 seconds or more in duration at intervals of 2 to 3 minutes; cervical dilatation is 6 cm or more for primigravidas, 4 cm or more for multiparas. If given too early in labor, the caudal block could interfere with the quality of the labor contractions. The patient is placed in a modified Sim's position. Caudal punctures are made with a thin-wall, 18-gauge needle with stylet. Vinyl tubing is inserted into the caudal canal. A small test dosage of the chosen drug is injected slowly through the vinyl tubing. The patient is then observed for signs of inadvertent spinal block.

Five to ten minutes later, if the catheter appears to be in the correct position, a full dosage of the drug is injected. It will cause a loss of feeling in the lower half of the woman's body within 15 to 20 minutes after injection, and the effect will last for 45 minutes to 1½ hours. If continuous, additional medications can be injected through the tubing as needed. This kind of anesthesia is helpful for easing the pain of uterine contractions, the pain in the vagina and rectum as the baby descends, and the pain of an episiotomy.

Lumbar Epidural Block. A **lumbar epidural block** is much like caudal anesthesia. It is performed by injecting a local anesthetic into the epidural space of the lumbar region, see Figure 13–3. This procedure blocks precisely the same anatomical area as the caudal block and is used for the same purpose.

There are several advantages of a spinal epidural block over a caudal block. Less anesthetic is required, and the onset of uterine pain relief is more rapid. There is less risk of infection, and there is no risk of puncturing the maternal rectum or the head of the fetus.

With modern techniques that use low doses of medication, most women can deliver normally with an epidural anesthetic. If the mother is very numb, however, it may be harder for her to bear down and help the baby

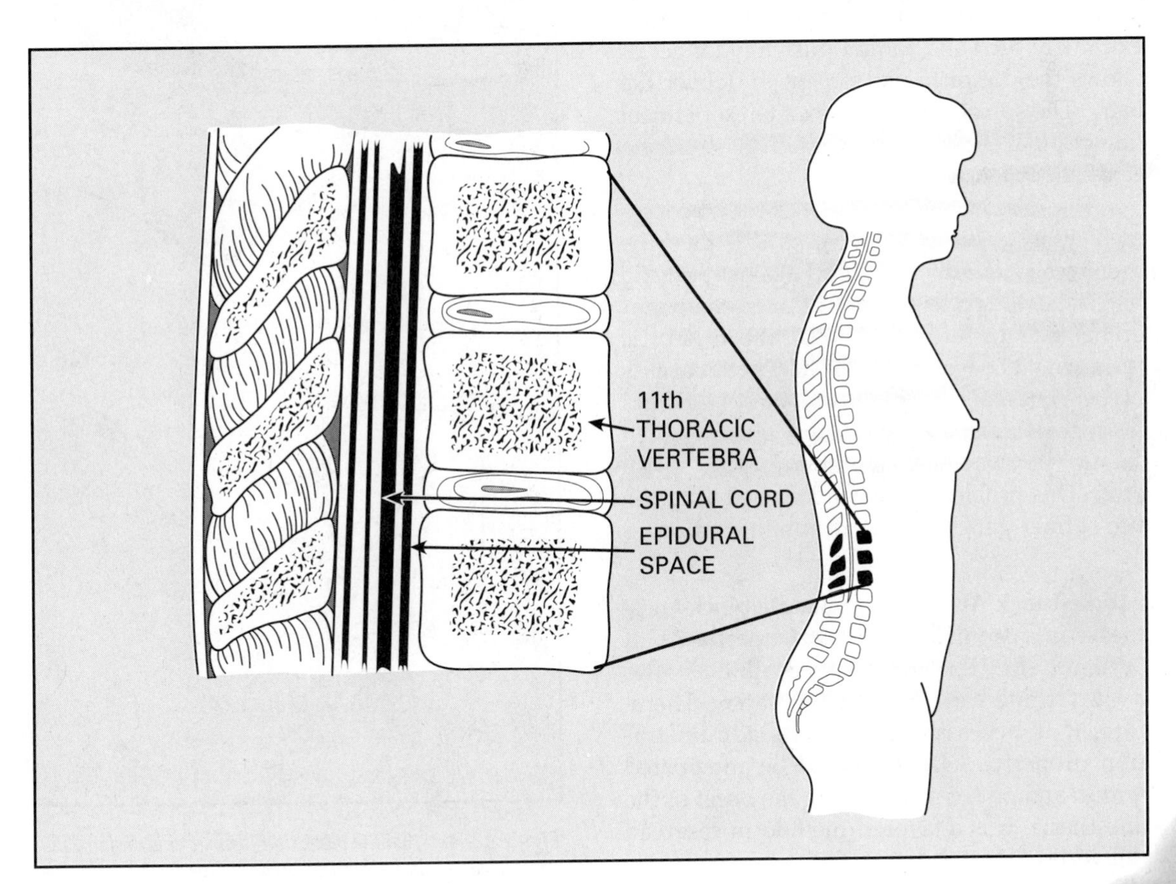

Figure 13–3 *Insertion points for epidural block anesthesia*

move through the birth canal. If this becomes a problem, low forceps or vacuum extraction may be indicated to help guide the baby's head out of the birth canal.

Epidural block can have some side effects. It may cause the mother's blood pressure to drop, which in turn, may slow the baby's heartbeat. Preventive measures are taken to avoid this problem. Before the mother receives the medication, fluids are given through an intravenous line, and she is positioned on her side to help circulation.

Spinal Anesthesia. The **spinal anesthetic** is injected into the spinal fluid. It is generally given after the cervix is fully dilated. The spinal is sometimes used for a mother who is extremely tired and cannot push any longer. It allows the doctor to use forceps to deliver the baby. The spinal can also relax a tense perineal floor. Spinal anesthesia most often is used for a cesarean delivery.

The mother's blood pressure may be lowered after a spinal is given, so she must be monitored carefully. To guard against possible headache, the patient is required to remain flat on her back for 4 to 8 hours after the anesthetic is given. The so-called **spinal headache** is caused because of the leakage of spinal fluid through the puncture in the dura, which causes pressure changes within the spinal cord. This problem has been lessened with the use of finer-gauge needles in administration.

Saddle Block Anesthesia. **Saddle block** anesthesia is a form of low spinal anesthesia. It becomes effective within 2 to 3 minutes after administration and is of short duration. Therefore, it is necessary to time its administration properly; delivery should be anticipated within an hour or so following the onset of the anesthesia. It is a favored method in cesarean deliveries.

The drug is introduced into the lowest part of the spinal canal, see Figure 13–4. It provides insensitivity to the area that would come in contact with a saddle if one were horseback riding; hence the name, saddle block. Headaches sometimes occur following anesthesia of this type; therefore, it is recommended that the patient be kept flat in bed 4 to 8 hours after delivery. Also, bladder dysfunction is fre-

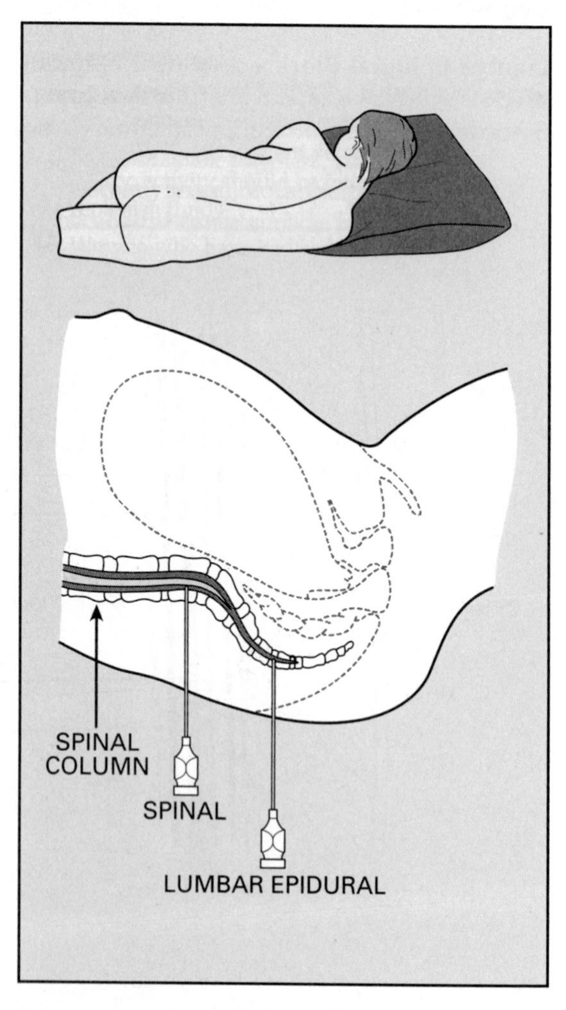

Figure 13–4 Saddle block and lumbar epidural are the anesthesias of choice for a cesarean delivery.

quent, so careful monitoring by the nurse is essential.

Pudendal Block Anesthesia. **Pudendal block** anesthesia affects the area of the perineum and vagina, Figure 13–5. It is given shortly before delivery and is helpful in numbing the perineum for the delivery, episiotomy, and repair. It relaxes the perineal muscles, but the patient is still able to aid contractions by bearing down. It can also aid a low-forceps delivery. The time of administration of pudendal anesthesia is important to its success. Once the presenting part of the fetus is distending the perineum, it is too late.

Local Anesthesia. **Local anesthesia** may be produced by injecting an anesthetic drug directly into the perineal area. This procedure numbs the perineum in preparation for the episiotomy. Local anesthesia is administered just before the baby is born. If the injection is not given before birth, it is given after the baby is born so that repair of the episiotomy will be painless. In many instances a natural anesthetic action is produced by the pressure of the baby's presenting part against the perineum. When this happens a local anesthetic may not be necessary until after the birth, when the natural anesthetic action is no longer in effect. See Figures 13–6 and 13–7.

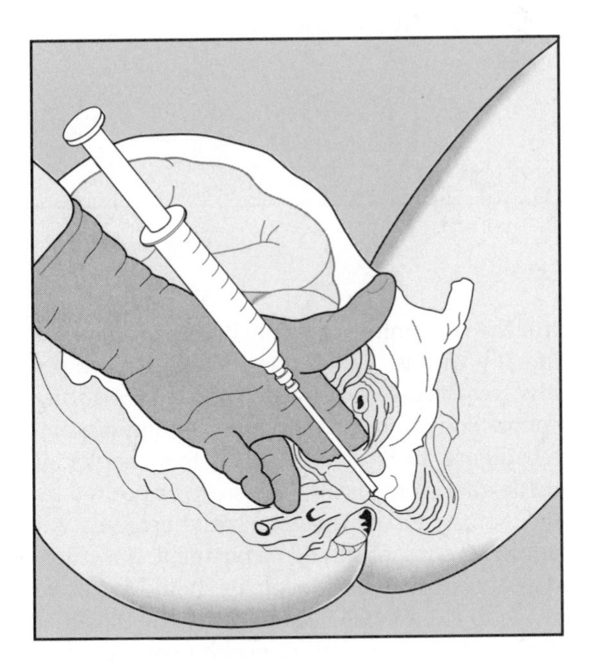

Figure 13–5 *Pudendal block*

SUPPORTIVE NURSING CARE

Much discomfort from labor and delivery can also be alleviated by a supportive nursing approach. The **fear-tension-pain syndrome** plays an major role in childbirth. If the nurse can keep the laboring woman and her immediate support person well informed of what is happening to the body during the labor process, then the expectant mother's fear level will diminish. With less fear, there is less tension. Therefore, pain is more easily kept under control. The nurse can also reinforce the principle that the body works effectively in the birthing process. The female body is designed to give birth. If the nurse can establish increased confidence that the sensations being felt are normal, then she can greatly reduce the fear and pain perception.

Along with education, the nurse can also help the laboring woman to find a comfortable position. A frequent change of position usually is helpful. The woman may wish to walk during part of her labor. The use of heat and cold are also effective tools in decreasing pain. Cool or warm compresses to the face, neck, or back may be comforting. Standing in a shower or sitting in a warm bath (if permitted) can enhance relaxation. Swabbing dry lips and giving sips of fluids or ice chips can also help. A

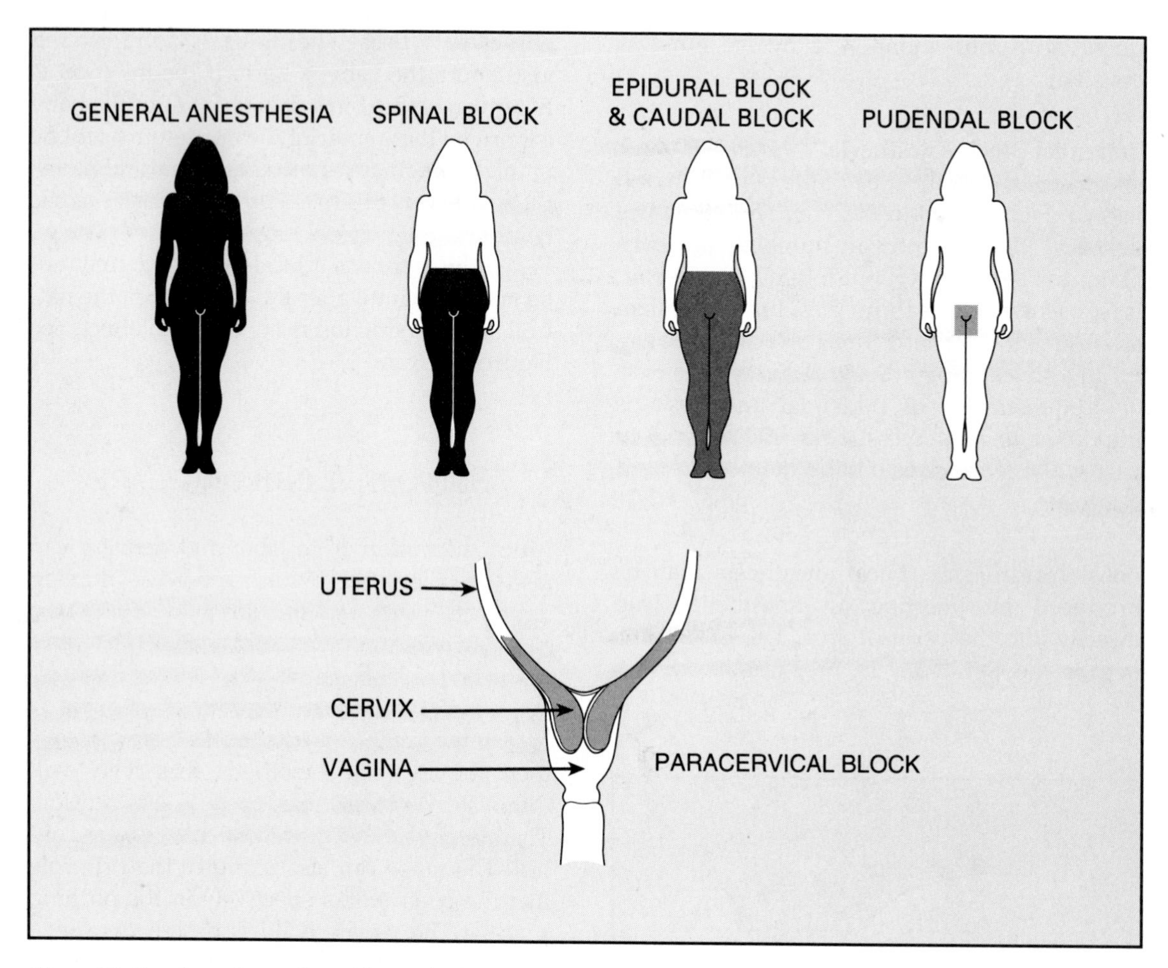

Figure 13–6 *Loss of sensation with anesthesia*

back massage can be effective in counteracting the pressure felt from a posterior positioned baby. The patient's partner or labor coach may wish to actively participate in some of these comforting measures. A caring attitude from the nurse can do much to decrease the laboring woman's pain sensations.

If the woman and her support person have attended childbirth preparation classes, they can be encouraged to breathe in the suggested pattern and to use the other concentration tools taught in class, Figure 13–8. Dr. Fernand Lamaze of France introduced psychoprophylaxis to control the discomfort of labor. Psychoprophylaxis literally means "mind prevention." It basically involves the use of distraction techniques during contractions to decrease the perception of pain, see Figure 13–9, at the end of this chapter. If medication is medically necessary or desired by the woman, an explanation should be given. An informed consent should be obtained. If medication is designated, the woman should never be made to feel that she has in some way failed at childbirth. The goal of all health care providers should be a healthy outcome and a joyous experience for the expectant parents.

REGIONAL ANESTHETICS

Type	Administration Site	Area Affected	May Be Given At	Takes Effect In	Effects Last For	Comments
Paracervical block	Into nerve trunks at both sides of cervix	Cervix and uterus	Dilatation of 4–9 cm	3–4 min	1–2 hr	Given by physician May be repeated as needed May cause slowing of fetal heart rate
Caudal block	Into caudal canal at base of sacrum	Below ribs to knees	Dilatation of greater than 5 cm	15–20 min	45 min–1½ hr	Repeat dose may be administered through catheter placed in caudal canal Given by an anesthesiologist May cause a drop in maternal blood pressure, resulting in a drop in fetal heart rate Diminishes urge to push
Lumbar epidural block	Lumbar spine region	Waist to knees	Dilatation of greater than 5 cm	10–15 min	45 min–1½ hr	Same as for caudal block
Spinal block	Between 3rd and 4th lumbar vertebrae	Breast to toes	2nd stage of labor	3–5 min	1½–2 hr	Often used for cesarean section Possible drop in maternal blood pressure

Figure 13–7

REGIONAL ANESTHETICS

Type	Administration Site	Area Affected	May Be Given At	Takes Effect In	Effects Last For	Comments
Saddle block	Between 3rd and 4th lumbar vertebrae	Inner thighs, perineum, and buttocks	2nd stage of labor	3–5 min	1½–2 hr	Used for discomfort during delivery or when forceps are indicated Given by physician or anesthesiologist Possible drop in maternal blood pressure
Pudendal block	Into pudendal nerve trunks via vagina	Vagina and perineum	2nd stage of labor	2–3 min	1 hr	Used for discomfort during delivery or when forceps are indicated Used for episiotomy and repair Fetal risks unknown
Local infiltration	Perineum	Perineum	2nd or 3rd stage of labor	5 min	20 min	Used for episiotomy and/or its repair

Figure 13–7 *continued*

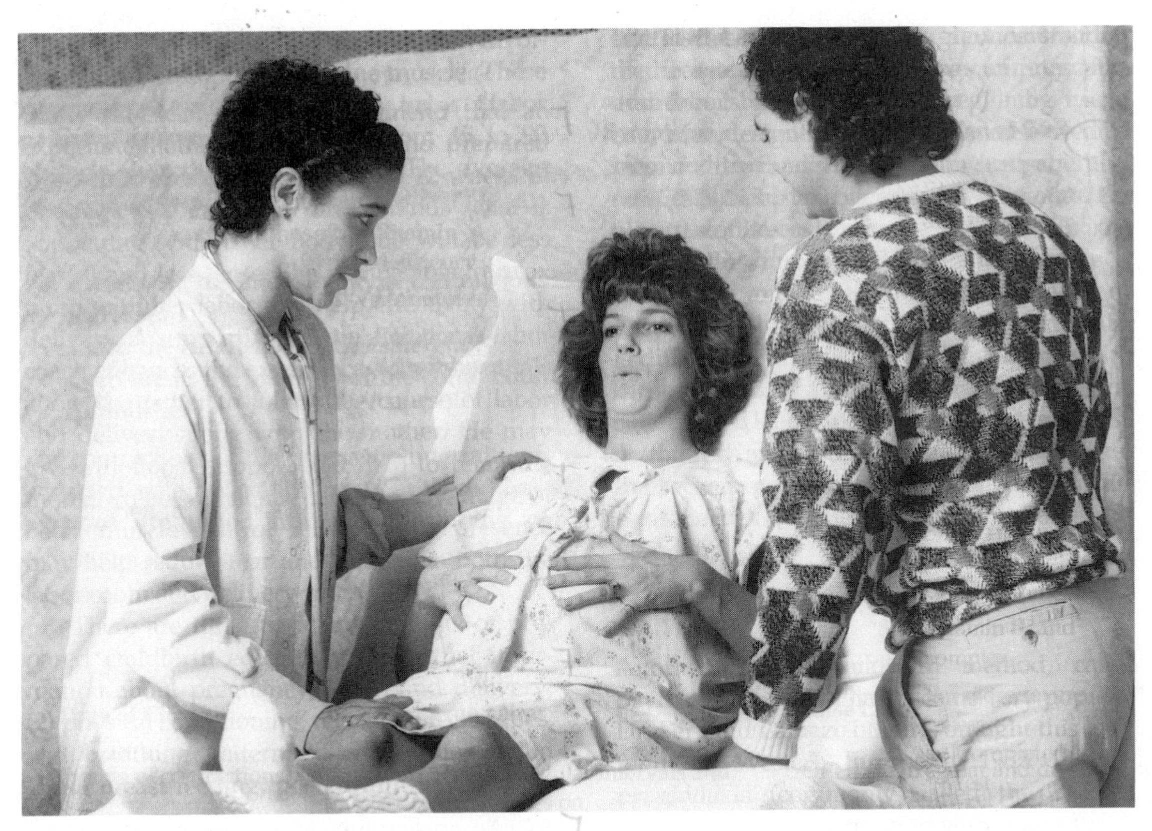

Figure 13–8 *Nurse and labor coach work with the laboring woman to help her stay relaxed through contractions.*

REVIEW QUESTIONS

A. Multiple choice. Select the best answer.

1. When saddle block anesthesia is used, the patient is kept flat in bed after delivery for
   a. 4 to 8 hours
   b. 3 to 4 hours
   c. 8 to 10 hours
   d. 12 to 24 hours

2. The mother's blood pressure must be taken frequently in
   a. caudal anesthesia
   b. epidural anesthesia
   c. analgesia
   d. all of the above

3. Medications that relieve anxiety are called
   a. barbiturates
   b. amnesiacs
   c. tranquilizers
   d. narcotics

4. Medications that relieve pain, produce sedation, and decrease anxiety are called
   a. barbiturates
   b. amnesiacs
   c. tranquilizers
   d. narcotics

5. Medication administered to reduce the pain caused by cervical dilatation is called
   a. pudendal block
   b. paracervical block
   c. caudal block
   d. epidural block

6. A caudal anesthetic is administered to a primigravida when the cervix is dilated
   a. 4 cm
   b. 8 cm
   c. 6 cm
   d. none of the above

7. The anesthesia used for repair of the perineum is called
   a. pudendal block
   b. paracervical block
   c. lumbar epidural block
   d. none of the above

8. The most helpful support the nurse can give the laboring mother is
   a. to explain what is happening during her labor
   b. to give a back massage and offer other comforting measures
   c. to encourage the laboring woman to change positions frequently
   d. all of the above

B. True or false. Briefly state the reason if the answer is false.

F 1. Some medications are completely safe for the laboring mother and fetus.

F 2. The mother does not need to know the risks of analgesia or anesthesia before it is administered.

T 3. Sedatives relieve anxiety and relax the patient but do not relieve pain.

F 4. Amnesic drugs are effective in reducing the pain of labor.

T 5. Inhalation agents such as nitrous oxide can be administered by the patient herself.

T 6. Regional anesthesia is the safest method of anesthetizing a patient because it involves only a localized area.

F 7. Pudendal blocks can be given at any time during labor.

T 8. There are advantages of the lumbar epidural block over the caudal block.

F 9. An episiotomy can be performed without the aid of local anesthesia and still not be painful for the woman if done during a contraction.

SUGGESTED ACTIVITIES

- Define psychoprophylaxis. Briefly describe its use in obstetrics.
- List at least three analgesics commonly used during the intrapartum period. Include indications and complications.
- Describe the procedures and list indications for and complications of the following modalities:
  - general anesthesia
  - regional anesthesia
  - spinal anesthesia
  - local anesthesia

BIBLIOGRAPHY

Hawkins, J. W., and L. Pierfedeici. *Maternity and Gynecological Nursing*. New York: J. B. Lippincott, 1981.

Oxorn, H. *Oxorn-Foote Human Labor and Birth*, 5th ed. E. Norwalk, CT: Appleton-Century-Crofts, 1986.

Pritchard, J. A., MacDonald, P. C., and N. F. Grant. *Williams Obstetrics*, 17th ed. E. Norwalk, CT: Appleton-Century-Crofts, 1985.

Simkin, P., Whalley, J., and A. Keppler. *Pregnancy, Childbirth and the Newborn*. Deephaven, MN: Meadowbrook Books, 1991.

PREPARED CHILDBIRTH LABOR GUIDE • LAMAZE TECHNIQUES © Childbirth Education Association of Seattle

Pre-Labor	Established Labor : Stage I : Effacement (%) & Dilatation of Cervix (cm)			Stage II	Stage III
Softening of Cervix	Remember : Lie on side Breathing : Deep Chest	Focal Point Accelerated	Effleurage Relax Transition	Birth of Baby	Delivery of placenta and immediate recovery
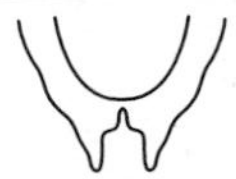	1 cm 2 cm 3 cm 4 cm	5 cm 6 cm 7 cm	8 cm 9 cm 10 cm	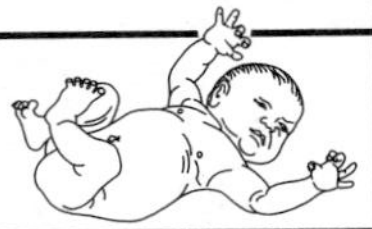	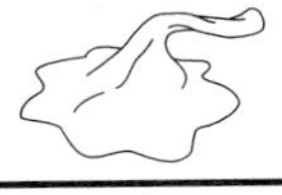
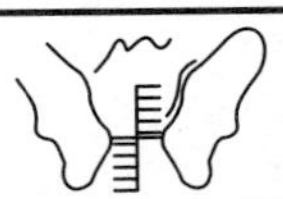	35-40 sec Rest 15-20 min	45-60 sec Rest 60-70 sec	Rest 2-3 min 60-90 sec	Rest 60 sec 2-3 min	Rest
Characteristic Signs: • Nesting urge • Preminitions • Sense of exhilaration • Bracton-Hicks contractions • False labor • Effacement Activity : • Prepare and pack for hospital for baby • Mild exercise may relieve contractions • Mild activity • Rest and nap	Characteristic Signs: • Bloody Show • Contractions become longer, stronger and more frequent • Membranes may rupture • Possible back pain • Excited, confident and talkative Activity : • Rest and nap if possible • Breathing techniques (if necessary) • Empty bladder every hour • Analyze & time contractions • Call doctor • Enter hospital • Perineal shave/ enema • Examinations Reminders for Coach: • Time contractions • Remind her to relax • Adjust physical environment as needed • Follows her lead	Signs: • Feel discoraged • Feel trapped • Contractions may be difficult to handle during exams • Doctor may rupture membranes (Labor will accelerate) • Monitoring device may be in place Activity : • Remain alert, eyes open • Try to anticipate contraction • Wipe brow • Chew ice, damp cloth or sponge • Empty bladder • Relax Coach : • Offer ice : do back massage/counter pressure for back pain; do effleurage; help with breathing techniques and relaxation • Offer reassurance	Signs: • Stong, irregular contractions • Pressure on rectum • Nausea • Cramps in thighs or legs • Sensitivity to touch • Uncontrollable shaking • Forgetfulness • Drowsiness • Irritability • Urge to push • Difficult to remain in control Activity : • Take each contraction individually • Remember that this phase is intense but short • Do not push without permission. Tell Doctor/Nurse Immediately Coach : • Do not leave her alone • Be alert to signs of transition • Help with relaxation between contractions • Ease back pain	Events : • Episiotomy • Crowning • Birth of head Activity : • Relax perineum • Push as directed • Be prepared to pant during delivery of head	Events : • Possible uncontrollable shaking • Possible injection to contract uterus • Lull in contractions • Episiotomy repair Activity : • Continue breathing patterns with contractions • Push to deliver placenta • Transfer of mother to recovery area • Transfer of baby to nursery • Uterine massage 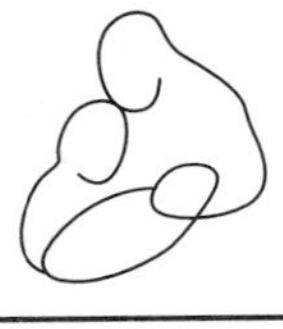

Figure 13–9 *Prepared childbirth labor guide (Courtesy Childbirth Education Association of Seattle)*

CHAPTER

14

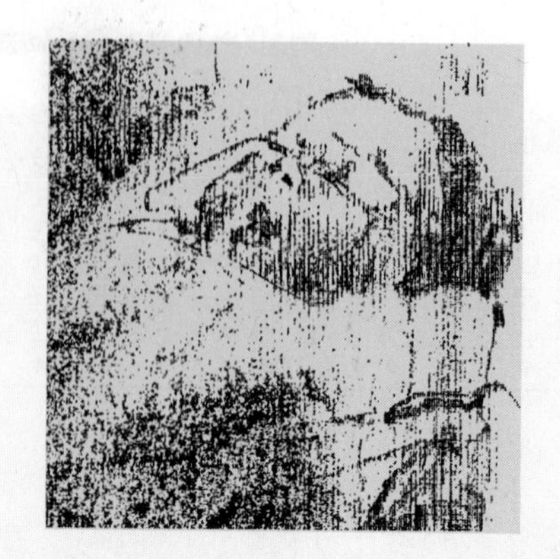

Nursing Care in Delivery

Objectives

After studying this chapter, the student should be able to:

- List six indications of the second stage of labor.
- Describe nursing care during the second, third, and fourth stages of labor.
- State how to prepare the patient for delivery.
- Explain the Apgar scoring system.
- Describe the immediate care of the newborn.
- List six factors that influence parent-infant bonding.

Key Terms

- crowning
- second stage of labor
- family-centered concept
- forceps
- vacuum extractor
- bonding
- Leboyer method
- extrauterine
- bulb syringe
- DeLee aspirator
- Moro reflex
- vernix caseosa
- Identabands
- Apgar scoring system
- resuscitation
- third stage of labor

While watching the progress of the patient in the first stage of labor, the nurse must be alert to the indications that the second stage of labor is beginning. The indications seen in most patients are:

- rectal bulging during a contraction
- urge to defecate or "bearing down" sensation
- rapid dilatation of cervix within a few contractions
- intense contractions that occur rapidly — 1 to 2 minutes apart lasting 60 to 90 seconds
- perspiration on the upper lip
- nausea with emesis (occasionally)
- sudden increase in show
- rupture of membranes (bag of waters)
- **crowning** (appearance of the fetal scalp at the vulva) or the appearance of the bag of waters if it hasn't ruptured

These signs are not infallible, and the condition of the cervix and station of the presenting part must be confirmed by rectal or vaginal exam. The **second stage of labor** lasts from the end of the first stage, when the cervix has reached full dilatation, to the birth of the baby, see Figure 14–1.

PREPARING FOR DELIVERY

Some hospitals still move women to a delivery room, but many hospitals nationwide have adopted a **family-centered concept.** The laboring woman is surrounded by her support team. She is left in the same bed that she has been in throughout the first stage of her labor. She is not moved to a different room for delivery. If a delivery room is to be used, there are some basic principles that underlie all common techniques. Procedure outlines are also followed for a cesarean birth.

HAND AND GOWN TECHNIQUE

Since the delivery room is an operating room, all personnel are required to scrub their hands according to surgical technique. Sterile caps, masks, and gowns are worn by personnel at the delivery table; circulating personnel wear scrub suits or dresses, masks, and caps.

DELIVERY ROOM SETUP

Before the patient is moved to the delivery room, it should be set up with the delivery table, sterile instrument table, sterile basins, and an infant warmer with resuscitation equipment for the baby. The sterile packs of linen and equipment should be in place and covered with sterile drapes. When everything is ready for delivery, the circulating nurse uncovers the sterile equipment, taking great care not to contaminate it. Adequate preparation eliminates last-minute hurry, confusion, and error.

If the hospital has family-centered birthing rooms, a proper setup for the delivery process will still need to be obtained and made available in the room for the physician. Clean technique is very important. Also, provisions for the newborn (an infant warmer, equipment for the immediate care and initial evaluation) will need to be readily available.

ASSISTING DURING DELIVERY

There are many ways the mother can be made more comfortable during the second stage of labor. Helping her to relax and at the same time to bear down with the contractions once the cervix is completely dilated helps to ease the delivery. It is futile to have the patient bear down before complete dilatation occurs; it is exhausting and could result in lacerating the

NURSING CARE PLAN: Second Stage of Labor

Second Stage of Labor: From complete dilatation of the cervix to the end of expulsion of the child (known as the "stage of expulsion"). It usually lasts 1 to 2 hours in the primipara; a few minutes to 1 hour in the multipara.

PATIENT PROBLEM	GOAL(S)
Desire to push; fear of soiling the bed	Woman uses abdominal muscles to push effectively as directed.
Leg cramps	Leg cramps are alleviated with hyperflexion or heat.
Dry lips	Lips are kept moist.
Profuse perspiration	Patient is kept comfortable and as dry as possible.
Distended bladder	Bladder is drained before labor is impeded.

Figure 14–1 *Nursing care plan for discomfort during the second stage of labor (Adapted from* Maternal and Child Health, *Littlefield, Adams & Co.)*

NURSING INTERVENTION	RATIONALE
Explain to the patient and reassure her that this is unavoidable and acceptable at this stage. Instruct her to bear down with each contraction until crowning, and then take short, quick breaths.	The baby gives the mother a feeling of pressure in the rectum as it enters the birth canal. Mother must use her abdominal muscles to expel baby. Mother should not push during crowning in order to avoid perineal lacerations and to allow the baby to be eased out slowly.
Advise the patient to stretch her leg out forcibly, pulling her foot toward her knee. If persistent, hot towels may be applied to the affected area.	Hyperflexion stretches the muscle and breaks the pain pathway. Heat will aid in muscle relaxation.
Apply oil or cold cream to lips.	Short, shallow breaths during labor tend to dry lips. Oil or cream will prevent cracking and will provide comfort to the patient.
Apply cool cloth to forehead and hands.	Provides soothing comfort to mother during the hard work of labor.
Assist the physician in catheterization.	A distended bladder impedes the progress of labor and causes the mother unnecessary discomfort.

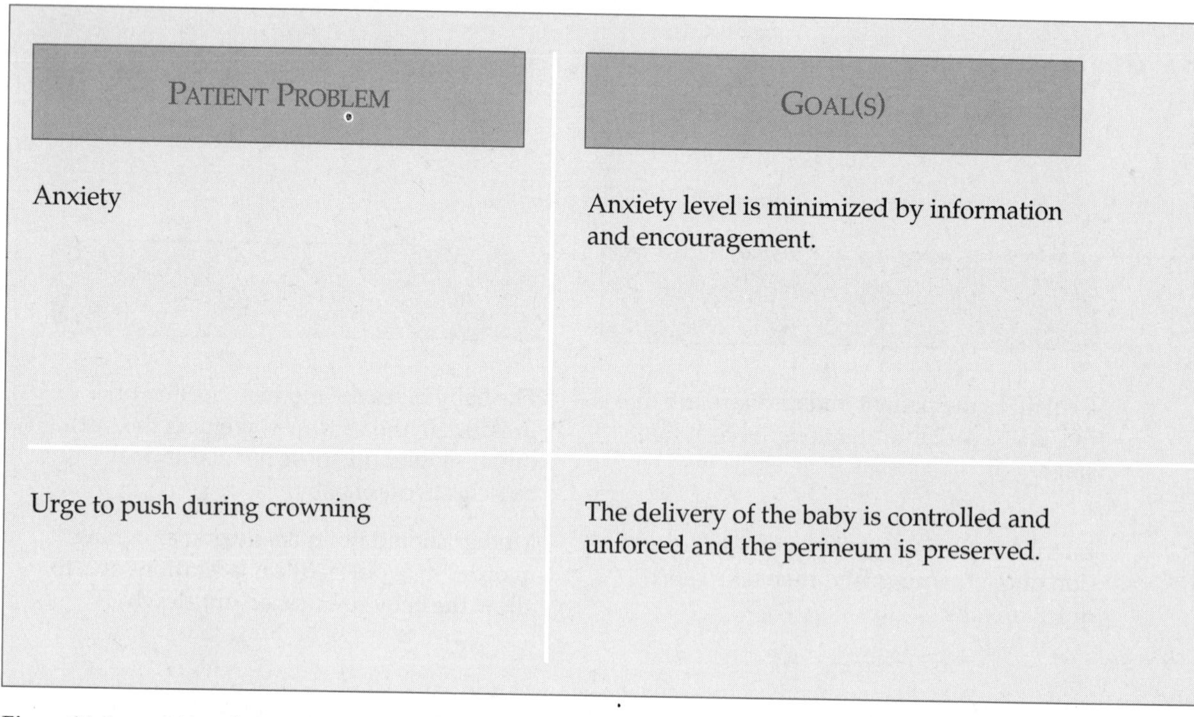

PATIENT PROBLEM	GOAL(S)
Anxiety	Anxiety level is minimized by information and encouragement.
Urge to push during crowning	The delivery of the baby is controlled and unforced and the perineum is preserved.

Figure 14–1 *continued*

cervix. The patient should be kept dry, clean, and as comfortable as possible. Two key concepts should guide the mother and her support team through the second stage of labor. One concept is the importance of not rushing. A woman should be encouraged to follow her own body signals, bearing down or pushing spontaneously as the urge demands. This approach allows the vaginal tissue to stretch open gently. During the early part of the second stage, the abdominal muscles, which are responsible for the bearing-down efforts, are under the patient's complete control. Later she sometimes finds it impossible to stop bearing down even if she wants to. Bearing down is more efficient if the patient braces herself against a solid object. When the contraction begins, the patient takes one or two deep breaths and then holds her breath to fix the diaphragm. She then pulls on the hand bars and at the same time bears down as hard and for as long a period as she can.

The second concept is the effective use of different positions. See Figure 14–2 for various birthing bed positions. The most common position in North America is semi-sitting with legs raised in stirrups, or with the feet in footrests or resting on the bed. If one position is uncomfortable or progress is slow, take advantage of the other positions that might use gravity to advantage or may aid progress and descent. As delivery approaches, a saddle block, local, or pudendal block may be given to numb the perineum.

NURSING INTERVENTION	RATIONALE
Keep mother and father informed of the progress of labor and encourage and reassure them.	The more knowledge the mother has of what is happening within her body, the less fear and anxiety she will have. The same holds true for the father or "coach," who will be able to offer additional encouragement and reassurance if he is assured that labor is progressing as it should.
Encourage panting	Concentrating on proper breathing techniques should help the mother to resist the urge to push during crowning. This will help prevent perineal lacerations, allowing the baby to ease out of the birth canal.

POSITIONS FOR THE SECOND STAGE OF LABOR

Semi-sitting

Advantages

1. Is convenient for birth attendant.
2. Is easy position to maintain for the laboring mother.

Disadvantages

1. May aggravate hemorrhoids.
2. May restrict sacrum movement when more room is needed in the pelvis.
3. May slow passage of head under pubic bone.

Side-lying, Figure 14–3:

Advantages

1. Gravity is neutral.
2. Is useful for slowing rapid labor.
3. Takes pressure off hemorrhoids.

Disadvantages

1. May not be familiar to birth attendant assisting in delivery.
2. Is unfavorable if you need to speed the second stage.

Hands and knees, Figure 14–4:

Advantages

1. Helps assist rotation of an O.P. baby.
2. May reduce backache.

Disadvantages

1. Is tiring for long periods.

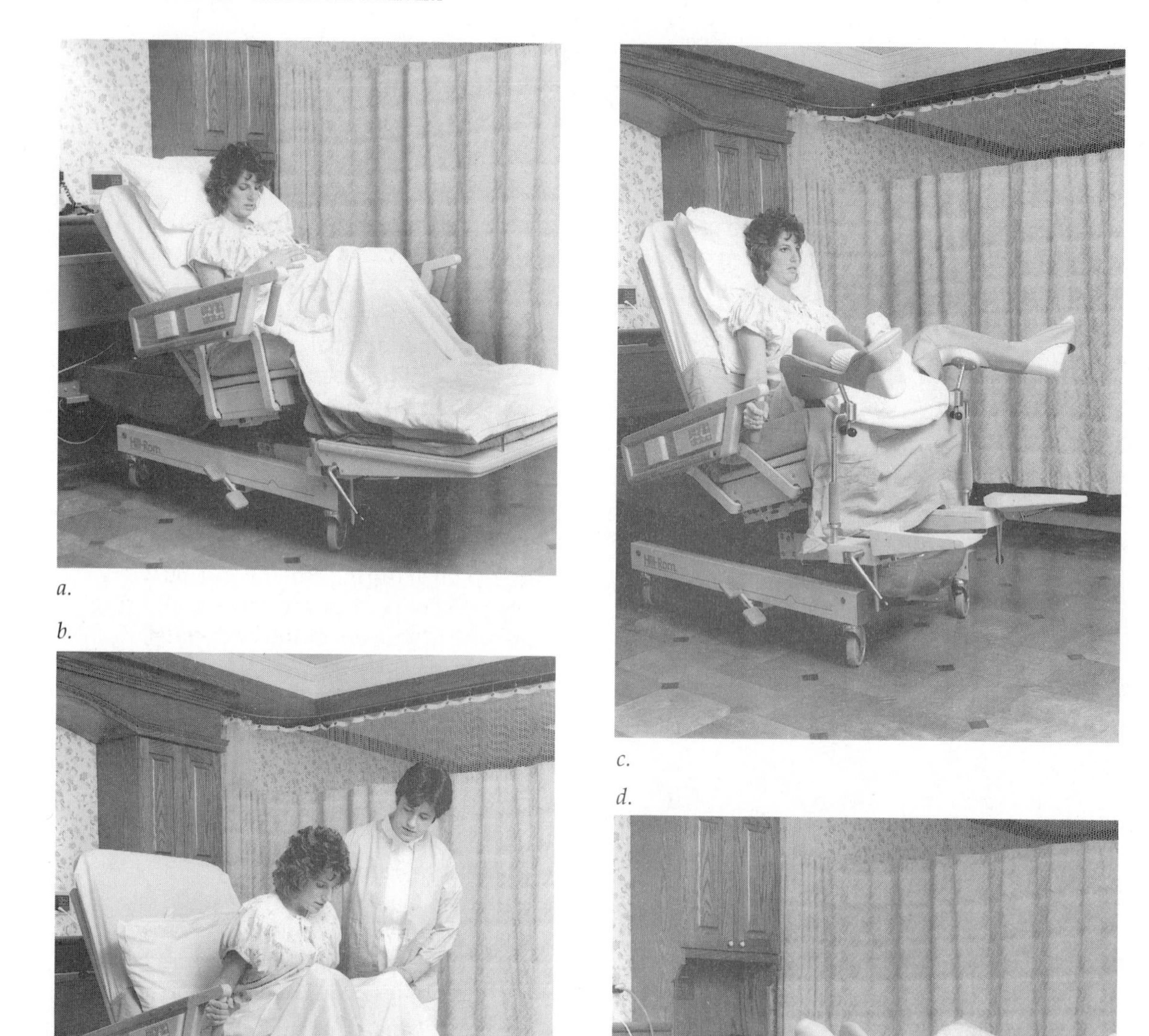

Figure 14–2 *A birthing bed is often used for all stages of labor and delivery. (a) Labor bed. (b) Birth chair. (c) Birth bed. (d) OB table. (e) Postpartum. (f) Critical-care transport surgery.*

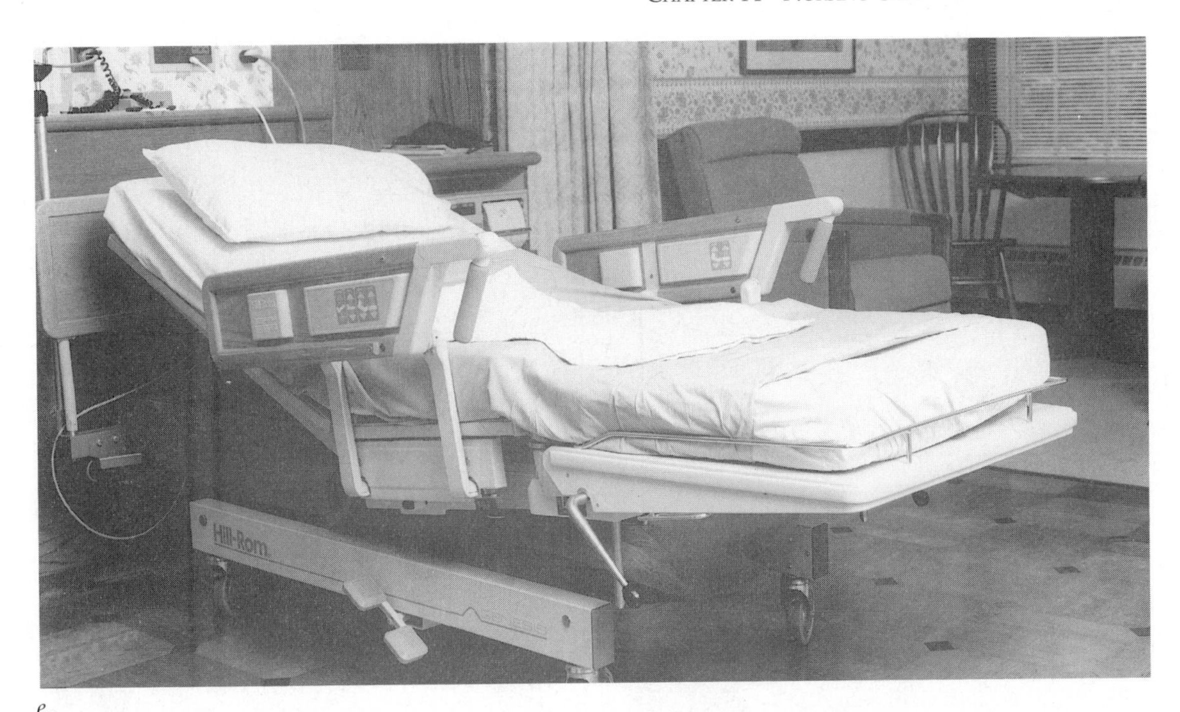

e.

f.

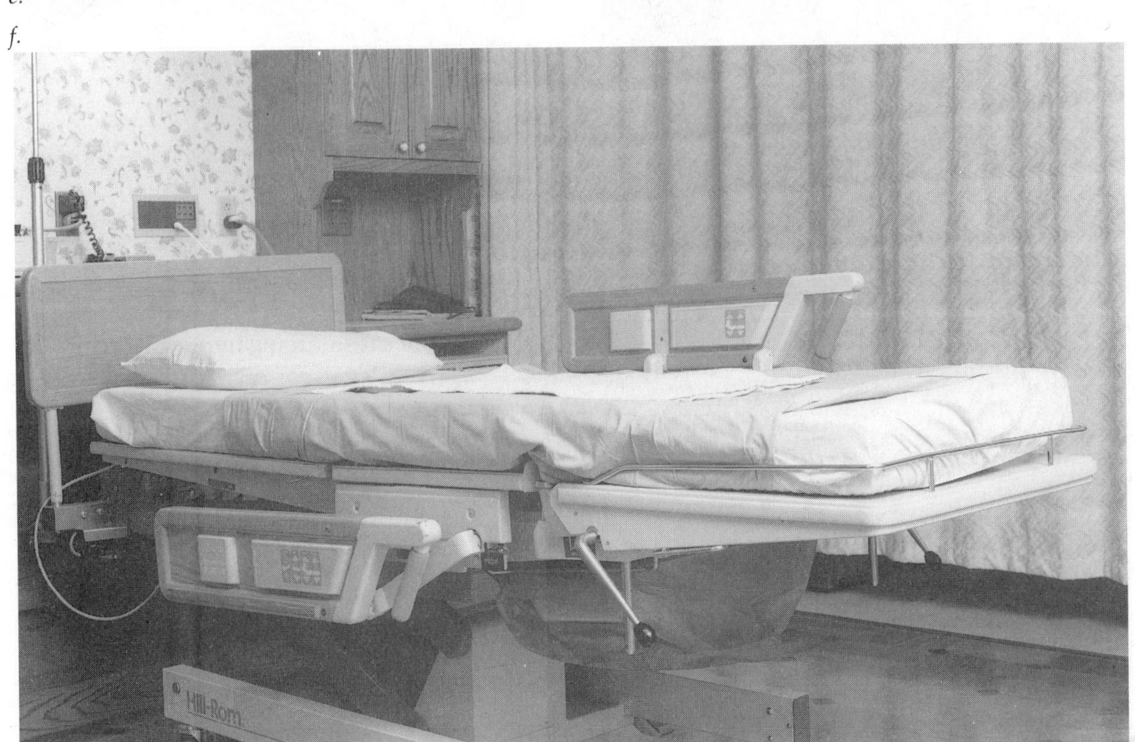

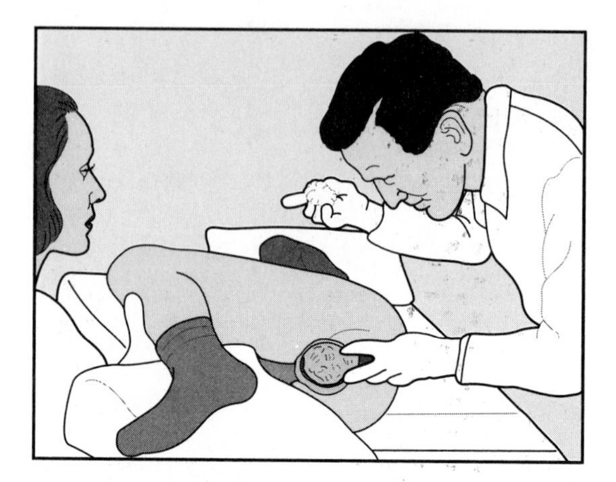

Figure 14–3 *Side-lying position*

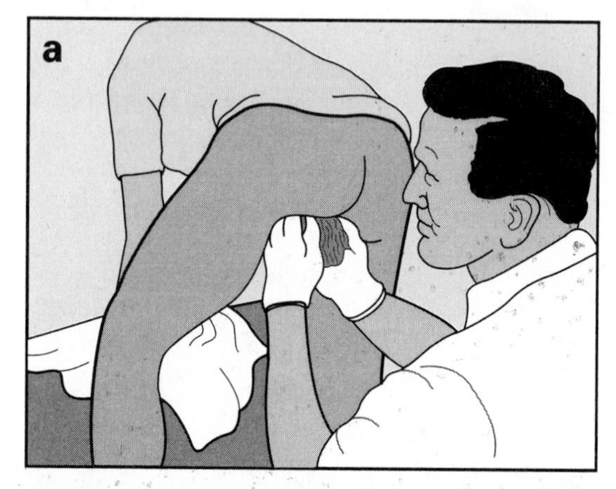

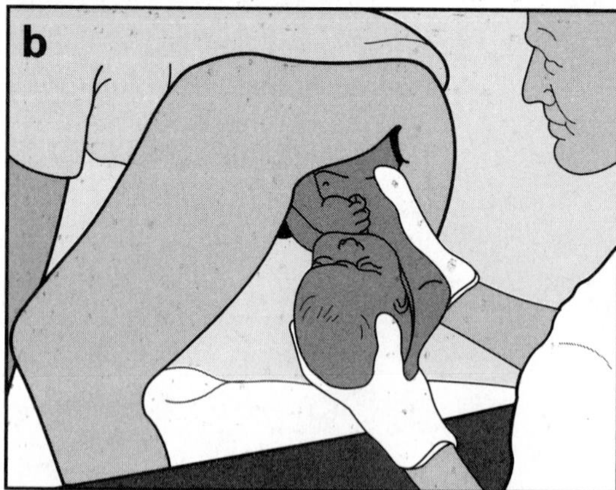

Figure 14–4 *Hands-and-knees position. (a) Delivery of the head is beginning. (b) Delivery of the infant's body.*

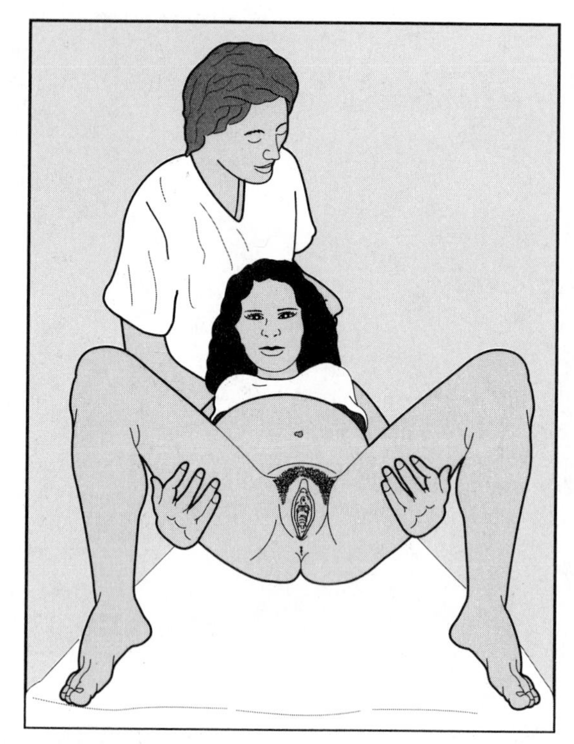

Figure 14–5 *Lying on back*

Lying on back (with legs pulled back, mother raises head to push), Figure 14–5:

Advantages

1. Pulling legs back and apart helps widen pelvic outlet.

Disadvantages

1. May cause supine hypotension.
2. Works against gravity.

Squatting

Advantages

1. Takes advantage of gravity.
2. Widens pelvic outlet to its maximum.
3. Requires less bearing-down effort.
4. May enhance rotation and descent in a difficult birth.
5. Helpful if an urge to push is not felt.

Disadvantages

1. Difficult to get into position on a bed without squat- bar.
2. Difficult for birth attendant to see perineum.

3. May result in too-rapid expulsion, leading to perineal tears.
4. May be uncomfortable.

Supported squat (mother leans with back against support person who holds her under the arms and takes all her weight)

Advantages
1. Allows the pelvis to spread as baby descends.
2. Provides a gravity advantage.

Disadvantages
1. Is hard work for support person.
2. Is difficult for birth attendant to assist in birth.

Semi-lithotomy (this back-lying position has head and shoulders elevated, legs in stirrups, and hips on edge of delivery table)

Advantages
1. Gives some gravity advantage.
2. Mother is able to see birth.
3. Is convenient for attendant.
4. May be necessary for interventions.

Disadvantages
1. Leg cramps are common.
2. Restricts sacral movement.
3. May cause supine hypotension.

Lithotomy

Advantages
1. Is convenient for attendant.
2. May be necessary for interventions.

Disadvantages
1. Works against gravity.
2. Leg cramps are common.
3. Is difficult to view birth.
4. May cause supine hypotension.

With each contraction, the head advances and then recedes as the uterus relaxes. Each time a little ground is gained. The head continues to advance and recede with the contractions until a strong one forces the largest diameter of the head through the vulva (crowning), see Figure 14–6. Sometimes it is necessary for the doctor to help the delivery process by using forceps or the vacuum extractor. These techniques are used when the fetal heartbeat slows or becomes irregular, when the baby's position makes delivery difficult, or when the mother is too tired to push any longer. Generally, an anesthetic is given before the use of forceps or vacuum extraction.

A **forceps** is a surgical instrument that looks like two large spoons, Figure 14–7. The doctor inserts the forceps into the birth canal, places them around the baby's head, and gently delivers the baby.

Vacuum extraction is similar to a forceps delivery, but in this technique a plastic cup is attached to the baby's head by using a vacuum pump, and the baby is gently pulled from the birth canal, Figure 14–8.

Anesthesia may also be given as the perineum bulges if the doctor performs an episiotomy. This procedure is done just before the head of the baby is delivered. An episiotomy is an incision of the perineum made to facilitate delivery. A straight, clean surgical incision is made in lieu of the ragged perineal laceration which might otherwise occur. The direction of the episiotomy can be controlled. It spares the baby from prolonged pushing of its head against the perineum, thus shortening the second stage of labor. If the doctor does an episiotomy, the nurse adds a suture pack and a

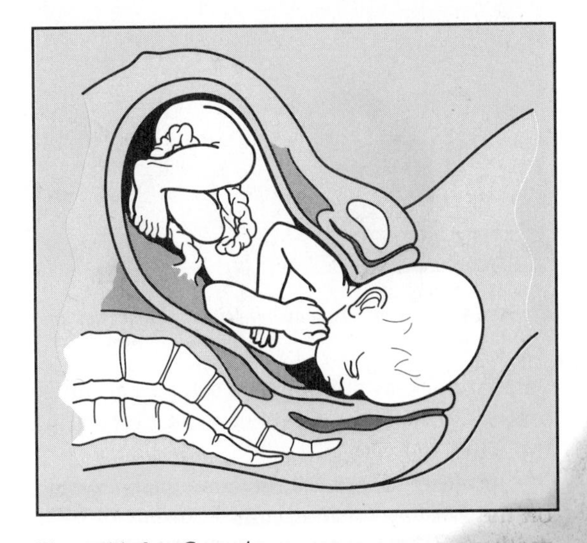

Figure 14–6 Crowning

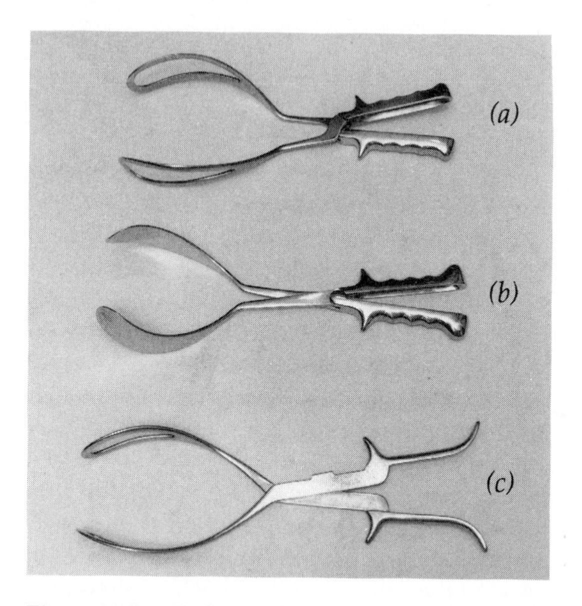

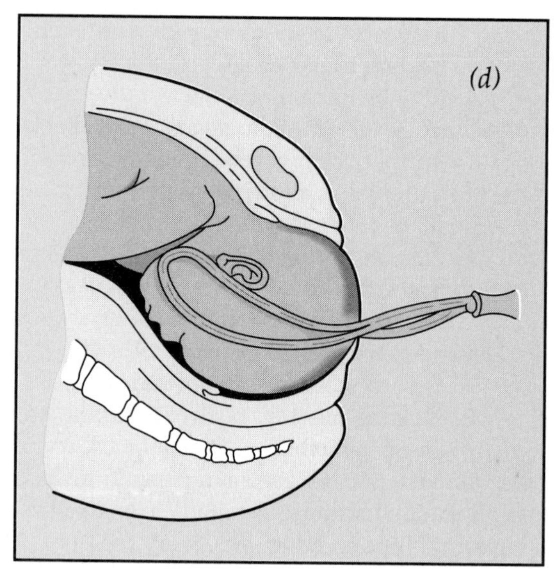

Figure 14–7 *Each type of forcep has its own application. (a) Simpson. (b) Tucker-McLean. (c) Kielland. (d) A baby being delivered with forceps.*

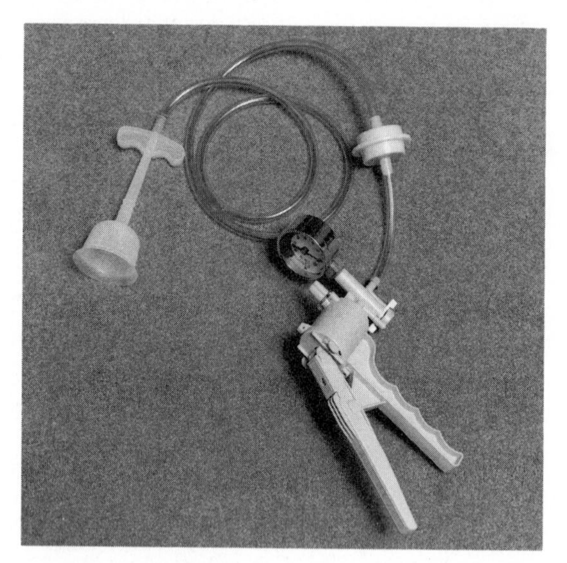

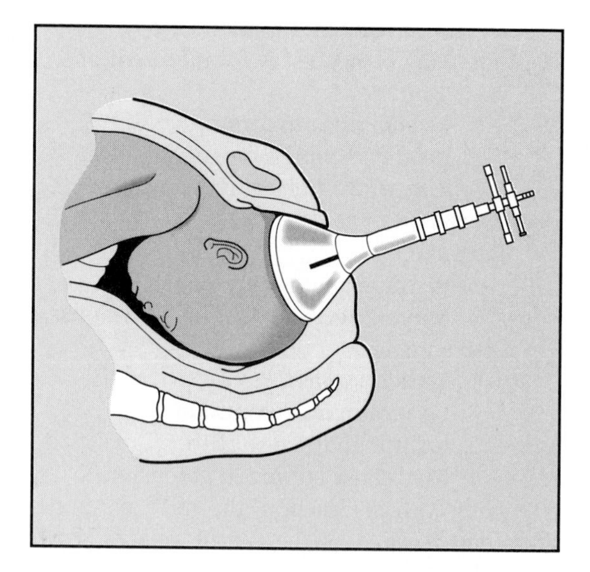

Figure 14–8 *Delivery may be assisted with a vacuum instrument.*

vaginal pack to the delivery setup. The nurse assists the doctor and patient as needed during the actual delivery.

Whether an episiotomy is needed depends on the elasticity of the perineal tissue and the mother's ability to control the pushing efforts. If the head is delivered slowly, the risk of tearing the perineum is reduced. If neither the baby nor the mother is in any distress, and the perineal tissue appears to be stretching adequately to accommodate the presenting part, a patient delivery team can avoid an episiotomy.

Catch baby c̄ towel

At birth, the infant takes its first breath and makes its first sound, a lusty cry. If it does not breathe immediately, the doctor may take measures to stimulate the baby's cry by holding the head downward and rubbing the baby's back or by flicking the soles of its feet. The respiratory system, which until now has been dormant, begins to function with this cry. The doctor wipes or suctions the mucus from the baby's mouth and checks its respiratory status. The cord is then clamped in two places — about 1½ inches and 2½ inches from the baby. When the doctor cuts the cord, the baby is physically separated from the mother. Figure 14–9 summarizes nursing care during the second stage of labor. After the cord has been cut and tied and the doctor has determined that there are no respiratory problems, the doctor may hand the newborn to the nurse and return to the care of the mother, Figure 14–10.

The nurse can then wrap the newborn snugly to ensure warmth before handing it to the parents to facilitate bonding. **Bonding** is a gradually unfolding relationship that begins during pregnancy. It blossoms with the baby's birth, as the parents and baby exchange messages and feelings through the meeting of their eyes, skin-to-skin contact, smell, and sound. The first few minutes and hours of life may be especially influential in the bonding process. During this period, the baby is alert and ready to respond to its environment. The mother and father are physically and emotionally attracted to their baby, and these reciprocal feelings may have long-lasting effects on the parent-child relationship, Figure 14–11.

The role of touch in maternal-infant bonding is fundamental. The mother may wish to have the newborn placed on her abdomen immediately after birth. To help maintain a warm temperature for the baby, the nurse may cover both mother and baby with a warm blanket. Giving the baby to the mother permits skin-to-skin contact, while helping the uterus to become firm through the stimulation of hormone release.

Nursing Care for Second Stage of Labor

- Keep the perineum cleansed.
- Place the patient's legs in stirrups when instructed to do so by the doctor.
- When the doctor is ready, coach the patient to take a couple of deep breaths as soon as the next contraction begins. Then with her breath held, head elevated, chin on chest, have her exert downward pressure exactly as though she were having a bowel movement. Effort should be as sustained as possible, with a quick breath taken every 6 to 12 seconds throughout the contraction. (This is to reoxygenate the bloodstream and keep pushing at a maximum effort.)
- At this time, have the patient push with her flexed legs against the table or stirrups.
- Check fetal heart tones frequently.
- Relieve muscular cramps, if necessary. Leg cramps are common in the second stage of labor because the baby's head exerts pressure on certain nerves in the pelvis. These cramps are relieved by changing the position of the legs and forcing the foot upward with pressure on the knees.
- Note exact time of birth.
- Receive the baby from the doctor with a sterile towel.
- Complete the records and stay in the room until the doctor has finished.
- After the doctor has finished, clean the patient; apply perineal pads and change the patient's gown, if indicated.
- Reextend the delivery table or birthing bed.
- Remove patient's legs from the stirrups, moving both legs at the same time.
- As soon as the delivery is completed, clean the delivery room and make it ready for the next delivery.

Figure 14–9

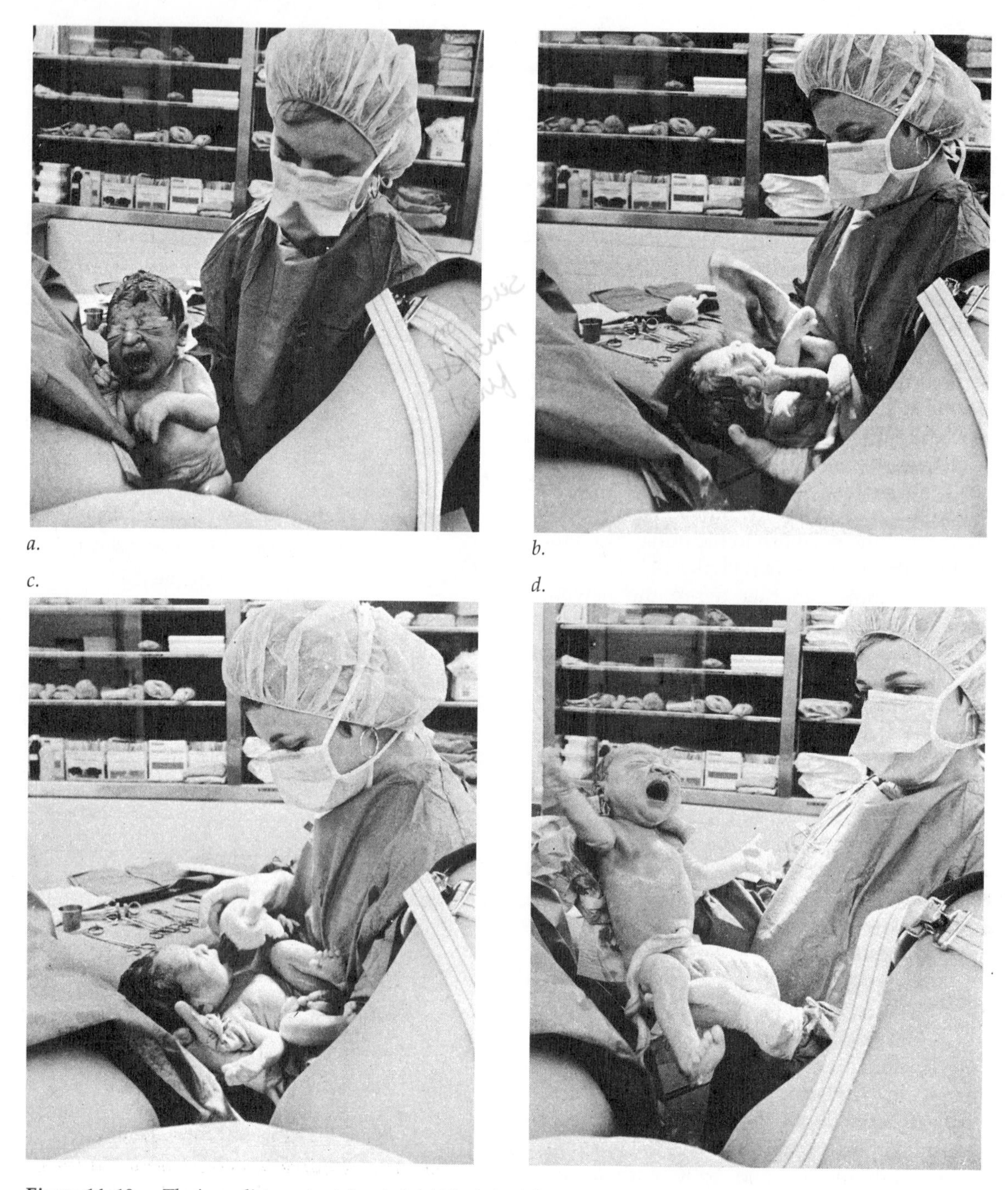

a.

b.

c.

d.

Figure 14–10 *The immediate postnatal period. (a) The baby is born. (b) He is wiped dry. (c) Mucus is removed. (d) Assessment is made.*

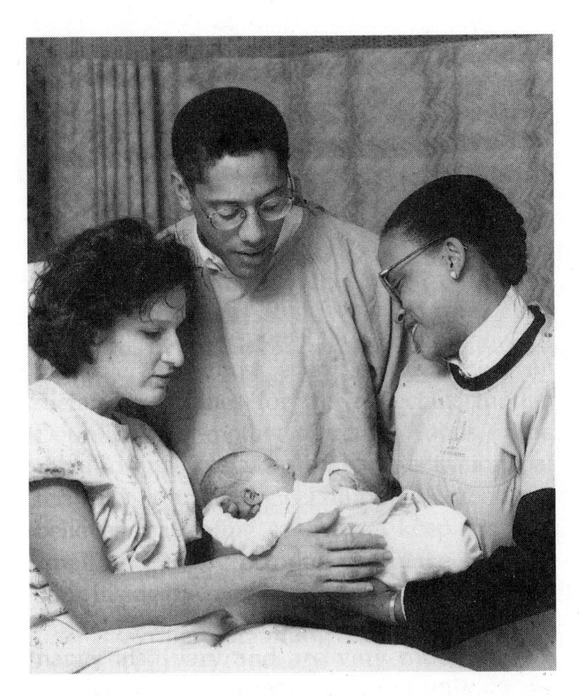

Figure 14–11 Mother, father, and newborn bonding after delivery

The nurse may be asked to administer intramuscular oxytocic drugs to the mother according to the doctor's orders. The drugs will increase uterine contractions and minimize bleeding. It is important for the nurse to record the exact time of placental delivery. The placenta is disposed of according to hospital policy.

The nurse should then complete the records, staying in the room until the doctor has finished caring for the mother. Then, the nurse may clean the patient, apply perineal pads, and change the patient's gown, if needed.

The delivery table is then reextended and both the patient's legs are removed from the stirrups at the same time. As soon as the delivery is completed, the delivery room must be cleaned up and made ready for the next delivery.

ALTERNATIVE BIRTHING CHOICES

Avoiding unnecessary interference with normal birth will provide the best opportunity for parents to respond spontaneously to the baby. Parents must decide in advance about being together during labor and birth; giving birth in a labor room, birthing room, or delivery room; the mother's desire for medication; breast feeding immediately after delivery; sharing the first minutes and hours with their baby; rooming-in privileges, and allowing siblings to visit the new baby at the hospital. In hospitals that provide a wide range of alternatives, including homelike birthing rooms, Leboyer-type births, father-attended cesarean births, and family recovery rooms, parents can choose the birth experience that satisfies their needs.

Some areas offer a birthing center as an alternative to a hospital or home birth. Many alternative birth centers are located within a hospital. The physical setup of the room differs from a standard labor room. The bed is larger, chairs and a dresser furnish the room, plants and pictures add decoration, and the standard equipment used for labor and delivery is stored away in cabinets until needed. The goal of the staff of an alternative birthing center is to meet the individual needs of the woman during a safe, normal childbirth while monitoring the progress of her labor. Enemas, pubic shaving, IVs, and electronic fetal monitoring are not routine procedures. The woman may choose the position that is most comfortable for delivery. The treatment of the newborn's eyes with an antibiotic ointment or silver nitrate may be delayed for a short period so that the infant can have eye-to-eye contact with the mother and father. It should be mentioned, however, that women considered to be high-risk mothers should be in a hospital environment with the equipment and staff available to provide the best possible care for the mother and baby.

LEBOYER METHOD

An approach to childbirth that gained popularity in the late 1970s and early 1980s is the **Leboyer method** instituted by Dr. Frederick Leboyer. This method teaches the physician to maintain a gentle, controlled delivery of the child, taking into consideration the emotional and physiological needs of both child and mother. A constant awareness of the infant as a uniquely sensitive human being is stressed. Leboyer recommends that all unnecessary stimuli in the delivery room be minimized and that the delivery be conducted with soft lights and with the least amount of trauma to both mother and baby. The four areas that are most important in the Leboyer method are:

- gentle, controlled delivery
- avoidance of stress on the craniosacral axis
- avoidance of overstimulating the newborn's sensorium (sensation center of the brain) or breathing
- importance of the maternal-infant bond

Leboyer felt that the ideal birth was one that takes place in a dark, quiet room. The baby is calmed by gentle massage and by being placed in a warm bath. Tying of the umbilical cord is delayed. Leboyer claimed that these infants grow up to be healthier and free of conflict. A recent study did not show that any clear-cut advantages were achieved by the use of this method. The infants were neither more responsive nor less irritable than the control infants during the neonatal period. There were also no differences found in temperament and development at 8 months of age. The conclusion was that the Leboyer method has no advantage over a gentle, conventional delivery. But Dr. Leboyer made many healthcare providers aware that the newborn is a separate human being who deserves consideration and gentleness in the birthing process.

IMMEDIATE CARE OF THE NEWBORN

The transition to **extrauterine** (outside the uterus) life is a critical time for the newborn. The earliest possible recognition of problems that may threaten the newborn's survival is extremely important. Because the nurse is usually the first health-care professional available to assess the newborn's adjustment during this transition, the nurse must possess both the knowledge and skills to evaluate comprehensively the baby's physical status.

PURPOSE

Immediate care is necessary in order to enhance the well-being of the newborn. The goals of this examination are to assess the newborn's ability to adapt to an extrauterine existence, to detect obvious congenital anomalies, to detect the effects of an adverse fetal environment, and to detect evidence of birth trauma. The four components of a comprehensive newborn assessment are initial assessment after birth, assessment after stabilization, ongoing, and discharge.

ASSESSMENT AFTER STABILIZATION

After respirations are sustained, the examination after stabilization should be performed rapidly but gently. The order of the examination is usually visual inspection; auscultation of the chest; palpation of the head, clavicles, abdomen, and extremities; and manipulation of the infant by passing catheters through various orifices, if necessary. This examination will give an immediate evaluation of the newborn to determine if any intervention is necessary.

Observe for obvious malformation of the head: for example, microcephaly, anencephaly, cleft lip or palate, malformed ears, and micrognathia (abnormal development of mandible).

PROCEDURE

Initial Assessment and Care of the Newborn

1. As soon as the baby is delivered, record the exact time of birth.
2. With a sterile towel, receive the baby from the doctor.
3. Rate the baby according to the Apgar scoring system (discussed later in this chapter); record the score.
4. Wipe the baby dry and wrap it in a warm blanket. It is vital that the newborn be kept warm. The infant should be protected from thermal stress, preferably by use of a radiant warming device.
5. If the immediate condition of the mother and baby permit, take the baby to the head of the table for the mother and father to see and hold for a period of time. This is an important time in the establishment of the parent-infant bond.
6. Place the baby on its side in the heated incubator or crib, with the head of the crib lowered; this position promotes drainage of mucus.
7. Suction the baby with the **bulb syringe** or a **DeLee aspirator** (mucus trap) to remove mucus or other secretions that may be present in the infant's mouth, nose, and pharynx. Positioning and suctioning are necessary so the infant does not aspirate this material. (*Caution:* If a bulb syringe is used, the bulb must be squeezed and all air expelled from the syringe before it is gently inserted. Otherwise, the material in the oropharynx will be forced into the bronchi and lungs when the bulb is collapsed.) Gentle suction is provided as the bulb regains its original shape, see Figure 14–12.

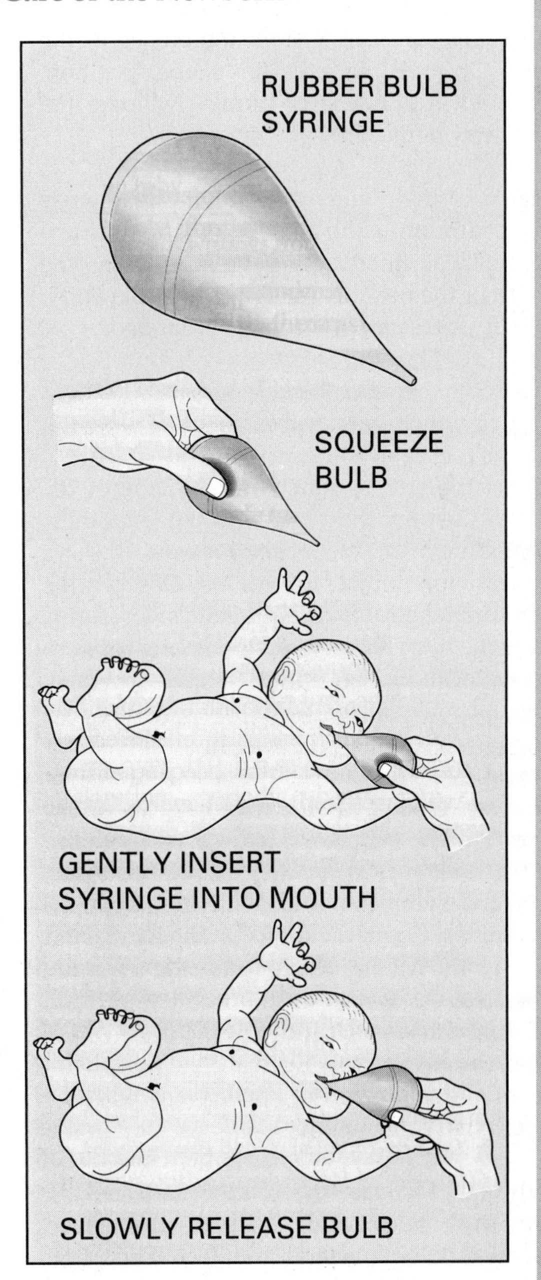

Figure 14–12 *Bulb syringe suctioning*

Also observe for excessive, frothy oral secretions that may suggest the presence of esophageal atresia. Palpate the fontanel and sutures for fullness, depression, overriding, and shape. Measure the circumference of the head. Observe the eyes for shape, position, size, and appearance of pupils. Evaluate the symmetry of the face.

Neck. Goiters and cystic lymphangiomas may compromise the airway, making immediate tracheal intubation necessary. Note the length of the neck, its relationship to the body, mobility, presence of webbing, or fat pads.

The Body. Record the baby's weight, length, head circumference, and chest circumference. Palpate the clavicles for masses and intactness. Inspect the size, symmetry, and shape of the thorax. Inspect the shape of the abdomen. Palpate the liver, spleen, and kidneys. Observe the cord for number of vessels. Observe the appropriateness of visible genitals for stated sex of the baby. Observe female babies for maturation of the labia and for vaginal discharge. Observe male babies for position of the urethral opening, presence of testes, and maturation of the scrotum. Note the elimination of urine and stool. Determine the patency of the anus. Palpate and inspect the spinal column for masses and symmetry of the vertebrae. Note the symmetry and ability to move all extremities. Count the digits on the hands and feet. Evaluate the rotation of the hips by abducting the thighs, rotate the hips through full range of motion, and observe the symmetry of the leg creases. Evaluate the peripheral pulses and compare the upper pulse with the lower pulse for strength.

Reflexes. Evaluate the rooting and sucking responses. Elicit and evaluate the grasp response in both hands and feet. Elicit and evaluate mobility to be pulled to a sitting position, noting head and arm position (traction reflex). Evaluate the Moro reflex, and the dance and stepping responses. To elicit the **Moro reflex**, grasp the infant's hands, extend and abduct the arms with just enough force to almost raise the head from the surface. Sudden release is normally accompanied by an embrace response. Absence of this reflex can indicate intracranial pathology. Asymmetry of the reflex suggests a fracture of the clavicle, the humerus, or a brachial plexus injury. Observe and evaluate tone, tremulousness, and jitteriness. If the infant is floppy, suspect a spinal cord injury or CNS depression.

Skin. **Vernix caseosa**, a white cheesy substance, is normally present on the skin of preterm infants. It is absent in post-term infants, and is present only in the skin folds of term infants. Cyanosis of the feet and hands can persist for some time after respirations have been adequately established. Pallor of the skin may indicate anemia, resulting from hemolysis or hemorrhage, or a state of shock with inadequate cardiac output. Yellow or stained skin, predominantly the nails, umbilical cord, and vernix, due to bile pigments from meconium-stained fluid, suggests previous fetal distress. Close observation for respiratory distress caused by meconium aspiration is indicated. Generalized petechiae and ecchymosis may be present in congenital viral infections such as that with rubella. Petechiae over the head and neck are common in rapid or difficult deliveries. Premature babies bruise easily and ecchymosis may appear in areas where they have been firmly grasped during delivery.

Auscultation of the Chest. The heart rate and rhythm should be noted. A rate of over 160 b.p.m. or under 120 b.p.m. usually indicates the need for diagnostic intervention. Coarse rales usually disappear in the first hours of life. The presence of bowel sounds in the chest may indicate a diaphragmatic hernia. Unilateral absence of breath sounds suggests a pneumothorax diaphragmatic hernia or lobar emphysema. Signs of respiratory distress include tachypnea (more than 50 breaths per minute), chest wall and sternal retractions, nasal flaring, and grunting. They indicate a need for close immediate observation. Slow respirations (fewer than 30 breaths per minute), if shallow, frequently suggest CNS depression.

Eyes. Gently wipe the infant's eyes. Instill the prescribed antibiotic ointment or 1% silver nitrate into the baby's eyes. This treatment protects the infant from any infectious organisms that may have been in the birth canal. It is required by law to prevent blindness caused by the gonococcus organism. The excess ointment may be gently wiped away approximately 15 minutes after application.

Temperature. Take the baby's temperature either axillary or rectally if patency of the rectum has been determined. Be careful not to chill the infant.

Identification and Recording. Fill out Identabands and attach to the infant. This must be done before mother and baby leave the delivery room. The **Identabands** are a wristband for the mother and a wristband and an ankleband for the baby. All three bands are printed with the same number. The mother's name, the doctor's name, the sex of the baby, and the date and time of birth are inserted into the bands. Some hospitals take footprints of the baby and fingerprints of the mother as a further identifying measure.

Complete the newborn record before the baby is taken to the nursery.

APGAR SCORING SYSTEM

The newborn is carefully observed for any signs of respiratory or circulatory distress at all times. One method of assessing the infant involves the use of the **Apgar scoring system**, Figure 14–13. The infant's condition is evaluated at birth on five signs: heart rate, respiratory effort, muscle tone, reflex response, and color. Each sign is graded as 0, 1, or 2. A total of 10 is a perfect composite score.

To score the baby in 1 minute as the test requires, the nurse or physician evaluating the baby should wait 55 seconds after birth and then appraise the baby and enter the score. The baby is evaluated again at 5 minutes after birth. Once a nurse has observed a number of births, the scoring can be done almost at a glance. A baby who is pink all over, howling, and clenching its fists has a 10 score almost automatically. On the other hand, a baby who is quiet and limp probably scores 0 to 1. A zero-rated baby has a better than 50% chance of survival. A stillborn has no score at all.

RESUSCITATION OF THE NEWBORN

The most important responsibility of the obstetrical nurse after a delivery is to observe the newborn closely and continuously for signs of respiratory or circulatory depression. Some infants who cry at birth subsequently develop apnea (temporary loss of breath) and may die unless appropriate resuscitative measures are taken. Therefore, the obstetrical nurse should observe a newborn continuously for at least 5 minutes after delivery and report any signs of depression to the obstetrician.

The responsibility for **resuscitating** (restoring to life) a newborn rests with the anesthetist and obstetrician. The routine measures — aspiration of the mouth, nose, and pharynx; stimulation by flicking of the feet; and administration of oxygen (not under pressure) — may be done by the nurse. Resuscitation of the newborn infant in distress is discussed in greater depth in Chapter 17.

APGAR SCORING SYSTEM

Sign	0	1	2
Heart Rate	Absent (initiate resuscitation)	Slow (below 100);	Good (over 100 b.p.m.)
Respiratory Effort	Absent (initiate resuscitation)	Weak cry; hypoventilation	Good strong cry; established respirations
Muscle Tone	Limp	Some flexion of extremities; weak or floppy resistance	Well flexed; strong resistance response; active motion
Reflex Response 1. Response to catheter in nostril (tested after oropharynx is clear)	No Response	Grimace	Cough or sneeze
2. Tangential foot slap	No Response	Grimace	Strong cry and with-drawal of foot
Color	Blue, pale	Body pink; extremities blue	Completely pink
Category Condition	0–3 poor, critical, severely depressed 4–6 moderately depressed 7–10 good		

Figure 14–13 *(Adapted from* Nursing Inservice Aid, No. 2, *Courtesy Ross Laboratories, published with permission of Dr. Virginia Apgar)*

THE THIRD STAGE OF LABOR

The **third stage of labor** begins after delivery of the baby and terminates with the discharge of the placenta, Figure 14–14. Nursing care given during the third stage of labor is shown in Figure 14–15. The nurse records the exact time the placenta is delivered. The mother is observed for hemorrhage and shock; the baby is observed for breathing, mucus, color, and cry.

The uterus is gently massaged to make it contract in order to expel the placenta. The

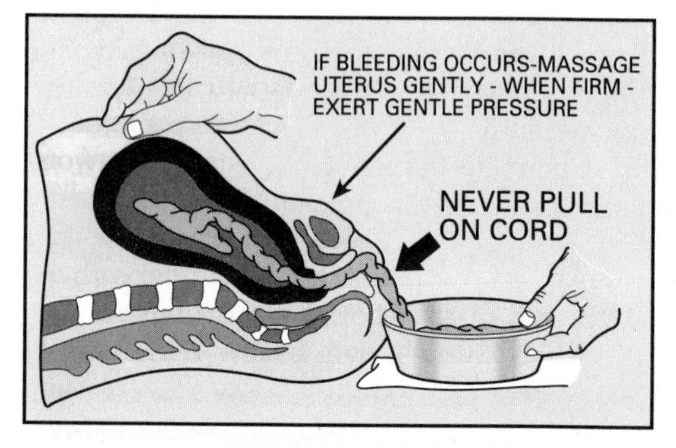

Figure 14–14 *Massaging the uterus aids in the delivery of the placenta.*

Nursing Care for Third Stage of Labor

- Observe the mother for hemorrhage and shock.
- Observe the baby for breathing, mucus, color, and cry.
- Palpate and massage the uterus as directed by the physician immediately after delivery of the infant to stimulate it to contract in order to expel the placenta.
- When a sudden gush of blood is seen and the umbilical cord lengthens, apply gentle pressure on the patient's lower abdomen to assist in expulsion of the placenta.
- Hold a container just below the vaginal opening to receive the placenta.
- Check the mother's pulse and watch for signs of impending shock (rapid pulse and cold perspiration).
- Massage the uterus, if it relaxes. A relaxed uterus is evident in cases of profuse bleeding or *uterine atony* (lack of normal tone of the uterus).
- Check frequently for excessive bleeding; make sure the uterus remains firm.
- Give medications as directed.
- Apply perineal pads to the mother after delivery is completed.
- Dispose of placenta according to hospital policy.
- Remove patient via stretcher to recovery room.
- Finish notes on chart concerning time and type of delivery and exact time of placental delivery.

Figure 14–15

physician may order medications at this time to aid in stimulating contractions of the uterine muscle. When the placenta has been delivered and the uterus is emptied, the fundus of the uterus is gently massaged until it is hard.

After the doctor has inspected the placenta carefully to be sure no afterbirth remains in the birth canal, the nurse disposes of the placenta. Many hospitals now take part in a placenta collection program. The placenta is processed for the recovery and purification of gamma globulin, a serum used in the prevention and treatment of a variety of diseases. The umbilical cord may also be saved. It has been used for femoral vein replacement. The nurse puts the placenta in the container provided for it and places the container in the freezer supplied. The processing company picks it up.

If the mother has had an episiotomy performed, it is repaired after delivery of the placenta. These sutures dissolve in about 3 weeks when the incision is healed.

Following delivery of the afterbirth, the mother must be observed closely for shock and hemorrhage. The average postpartum blood loss is 300 mL. Blood loss of 500 mL or more is considered a hemorrhage. Should this occur, grasp the uterus and massage it gently but firmly until it becomes hard, Figure 14–16. The fundus of the uterus lies just below the umbilicus as soon as delivery is complete.

THE FOURTH STAGE OF LABOR

The first few hours after delivery are vital to the well-being of the new mother. She should be observed closely for any adverse reactions, Figure 14–17. Blood flow, pulse, temperature, and blood pressure should be checked every 15 to 20 minutes for possible hemorrhage, shock, and infections. The fundus of the uterus should be checked for hardness and location. Check to be sure the patient is warm. Many women experience a chill after giving birth. If the woman has an episiotomy, ice to the area during the fourth stage can often reduce swelling and thereby decrease the discomfort that may follow this procedure.

The nurse should keep a written record of all observations so that the physician may be

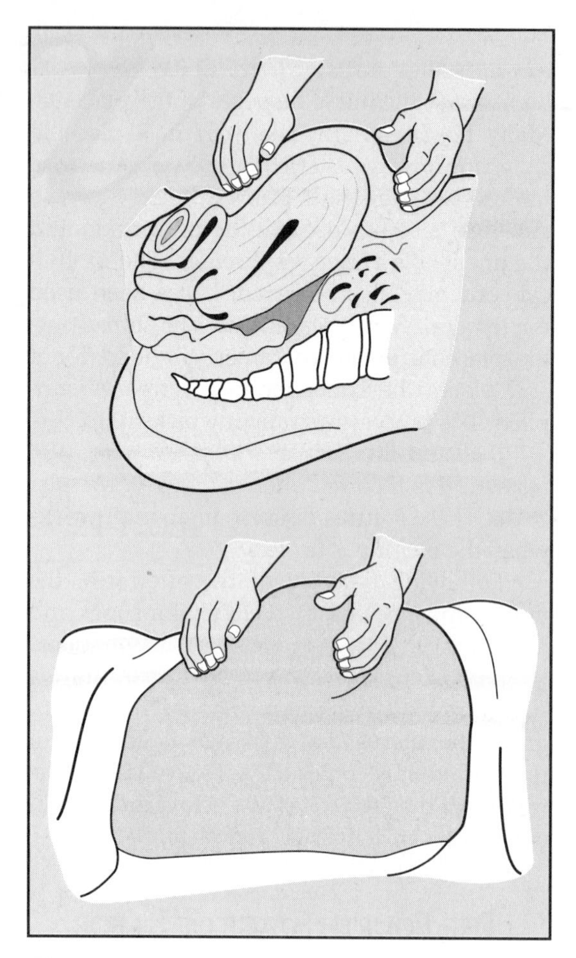

Figure 14–16 *Massaging the uterus to prevent hemorrhage*

Nursing Care for Fourth Stage of Labor

Check Patient for the Following:

- Vaginal drainage. If more than two sanitary napkins are saturated with bloody drainage during the first hour after delivery, there is excessive bleeding. The normal flow of vaginal blood within the first 2 hours after delivery is about 2 ounces. There should be no clots in the blood. If the blood flow increases, the uterus should be massaged until it becomes firm.
- Pulse. After delivery, there may be a slight drop in the pulse rate; it may be 60 to 80 b.p.m. A fast pulse may be a sign of shock or concealed hemorrhage. The nurse should notify the doctor immediately.
- Temperature. Slight rises in temperature may occur following delivery. In general, the temperature should remain within normal limits.
- Blood pressure. The blood pressure should be taken frequently and noted. Any extreme variation should be reported. It is not uncommon for a new mother to complain of a headache. Lying flat may give relief.
- Fundus. The top of the uterus should be hard and firm. It should be located below the navel. If the fundus is soft or large, massage it gently with a circular motion until it is firm. Normally the uterus quickly responds to massage. Do not overmassage.

Figure 14–17

informed of the progress and condition of the new mother.

If the baby's condition is good, many hospitals allow the baby to remain with the mother during this time. Many mothers wish to nurse their baby for a short time. The mother and father may feel like cuddling, holding, talking to and getting to know their infant. Research has shown that the infant is in a heightened state of alertness and responsiveness in the first hours after birth. The infant may be intrigued with nuzzling or sucking at the breast, making eye contact with the parents and responding to verbal and touching contact. This reciprocal responsiveness is the first step in the parent-infant attachment called bonding (see section on bonding in Chapter 15).

New techniques for measuring newborn behavior have been developed that show that newborn infants are much more discriminating and responsive than was previously realized. At birth, the alert newborn is attracted by a variety of visual, sound, and other stimuli. The infant is particularly intrigued by the eyes and other features of the human face. When the baby is in a state of quiet alertness, he will respond to these stimuli with behavior such as gazing, imitating, following with his eyes, and clinging. These reciprocal, synchronized responses between the newborn and his parents reinforce their developing relationship.

Many factors can influence the outcome of birth and the quality of the parent-infant bond. Among these factors are the parents' cultural and socioeconomic backgrounds; their personalities; their previous experience with pregnancy; their attitudes toward pregnancy, parenting, the birth process, and the newborn; and any complications of pregnancy or birth. The physical and mental health of the mother before and during pregnancy can affect the health and development of the fetus, as well as the capacity for the mother and baby to interact at birth. A positive childbirth experience appears to create in the mother and father an increased self-esteem and self-confidence that may foster parental bonding.

The nurse can help facilitate the bonding process by pointing out and reinforcing the parents' perceptions of their baby's ability to interact with them. A father should be encouraged to touch, hold, and interact with his baby. Because early father-baby interactions may be basic to the development of a strong father-child relationship later in life, the nurse's support of the father's role in childbearing and child care after birth is essential. Mother, father, and baby are acutely sensitive to their surroundings and to each other immediately after birth. Therefore, the care, actions, comments, and attitudes of the hospital staff can profoundly influence the early establishment of the parent-infant bond.

ONGOING ASSESSMENT

Hospital stays vary from a short stay of 6 to 12 hours after delivery to 5 or more days after a cesarean section. Both the mother and the newborn need continued assessment for the identification of early problems. If the initial assessment of the newborn is normal, the following should be assessed daily:

- vital signs
- weight (evaluate according to birth weight)
- general changes in color or activity
- feeding status
- elimination
- parent-newborn interaction
- health education needs for the parents

The new mother should be monitored daily for:

- amount of bleeding
- temperature, blood pressure, pulse
- condition of breasts and milk production
- urinary output and bowel movement
- condition of perineum (hemorrhoids or episiotomy or both), or cesarean section incision status
- psychological well-being

The initial and continuing assessment becomes the basis for all discharge planning.

DISCHARGE PLANNING

If possible, the nurse should do the physical and behavioral assessments in the presence of the parents because the assessments present a good opportunity for discussion. Topics might include:

- health education and well-baby care
- parent-newborn interaction — infant cues, behavioral capabilities, and implications to caregiver

- community resources for information and support
- appointment to return to the physician for both a postpartum check for mother and continued infant evaluation and immunizations

Because the transition to extrauterine life is a critical event for the infant, the nurse must possess the knowledge and skills to evaluate both the mother's and the newborn's status initially, daily, at discharge, and during postpartum follow-up visits. Early recognition of problems not only affects whether the infant successfully survives the transition but also may affect the newborn's later growth and development.

REVIEW QUESTIONS

A. Multiple choice. Select the best answer.

1. The Apgar system of evaluating the newborn must first be done at
   a. 1 minute after delivery
   b. 5 minutes after delivery
   c. anytime before the newborn is taken to the nursery
   d. within 24 hours after delivery
2. Placenta collection programs process the placenta for the recovery of
   a. red blood cells
   b. white blood cells
   c. hemoglobin
   d. gamma globulin
3. The purpose of an antibiotic ointment being placed in the eyes of the newborn is to
   a. help the baby see better
   b. prevent infection that may have been transmitted in passage through the birth canal
   c. prevent infection that may have been transmitted during the pregnancy
   d. help prevent jaundice
4. The person placing the patient's legs in stirrups must lift both legs at the same time in order to prevent
   a. rupturing the membranes
   b. straining the patient's back
   c. straining the ligaments of the patient's pelvis
   d. blocking blood flow to the uterus and fetus
5. Leg cramps may be relieved by
   a. applying cold compresses to the legs
   b. stretching the leg out forcibly and pulling the foot toward the knee
   c. taking the legs out of the stirrups momentarily
   d. giving pain-relieving medication
6. Nursing care during delivery includes
   a. coaching the patient
   b. checking fetal heart tones
   c. recording exact time of birth
   d. all of the above
7. Immediate care of the newborn includes all except
   a. suctioning the mouth, nose, and pharynx to remove mucus
   b. observing for signs of respiratory or circulatory distress
   c. bathing the newborn
   d. instilling eye drops or ointment
8. During the fourth stage of labor, it is important for the nurse to monitor the mother's
   a. vaginal discharge
   b. pulse, blood pressure, and temperature
   c. firmness of uterine fundus
   d. all of the above

B. Briefly answer the following questions.

1. List six signs that indicate that the second stage of labor is beginning.
2. Name the five signs scored in the Apgar scoring system for evaluating the newborn.
3. List six factors that may influence parent-infant bonding.
4. Name the different positions a woman may use in the second stage of labor. Give one advantage and disadvantage of each.

SUGGESTED ACTIVITIES

- Describe the various positions for the second stage of labor. List the advantages and disadvantages of each.
- Identify components to be included in a newborn screening physical exam. Differentiate normal from abnormal findings.
- Describe and chart normal and abnormal findings in the neonate.
- Discuss the advantages and disadvantages of prepared childbirth. Discuss medicated versus nonmedicated labor and birth.
- Discuss the pros and cons of in-hospital birth versus out-of-hospital birth as they are related to:
  - safety
  - family-centered care
  - sibling involvement
  - immediate postpartum management
- Role play assisting with a delivery and immediate care of the newborn.
- Discuss the complications that might occur during the second stage of labor such as prolapsed cord, precipitate delivery, ruptured uterus, uterine inertia, severe dehydration of mother, drop in fetal heart tones or irregularities of tone, and premature separation of placenta. Investigate each complication and discuss the nursing care required for each.
- Write a complete examination of a healthy newborn in the delivery room. Include observations and significance of findings.

BIBLIOGRAPHY

Hamilton, P. M. *Basic Maternity Nursing*, 6th ed. St. Louis, MO: C. V. Mosby, 1989.

Hassid, P. *A Textbook for Childbirth Educators*. New York: Harper and Row, 1978.

Hawkins, J. W., and L. Pierfedeici. *Maternity and Gynecological Nursing*. New York: J. B. Lippincott, 1981.

Jenson, M. D., Benson, R., and I. Bobsk, *Maternity Care: The Nurse and the Family*, 3rd ed. St. Louis, MO: C. V. Mosby, 1985.

McNall, L. K. *Obstetric and Gynecologic Nursing*. St. Louis, MO: C. V. Mosby, 1980.

Oxorn, H. *Oxorn-Foote Human Labor and Birth*, 5th ed. E. Norwalk, CT: Appleton-Century-Crofts, 1986.

Pillitteri, A. *Maternal-Newborn Nursing: Care of the Growing Family*, 2nd ed. Boston: Little, Brown and Co., 1981.

Pritchard, J. A., MacDonald, P. C., and N. F. Grant. *Williams Obstetrics*, 17th ed. E. Norwalk, CT: Appleton-Century-Crofts, 1985.

Reeder, S., Mastroianni, L., Jr., and L. Martin. *Maternity Nursing*, 16th ed. New York: J. B Lippincott, 1987.

Tucker, S. M., et al. *Patient Care Standards: Nursing Process, Diagnosis, and Outcome*, 5th ed. St. Louis, MO: C. V. Mosby, 1992.

CHAPTER

15

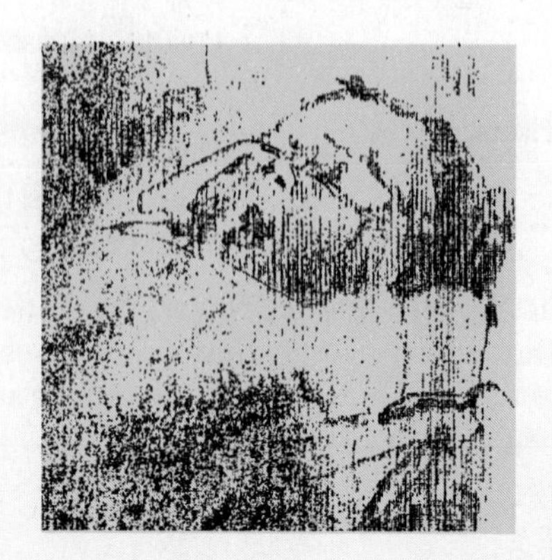

Complications of Labor and Delivery

OBJECTIVES

AFTER STUDYING THIS CHAPTER, THE STUDENT SHOULD BE ABLE TO:

- DIFFERENTIATE BETWEEN PREMATURE, PROLONGED, AND PRECIPITOUS LABOR.
- IDENTIFY COMPLICATIONS CAUSED BY THE FORCES, THE PASSENGER, AND THE PASSAGE.
- DESCRIBE ABNORMAL FETAL POSITIONS.
- LIST THE REASONS FOR A CESAREAN DELIVERY.
- DESCRIBE THE CARE GIVEN IF THE MOTHER IS UNCONSCIOUS.

KEY TERMS

PREMATURE LABOR
TOCOLYTIC TREATMENT
PROM
CHORIOAMNIONITIS
RDS
PRECIPITOUS LABOR
PRECIPITATE DELIVERY
DYSTOCIA
UTERINE DYSFUNCTION (FORCES)
FRANK BREECH

COMPLETE BREECH
FOOTLING BREECH
VERSION
CEPHALOPELVIC DISPROPORTION
SHOULDER PRESENTATION
BROW PRESENTATION
FACE PRESENTATION
FETOPELVIC DISPROPORTION
CESAREAN SECTION
MIDLINE INCISION
BIKINI CUT
VBAC
PROLAPSED CORD
NUCHAL CORD
PLACENTA PREVIA
PLACENTA ABRUPTIO
POSTPARTUM HEMORRHAGE
STILLBIRTH

About 85% of all births are vaginal deliveries. Some situations, however, can threaten the life of both the mother and the baby. A labor complication presents problems to the mother or the baby that require medical assistance and intervention to ensure an optimal outcome. Observation, reporting, technical skill, and physical and emotional supportive measures must all be carried out with a fine degree of competency.

Premature Labor

Gestational age appears to have a more significant effect than weight on the survival of the baby. Labor that begins three or more weeks before the expected date is termed **premature labor**. It is difficult to make a cut-off point for survival; babies born at 24 weeks of gestation have survived. Optimal outcome depends on closely coordinated care.

If a woman appears to have started her labor too early, active therapy is often indicated to try to arrest the uterine contractions as long as there is no evidence of fetal distress. Sometimes bed rest in the left lateral position is successful in reducing the frequency and intensity of contractions. Hydration with Ringer lactate may also help arrest the labor process. The decision of whether to use medication to stop the labor is based on the likelihood that prolonging the pregnancy will benefit the baby and not risk the health of the mother. Stopping premature labor with medications is known as **tocolytic treatment**. The most common cause of morbidity and mortality in premature infants is lung immaturity. As a rule, the lungs mature at approximately 35 weeks of gestation. At 35 weeks there is a large increase of pulmonary surfactant resulting in the lecithin-sphingomyelin (L-S) ratio in the amniotic fluid reaching 2 or more. Lung maturity can be diagnosed by amniocentesis to determine the L-S ratio. If the lungs are immature, therapy with steroids is considered to induce the baby's lungs to mature.

Because the baby is small, medications that tend to depress the baby are avoided during labor. If the baby is premature, special attention should be focused in four basic areas. The infant should be helped to breathe, kept warm and dry, handled with care, and protected from infection, see Figure 15–1.

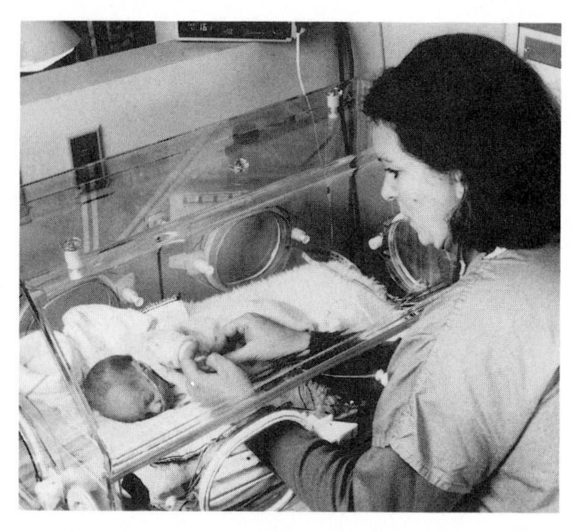

Figure 15–1 *Caring for the premature infant requires special attention.*

PREMATURE RUPTURE OF MEMBRANES

Spontaneous rupture of the membranes one hour or more before the onset of labor is defined as **premature rupture of membranes (PROM)**. PROM complicates about 10% of term pregnancies and as high as 30% of preterm pregnancies. The cause of PROM is usually unknown. The most common known risk factors are trauma (coitus or pelvic exam), incompetent cervix, infection, or polyhydramnios (excessive amniotic fluid). If the expectant mother reports a leak or gush of fluid from the vagina, further tests are indicated to confirm a rupture of the membranes. The mother should be asked to describe the color of the fluid and to report any foul odor. Diagnosis should not be based on history alone. Further investigation is necessary before a definitive diagnosis of PROM is made. One of the easiest ways to determine ruptured membranes is the nitrazine test. Amniotic fluid is more alkaline than vaginal or cervical secretions. When the membranes rupture, the vagina is bathed with amniotic fluid, which alters the pH. If the vaginal fluid is acid on the nitrazine test (paper strip sensitive to pH values), the membranes are definitely intact. If the fluid is alkaline on the nitrazine test, the membranes are probably ruptured. Nitrazine paper, however, will give an alkaline result if it is contaminated with blood, urine, or secretions caused by a vaginal infection. A positive nitrazine test should be confirmed by a fern test.

A drop of vaginal fluid is placed on a slide and allowed to dry. It is then examined under the microscope. Sodium chloride from the amniotic fluid, when allowed to dry on a clean slide, will crystallize and will show a characteristic fern pattern. This pattern indicates that the membranes have ruptured.

The major complication following premature rupture of membranes is **chorioamnionitis,** or an infection within the amniotic sac. The longer the duration of PROM, the greater is the likelihood of development of maternal sepsis. There are also numerous risks to the baby, depending on maturity, including infection and prolapsed cord.

Management of PROM depends on when in the pregnancy it occurs and the health of both the mother and the baby. If the pregnancy is more than 36 weeks, the greater the duration of PROM the higher the risk of infectious morbidity and mortality for both the mother and the baby. If the baby is close to term, the incidence of serious **respiratory distress syndrome (RDS)** is rare and the risk of infection becomes much more significant. Induction (starting labor) is the management of choice in this gestational age group.

PRECIPITOUS LABOR

A **precipitous labor** is spontaneous labor that progresses very rapidly and usually lasts less than 3 hours. A labor of this sort usually starts out almost immediately with very strong, frequent contractions. Things happen so fast that it is often difficult for the mother to handle the contractions.

Conditions that predispose to or contribute to the etiology of precipitous labor include:

- multiparity
- large pelvis
- lax and unresistant soft tissues
- strong uterine contractions
- small baby in a good position
- induction of labor
- previous precipitous labor

The distinction should be made between a precipitous labor and a precipitate delivery. A **precipitate delivery**, if sudden and unexpected, may mean an unattended delivery. Any delivery should be gentle and controlled because it lessens the chance of cerebral trauma in the infant and vaginal laceration in the mother. But a gentle, controlled delivery may be difficult with a precipitate delivery. Doctors sometimes attempt to slow the progress of labor through the use of medication, depending on how well the mother and baby are coping with the labor process.

PROLONGED LABOR

Occasionally, the nurse might observe that a woman is in labor for hours and hours without progress. There is obviously something wrong with the mechanism of labor. This situation is termed **dystocia** (difficult labor). The cause could be related to three factors: the forces, the passenger, or the passageway.

THE FORCES: UTERINE DYSFUNCTION

A delay in any of the phases of labor is known as **uterine dysfunction**. This delay could be due to the poor quality of uterine contractions or to maternal exhaustion. The chief causes of uterine dysfunction are:

- weak, irregular, uncoordinated uterine contractions
- minor degrees of pelvic contraction
- slight extension of the fetal head
- unwise use of analgesia

Other contributing factors include overdistention of the uterus, maternal age, successive pregnancies at close intervals, uterine fibroids interfering with uterine muscle coordination, and rigidity of the cervix. Sometimes the actual cause is unknown. The complications can be unfortunate. Fetal injury or death are the most serious outcomes. For the mother, exhaustion and dehydration occur if labor goes on too long. Intervention can be effective in preventing these serious problems if good observation and support are given by the nurse and the attending physician is kept notified of the patient's condition. A prolonged latent phase may be managed in one of two ways: Either the mother may be sedated to allow her to rest for a period of 4–6 hours or the contractions may be stimulated to facilitate progress. The choice of treatment depends on the status of the mother and her baby.

THE PASSENGER: ABNORMAL FETAL POSITION

Positions and presentations that are not normal often cause dystocia and subsequent complications. It is difficult for the baby to move forward.

Persistent Occiput Posterior Position. The occiput posterior (O.P.) position prolongs labor whenever the fetal head enters the pelvis with the occiput directed diagonally posterior (in either the R.O.P. or L.O.P. position). Under these circumstances, the head must rotate through an arc of 135 degrees of the process of internal rotation instead of the normal 45 to 90 degree arc. With good contractions, adequate flexion, and an average-size baby, most of these infants spontaneously rotate through the 135 degree arc as soon as the head reaches the pelvic floor. However, the fetus may rotate only partially and be born with its face upward. The mother may experience a great deal of discomfort in her back as the baby's head presses against the sacrum during the rotation. Sacral counterpressure, back rubs, and frequent change of position from side to side can be helpful.

Breech. Breech occurs in about 3% of all term deliveries; the breech instead of the vertex (top of the head) presents at the pelvic outlet. There are three classifications of breech position (see Figure 15–2):

- **Frank breech**: the buttocks present, the legs are extended up and are pressed against the abdomen and chest
- **Complete breech**: the buttocks and feet present, and the knees are drawn up
- **Footling breech**: one or both feet present

In a breech position, the baby often passes meconium (a greenish black to light brown tar-like material) from his rectum after the rupture of the membranes. Upon seeing this substance coming from the birth canal, the nurse must be sure that the baby is, in fact, in the breech position. This diagnosis is made by a pelvic exam. The soft, palpable buttocks with genitals, ischial tuberosities, and sacrum are felt with increased ease as cervical dilation proceeds. If a complete or footling breech is present, an extremity can often be felt. If the baby is in the vertex position, discharge of meconium is an indication of fetal distress.

The management of breech presentation is in a state of flux at the present time. The use

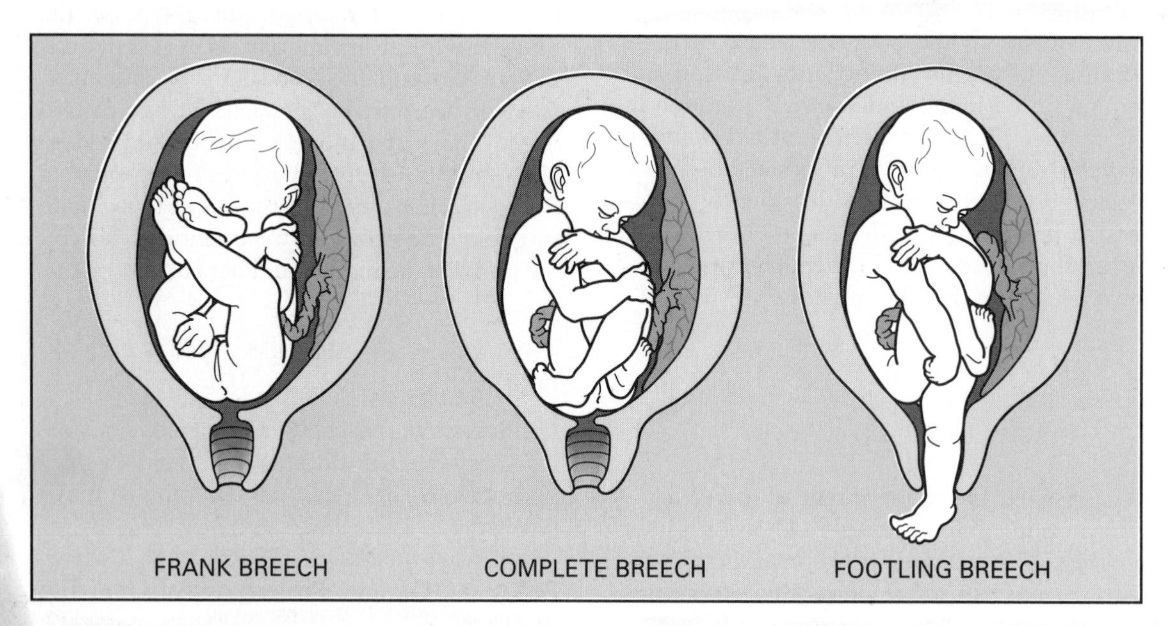

Figure 15–2 Types of breech presentations

of cesarean section is increasing. Attempting external **version** (turning a breech to a vertex position) with the use of tocolytic agents for uterine relaxation has been advocated. Version is aided with the use of ultrasound to monitor the baby's position.

Certain criteria should be met if breech-positioned babies are to be delivered vaginally. The position should be a frank breech. Complete and footling breeches are associated with a higher incidence of prolapsed cord and thus should be delivered by cesarean section. The estimated fetal weight should be between 2,500 and 3,500 g (5½ lb–7 lb 11 oz). If the baby is under 2,500 g and premature, there is a greater risk of morbidity and mortality. The risk that the cervix will entrap the fetal head is also higher because of the smaller trunk-to-head ratio in prematurity. If the estimated weight is over 3,500 g, a cesarean section is performed because of the risk of **cephalopelvic disproportion** (the baby's head is too large for the pelvis). The mother's pelvis should be gynecoid and adequate in size to accommodate an infant of this size. The labor should progress, with both cervical dilatation and descent occurring within a normal range of time (under 18 hours). There can be no evidence of abnormal fetal heart rate patterns, and continuous fetal monitoring must be maintained. The risks of breech delivery should always be explained to the parents so that they may be involved in the decision-making process.

Shoulder, Brow, and Face Presentations. In **shoulder presentations** the infant lies crosswise, Figure 15–3. This is a serious complication. Rupture of the membranes poses a considerable risk of prolapsed cord. Sometimes, an extremity prolapses alongside the presenting part and the two enter the pelvis simultaneously. This complication is not seen commonly, with greater frequency associated with birth weights of less than 1,500 g and with multiple gestations. The diagnosis is made with abdominal palpation and pelvic exam. An arm, shoulder, or rib cage is felt vaginally. Also, the fundus is usually lower

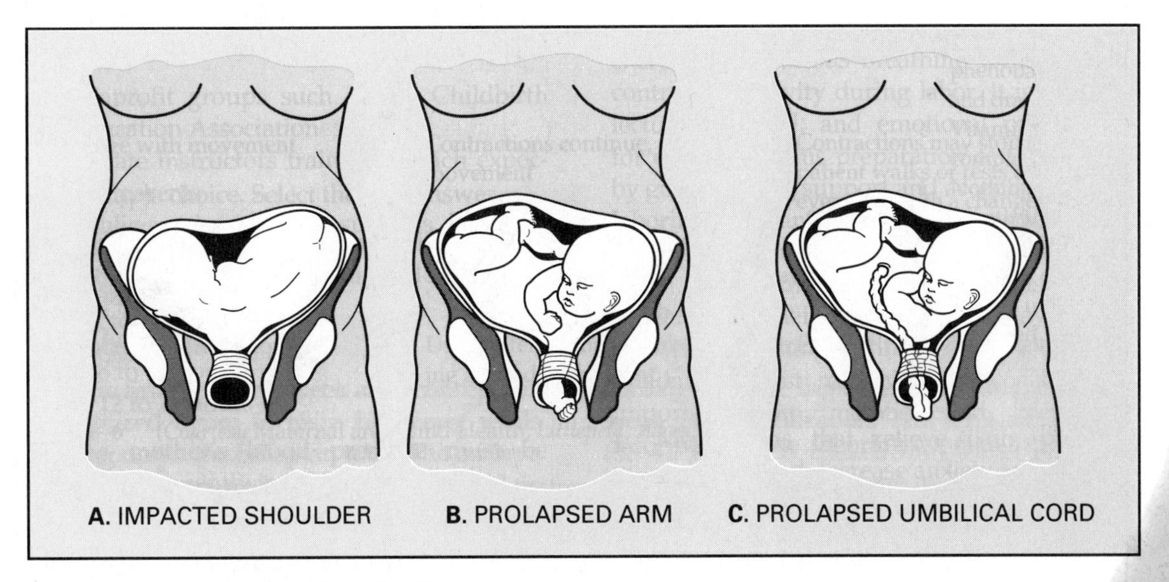

Figure 15–3 Abnormal positions: shoulder presentations

than expected for the length of gestation. The physician may try to turn the baby under tocolysis to a vertex position. (Altering the fetal position in utero in order to facilitate delivery is known as version.) Ultrasound to confirm the baby's position is helpful in versions. More frequently, a cesarean section is necessary.

Brow presentation is an attitude of partial or halfway extension. In **face presentation**, the extension is complete, see Figure 15–4. Brow presentation, fortunately, is rare; it occurs in fewer than 1 in 1,000 deliveries. The usual course of labor with brow presentation is conversion to an occiput or a face presentation. Face presentation occurs approximately once

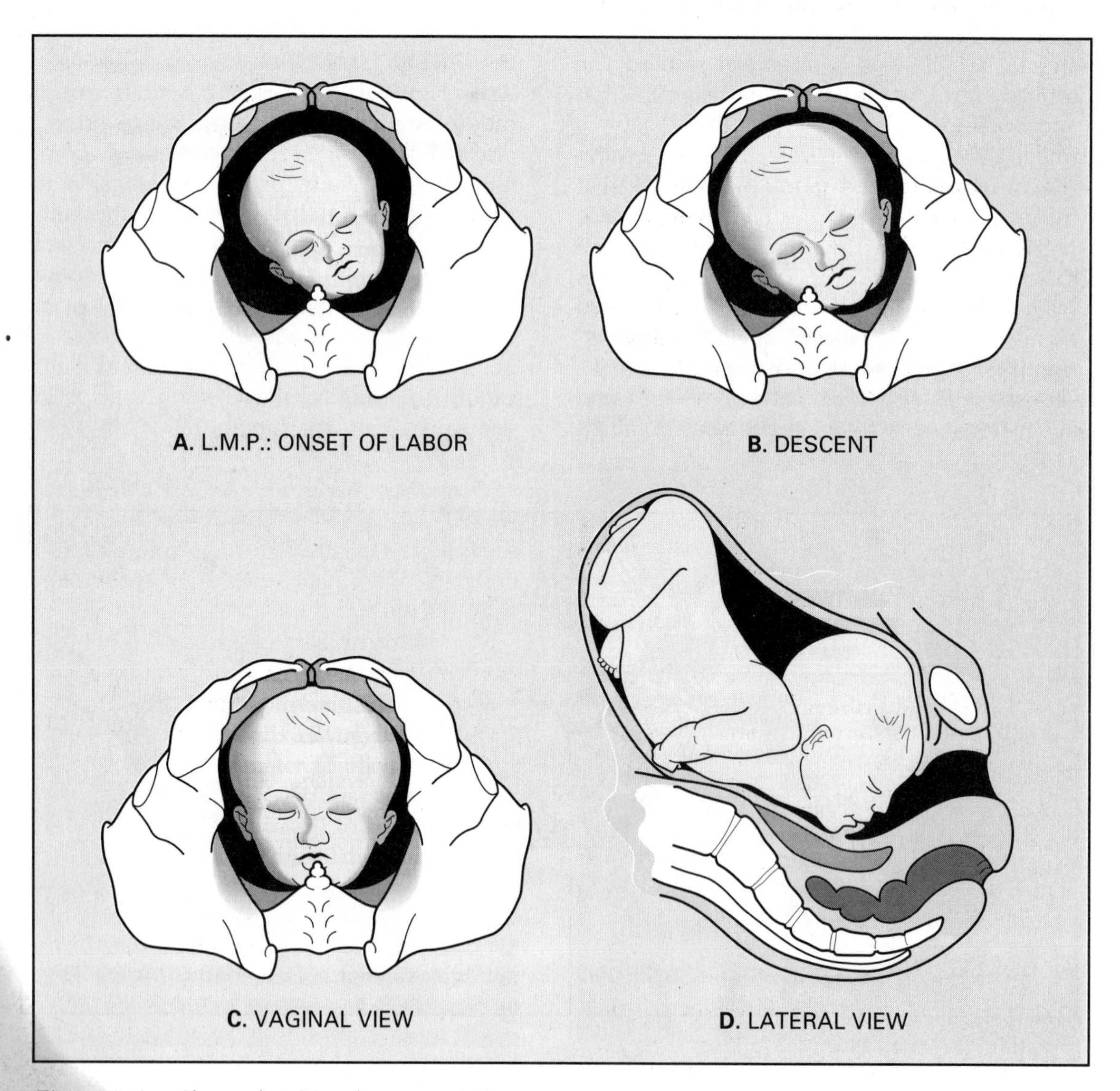

Figure 15–4 Abnormal positions: brow presentations

in 500 deliveries and results, in most instances, from an initial brow presentation that extends to the face presentation at the pelvic inlet. The diagnosis is made by pelvic exam. The frontal sutures, large anterior fontanelle, orbital ridges, eyes, and nose may be felt on vaginal examination. Usually there is a delay in descent. The diagnosis may be confirmed by abdominal roentgenography or ultrasound. Management of these positions is usually cesarean section unless the baby changes its position early in labor.

THE PASSAGEWAY: DISPROPORTION

Fetopelvic disproportion arises when the infant is too large to pass through a small contracted pelvis at either the inlet, the midpelvis, or the outlet, see Figure 15–5. A small pelvis is often detected during antepartal care. The infant size at the time of delivery is also important. One of the common causes of a large for gestational age baby is diabetes. Prolonged pregnancy can also be a factor.

Minor degrees of pelvic contraction can be overcome by efficient uterine contractions, the ability of expansion of the soft tissues, favorable attitude, presentation and position of the baby, and the moldability of the fetal head. If contractions are poor, soft parts are rigid, the position is abnormal, or the head does not mold properly, vaginal birth is impossible. When a labor is not progressing, the physician will evaluate by doing a pelvic exam and sometimes using x-ray pelvimetry. If fetopelvic disproportion is only suspected but not confirmed, amniotomy (breaking the bag of waters) and oxytocin stimulation may be started. The rationale is simply that if the pelvis is not adequate, delivery will not occur. Careful monitoring and close observation are essential to be sure the baby is not compromised. If labor does not progress with these interventions, or if the fetus is showing any sign of distress with prolonged labor, a cesarean section will be performed.

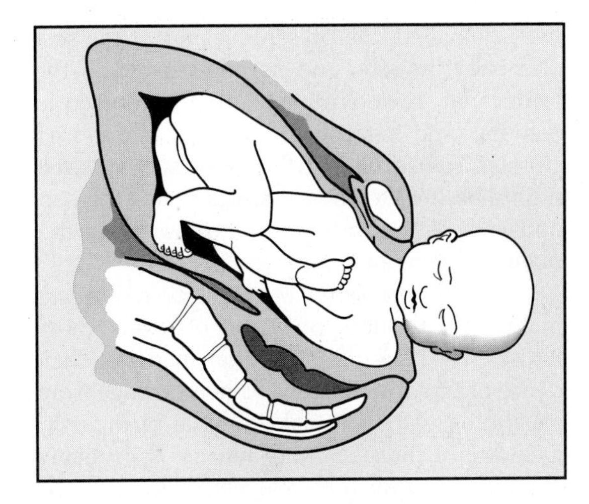

Figure 15–5 *Shoulder dystocia*

MULTIPLE PREGNANCY

Multiple pregnancy, or multiple gestation, is usually diagnosed when the uterus is found to be larger than expected. Two or more fetal heart beats may also be discovered during prenatal care. The diagnosis is confirmed by ultrasound. The mother usually experiences greater discomforts and higher risks than the woman with a single pregnancy. Because multiple births are associated with an increased risk of PIH, preeclampsia, anemia, postpartum hemorrhage, abruptio placenta, placenta previa, hydramnios, premature labor, and dysfunctional labor, close prenatal care from the 25th week is indicated.

If the first baby is breech, a cesarean section is usually performed. Some physicians advocate cesarean section for all pregnancies of less than 32 weeks gestation regardless of presentation. When the first baby is presenting in a vertex position, a trial of labor is often given with indications for cesarean section or oxytocin being the same as for a single pregnancy. Anesthesia is usually desired in case manipulative procedures are necessary for the second baby. As soon as the first baby has been delivered, the presenting part of the second baby, its size, and its relationship to the birth canal are determined. Labor is allowed to resume, and fetal heart rate is monitored closely. The second baby is usually delivered within 30 minutes of the first. Even if the second baby is not in a vertex position, it is frequently delivered vaginally.

All the problems of twin gestation are intensified by the presence of even more fetuses. The risks of malposition, increased incidence of prolapsed cord, and hemorrhage from separating placentas make vaginal birth risky. Delivery of three or more fetuses is probably better accomplished by cesarean section.

At delivery, the nurse has the responsibility of supportive care and assisting the doctor. In multiple births, the infants are likely to be small, and oxygen and resuscitative measures may be necessary. The care is similar to that of the premature infant. The nurse must realize that it may be difficult for the parents to adjust to the birth of more than one child, both emotionally and financially. Problems may also be compounded in feeding, especially if the mother wants to breast feed the babies. None of these problems is insurmountable, but some parents may need an understanding person to help them through this initial adjustment period.

CESAREAN SECTION

Under certain conditions it is necessary that the baby be delivered through the abdominal wall by a surgical procedure called a **cesarean section**, Figure 15–6. The cesarean birth is becoming more common. Approximately 10% to 20% of hospital births are cesarean deliveries, with a higher rate in medical centers that treat high-risk mothers. There are numerous reasons for cesarean deliveries:

- fetopelvic disproportion
- malpresentation
- failure to progress through labor (little or no cervical dilatation)
- fetal distress
- prolapsed cord
- placenta previa
- abruptio placenta
- maternal disease (preeclampsia, diabetes, high blood pressure, acute case of genital herpes)

In some hospitals, cesarean deliveries are performed in the operating room because it is considered major surgery. The surgical area is connected to the labor and delivery unit in most hospitals, so the woman stays in the same area, cared for by the specially trained delivery staff. The setup is for major surgery, and the obstetrical technician or nurse acts as scrub nurse in such operations. The routine in preparation for a cesarean delivery is similar to the usual surgical procedure, but the setup pack is different because of the special instruments used. If the operation is elective (not an emergency), the physician may schedule it one or two weeks before the due date to avoid the beginning of spontaneous labor.

The procedure takes about 1 to 2 hours, but often the baby is born only 5 to 10 minutes after the surgery begins. Anesthesia is necessary for the procedure. Regional anesthesia, which allows the mother to be awake without feeling pain, is most often used. A spinal anesthetic makes the mother numb from the chest to the toes. Some women report a sensation of tugging or pulling, shoulder pain, pressure, burning sensations, nausea, or shortness of breath during the surgery. A general anesthetic is occasionally used for cesarean births when the anesthesiologist deems it necessary or in an emergency.

There are two types of skin incisions for a cesarean birth. The **midline incision** is vertical between the navel and the pubic bone. It allows for a quicker delivery in an emergency. The reasons for using the midline incision include:

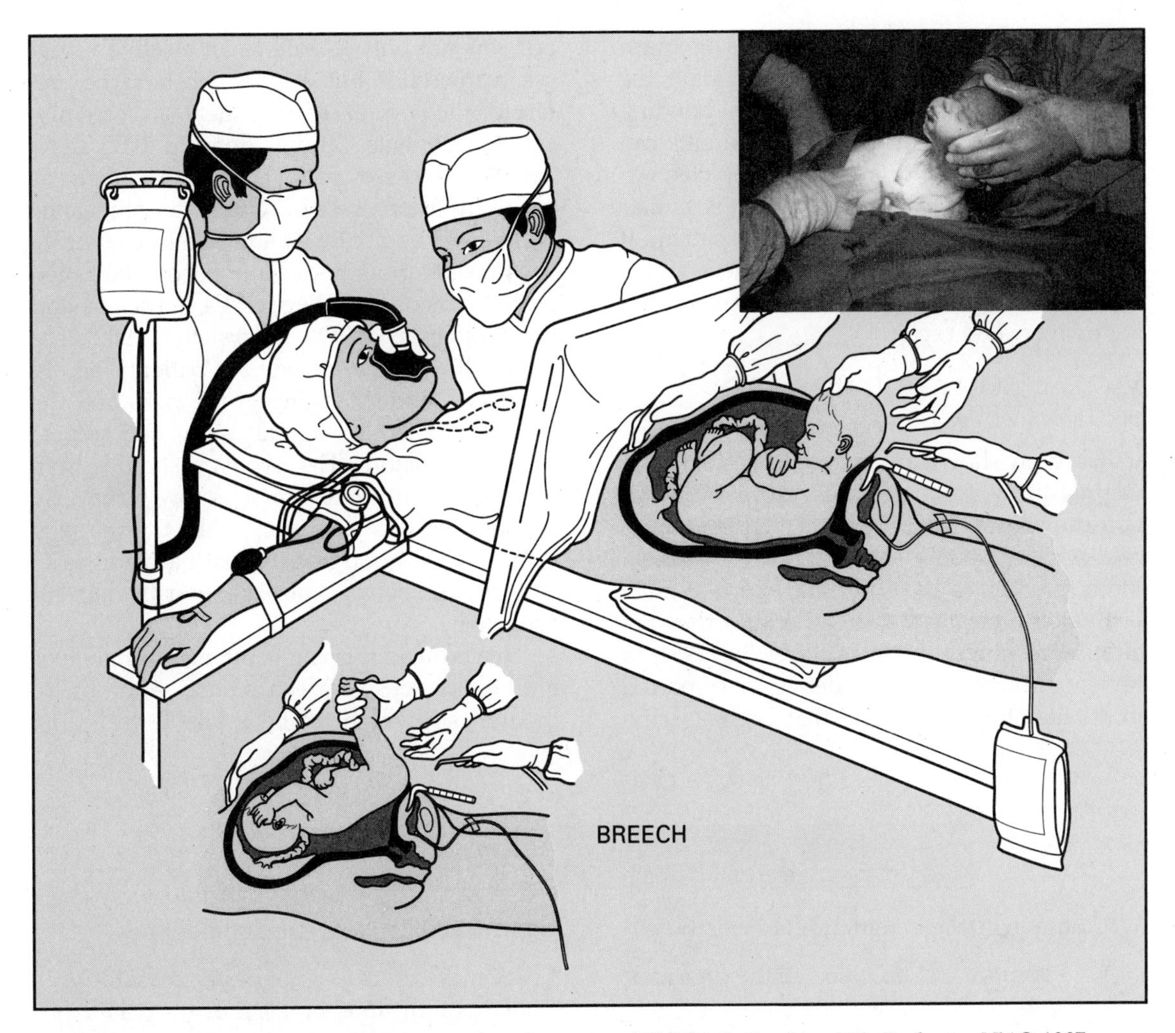

Figure 15–6 *Cesarean section (Illustration adapted courtesy of Childbirth Graphics, Ltd., Rochester, NY © 1987; Photo by Marjorie Pyle, © LIFECIRCLE)*

- the lower uterine segment cannot be exposed or entered safely because of the bladder
- a large fetus is in a transverse lie, and the shoulder is impacted in the birth canal
- there is an anterior placenta previa implantation
- there are certain uterine malformations

The transverse skin incision (Pfanaenstiel transverse suprasymphyseal incision), or **"bikini cut,"** is made just above the pubic bone. This type of incision is associated with less blood loss and reduced postpartum infection. After a lower uterine segment transverse incision, a future vaginal birth is possible.

The majority of hospitals permit the father to remain with the mother during the surgery. He will be required to dress in a surgical scrub suit with cap, foot coverings, and mask. He will be asked not to touch any sterile trays or equipment. After the initial newborn evaluation, the father may hold his baby. The initial bonding process between the baby and its parents can begin while the surgical repair is completed.

Postoperative care of this patient is similar to that given any abdominal surgery patient. If the woman is given a general anesthetic and is unconscious, special care must be given after her delivery and repair.

VAGINAL BIRTH AFTER A CESAREAN SECTION (VBAC)

It has been shown in various studies that a **vaginal birth after a cesarean section (VBAC)** will prove safe if the previous cesarean surgical incision was a low transverse incision. Many physicians have not allowed a vaginal birth after a cesarean section because they are afraid the uterus will rupture. In 1981, a review of more than 8,000 deliveries (reported in the literature) concluded that vaginal delivery was not only as safe as an elective repeat cesarean section but was also, in fact, the preferred method of management in carefully selected patients. Studies done in 1985 show that two-thirds of patients with the diagnosis of failure to progress in a previous pregnancy will deliver vaginally if allowed a trial labor.

Specific guidelines have been established by the American College of Obstetricians and Gynecologists (ACOG Newsletter 1982), see Figure 15–7. They include the patient's acceptance and understanding of the risks and the benefits of both vaginal birth and repeat cesarean section. The woman should have undergone only one previous low transverse incision with no extension of the uterine incision. Finally, a judgment must be made as to whether the pelvis is adequate for the current pregnancy.

If a woman is going to attempt a trial labor after a previous cesarean section, appropriate medical support must be available including

MANAGEMENT OF VBAC

Common management guidelines

1. Parents have discussed all the pros and cons of a VBAC with their doctor.
2. The present pregnancy has no indications for recommending a cesarean section.
3. A low transverse incision was used in the previous cesarean section.
4. The mother is admitted to the hospital early in labor, so that her progress can be carefully monitored.
5. Backup facilities for an immediate cesarean section are available.

Controversial management guidelines

1. Some doctors will not permit a trial labor if the mother has previously had a cesarean section because of too small a pelvis.
2. Some doctors won't use drugs that stimulate labor if the mother has had a previous cesarean.
3. Some doctors don't recommend regional anesthesia during a vaginal delivery after a cesarean because they believe it could mask rupture problems.
4. Some doctors recommend the routine use of low forceps to shorten labor if the woman has previously had a cesarean.

Figure 15–7 *Prerequisites for a safe vaginal birth after a cesarean section (VBAC)* in-hospital obstetrician, pediatrician, anesthesiologist, and skilled nursing staff. An adequate blood bank should be available. Electronic fetal heart rate monitoring is advisable during labor. There must also be an appropriately staffed operating room available in case a repeat cesarean is indicated.

PROLAPSED CORD

A **prolapsed cord** has occurred if the umbilical cord can be seen beside the presenting part of the baby as it appears at the vaginal opening or if the cord is seen coming out of the vaginal opening, Figure 15–8. This complication is not

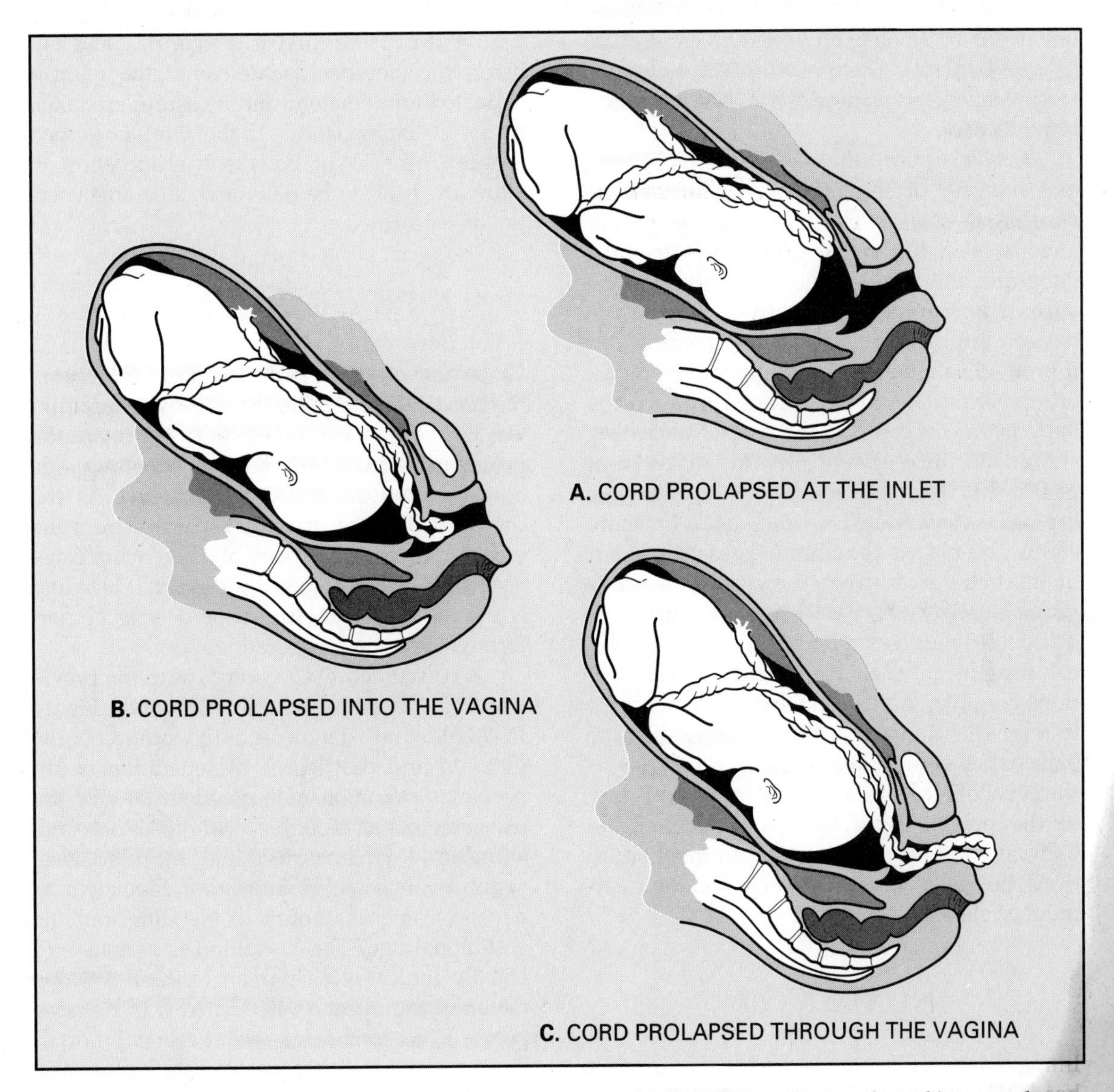

Figure 15–8 *If the umbilical cord emerges before the baby, the baby's life is in danger because the cord is squeezed between the baby and the mother's bony pelvis.*

common; it happens only about once out of every 400 births. The cause for cord prolapse is simply that the presenting part does not completely occupy the lower segment of the uterus. When the membranes rupture, the cord can prolapse between the maternal pelvis and the presenting part of the baby. Prolapsed cord is more likely to occur in pregnancies with malpresentations such as breech, transverse lie, or brow or face presentation; premature or small infants; twins; contracted pelvic or fetopelvic disproportion; and low placenta implantation.

This complication, however, is very serious because of the high infant death rate associated with it. The baby's life is threatened because the cord is pressed between the baby and the bony pelvis. The baby's blood supply is shut off and with it, the baby's oxygen supply. The baby quickly suffocates if immediate attention is not given. The mother's position should be changed to keep the baby from compressing the cord. The mother should be immediately put in a knee-chest position or Trendelenburg position, with the hips elevated and the head low. Pressure should be placed against the presenting part of the baby away from the cord. Oxygen is given to the mother by mask. Because it is difficult to reduce the pressure on the umbilical cord as long as strong uterine contractions continue, a tocolytic drug may be given to relax the uterus. Immediate delivery of the baby is, of course, the optimal treatment. If the cervix is fully dilated and the head is low in the pelvis, using forceps to deliver the baby quickly may be possible. In most situations, however, a cesarean section is the treatment of choice.

NUCHAL CORD

Immediately after the birth of the infant's head, the physician checks for a **nuchal cord** (around the neck). The fingers are passed along the occiput to the infant's neck to determine whether one or more loops of umbilical cord encircle the neck. If the cord is coiled around the neck, it is gently drawn down and, if loose enough, slipped over the baby's head. This is done to prevent any interference with the baby's oxygen supply as the shoulders are delivered. If the cord is coiled too tightly to permit this procedure, it is clamped and cut before the shoulders are delivered; the infant is extracted immediately, and measures are taken to avoid asphyxiation. If the cord is looped around the neck or body and is too short to allow the head to be delivered, a cesarean section is performed.

PLACENTA PREVIA

When the placenta covers or partially covers the cervix, the condition is called **placenta previa**, Figure 15–9. The placenta is in front of the presenting part of the baby. Placenta previa occurs in 1 out of 200 pregnancies. As the cervix dilates, the placenta separates from the uterus, depriving the baby of oxygen and causing painless bleeding in the mother. If bleeding is present, a pelvic exam should *never* be performed unless in an operating room.

As discussed in Chapter 8, placenta previa may be marginal, partial, or total, Figure 15–10. Accurate diagnosis of the location of the placenta and the degree of separation is important. Separation of more than 50% of the placenta is incompatible with fetal survival. Ultrasound is the safest and most accurate means to obtain this information. Management depends on the amount of bleeding and the gestational age. This condition is serious and usually indicates a cesarean birth. The major maternal complication associated with placenta previa is hemorrhagic shock. Perinatal mortality in recent studies is reported to be low and usually is caused by prematurity.

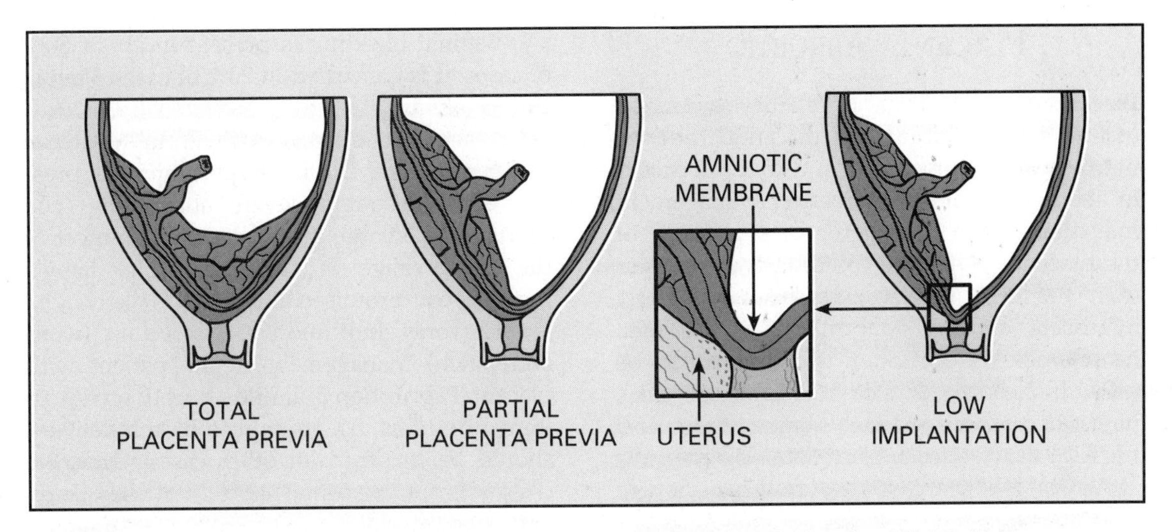

Figure 15–9 *Placenta previa — abnormal implantation (Adapted from Clinical Education Aid, No. 12, Ross Laboratories)*

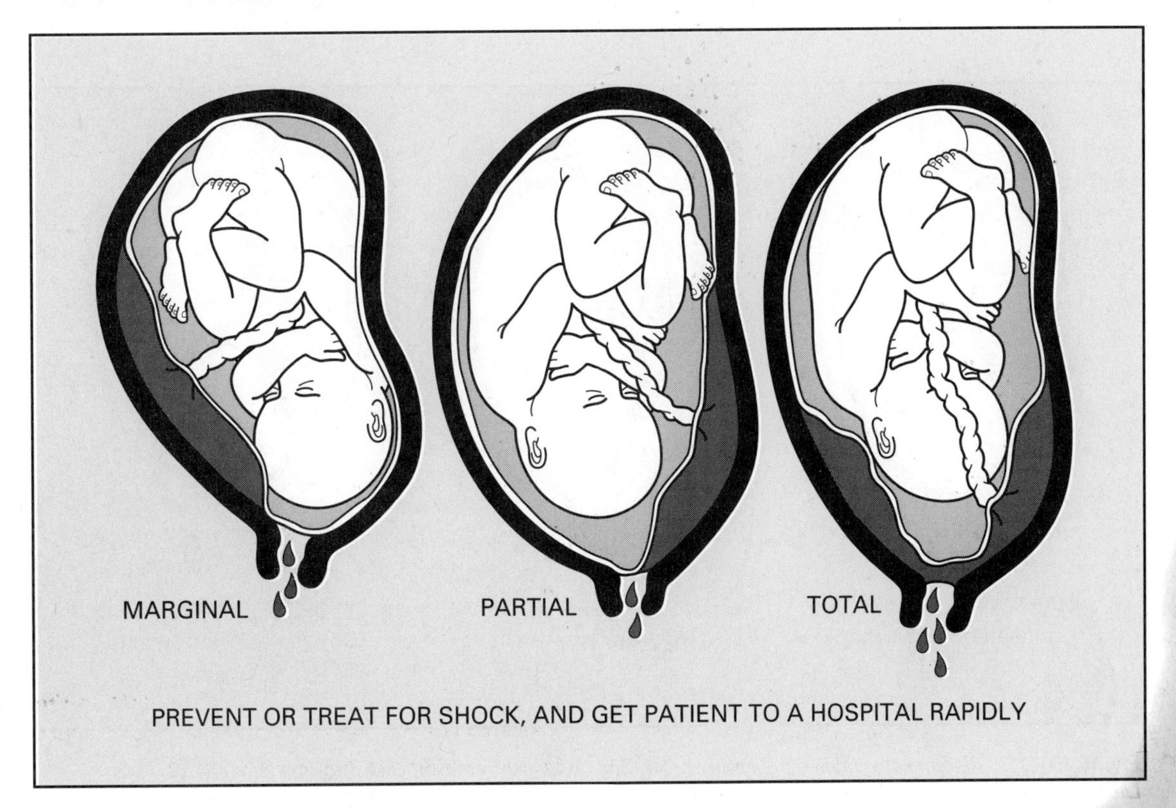

Figure 15–10 *Placenta previa and the fetus*

PLACENTA ABRUPTIO

Placenta abruptio is the premature separation of the normally implanted placenta from the uterine wall, Figures 15–11 and 15–12. It occurs in about 1 out of 100 deliveries. Management may depend on the degree of separation of the placenta. If vaginal bleeding is slight (less than 100 mL), uterine activity only slightly increased, and no abnormality in the fetal heart tones, the abruption is considered to be mild. If bleeding is moderate (100–500 mL), uterine tone increased and hypersensitive, and the fetal heart tones suggest some distress, the abruption is considered to be moderate. Severe abruption is categorized by moderate to excessive bleeding (greater than 500 mL), a uterus that is tetanic and very reactive to palpation, and evident fetal distress.

Vaginal bleeding is present in about 80% of cases; it is concealed in 20% of cases. Pain is almost always present and is usually of sudden onset, constant, and localized to the uterus and lower back. Uterine hypertonicity is present with the more severe abruptions. The uterus may enlarge, particularly when most of the hemorrhage is concealed. The baby's health is compromised and shock is likely.

The only indication for expectant (wait-and-watch) management of the patient with placental abruption is a mild abruption with an immature fetus. An attempt to hasten delivery should be made in all other cases. Once the diagnosis of placental abruption has been made, amniotomy (rupturing the membranes) should be performed, since it may facilitate labor. Oxytocin may be initiated to augment the labor as needed. A vaginal delivery is pre-

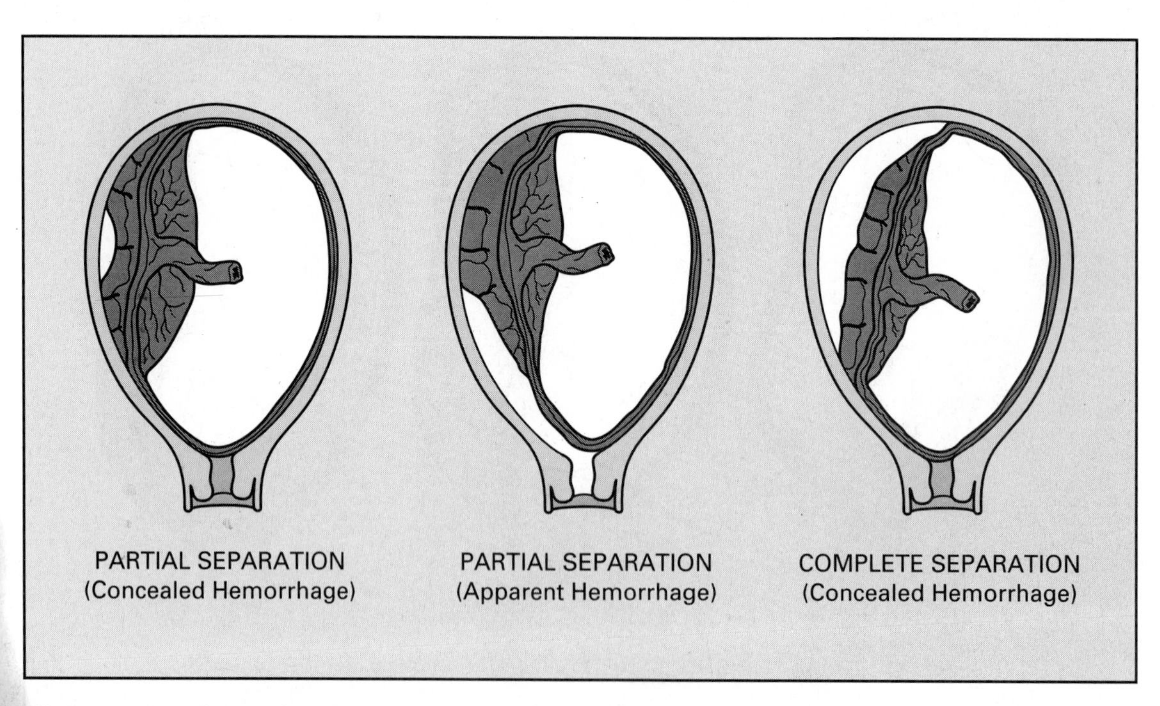

Figure 15–11 *Placenta abruptio — premature separation (Adapted from Clinical Education Aid, No. 12, Ross Laboratories)*

ferred, but a cesarean section is indicated when vaginal delivery is not imminent; when fetal distress develops; in cases of severe abruption with a viable fetus; when hemorrhage is severe enough to jeopardize the life of the mother; and in patients who have failed a trial labor.

POSTPARTUM HEMORRHAGE

Postpartum hemorrhage can be defined as bleeding after the birth of the baby. Bleeding can be before, during, or after the delivery of the placenta. By definition, loss of more than 500 mL of blood during the first 24 hours constitutes postpartum hemorrhage. The incidence of postpartum hemorrhage is around 10%.

In a normal vaginal delivery, approximately 200–300 mL of blood are lost. If an episiotomy is necessary, an additional 100 mL of blood or more may be lost. Because pregnant women have an increased blood volume, a loss of 500 mL of blood may not have a serious effect. But an even smaller amount of bleeding can be dangerous if the patient is anemic.

Clinically, postpartum hemorrhage involves:

- continuing bleeding
- rapid and weak pulse

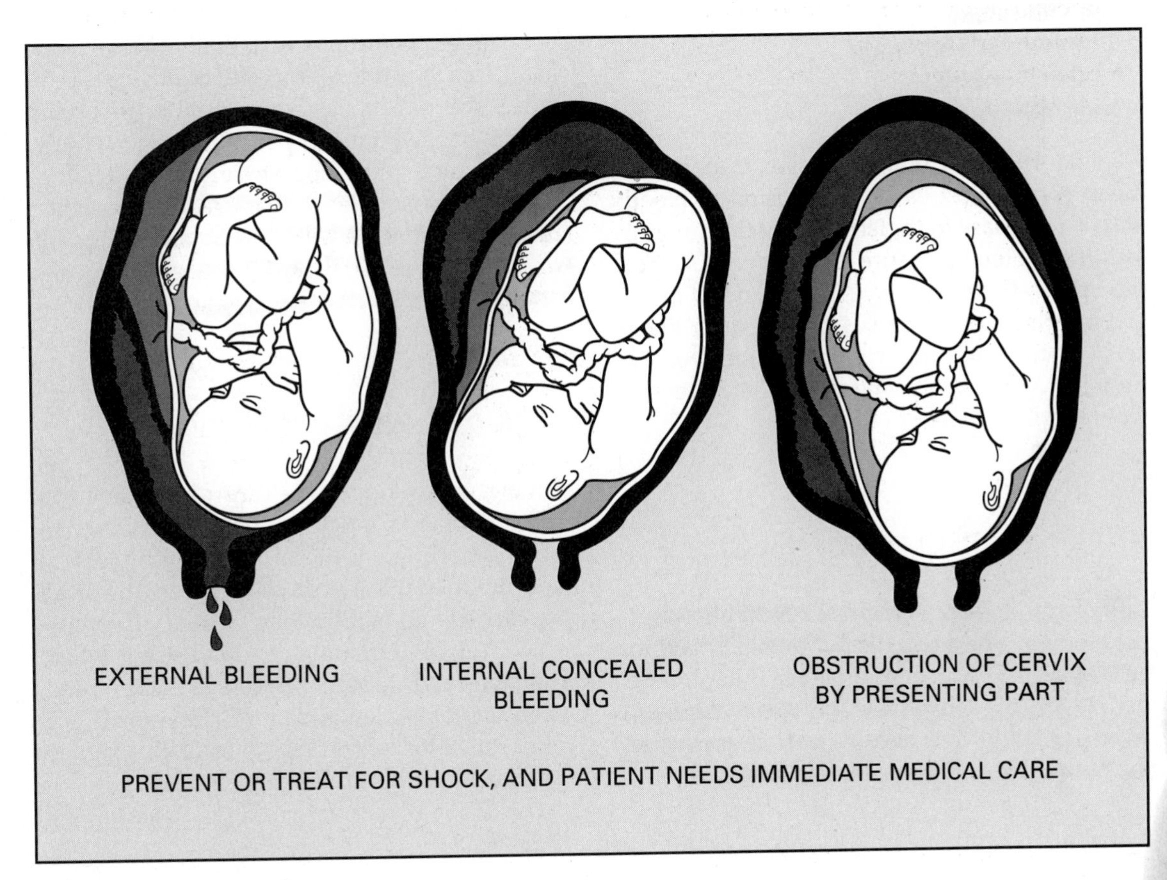

Figure 15–12 *Placenta abruptio and the fetus*

- falling blood pressure
- shortness of breath
- pale, cold appearance of patient

A treacherous feature of postpartum hemorrhage is that these signs can appear suddenly even though the blood loss has been occurring all along. The danger of this condition is twofold. First, the anemia that ultimately results from hemorrhage weakens the patient, lowers her resistance, and predisposes her to puerperal infection. Second, if the loss of blood is not stopped, death can result.

The four main causes of postpartum hemorrhage are:

- uterine atony
- trauma and lacerations
- retained placenta
- bleeding disorders

The treatment will, of course, depend on the cause. In most cases, transfusion of blood will be necessary to replace at least the amount lost. If the blood pressure is falling, the foot of the bed is elevated. Oxygen may need to be given by mask. Warmth is provided by blankets. If the bleeding cannot be stopped, a hysterectomy may be necessary to save the woman's life.

STILLBIRTH

If the baby does not breathe at birth and does not respond to resuscitative efforts, it is said to be stillborn. **Stillbirth** and neonatal loss occur in 2%–8% of deliveries. The most common cause for stillbirth is anoxia (lack of oxygen to the baby). Anoxia can be associated with:

- placental insufficiency (placenta is small and its functioning is impaired)
- antepartum hemorrhage (placenta abruptio)
- umbilical cord problems
- abnormalities of labor and delivery (breech presentations and prolonged labor)
- maternal disease, especially diabetes

Early neonatal deaths are most commonly related to:

- preterm labor and their complications, especially respiratory distress syndrome
- congenital malformations
- infection
- intrapartum asphyxia or trauma

The emotional stress of stillbirth and neonatal loss is difficult for the health-care provider, the patient, and her family. Important aspects in helping the patient and her family cope include providing straightforward information, allowing the patient to see or touch her infant, providing a description or photograph of the baby, referring to local support groups and, in general, facilitating grieving.

NURSING CARE

Giving good supportive care to a woman in labor demands much of the nurse. Observation, reporting, technical skill, and physical and emotional supportive measures must all be carried out with a fine degree of competence. Yet, in a situation of added stress, where the labor and delivery process is complicated, even more is demanded of the nurse. The importance of supportive care of the highest caliber cannot be emphasized enough.

PROCEDURE

Care of the Unconscious Mother

Purpose: Care involves protecting and observing the unconscious mother closely at all times to prevent postdelivery complications such as shock, hemorrhage, pneumonia, or injury.

Equipment:

- Postdelivery bed
- Bedside table
- Sphygmomanometer and stethoscope
- Tongue blades
- Tissue wipes
- Emesis basin covered with towel
- Paper and pencil
- Suction machine, if patient has had a general anesthesia
- Oxygen setup
- IV standard

Precautions:

1. Never leave an unconscious patient alone.
2. Examine dressings and watch body openings for hemorrhage.
3. Be sure that air passages are kept open and that respiration is adequate.
4. Watch closely for symptoms of oncoming shock (pulse, respiration, blood pressure, perspiration).
5. Keep the patient warm. Maintain quiet.
6. Be sure the room is warm and free from drafts.
7. Frequently check fundus for firmness.

Procedure:

1. When the patient returns to the ward or recovery room, roll the bed covers to the side of the bed away from the stretcher.
2. Give assistance in transferring the patient to the bed and cover the patient with rolled covers.
3. Tuck in bed covers as soon as possible.
4. Obtain chart from anesthetist. Learn patient's condition, type of anesthetic given, drains used, and parenteral solutions administered from anesthetist. Check the postdelivery orders carefully.
5. Check and record the following:
   rate and character of respirations
   state of consciousness
   color and condition of skin
   rate and quality of pulse
   blood pressure
   amount of flow
   presence of packing
   firmness and position of fundus
   time of return from delivery room
6. Make patient comfortable. Place bedrails in position.
7. Carry out orders and record them.
8. Count and record pulse, respirations, and blood pressure every 15 minutes until stabilized. Count and record more frequently, if indicated.
9. If the patient vomits:
   Turn the patient's head to one side, supporting the head and angle of the jaw with hands.
   Clear air passages by suctioning, if necessary.

PROCEDURE

Care of the Unconscious Mother *continued*

If air passage cannot be cleared immediately, obtain assistance of anesthetist.

If patient aspirates vomitus, suction and notify anesthetist and doctor immediately. Have oxygen ready to administer when air passages are clear.

10. Report immediately to charge nurse or doctor any signs of inadequate or obstructed respiration, shock, or hemorrhage or any other untoward symptom.
11. Remain with the patient as long as she is unconscious.
12. When the patient has fully reacted and is ready to be returned to her room, she should be accompanied by an RN or LPN and one other person.
13. When the patient is settled in her unit she is checked by an RN; at the transfer of responsibility for the patient, the patient's condition is ascertained to the satisfaction of both nurses.
14. The delivery room nurse gives the report to one of the RNs on the floor (to the charge nurse, if possible).
15. The recovery room notes are continued until the patient is returned to the ward. Detailed nurse's notes should be continued as long as the patient's condition indicates a need for detailed records. Include all medication, treatment, blood and lab tests, and intravenous therapy while in the recovery room. The first voiding should be noted.

REVIEW QUESTIONS

A. Multiple choice. Select the best answer.

1. Premature labor is defined as labor that
   a. begins one week before the expected date
   b. begins three or more weeks before the expected date
   c. is spontaneous and progresses rapidly
2. Precipitous labor is defined as
   a. labor lasting many hours without progress
   b. labor pains without dilatation of the cervix
   c. spontaneous labor that progresses very rapidly
   d. none of the above
3. The term *uterine dysfunction* refers to a delay in any phase of labor. It may be caused by
   a. poor-quality uterine contractions
   b. maternal exhaustion
   c. unwise use of analgesia
   d. all of the above
4. The term *dystocia* means
   a. abnormal fetal position
   b. difficult labor
   c. disproportionate passageway
   d. short labor

5. A frank breech birth is one in which
   a. the buttocks and feet present and the knees are drawn up
   b. one or both feet present
   c. the buttocks present; the legs are extended up and are pressed against the abdomen and chest
   d. the occiput is directed diagonally and posterior

6. The major risk in PROM is
   a. chorioamnionitis and prolapsed cord
   b. prolonged labor and maternal exhaustion
   c. precipitous labor
   d. respiratory distress syndrome

7. The term used when an infant is too large to pass through a small contracted pelvis at either the inlet, the midpelvis, or the outlet is
   a. face presentation
   b. breech presentation
   c. persistent occiput posterior position
   d. fetopelvic disproportion

8. When the placenta covers or partially covers the cervix, the condition is known as
   a. placenta previa
   b. placenta abruptio
   c. prolapsed placenta
   d. malpositioned placenta

9. Postpartum hemorrhage is dangerous for the mother because
   a. it can cause anemia
   b. it predisposes her to puerperal infection
   c. it can cause death
   d. all of the above

10. Which of the following precautions is taken when delivering a premature infant?
    a. medication is used to sedate the mother
    b. medications are avoided or used sparingly
    c. a cesarean section is considered to prevent fetal trauma
    d. no episiotomy is done

11. Which of the following is not a good reason for doing a cesarean section?
    a. fetopelvic disproportion
    b. failure to progress
    c. prolapsed cord
    d. severe pain in the first stage of labor

12. A woman having a cesarean section under regional anesthesia may feel
    a. a tugging or pulling sensation
    b. shortness of breath
    c. a burning sensation and shoulder pain
    d. all of the above

SUGGESTED ACTIVITIES

- Investigate the problems that may arise in labor if the baby's head fails to rotate normally.
- Discuss the problems of a premature birth for both parents and baby.
- Briefly describe the presentation and management of prolapsed cord.
- Outline the rationale and the procedure for breech delivery.
- Describe clinical signs that reflect labor complications.
- Identify the causes of predisposing factors and management of third-stage hemorrhage.
- Role play how you would be supportive to a couple who just delivered a stillborn infant.

BIBLIOGRAPHY

Benson, R. C. *Current Obstetric and Gynecologic Diagnosis and Treatment*, 5th ed. Los Altos, CA: Lange Medical Publications, 1984.

Morrison, J. "Preterm Birth: A Puzzle Worth Solving." *Maternal-Fetal Medicine* 76(1):Supplement, July, 1990.

Oxorn, H. *Oxorn-Foote Human Labor and Birth*, 5th ed. E. Norwalk, CT: Appleton-Century-Crofts, 1986.

Pritchard, J. A., MacDonald, P. C., and N. F. Grant. *Williams Obstetrics*, 17th ed. E. Norwalk, CT: Appleton-Century-Crofts, 1985.

Reeder, S., Mastroianni, L., Jr., and L. Martin. *Maternity Nursing*, 16th ed. New York: J. B. Lippincott, 1987.

UNIT

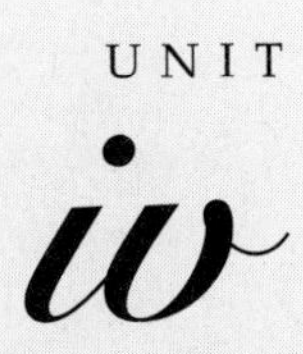

The Postpartum Period

CHAPTER

16

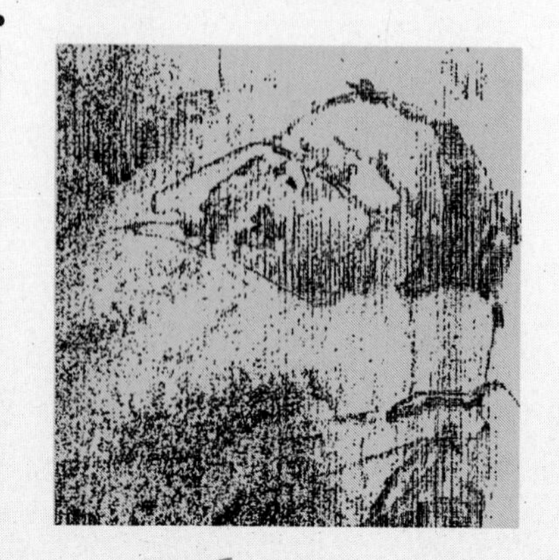

Postpartum Care

Objectives

After studying this chapter, the student should be able to:

- Identify principles of nursing care during the postpartum period.
- Explain the process of involution.
- Identify complications that may occur during the puerperium.
- Cite causes for postpartum depression.
- State why sleep is an essential part of postpartum care.
- State measures of self-care for the patient.
- Define bonding and attachment.

Key Terms

puerperium
involution
striae
afterpains
lochia rubra
lochia serosa
lochia alba
hemorrhoids
venous thrombosis
colostrum
engorgement
let-down reflex

MASTITIS

STASIS

PUERPERAL INFECTION

PUERPERAL THROMBOSIS

THROMBOPHLEBITIS

HOMANS' SIGN

EMBOLUS

POSTPARTUM HEMORRHAGE

UTERINE ATONY

CYSTITIS

POSTPARTUM DEPRESSION

PROLACTIN

PAPANICOLAOU (PAP) SMEAR

ATTACHMENT

BONDING

The six-week period immediately after childbirth is called the **puerperium**. The term is taken from the Latin words *puer*, meaning child, and *parare*, to bring forth. It takes about six weeks for the organs to return to their normal size and condition. This process is known as **involution**.

The principles of nursing care during the puerperium, or postpartum period, include:

- promoting a revitalization of physical and emotional energy
- encouraging normal involution of the reproductive organs
- preventing infection of the reproductive and urinary systems
- promoting healing of tissue damaged during pregnancy and delivery
- encouraging normal lactation or suppression of lactation with minimal discomfort

IMMEDIATE POSTPARTUM CARE

After the woman has delivered, she is encouraged to hold her infant, attempt to breast feed, if she chooses, and bond with her newborn. The father is also encouraged to participate in this process. The new family will stay together as a unit during this initial postpartum time, Figure 16–1. They should be supported as needed. The new mother is usually both exhilarated and physically exhausted after the birth of her baby. The first few hours after delivery are known as the fourth stage of labor. The nurse should be knowledgeable of this stage.

The patient should be placed in the dorsal recumbent position and advised to lie quietly. Her pulse may drop, probably because of the lessening of arterial tension; the pulse rate may be 60 to 80 beats per minute. A rapid pulse may be an indication of shock or concealed hemorrhage. Generally the body temperature does not rise after delivery; however, it may rise to above 37.2°C (99°F) without ill effects. The pulse is the best guide to use in judging the significance of temperature.

A slow pulse with a slightly elevated temperature is not likely to indicate a complication. Nevertheless, the nurse should report any rise in temperature at once. The normal flow of

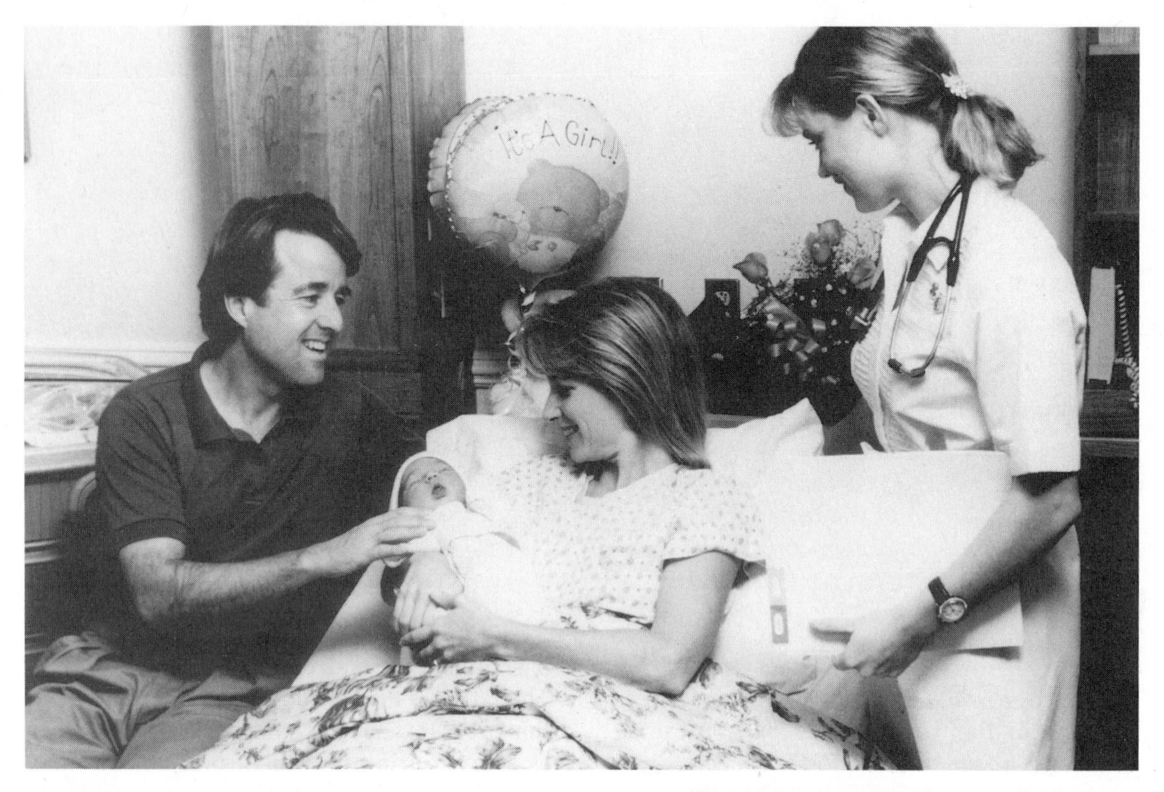

Figure 16–1 *The new family together as a unit (Courtesy of Evergreen Hospital Medical Center, Kirkland, WA)*

vaginal blood within the first two hours after delivery is approximately two ounces. There are no clots at this time. If the discharge increases the nurse should massage the uterus. She should also check for a full or distended bladder and monitor urinary output. If the new mother is unable to empty her bladder and there is tenderness and fullness at the bladder site or if the uterus feels displaced by the bladder catheterization may be necessary. General hygienic care of the skin and mouth is essential to promote comfort and prevent odor. The patient should be encouraged to rest and sleep as much as possible. The diet is usually regular unless there have been complications.

It is not uncommon for the mother to experience a chill immediately after labor. This chill is usually caused by a nervous reaction — a disturbance of internal and external temperature due to the excessive perspiration that occurs during labor and ceases abruptly after delivery. A warm bed and the application of external heat help to avoid this reaction. The patient may also complain of a headache. A headache is an important symptom and must be reported because it can indicate a change of pressure within the spinal column. The blood pressure should be taken and given in the report to the head nurse and doctor.

THE IMPORTANCE OF SLEEP

Rest and repair of body tissue require a recovery period of six weeks during which the mother must maintain normal sleep requirements. Fatigue, one of the earliest presumptive signs of pregnancy, shows the increased need for sleep because of increased metabolic requirements. In addition, the hard physical work of labor requires adequate energy reserves; restoration of this physical and emotional energy depletion can be secured through rest and sleep.

Although sleep is a psychophysiological phenomenon essential for maintaining both physical and emotional health, the exact metabolic or physiological need has not been clearly explained. It is more crucial for emotional well-being than physical. When a person is deprived of sleep, psychological disturbances appear first and can be more disabling than physical manifestations. Chronic loss of sleep may lead to personality changes and may be the first warning of an impending emotional disorder. According to some theories, there may be some relationship between sleep deprivation and emotional disturbance in the development of postpartum depression.

The nurse can be of great value if she understands the importance of sleep, what prevents sleep, and consequences of lack of sleep. From admission through delivery, the nurse should be alert for signs of undue excitement or apprehension and gear nursing care to provide maximum relaxation. These efforts will reduce fear, tension, and exhaustion. After delivery, if the mother is not ready for sleep — if she is excited, talkative, or hungry — the nurse should alleviate the cause and explain why sleep is so important, thus preparing the patient and her environment.

THE PROCESS OF INVOLUTION

Immediately after labor the uterus weighs about two pounds, Figure 16–2. It can be felt through the abdominal wall at the level of the umbilicus. Immediately after delivery it begins to return to its normal position. Complete involution requires several weeks. By the time involution is complete, the uterus has shrunk

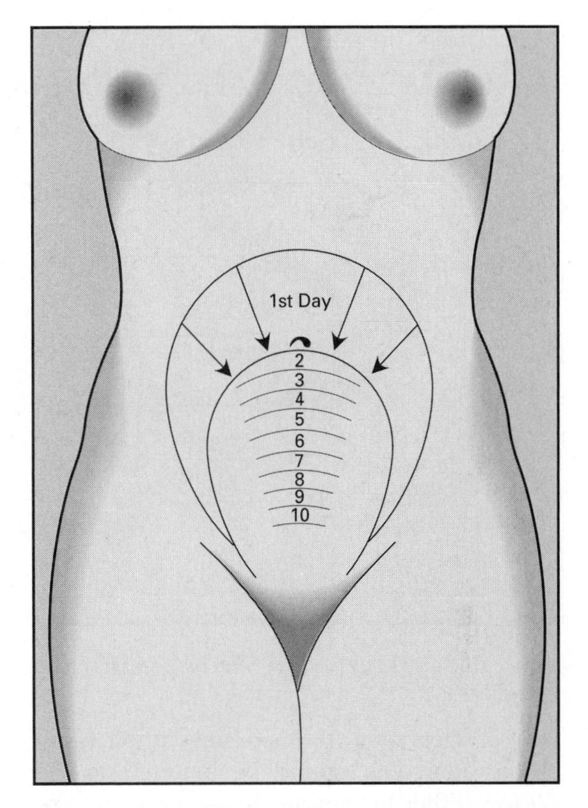

Figure 16–2 *Changes in height of fundus during first 10 days postpartum*

so much that it lies entirely in the pelvis and it should weigh only a few ounces, Figure 16–3. The vaginal walls, the vulva, and all other tissues that became enlarged during pregnancy also undergo a process of involution. The abdominal walls recover from overstretching, but the **striae** (stretch marks) usually remain. The redness will fade away in time, leaving silvery white markings where the tissue was stretched during pregnancy.

Multiparas may be bothered by uncomfortable contractions of the uterus known as **afterpains**. Afterpains may become more noticeable at the beginning of each breast feeding. They usually last only a few minutes. The contractions are useful because they keep the uterus

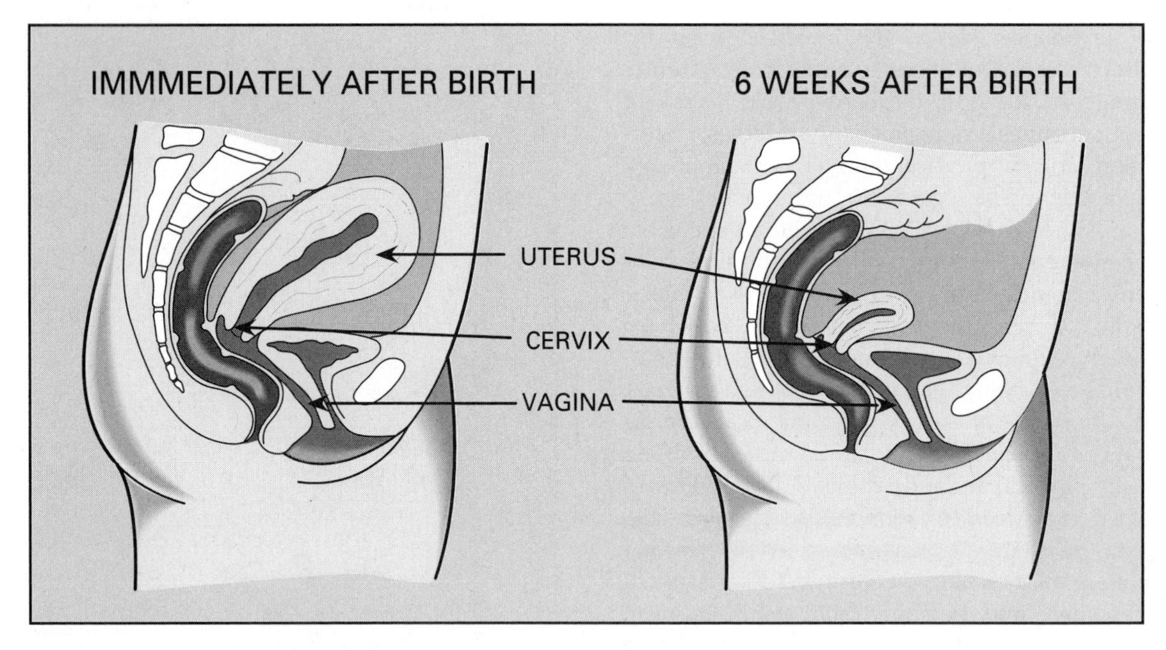

Figure 16–3 *The uterus lies within the pelvis and weighs only a few ounces by 6 weeks.*

free of clots and promote involution. Any severe afterpains should be reported to the doctor. If they are severe, an analgesic may be prescribed.

The uterine and vaginal discharge after delivery is called the lochia. It is red from the 1st to 4th day postpartum and is called **lochia rubra**. The discharge is referred to as **lochia serosa** when it changes to a dark brownish red and then to a yellowish brown from the 4th to the 14th day. From the 14th day to the end of puerperium, the secretion is less profuse and whitish. It is called **lochia alba**.

The nurse must observe the patient carefully to make sure that involution and lactation are progressing normally. Many complications of the postpartum period can be avoided or prevented by early treatment. The nurse should check daily the following and report any unusual changes to the supervising nurse or physician.

- bladder and bowel: emptying regularly, painful, pressure, presence of hemorrhoids
- fundus: firmness, distance (fingerbreadths) from umbilicus
- lochia: amount and characteristics such as color and odor
- episiotomy: clean, healing, irritated, inflamed
- breasts: soft, firm, engorged, painful
- nipples: erect, flat, inverted, cracked, painful

THE PERINEUM

The procedures used for perineal care depend on the policy of the hospital. The patient is instructed in the procedure. When the patient is allowed to take showers and have bathroom privileges she administers perineal care herself. The various procedures have the following characteristics in common:

- Perineal care is given during the bed bath or shower and after elimination.
- The soiled perineal pad is removed from front to back to prevent contamination.
- The perineum is cleansed from front to back to prevent contamination.

BUBBLEHE

- After the perineum has been cleansed, the clean pad is applied from front to back.

Healing of the episiotomy may cause the patient some discomfort. Tissue surrounding the sutures may become edematous and cause pressure on the sutures. **Hemorrhoids** (swollen vessels in the rectum), caused or enlarged during the delivery process, can also cause pain. The doctor may order the application of an ice bag immediately after delivery to minimize the swelling. The doctor also may order a topical or oral analgesic, a sitz bath, or witch hazel (Tucks pads) to be applied to relieve pain. Cleanliness and perineal care after each voiding are most important. Also avoiding constipation is important for the healing of hemorrhoids. The pelvic floor contraction (Kegel) exercise (Chapter 7) can also promote the healing process.

THE URINARY SYSTEM

During the puerperium, strain is put on the urinary system because the body is eliminating unusually large amounts of fluid to return to the normal fluid balance. The process of labor may have bruised the urethra and bladder and weakened the abdominal wall. Therefore the patient may have difficulty voiding in spite of the increased necessity of voiding frequently. If ordinary means have not been effective within six hours after the delivery, the doctor may order catheterization. The nurse should be alert for signs of urinary retention and residual urine. A full bladder will keep the uterus from staying contracted and will displace it from the midline.

THE BOWELS

Constipation is a common problem during the puerperium. Loss of muscle tone after delivery and inactivity are predisposing causes. The doctor may order a mild laxative or stool softener or an enema if the condition persists and is causing distress.

RECOVERING FROM A CESAREAN DELIVERY

A woman who has had a cesarean delivery will be evaluated at least hourly for the first four hours. Her blood pressure, pulse, urine flow, amount of bleeding and status of the uterine fundus are checked at these times. Abnormalities are reported immediately. Thereafter, for the first 24 hours, these are checked at four-hour intervals, along with the temperature.

Medication will be ordered by the doctor to help keep the new mother more comfortable after her surgery. Most women can tolerate oral fluids the day after surgery and a general diet by the second day. The catheter is usually removed from the bladder by 12 hours after the operation. Monitoring urine output to avoid overdistention of the bladder is important as with a vaginal birth. Gas pains from incoordinate bowel action may cause discomfort. A rectal suppository may offer relief.

By the first day after surgery, the patient should get out of bed briefly at least twice, assisted by the nurse. Ambulation can be timed so that recently administered analgesics will decrease any discomfort. She should be encouraged to stand tall and move around. Movement helps to alleviate gas pains and speeds recovery. By the second day, the patient should be able to walk to the bathroom with assistance. With early ambulation, **venous thrombosis** (blood clots in the legs) and pulmonary embolism are uncommon.

The incision is inspected every day. Normally, the skin sutures or skin clips are removed by the fourth day. Bathing in a tub or shower will not be harmful to the incision by the third day after surgery. Any signs of infection at the wound site should be reported immediately.

Unless there are complications during the puerperium, the mother may be discharged from the hospital on the third to sixth day postpartum. The mother's activities should be restricted to self-care and care of her newborn for the first week she is home. Usually the woman who has had a cesarean birth is seen three weeks after delivery in the doctor's office and again at the traditional six weeks postpartum time.

CONDITION OF THE BREASTS

The breasts change rapidly after delivery to prepare for the nourishment of the newborn. They secrete a small amount of colostrum during the first day postpartum. **Colostrum** provides the newborn with immune bodies and a large amount of vitamin A. It also acts as a laxative for the newborn. Milk is present on the second or third day postpartum depending upon how early after birth the baby is allowed to nurse.

ENGORGEMENT

On the second or third day after delivery there is usually a rush of blood and lymph into the breasts, known as **engorgement**. Engorgement results from congestion and increased vascularity in the breasts as well as from accumulation of milk. It precedes true lactation and lasts about 48 hours. The breasts become swollen, hard, and painful because of the increased blood and lymph supply.

If the mother decides not to nurse her baby, application of ice packs to each breast for at least an hour three or four times a day controls breast discomfort. The mother should wear a well-fitted bra that gives adequate support 24 hours a day. If the breasts are pendulous, a breast binder may be applied. The doctor may order a hormonal medication to inhibit milk production and an analgesic medication to relieve discomfort. Engorgement should subside in 24 to 48 hours. Occasionally, milk may reappear in the breasts in 10 or 12 days, and the same treatment is indicated. Pills or hormone injections may not help at this time. If there is an area on either breast that becomes red, hot, and tender, the physician should be notified without delay.

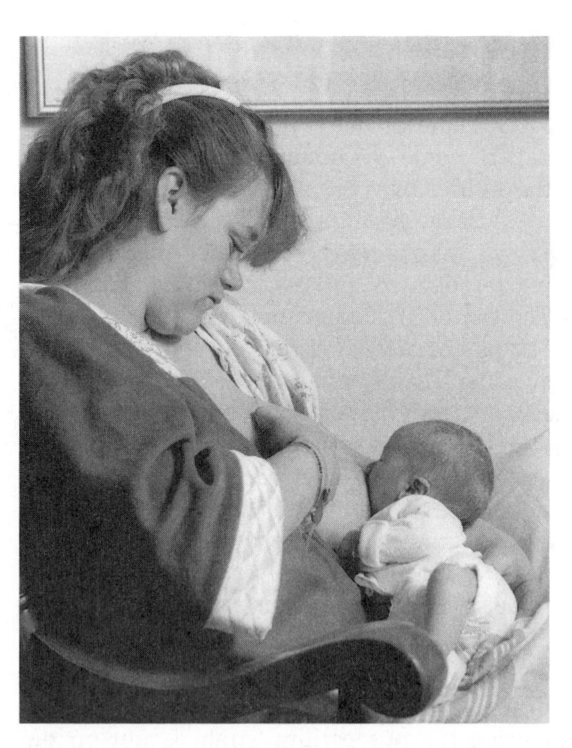

Figure 16–4 *Breast feeding*

If the mother is breast feeding her baby, she should not decrease nursing time, as this only increases the discomfort from engorgement, Figure 16–4. Once the baby begins to nurse vigorously and regularly, engorgement seldom is a problem. The following steps may help relieve the discomfort of engorgement.

- The mother should express milk from the engorged breasts manually before nursing. In this way, the pain is lessened because the breasts become less full and softer. The baby is then able to take the nipple more easily and empty the breast of still more milk.

- Both heat and ice packs may help relieve the discomfort of engorgement. Hot packs placed on the breasts or a hot shower stimulates the breast to leak milk. Ice packs on the breasts constrict the blood vessels and decrease engorgement. The mother may try either approach or both at different times.
- Massaging the breasts may help open any obstructed ducts that are causing the accumulation of milk. If breasts are too tender to massage, manual expression of milk from the breasts during a hot shower may help.
- A nursing bra that supports the breasts firmly but does not fit too tightly will make the mother more comfortable. A bra that is too tight can cut off circulation and actually causes plugged ducts.

SORE OR CRACKED NIPPLES

Some discomfort of the nipples is common when a woman first begins to nurse. The soreness usually disappears after the breasts become accustomed to nursing. The mother may express a small amount of milk from the breasts before nursing. The milk will flow more readily, and the baby can nurse with less effort. Also, letting the baby nurse more often for shorter periods puts less strain on sore nipples. The mother can offer the less-sore nipple first so that the baby is less hungry by the time he nurses on the sore nipple. Nursing in different positions helps relieve the problem as it puts pressure on different parts of the nipple.

The breasts should be washed first during the daily shower to prevent contamination from other parts of the body. The nipple is washed first, and the rest of the breast is cleansed by using circular motions upward from the nipple. Gentle handling and cleanliness are necessary to prevent cracks in the nipple and possible infection. Soap on the nipple area should be used sparingly and rinsed thoroughly because soap dries the skin and increases the risk of cracks in the nipple. Petroleum jelly, alcohol, or any other irritating substance should not be used on the nipples. Only a mild emollient cream such as lanolin should be used. The nipples should be kept clean and dry and exposed to the air as much as possible. Heat from an electric lamp (60-watt bulb) at a distance of at least 18 inches for 20 minutes two or three times a day will help heal sore nipples. Sore nipples should be examined by the physician.

LUMPS

Lactating breasts are lumpy; the lumps may shift from day to day. The breasts may become especially lumpy if a woman goes too long between breast feedings. Breasts also may feel lumpy if engorgement is present. The nursing mother can be reassured that any lumps she may feel are most likely harmless. Examination of the breasts by a physician can allay the mother's concern.

LET-DOWN REFLEX

The **let-down reflex** is caused by the release of oxytocin (hormone from the posterior pituitary gland) released into the bloodstream in response to the baby's suckling. Oxytocin causes the small muscles around the milk-producing cells to contract, releasing milk. The woman may feel this as a tingling, itching, or burning sensation in the breast tissue, or she may feel no sensation at all.

LEAKING

Leaking of milk from the breasts is a common problem at first for nursing mothers. However, leaking usually decreases as nursing is established. Generally, a woman feels a tingling in her breasts that signals that the rush of milk is imminent. If this let-down sensation occurs when she is not ready to nurse, pressing the heels of her hands firmly against her breasts may check the flow of milk. The breasts also may begin to leak two or three hours after the last feeding without any warning signals. It may be necessary for the mother to wear breast pads if the nipples leak. Breast pads should be changed when they become damp and soiled. Some women do not tolerate continuous moisture around the nipple and should be cautioned not to wear plastic liners continually.

SAGGING

Changes in the breasts take place as a result of pregnancy. Generally, the more weight gained during pregnancy, the more the breasts sag afterward. The firmness and contour of the breasts before and after pregnancy are influenced largely by heredity. Aging is the most common cause of sagging because it robs the skin of its elasticity. Sagging of the breasts is not caused by lactation.

MASTITIS

Mastitis (inflammation of the breast) may occur during lactation. A duct becomes plugged or the let-down is incomplete for a few feedings or for some other reason the milk fails to flow from one section of a breast. **Stasis** (stoppage or slowing of normal flow of fluid) occurs, the milk backs up, the area becomes tender to the touch or slightly reddened and infection begins to develop. Symptoms may include nausea, fatigue, chills, and fever. It is important to get the affected area flowing again. The mother should be helped to relax so that her let-down reflex will function well. Hot compresses on the sore area and frequent nursing on the affected breast are often recommended.

The physician should be notified immediately and may order antibiotic therapy. Some physicians believe that the mother should stop nursing on the affected breast and continue to express milk from the breast manually or with a breast pump. Other physicians believe that it is necessary to stop nursing on the affected breast only if there is a purulent discharge from the nipple or an actual abscess. Other authorities stress the importance of emptying the breasts regularly and feel mothers should nurse their baby frequently in the treatment of mastitis. Not emptying the breast aggravates the backed-up milk problem and can make the situation worse. If antibiotic therapy is started immediately and the breasts are emptied regularly, mastitis can subside in a day or two.

COMPLICATIONS DURING THE PUERPERIUM

Some of the most common organisms that invade the reproductive system during the puerperium are streptococci, staphylococci, gonococci, pneumococci, and bacteria native to the bowel. In the nineteenth century, puerperal infection was commonly known as childbed fever.

PUERPERAL INFECTION

Puerperal infection, a term that refers to the infection of any part of the reproductive system after delivery, has been largely prevented in modern medicine by aseptic technique and effectively treated with antibiotic drugs.

Puerperal infection is suspected in any patient who is feverish during labor, delivery, or in the postpartum period. The symptoms vary according to the location and severity of the infection. Symptoms of local infection include a slight rise in temperature, edema, inflammation, and tenderness of the part affected. Indications of a severe infection are malaise, fever, chills, lower abdominal tenderness, faulty regression of the uterus, and purulent lochia. It is important for the nurse to note the height of the fundus, characteristics of the lochia, and healing of the episiotomy so that medical attention can be given at the first sign of infection and proper isolation measures taken.

Treatment consists of the administration of antibiotic or sulfonamide drugs after the causative organism has been determined and comfort measures taken to relieve the symptoms of fever.

PUERPERAL THROMBOSIS (THROMBOPHLEBITIS)

A slowdown in circulation during the postpartum period may cause thrombi (blood clots) to form in the legs or pelvis, a condition called **puerperal thrombosis**. The inflammation of a vein that results in a blood clot is called **thrombophlebitis**. The most common site for this condition is the patient's legs. Signs of the condition may include a slight rise in temperature, swelling, areas of redness or whiteness of the leg or thigh (sometimes called "milk leg"), and pain. Pain or discomfort behind the knee or in the calf may be noted upon flexion of the foot when the leg is extended. This condition is known as a positive **Homans' sign**. The swelling may disappear after about two weeks, but it sometimes lasts for several months. The condition must be treated carefully. If a portion of a thrombus is dislodged into the circulation, it becomes an **embolus**. This embolus may be fatal if it is carried by the bloodstream into the heart, lungs, or brain.

The treatment for thrombophlebitis is to elevate the leg and use a heat cradle to protect the leg from the irritation of bed linen and to apply dry heat. Anticoagulants are usually administered to lessen the danger of embolism. The patient usually remains in bed at least one week after the temperature has returned to normal.

POSTPARTUM HEMORRHAGE

The average blood loss after giving birth is about 300 mL. **Postpartum hemorrhage** is bleeding in excess of 500 mL (1 pint).

Uterine atony is the most common cause of postpartum hemorrhage. The uterus must stay contracted after delivery. Relaxation of the uterus allows the vessels in the uterus to bleed freely, particularly at the site of the placenta. Frequent massage of the uterus helps it to stay contracted. Also, oxytocics may be given to prevent **uterine atony** (lack of muscle tone).

Laceration of the perineum, the vagina, or the cervix is sometimes the cause of postpartum hemorrhage. After delivery, the physician inspects the mother for any lacerations and repairs any that are present.

Retained placental fragments are an uncommon cause of postpartum hemorrhage. If the fragment is large, it will prevent the uterus from contracting, thereby causing hemorrhage shortly after expulsion of the placenta. If the retained fragments are small, hemorrhage may not occur until the fragments separate from the uterine wall, leaving open blood vessels to cause hemorrhage. The placenta must be inspected carefully when it is expelled to be sure it is intact and no fragments are left within the uterus. If placental fragments are retained, they may be removed by dilatation and curettage.

Because of the risk of postpartum hemorrhage, the mother's vital signs should be monitored frequently (every 10–15 minutes) along with the quantity of blood loss for several hours after delivery.

CYSTITIS

Cystitis (inflammation of the bladder) is an occasional complication of the puerperium. If aseptic technique is carried out at all times and the bladder is emptied regularly and completely, inflammation can be avoided.

Symptoms of cystitis are painful and frequent urination, pain over the bladder, and the presence of blood and pus in the urine upon microscopic examination. Diagnosis is made from a clean-catch specimen or a catheterized specimen.

The doctor usually orders an antibiotic that is specific for common organisms that can cause cystitis. Increased fluids are encouraged. An indwelling catheter is ordered only if the patient cannot void.

POSTPARTUM DEPRESSION

It is not unusual for the mother to experience feelings of depression after her baby is born. **Postpartum depression** is caused by the physiological changes that are rapidly taking place, by exhaustion after the process of delivery, and by the fact that the long-awaited birth has occurred. After the delivery, the new mother may doubt her ability to care for her baby. She may worry about the changes that may occur in the relationship between her partner and herself. The mother of a family may be uncertain of the reaction of the older children to the new baby.

The nurse may help the patient during this period by listening attentively, encouraging the patient to talk about her problems, and answering questions regarding daily health care. The nurse should not attempt to give information of a medical nature, and she should not try to advise a troubled patient. There are a number of signs and symptoms of postpartum depression:

- "baby blues" that don't go away after two weeks, or strong feelings of depression and anger that begin to surface a month or two after childbirth
- feelings of sadness, doubt, guilt, helplessness, or hopelessness that seem to increase with each week and begin to disrupt a woman's normal functioning
- sleeplessness even when tired, or sleeping most of the time even when the baby is awake
- marked changes in appetite
- extreme concern about the baby or lack of interest in the baby or other members of her family
- panic or anxiety attacks
- fear of harming the baby or thoughts of self-harm

The nurse should immediately report any of these symptoms to the physician. These symptoms may be a sign of a more serious postpartum psychosis and will need special attention.

Figure 16–5 provides an overview of postpartum nursing care.

SELF-CARE INSTRUCTIONS

Under normal circumstances, most women leave the hospital two to four days after delivery. The woman is given a physical examination before discharge. She should also be given the opportunity to ask questions and discuss any problems or concerns that she may have. The mother is given instructions for her self-care at home during the puerperium and told to return to her obstetrician for a checkup within six weeks. Some obstetricians want to see the woman as soon as three weeks after delivery.

By the time the mother leaves the hospital, the lochia will be rapidly diminishing in amount and changing in color. Sometimes, because of excessive activity, the lochia may again became red for several days. In about 10 to 14 days, the discharge becomes white or yellow and gradually stops. The length of time of the discharge differs for each woman. Douching is not necessary, and in no case should it be started before the discharge stops or before at least three weeks postpartum. Consultation with her physician is recommended.

POSTPARTUM NURSING CARE

Parameter for Assessment	Expected Changes	Abnormal Findings	Nursing Intervention
Pulse	May drop at first before returning to normal	Rapid pulse may indicate shock or hemorrhage.	Investigate cause. Report findings to the physician immediately.
Vaginal bleeding	Approximately 2 ounces in the first 2 hours after delivery	Profuse bleeding Clots	Massage the uterus. Report finding to the physician.
Temperature	Mild elevation before returning to normal Patient may experience chill	Elevation indicative of infection	Report to physician. Administer antibiotic, if ordered.
Blood pressure	Mild hypotension, after which BP returns to normal	Low blood pressure may indicate shock High blood pressure may indicate preeclampsia	Report to physician. Monitor blood pressure often.
Sleep	Mother will initially be excited and talkative before fatigue from labor and delivery efforts becomes evident	Unable to relax in order to sleep	Explain the need for sleep. Prepare the patient and her environment in order to promote sleep.
Uterus	Gradual involution	Uterus fails to descend	Check involution each day. Remind the patient to empty her bladder regularly. Report findings.
Afterpains	Uterine contractions cause afterpains in the process of accomplishing involution Pain increases with breast feeding	Severe afterpain	Report findings to physician. An analgesic may be administered.
Perineum	Swollen and discolored; episiotomy healing	Infection indicated by pus Foul odor with lochia	Report findings to physician. Analgesics or antibiotics may be administered. Careful aseptic techniques. Dry heat or sitz baths to promote comfort.

Figure 16–5

POSTPARTUM NURSING CARE

Parameter for Assessment	Expected Changes	Abnormal Findings	Nursing Intervention
Bladder	Return to normal	Pain and frequent urgency, or an inability to urinate	Report findings to physician. Catheterize the patient prn. Force fluids. Obtain a urine culture. An antibiotic may be administered, if ordered.
Bowel	Normal function	Constipation	A mild laxative or enema may be administered, if ordered by the physician.
Breasts	Secrete colostrum until milk comes in	Breast becomes hot, red, or tender Nipples become cracked and/or infected	Apply heat or ice packs to affected breast. Teach mother how to massage breast. Report findings to physician if mastitis is suspected. An antibiotic may be administered, if ordered. Advise patient to use mild emollient cream on nipples. Apply dry heat to nipples. Instruct mother in use of nipple shield for nursing.
Postpartum depression	Possibility of mood swings	Severe depression	Listen attentively to patient. Encourage patient to talk about her problem. Report any severe symptoms such as insomnia, apathy, anorexia, delusions, or severe anxiety.

Figure 16–5 *continued*

RESUMPTION OF MENSES

The return of the menses after childbirth is quite variable and may take up to three months or longer. The nursing mother may expect menses to reappear in two or three months, or it may be delayed until breast feeding has been stopped completely. Nonnursing mothers usually start to menstruate within seven to nine weeks. Many women do not menstruate while breast milk is their baby's sole supply of food. When formula or solid foods are used to supplement breast milk, menses may resume. The mother's body produces less of the hormone **prolactin** when the baby sucks less often or less vigorously. As the amount of prolactin diminishes, its inhibitory effect on the ovaries decreases and ovulation and menses can develop. Some women do not resume their periods until their babies are completely weaned. Some women, however, begin menstruating even though they are breast feeding and their babies are receiving no other food.

The first menstrual period is often abnormal; profuse clots may be noted, and it may stop and start again. The second period is usually quite normal. But it may take a few months for a regular cycle to be reestablished. The cycle may differ somewhat in length from previous cycles.

CONCEPTION

The mother should realize that the possibility of conception exists at any time after childbirth, regardless of whether menses have recurred or not. She should not engage in sexual intercourse until the doctor indicates that she has recovered from the delivery process (usually after the first checkup). The nurse should offer information about methods of contraception with other discharge instructions. (See Chapter 16 for information on contraception.)

Lactation influences the return of menses and ovulation. During lactation, ovulation may be suppressed for as long as 12 to 16 months. But not all women maintain an anovulatory state during lactation, and ovulation may start before menses. Therefore, it is not safe for a woman to assume that she cannot become pregnant just because she is not having her menstrual periods.

BREAST FEEDING DURING MENSTRUATION

There is no reason why a woman should not nurse her baby while she is menstruating. Hormonal changes connected with the menstrual cycle may cause the milk supply to lessen temporarily. Production of less milk is not a problem if the mother allows the baby to nurse more frequently. Some infants may not nurse as well during menstruation, and may tend to be more irritable at this time. This irritability is a transient, and normal lactation will resume after menstruation.

PERSONAL HYGIENE

The mother should continue the perineal care she learned in the hospital until after the episiotomy has healed. After a bowel movement, as always, wiping should be directed upward and away from the vagina. After each bowel movement or urination, the mother should pour warm water from a clean pitcher or a peri bottle over the genitals. She should then gently pat the area dry.

If the sutures continue to be uncomfortable, she may soak in a tub of warm water for 20 minutes and apply medication locally. Over the weeks after the birth, the perineal muscles will begin to regain some of their tone. The new mother can help this process along by doing Kegel muscle exercises (discussed in Chapter 7), which can be started as soon as it is comfortable to do them.

The mother should take a shower daily. For three to five days after delivery, her body may perspire more than usual as a means of ridding it of some fluids that were retained by the tissues during pregnancy.

ELIMINATION

Hemorrhoids that appear for the first time in late pregnancy or as a result of delivery usually disappear. In the acute stage they respond well to cold witch hazel compresses and sitz baths. Occasionally, local medication may be ordered. The patient should avoid straining with stool, and she should drink six to eight glasses of water a day. A stool softener, if prescribed by the physician, may be taken daily in the acute stages.

There may be a tendency toward constipation during the first few weeks postpartum. The condition usually responds to dietary measures such as six to eight glasses of water daily, roughage such as celery, lettuce, and greens, and adequate intake of citrus fruits, figs, dates, and prunes. A mild laxative may be ordered if necessary.

ABDOMEN

Many women are surprised and disappointed that their abdomens are flabby after delivery, making them look as if they are still pregnant. During pregnancy, the abdominal muscles stretch, and the return of good muscle tone takes time. Exercise to improve muscle tone may be started two weeks postpartum. The new mother should begin her program of exercise gradually and should be cautioned about overexertion. A backache is not uncommon until the abdominal muscles tighten up and work with back muscles to help maintain an erect posture.

Afterbirth pains are caused by the uterus contracting and relaxing as it returns to its normal state. The contractions are usually mild with first babies and stronger with subsequent babies and with nursing, but they last only a few days. Changing position, lying on the abdomen, and keeping the bladder empty will help ease the discomfort. The physician may order a mild analgesic, if indicated.

DIET

A sensible diet continues to be important. If fewer than 25 pounds were gained during pregnancy, the mother should not have a weight problem now. The new mother will lose about 18–20 pounds within 10 days after delivery. It is best to lose about ½ pound per week after this. With a well-balanced diet, she will return to her normal weight within two months after delivery. If she gained considerably more than the recommended weight during her pregnancy, the only way to lose weight is by strict adherence to a reducing diet. A gradual increase in exercise will also aid the reducing program and will tone the muscles. If a diet is necessary, the physician prescribes the type of diet to be followed and supervises the mother's progress. If she is nursing her baby, she must increase the amount of calories in her diet as during pregnancy. She should drink the nutritional equivalent of one quart of milk daily and maintain a high-protein intake. The mother may notice that her infant reacts adversely to certain foods she consumes. The most common offending foods include food dyes, additives, certain spices, eggs, chocolate, cola, corn, citrus fruits, peas, broccoli, cabbage, beans, wheat, nuts, tomatoes, shellfish, and certain meats, onions, garlic, and any foods to which the mother herself may be allergic. Cow's milk and milk products may also cause adverse reactions in the infant such as rash, stuffy nose, or diarrhea. Eliminating these foods for a while if the infant is reacting adversely is recommended.

ACTIVITIES

It is important to do things in moderation after the birth of a child. Usually it takes from six to eight weeks before a mother returns to her normal schedule of activity. Her return to normal is progressive; she begins to feel stronger day by day. Rest is extremely important. She should be encouraged to take naps during the day while her baby is sleeping. Strenuous work, heavy lifting, and excessive social activity should be avoided. Daily exercise can help restore muscle strength and return her body to its prepregnancy shape, Figure 16–6. A mild exercise program can actually help decrease fatigue and increase energy level. If the baby was born by cesarean delivery or if the delivery was complicated, an exercise program should be delayed until the physician has approved it. Otherwise, exercise may be started when the mother feels ready. Walking briskly is a good way to return to an exercise program. Swimming is also an excellent postpartum exercise.

After the baby is a week or two old, there are no contraindications to travel except for possible overexertion and fatigue. If a long automobile trip is necessary, the mother is advised to get out of the car at frequent intervals and walk for several minutes to maintain adequate circulation.

Returning to work outside the home is also a consideration for many new mothers. The financial factors as well as costs and availability of child care have to be considered. If the mother is breast feeding, the number of feedings from the breast may need to be decreased before the woman can comfortably return to full-time work. Many employers are becoming more flexible and offering options to working mothers. Many women can work part-time or share a full-time position. The physician may recommend that a new mother stay home for a certain period of time to recover strength before returning to work.

POSTPARTUM CARE

The mother should return to the obstetrician within six weeks for a postpartum checkup. At this time, she is examined and has the opportunity to discuss with the doctor any problems she may wish to bring up. Instruction in family planning may be given if the patient desires (see Chapter 17). The cervix is inspected. It is essential in terms of future health that the cervix be completely healed before discharge from medical care for this pregnancy.

If the effects of childbirth on the cervix require treatment, the patient is instructed to return regularly until full healing has occurred. The importance of complete healing cannot be overemphasized. It is also recommended that sexual intercourse be delayed until the healing process is complete to avoid hurting delicate tissues. Healing usually takes about three to four weeks.

DISCHARGE PLANNING

Discharge planning should include written instructions for observing and reporting signs and symptoms of complications and the type of recovery to be expected. Contraception information should also be offered. The date and time for a follow-up appointment and referrals to other community resources when appropriate should be given to the mother.

When the patient is discharged, the obstetrician suggests that she have a yearly physical examination, which includes a **Papanicolaou (Pap) smear** for the detection of cancer of the cervix. These tests should be scheduled yearly.

ATTACHMENT AND BONDING

Attachment can be defined as an enduring affectional tie that one person forms to another individual. **Bonding** can be defined as the development of attachment. In 1972, Klaus and Kennell performed a landmark study that provided the earliest evidence for the existence of a sensitive period in human maternal-infant bonding. Klaus and Kennell defined the sensitive period as the time "during which the parents' attachment to their infant blossoms . . . [and during which] complex interactions between mother and infant help lock them together." Between 1972 and 1982, 17 additional studies were done on the effects of sepa-

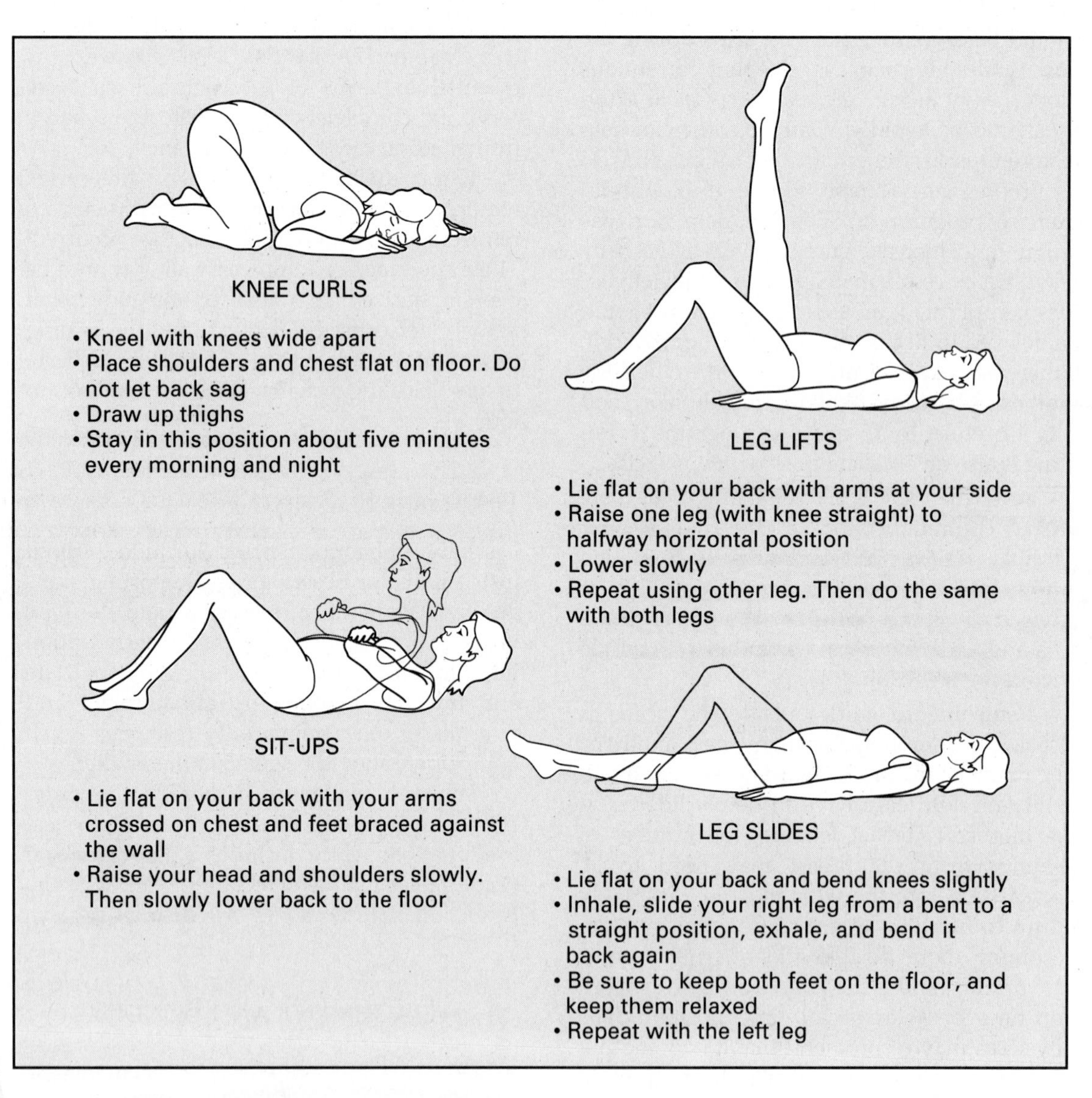

KNEE CURLS
• Kneel with knees wide apart
• Place shoulders and chest flat on floor. Do not let back sag
• Draw up thighs
• Stay in this position about five minutes every morning and night
LEG LIFTS
• Lie flat on your back with arms at your side
• Raise one leg (with knee straight) to halfway horizontal position
• Lower slowly
• Repeat using other leg. Then do the same with both legs
SIT-UPS
• Lie flat on your back with your arms crossed on chest and feet braced against the wall
• Raise your head and shoulders slowly. Then slowly lower back to the floor
LEG SLIDES
• Lie flat on your back and bend knees slightly
• Inhale, slide your right leg from a bent to a straight position, exhale, and bend it back again
• Be sure to keep both feet on the floor, and keep them relaxed
• Repeat with the left leg

Figure 16–6 Postpartum exercises (Adapted from the Maternity Center Association)

rating babies from their mothers directly after birth. Klaus and Kennell's initial findings corroborated that extra contact in the first several days led to more physical contact and affectionate displays between mothers and their infants. Several other studies tend to broaden the definition of bonding. Other factors affecting the process include the mother's economic status, race, housing, education, number of previous children, and age.

Klaus describes a bond as "a unique relationship between two people that is specific

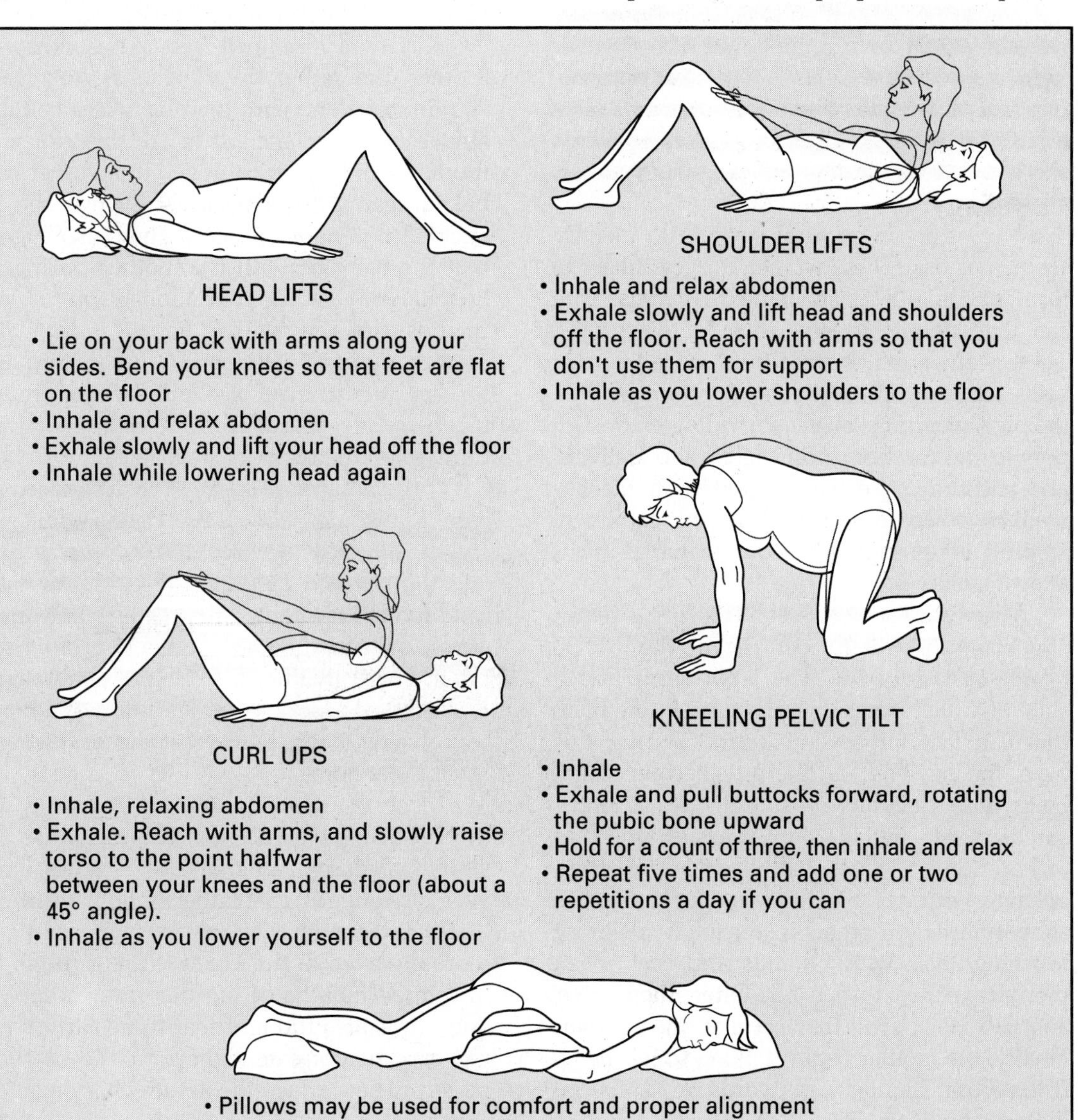

HEAD LIFTS
• Lie on your back with arms along your sides. Bend your knees so that feet are flat on the floor
• Inhale and relax abdomen
• Exhale slowly and lift your head off the floor
• Inhale while lowering head again
SHOULDER LIFTS
• Inhale and relax abdomen
• Exhale slowly and lift head and shoulders off the floor. Reach with arms so that you don't use them for support
• Inhale as you lower shoulders to the floor
CURL UPS
• Inhale, relaxing abdomen
• Exhale. Reach with arms, and slowly raise torso to the point halfwar
between your knees and the floor (about a 45° angle).
• Inhale as you lower yourself to the floor
KNEELING PELVIC TILT
• Inhale
• Exhale and pull buttocks forward, rotating the pubic bone upward
• Hold for a count of three, then inhale and relax
• Repeat five times and add one or two repetitions a day if you can
• Pillows may be used for comfort and proper alignment

Figure 16–6 continued

and endures through time." He considers fondling, kissing, cuddling, and prolonged gazing to be behaviors that indicate parental-newborn attachment. Klaus also divides the factors that produce a bond into two types: internal and external. Internal factors include not only how the mother and father were raised by their own parents but also the cultural influences as they were growing up. External factors affecting a new mother's reaction to her newborn include the way in which she is cared for during her pregnancy, labor, and delivery.

Nurses are in an ideal position to identify women at risk. These women are less likely to form maternal-fetal attachment. Prenatal care can then be altered according to these risks. These women may benefit from more frequent visits, focusing on the psychological rather than the physiological changes. Providing extra support to the mother during labor and delivery and encouraging extended contact in the immediate postpartum period can be extremely helpful in promoting good maternal-infant attachment.

There are many reasons that parent-infant attachment is strengthened during the first 30 to 60 minutes of life. The labor stimulates a state of wakefulness and alertness in the baby that can last for several hours. During this time, the newborn is likely to become calm, begin observing, and sensing the new sounds, smells, sights, touches, and tastes around him or her. Klaus believes that the most important behavior during this time is touch. Studies show that new mothers instinctively begin by touching their baby's hands and feet. Then they stroke the baby's trunk. Often, the mother and baby lock eyes; they stare at one another. Finally, the mother begins talking to her baby, using both sounds and words in a special high-pitched voice.

Awareness of bonding-attachment has led to dramatic changes in the hospital environment. Klaus and Kennell's goal was to produce "conditions that are optimal for the development of parent-infant attachment in the first days of life." They recommend that during labor, the mother never be left alone. She should be attended constantly by someone giving guidance and reassurance.

Klaus and Kennell also advise that the mother and father be allowed at least 15 to 20 minutes alone with their baby in a comfortable room after the birth. At this time, the mother should be encouraged to hold her baby naked against her bare chest even if she has decided not to breast feed. They also suggest that the baby be with the mother during the hospital stay either continuously or for long periods (minimum five hours a day). The mother should be the primary care provider for her infant, even if the baby requires an incubator for extra warmth or is receiving ultraviolet treatment for neonatal jaundice.

If the newborn is very ill or is in intensive care, Klaus and Kennell recommend that parents be allowed to visit the baby at any time, and they should be encouraged to touch and care for their infant. This contact and interaction will strengthen a mother's sense of confidence and give her a feeling of competence. A great deal of anxiety will be alleviated in this way during the first days that she is alone with her baby at home.

Most of the research on bonding has involved mothers and their babies. Only a few studies focus on fathers. These studies, however, also suggest that fathers who have immediate contact with their newborn after birth are more involved in the infant's care through the first three months of life than are those who don't. It is also thought that these early bonding experiences extend beyond the newborn period. They affect the father-child relationship in later years.

With regard to breast feeding, Klaus and Kennell recommend total on-demand feeding.

They also suggest that fathers and siblings be encouraged to visit with mother and baby for long periods while they are in the hospital in order to strengthen intrafamily relationships.

In most hospitals, the father is at hand during the birth of the baby; in others, he is able to see the mother and child immediately after the delivery. The father is able to hold his baby and become acquainted with the newborn. Rooming-in helps to make obstetrical care a family affair, Figure 16–7. By participating in the care of his child, the father is more likely to accept his new role and become aware of his unique position as a father. The nurse and all other health personnel should consider both mother and father throughout the perinatal and postpartum period. Decisions regarding the pregnancy and plans for the new member of the family should be discussed with the mother and father. In addition, any questions regarding family planning can be presented and referrals can be made by the nurse.

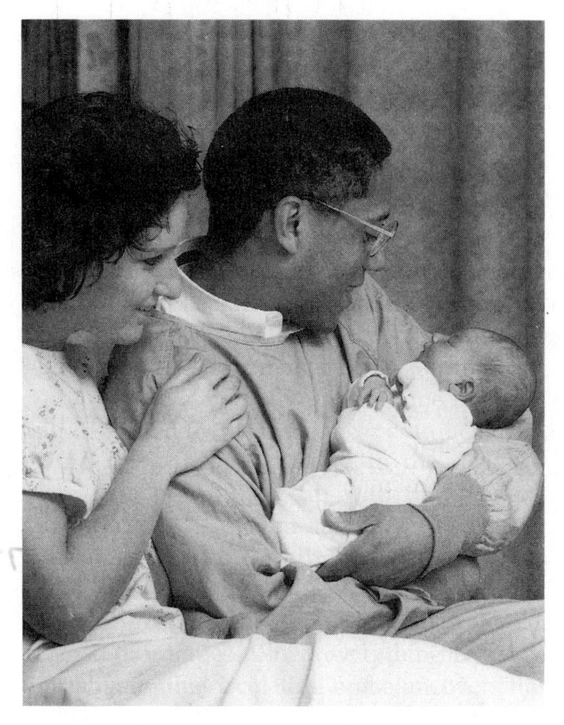

Figure 16–7 *Father bonding with his newborn*

REVIEW QUESTIONS

A. Match the principle of nursing care in Column I to the correct action in Column II.

Column I	Column II
1. encouraging normal involution of the reproductive organs	a. applying dry heat and a topical analgesic to the perineal area
2. preventing infection of the reproductive and urinary system	b. fastidious perineal care during the daily shower and after each elimination
3. promoting healing of tissue damaged during pregnancy and delivery	c. preparing the patient and her environment to promote sleep
4. encouraging normal lactation or suppression of lactation with minimal discomfort	d. applying a breast binder and administering a hormonal medication
5. promoting a revitalization of physical and emotional energy	e. massaging the uterus

B. Match the obstetrical term in column I to the correct description in column II.

Column I

1. perineum
2. embolus
3. cystitis
4. puerperium
5. thrombophlebitis
6. lochia alba
7. mastitis
8. engorgement
9. lochia serosa
10. colostrum
11. lochia rubra
12. involution
13. stasis
14. afterpains

Column II

a. six-week period immediately after childbirth
b. discharge 4–14 days postpartum
c. provides newborn with immune bodies and vitamin A
d. area between vulva and anus
e. discharge 14 days to end of puerperium
f. thrombus traveling in the circulatory system
g. inflammation of a vein resulting in a blood clot
h. return of organs to normal size and condition after delivery
i. inflammation of the breast
j. filling of breast with blood and lymph
k. inflammation of the breast
l. discharge 1–4 days postpartum
m. uncomfortable uterine contractions during the puerperium
n. stoppage or slowing of normal flow of fluid

C. Multiple choice. Select the best answer.

1. Mrs. Jones tells her nurse that she is afraid of her baby and that she doubts she will be able to love the baby. The nurse should
   a. ask Mrs. Jones what aspects of baby care she does not feel capable of handling and advise her
   b. encourage Mrs. Jones to talk about her feelings and avoid giving her advice or criticizing her emotions
   c. report the results of her conversation with Mrs. Jones to her attending physician
   d. all of the above

2. A program of proper exercise
   a. helps the process of involution and improves muscle tone of the abdomen
   b. may be started two weeks postpartum with physician's permission
   c. is supplemented by lying on the abdomen while sleeping
   d. all of the above

3. Recommended care of the perineum after discharge from the hospital includes all of the following *except*:
   a. wiping from front to back after each bowel movement and urination
   b. pouring warm water over the genitals after bladder and bowel elimination
   c. changing the perineal pad frequently
   d. taking tub baths

4. Some activities permitted during the first month postpartum include all of the following *except*:
   a. short-distance traveling
   b. marital relations
   c. caring for other children
   d. mild exercise and light housework

5. What must be completely healed before the patient is discharged from the doctor's care?
   a. episiotomy
   b. uterus
   c. cervix
   d. breasts

6. A papanicolaou smear is a test for
   a. syphilis
   b. cancer of the cervix
   c. cancer of the uterus
   d. gonorrhea
   e. all of the above

7. Postpartum depression may occur in some women because of
   a. hormonal changes
   b. physiological changes
   c. physical exhaustion
   d. all of the above

SUGGESTED ACTIVITIES

Postpartum

- Practice applying a breast binder.
- Demonstrate postpartum exercises that improve abdominal muscle tone.
- Discuss the effect that lack of sleep can have on the body.
- Make a chart listing complications during the puerperium, their signs and symptoms, and nursing care to be given.
- Develop a plan to teach the patient about self-care during the postpartum period.
- Identify indications and medical management of a retained placenta.
- Develop a care plan with short- and long-term goals for the new mother in the postpartum period. Include nursing goals and assessment.

Attachment and Bonding

- List the variables that influence mother-infant interactions.
- List factors that enhance bonding.
- Describe observations of the mother with her baby that reflect the bonding process.
- Discuss the needs of the father during the immediate postpartum period.
- Identify the support measures that the nurse can provide to enhance the experience.

BIBLIOGRAPHY

Hamilton, P. M. *Basic Maternity Nursing*, 6th ed. St. Louis, MO: C. V. Mosby, 1989.

Hawkins, J. W., and L. Pierfedeici. *Maternity and Gynecological Nursing.* New York: J. B. Lippincott, 1981.

Jenson, M. D., Benson, R., and I. Bobsk. *Maternity Care: The Nurse and the Family*, 3rd ed. St. Louis, MO: C. V. Mosby, 1985.

McNall, L. K. *Obstetric and Gynecologic Nursing*. St. Louis, MO: C. V. Mosby, 1980.

Pillitteri, A. *Maternal-Newborn Nursing: Care of the Growing Family*, 2nd ed. Boston: Little, Brown and Co., 1981.

Pritchard, J. A., MacDonald, P. C., and N. F. Grant. *Williams Obstetrics*, 17th ed. E. Norwalk, CT: Appleton-Century-Crofts, 1985.

Reeder, S., Mastroianni, L., Jr., and L. Martin. *Maternity Nursing*, 16th ed. New York: J. B. Lippincott, 1987.

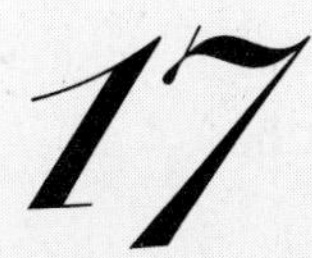

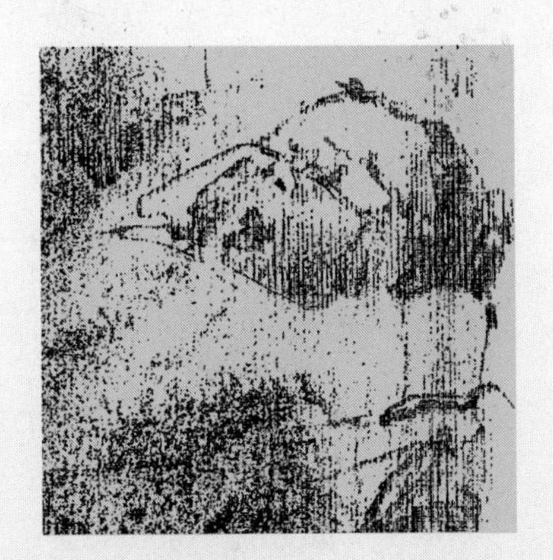

Family Planning

OBJECTIVES

AFTER STUDYING THIS CHAPTER, THE STUDENT SHOULD BE ABLE TO:

- LIST THREE AREAS THAT MAKE DEMANDS ON THE NEW FATHER.
- EXPLAIN WHY THE NEW FATHER SHOULD BE INCLUDED IN PLANS FOR THE NEW BABY.
- DEFINE THE ACRONYM BRAIDED AND ITS IMPORTANCE IN CHOOSING A CONTRACEPTIVE.
- EXPLAIN THE VARIOUS METHODS OF BIRTH CONTROL, THEIR ACTIONS AND LIMITATIONS.
- EXPLAIN THE DIFFERENCES BETWEEN VARIOUS HORMONAL CONTRACEPTIVES AND THEIR EFFECTS ON THE BODY.
- DESCRIBE TWO STERILIZATION PROCEDURES.
- EXPLAIN THE VARYING VIEWPOINTS OF THE ABORTION ISSUE.

KEY TERMS

CONTRACEPTION
BRAIDED
THEORETICAL EFFECTIVENESS RATE
ACTUAL EFFECTIVENESS RATE
NATURAL FAMILY PLANNING (NFP)
SYMPTOTHERMAL METHOD
BASAL TEMPERATURE METHOD
OVULATION METHOD

COITUS INTERRUPTUS

SPERMICIDALS

SPONGE

NONOXYNOL-9

DIAPHRAGM

CERVICAL CAP

CONDOM

INTRAUTERINE DEVICE (IUD)

COMBINED ORAL CONTRACEPTIVES

NORPLANT SYSTEM

MINIPILL

DEPO-PROVERA (DMPA) INJECTION

STERILIZATION

BILATERAL TUBAL LIGATION

VASECTOMY

VACUUM CURETTAGE

DILATION AND CURETTAGE (D&C)

DILATION AND EVACUATION (D&E)

RU-486

Pregnancy is a family affair. It is a biological event and an emotional experience beginning with a relationship between two people that develops into a new relationship between them and their offspring. Both the expectant mother and the father have a tremendous investment in the pregnancy. The expectant father is facing new financial, emotional, and social demands. He is also having to learn new skills to be able to contribute to the care of his new baby. A new dimension is added to the relationship between this man and woman. They are no longer simply a couple, but now have to interact with one another as "mother" and "father" in the rearing of their new baby.

THE FATHER'S ROLE

Usually, involved fatherhood begins during the prenatal period. At that time, well-planned instruction prepares the father for meaningful participation in the labor and delivery room. Instruction, however, should not be restricted to the mechanics of labor and the immediate environment of the hospital. Social pressures exerted on the father show up in his relationships with male friends, close members of the extended family, and with people at work. Therefore, he needs to understand the psychological changes taking place within himself and the pregnant woman. A person's attitude toward fatherhood and its responsibilities has its roots in early childhood and the interpersonal family relationships. How a new father feels affects the kind of influence and support he is able to give throughout the pregnancy. His feelings also determine the kind of relationship he is able to establish with his child when the baby is born.

Pregnancy is a time of increasing dependence in which the woman may experience a great need to be protected. Support, acceptance, and understanding are extremely important. If the father understands that somatic (body) changes of the mother may bring about withdrawal from him and a concentration on herself and the child, his anxiety is less marked. He needs to know that these changes are temporary and normal; they are not the result of something he has or has not done.

The expectant father should share the entire experience. Being prepared helps relieve any feelings of inadequacy in his supportive role. He needs to understand pregnancy and labor and how he can participate effectively in the birth of his child. Whenever plans are being made for the care of the mother and child, the father should be included. If he is helped to understand how vital his role is during the neonatal period, he is better able to meet the responsibilities of the postpartum period and beyond. A readiness to assist with household chores is not the only demonstration of cooperation and love. Of even more importance is the willingness to give encouragement and support. This attitude provides the foundation upon which the parent-child relationship is built.

FAMILY PLANNING

Nurses have an ideal opportunity to discuss family planning with the parents. Since family planning is an integral part of comprehensive maternity care, counseling in **contraception** (preventing pregnancy) is appropriate. If the new mother used a method of contraception before pregnancy, it must be reevaluated in view of the physical changes of childbearing. The patient's freedom to choose requires a knowledge of the choices. It is the responsibility of every nurse to be aware of all methods of contraception so that the method selected is acceptable to both father and mother. The nursing mother should be counseled that the reproductive organs will soon return to the menstrual cycle and ovulation can occur at regular intervals. She should also be reminded that breast feeding is *not* a dependable means of contraception and that she could become pregnant again.

Although birth control is an important element in preventive medicine, it is profoundly objectionable to many people. Individual views must be fully respected, whether expressed by patients, nurses, or physicians. When the personal convictions of the physician or nurse prevent providing medical supervision and information on family planning, referrals should be made. Whenever there are clearly defined conditions in which the health of the woman may be jeopardized by pregnancy, it is generally recognized by the medical profession that contraceptive measures are proper medical practice.

METHODS OF BIRTH CONTROL

Before a couple can decide on which method might be best for them, they need information on which to base their choice. The acronym **BRAIDED** helps nurses to be sure that they have covered the appropriate information with the couple in helping them to choose an appropriate contraceptive method.

B — benefits of each method, including effectiveness rates

R — risks of each method and danger signs to watch for

A — alternatives, reviewing all methods available

I — inquiries from the couple about each method are encouraged

D — decision of contraception is the patient's right

E — explanation of the chosen method needs complete review

D — document all that has happened in the counseling session

Thanks to advances in medical technology, more choices of birth control are available now than ever before, see Figure 17–1. The couple needs to consider the success rate of each method. There is a difference between the theoretical effectiveness rate and the actual effectiveness rate. The **theoretical effectiveness rate** implies that the method is used correctly at all times with no "user" mistakes or product failure. The **actual effectiveness rate** is more realistic. There are both personal considerations and health considerations in choosing a contraceptive. Most couples will prefer an easy method that fits personal needs. If a couple is having intercourse often, for example, they may prefer a method that works around the clock without interruption, such as the pill, IUD, or Norplant system. Some methods carry health risks and side effects that also need to be considered. It must be kept in mind, however, that pregnancy is a greater health risk than all forms of birth control combined. The best birth control method is the one that the couple is most comfortable with, will use correctly each and every time, and is safest for overall health.

NATURAL FAMILY PLANNING

Natural family planning (NFP), also known as the rhythm method, is based on fertility awareness, that is, knowledge of the natural cycle of fertility and infertility individual to each woman. It is based on the fact that conception occurs near the time of ovulation. Ovulation occurs about 14 days before the beginning of a menstrual period. In a regular monthly cycle of 28 days, the fertile period is from about the 10th to the 17th day after the beginning of the menstrual period; sexual intercourse is avoided during those days.

The theoretical effectiveness rate of this method of contraception is 90%–97%, but the actual effectiveness rate is closer to 80%. The symptothermal method of NFP along with watching the calendar will increase the effectiveness rate. The **symptothermal method** uses changes in the basal body temperature and cervical mucus that occur at the time of ovulation to help predict the fertile time in a cycle, see Figures 17–2 and 17–3.

When using the **basal temperature method**, the woman measures her body temperature every morning after at least six hours of sleep. The temperature during the first part of the menstrual cycle will be lower than that during the later part. Near the middle of the cycle there is a further slight temperature drop. The midcycle temperature drop is about the time of ovulation. One or two days after ovulation, the body temperature rises about 3/10 to 1 degree higher and remains there until the beginning of menstruation. Starting from the day of temperature rise and allowing two to three safety days, conception should no longer be possible.

The **ovulation method** was developed by two physicians, John and Evelyn Billings. This method is based on the changes that occur in the cervical mucus during the menstrual cycle and the action of the mucus on sperm. This method can be used by women with irregular cycles. It relies upon observing and understanding vaginal secretions. Clear slippery mucus that appears at the time of ovulation is thought to keep the sperm alive and potent and also facilitates their progress through the vagina and cervix and penetration of the ovum. When vaginal secretions are clear, the couple avoids intercourse or takes additional precautions to avoid pregnancy. This method takes a certain amount of time to learn and requires a commitment to daily observation and charting. Ovulation can be affected by stress, illness, medications, or breast feeding. Also, some couples may consider the time of abstinence from intercourse a disadvantage.

METHODS OF CONTRACEPTION			
Method	Percentage of Couples Using Method	Percentage of Women Who Avoid Pregnancy in a Given Year	Percentage of Women Experiencing Accidental Pregnancy during 1st Year of Use
Oral contraceptive	18.5	97	3
Female sterilization	16.6	99.6	0.4
Male condom	8.8	86	12
Male sterilization	7	99.8	0.15
IUD	1.2	94	3
Sponge	0.7	72 – 82	18 – 28
Spermicide	0.6	79	21
Rhythm/chance	1.8	80	85
Cervical cap	1	73 – 92	18
Diaphragm	1	84	18
Depro-Provera (injectable progestogen)	Statistics unavailable		0.3
Implants Norplant capsules	Statistics unavailable		0.04

Figure 17–1 *Birth control options and their effectiveness rates*

1. Enter the date of the month in the space provided on the graph.
2. Place a thermometer under the tongue for at least two minutes upon awakening each morning and before getting out of bed. Do this every morning even during menstruation. Do not eat, drink or smoke before taking the temperature.
3. Record the temperature reading on the graph by placing a dot in the proper place.
4. Indicate days of coitus (intercourse) by placing an arrow in the appropriate space.
5. The first day of the menstrual flow is the start of a cycle. Indicate each day of flow by shading the appropriate square on the graph.
6. Note any obvious reasons for temperature variation (such as medications, infection, colds, indigestion, etc.) on the graph above the reading for that day.
7. Some women may have a slight pain in the lower abdomen when ovulation occurs. If this is noticed, indicate the day it occurred on the graph.
8. Start a new cycle on another graph.

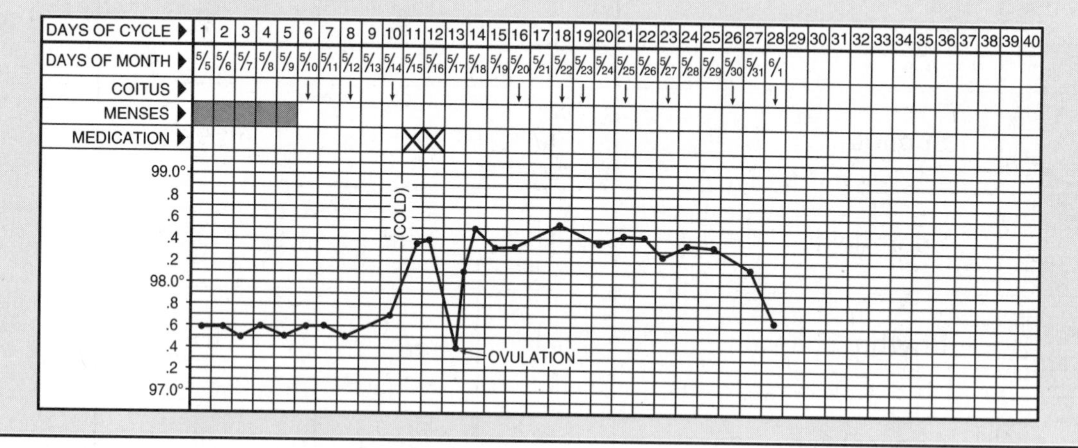

Figure 17–2 *Basal temperature chart and instructions*

COITUS INTERRUPTUS

Coitus interruptus (withdrawal) is an interruption of sexual intercourse. The man withdraws his penis from the woman's vagina before ejaculation of seminal fluid. As a method of birth control, withdrawal has several advantages. It requires no devices, involves no chemicals, and is available in any situation at no cost. It does, however, have one major disadvantage: It is very unreliable. A first-year failure rate among typical users is approximately 16%–23%. Preejaculatory fluid, which contains active sperm in the seminal fluid, can escape at any time before ejaculation. In addition, this method requires self-control

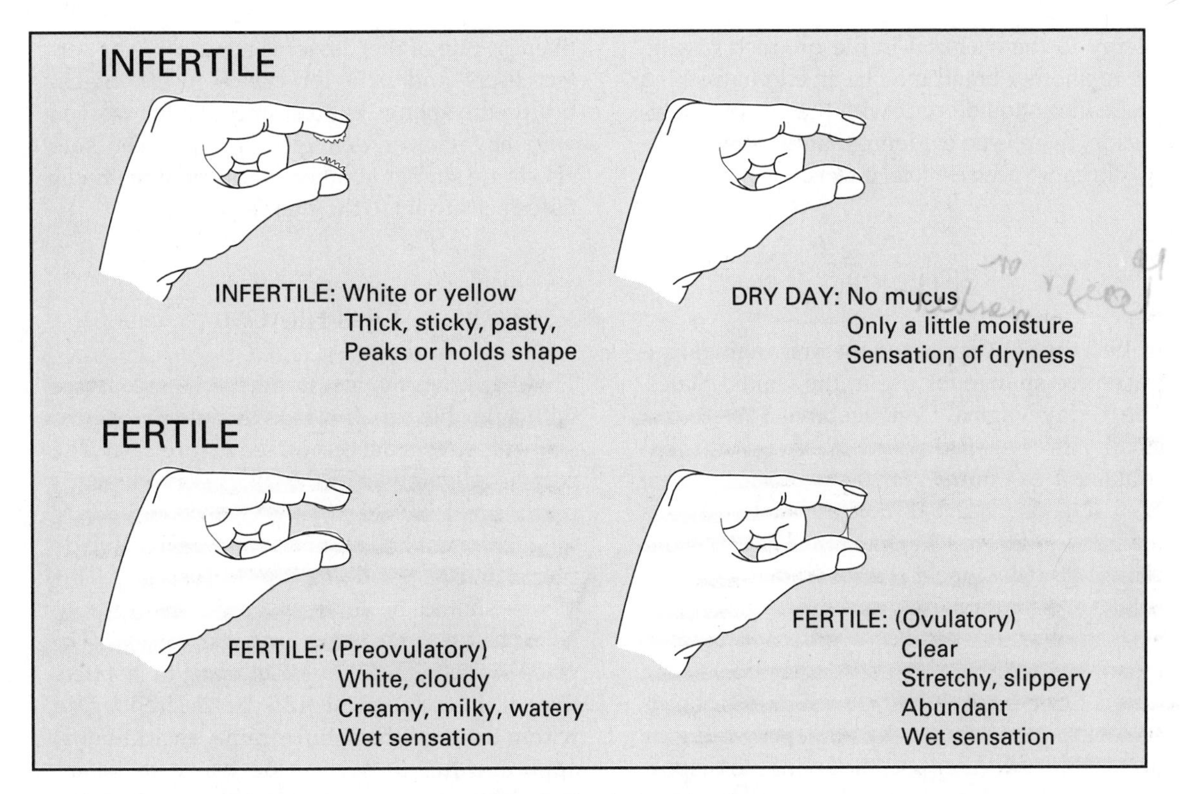

Figure 17–3 *Checking ovulatory mucus to determine fertile time of cycle*

which many people lack. Although coitus interruptus has no medical side effects, interruption of the excitement phase of the sexual response cycle can markedly diminish the pleasure for the couple.

SPERMICIDALS

Spermicidals (foams, tablets, creams, jellies, suppositories, or films) introduced into the vagina 10 to 15 minutes before intercourse produce a reaction destructive to spermatozoa, Figure 17–4. Spermicidals have several important advantages. They are simple, medically safe, available without prescription, and can reduce sexually transmitted disease (STD) transmission rates. The effectiveness rate among perfect users would be about 97%. The rate for the typical user is about 79%. The most common side effect is a temporary skin irritation involving the vulva or penis caused by sensitivity or

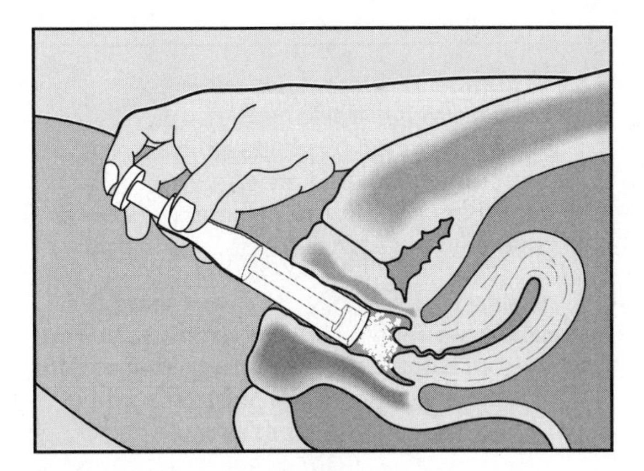

Figure 17–4 *Spermicidals*

allergy to the chemical in the product. Changing to another brand may be an alternative. If a pregnancy should occur with the use of a spermicide, there is no evidence that the spermicide would cause adverse fetal effects.

SPONGE

In 1983 the FDA approved the first vaginal contraceptive **sponge** for use in the United States. The Today Vaginal Contraceptive Sponge is a small, pillow-shaped polyurethane sponge that contains 1 g of **nonoxynol-9** spermicide, Figure 17–5. It has a concave dimple on one side that is intended to fit over the cervix and decrease the chance of dislodgment during intercourse. It is available in one size only and can be purchased over the counter without a prescription. It is moistened with water and placed close to the cervix. Once in place, the sponge provides continuous protection by releasing spermicide for up to 24 hours. After use, the sponge is disposable and should not be used again. The effectiveness rate of this device is about 88% for perfect users and 82% for typical users. Statistically, the sponge is most effective for women who have never delivered a baby. The side effects are similar to other spermicidal methods: tissue sensitivity to the chemicals used.

DIAPHRAGM

The **diaphragm** is a soft, dome-shaped device with a flexible rim. It is inserted into the vagina so that it covers the cervix, see Figure 17–6. The contraceptive effect of the diaphragm depends partly on its function as a barrier and partly on the sperm-killing effect of the spermicide placed inside the dome before insertion. This device should be inserted no more than two hours before intercourse, and it must be left in place at least eight hours afterward to be effective. If intercourse should be desired again within the eight-hour time frame, an additional applicator-full of spermicide needs to be inserted into the vagina, without removing the

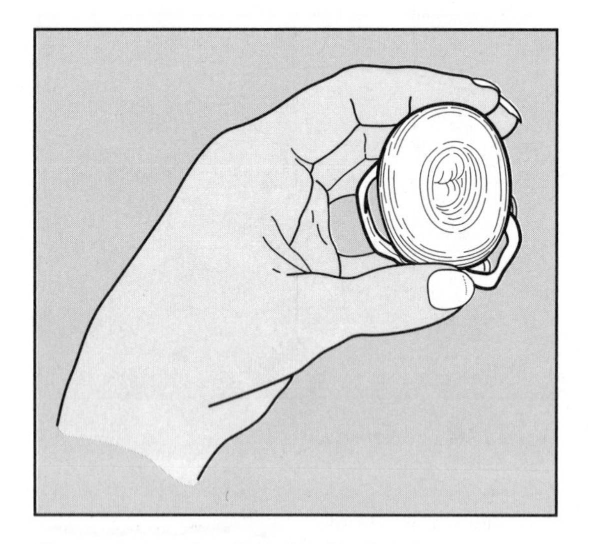

Figure 17–5 *Contraceptive sponge*

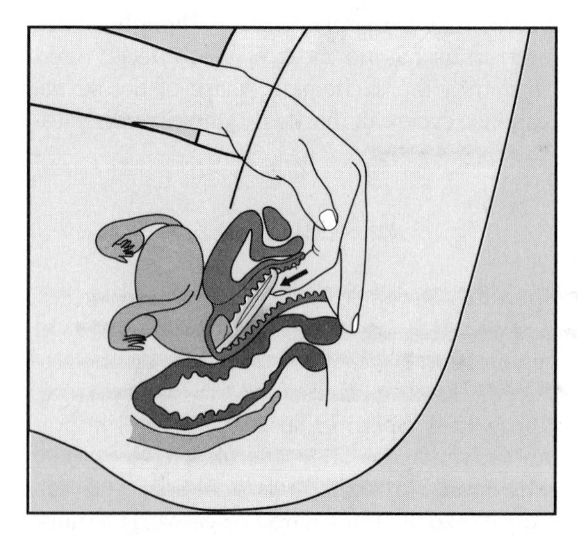

Figure 17–6 *Diaphragm placement*

diaphragm. The theoretical effectiveness rate is about 94%; the typical effectiveness rate is closer to 82% because it is not always used consistently or correctly. It offers the advantages of some protection against STDs; there is no hormonal influence on the system; contraception is immediately reversible when pregnancy is desired; and it is easy to use. The disadvantages are few. Sensitivity to spermicides is again a factor for some; compliance and decrease in spontaneity may be a disadvantage; and some women experience frequent urinary tract infections due to pressure of the diaphragm on the urethra.

CERVICAL CAP

In April 1988, the FDA approved the Prentif Cervical Cap as an effective and safe method of contraception. The **cervical cap** looks like a large rubber thimble with a soft latex dome and a firm rim, Figure 17–7. A small amount of spermicide is placed in the dome, and the cap is fitted over the cervix. It stays firmly in place by gripping the cervix and forming a strong suction. The cap itself provides a physical barrier to sperm, while the spermicide affords an additional chemical barrier.

Because it is smaller than the diaphragm, the Prentif cap has several advantages. It is more comfortable than the diaphragm and can be left in place for 48 hours. The cap stays snugly on the cervix, requiring no additional spermicidal cream or jelly with additional coitus. Consequently it is less messy and does not need to interfere in spontaneity because it can be inserted at any time before intercourse. Like the diaphragm, the cervical cap must be left in place for at least eight hours after the last intercourse to be effective. Used correctly, this method proved to be 82% to 94% effective in 90 study sites nationwide since cervical cap research began in 1977.

CONDOM

Condoms date back to 1350 B.C. and have recently gained in popularity because of their reported protection against various sexually transmitted diseases. The **condom** is a rubber sheath that may be put on the erect penis before it enters the vagina. Some condoms are coated with spermicide, and they vary also in size, shape, thickness, and presence or absence of lubricants.

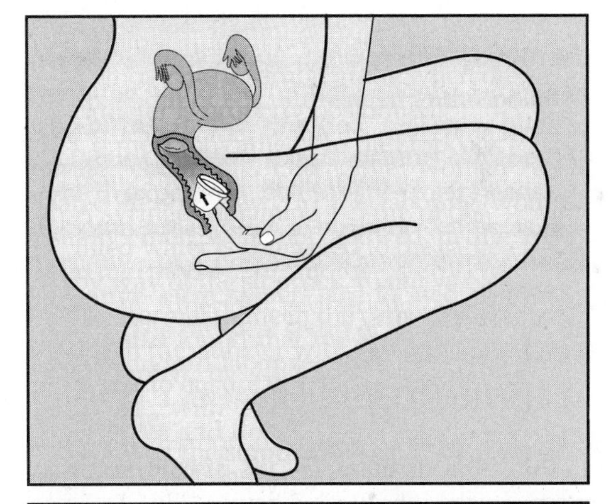

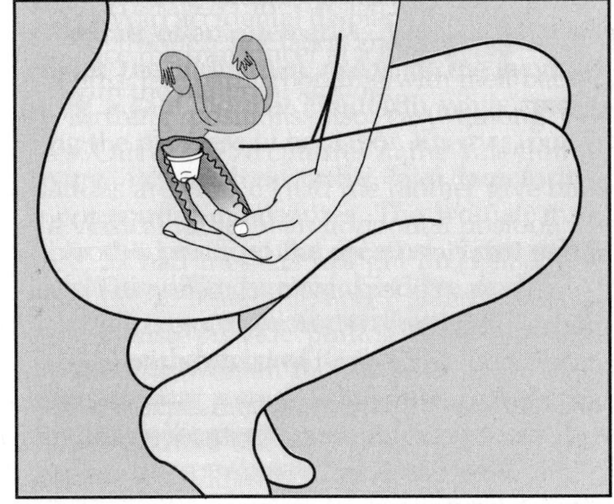

Figure 17–7 *Cervical cap placement*

Condoms, used carefully each and every time, are thought to be 98% effective in preventing pregnancy. The actual effectiveness rate, however, is about 88%. The lower rate may be due to inconsistent use or condom breakage. Condoms are readily accessible without a prescription and relatively inexpensive. They may be contraindicated for men or women with an allergy to the material used in condoms. Natural-skin condoms do not offer the same protection as latex condoms against some sexually transmitted diseases such as the human immunodeficiency virus (HIV).

The female condom is a pouch connected by two rings, Figure 17–8. The inner ring, much like a diaphragm, is 2 in. in diameter and is inserted inside the vagina. The pouch is approximately 7 in. long and lines the vaginal walls. The female condom offers more protection against STDs than other barrier methods. The outer ring is 2¾ in. in diameter and remains outside the vaginal opening when in place.

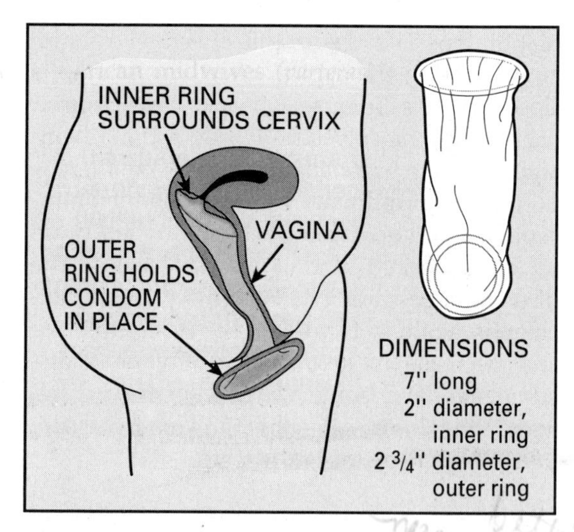

Figure 17–8 *The female condom*

INTRAUTERINE DEVICE (IUD)

In the 1970s, as many as 10% of contracepting women used intrauterine devices. But, because the IUD was linked to a high rate of pelvic infections and an increased incidence of septic abortions, manufacturers could no longer afford to market IUDs. There were only two brands of IUD available in the United States in 1991: the TCu 380A (ParaGard) and the progesterone T device (Progestasert).

The exact mechanism of action of **intrauterine devices (IUDs)** is not completely understood. Properly positioned, the IUD is thought to immobilize sperm and interfere with the migration of sperm from the vagina to the fallopian tubes (Figure 17–9). It may speed the transport of the ovum through the fallopian tubes. It inhibits fertilization and prevents implantation by interfering with the endometrium (lining of the uterus).

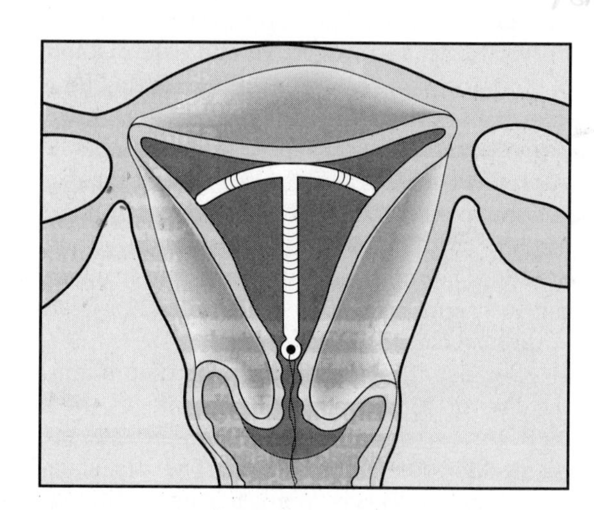

Figure 17–9 *IUD placement*

The effectiveness rate of the IUD is 98%–99%. It does not depend on compliance of use, but effectiveness rates are influenced by the woman's age, parity, and the individual characteristics of the different IUDs.

Two absolute contraindications for IUD use are:

- active, recent, or recurrent pelvic infections
- pregnancy

Strong relative contraindications are:

- risk factors for PID (pelvic inflammatory disease)
- irregular or abnormal uterine bleeding
- risk factors for exposure to HIV
- cervical or uterine malignancy, including unresolved abnormal Pap smears
- history of ectopic pregnancy
- previous problems with IUD pregnancies or expulsion
- impaired ability to check for danger signals
- history of severe vasovagal reactivity or fainting
- emergency treatment difficult to obtain

The IUD may also increase menstrual flow, cramps, and backaches. It is recommended only for women who have had at least one child; women who have only one sexual partner and he has no other partners; women who do not have a history of pelvic infection; and women who do not have problems with their periods. The IUD does not interfere with sexual spontaneity and is highly effective in preventing pregnancy. In the right woman, it may have many more benefits than risks. The IUD should be changed every 4 to 6 years, depending on the manufacturer's directions.

ORAL CONTRACEPTIVES (THE PILL)

The **combined oral contraceptive**, more commonly known as the birth control pill, is a safe and effective method, offering 99.9% protection against pregnancy for the "perfect" user. The "typical" user effectiveness rate is 97%. Failure is usually due to keeping an improper schedule of taking the pill. The oral contraceptive contains two synthetic hormones that mimic the action of two natural hormones, estrogen and progesterone. The two synthetic hormones in each pill effectively prevent ovulation or release of any ovum from either ovary during the time the pills are taken. Since no ovum is available to be fertilized, pregnancy cannot be achieved.

Oral contraceptives today are extremely safe for young women. The noncontraceptive benefits of the pill have been widely underpublished. It has a protective effect not only against menstrual disorders, ectopic pregnancy, benign breast disease, dysmenorrhea, anemia, and ovarian cysts but also offers protection against cancer of the ovary and endometrium. These positive effects have been overshadowed by publicity about the occurrence of heart attack, stroke, thromboembolism, liver tumors, and deep vein thrombosis. These concerns were much higher when the oral contraceptive was prescribed in much higher dosage. Recent studies have investigated the relationship between the birth control pill and breast cancer. To date, there is no valid evidence that oral contraceptives cause breast cancer.

There are approximately five pill-related deaths per 100,000 users per year. Most of these are among either pill users 40 years or older or pill users 35 years or older who smoke. Maternal mortality from obstetrical causes is about 10 per 100,000 births. Maternal mortality from all causes is nearly twice that rate. The mortality risk from driving a car is 19 per 100,000 drivers per year and from smoking a pack of cigarettes a day, 500 per 100,000 smokers. The birth control pill is clearly safer than many other risks that women are subjected to during their reproductive life.

Some women cannot take the birth control pill because of undesirable side effects, including missed periods, spotting or breakthrough bleeding, nausea, breast fullness and tenderness, mood changes, weight change, chloasma or other skin changes, and headaches. The birth control pill also offers little or no protection against sexually transmitted diseases. Women using birth control pills should also use condoms if they are at risk for getting a sexually transmitted disease. The pill is somewhat expensive unless obtained through a local family planning clinic with government funding. It must be taken daily at approximately the same time each day to be highly effective. And certain medications may affect the contraceptive value of the pill (for example, Rifampin and certain antibiotics may decrease the contraceptive effect). See Figure 17–10 for the contraindications for birth control pills.

NORPLANT SYSTEM

Early in 1991, the FDA approved a new method of contraception in the United States called the Norplant system. The **Norplant system** consists of six silicone, matchstick-sized capsules filled with a powdered synthetic progesterone, see Figure 17–11. These rods are implanted surgically just beneath the skin in the upper inside arm. The procedure is performed under a local anesthetic. The synthetic progesterone begins to leak through the semiporous walls of the capsules at a slow, controlled rate into the bloodstream and is carried to the pituitary gland in the brain. Within 24 to 48 hours, the pituitary completely stops producing the luteinizing hormone and follicle-stimulating hormone. Without their hormonal cue, the ovaries will not release an ovum for fertilization. The Norplant system offers 99.9% protection for a continuous period of 5 years. If a pregnancy is desired, the rods may be surgically removed, and fertility resumes within 24 hours.

The Norplant system has several disadvantages. It is more expensive than short-term methods; minor surgery is required to implant and remove the system; the implants may be slightly visible; users are likely to experience alterations in bleeding patterns, including prolonged menstrual bleeding, spotting between periods, very scanty menses, or no menses at all; and weight changes, headaches, and mood changes are also possible side effects.

Norplant implants may be used by almost all women in good health. It is particularly suited for women who want continuous contraception and long-term spacing between their children. It is also indicated for women who desire a method not related to intercourse and one that does not have to be remembered every day. Contraindications for use include acute liver disease; jaundice; unexplained vaginal bleeding; a history of blood clots in the legs, lungs, or eyes; and a history of heart attack, chest pain due to diagnosed heart disease, or stroke.

PROGESTIN-ONLY PILL (MINIPILL)

Historically, the **minipill**, or progestin-only pill, followed the combined oral contraceptives by about 10 years. The progestin-only pills are taken every day with no pill-free interval. They differ from the combined pill in that they do not consistently suppress ovulation. Rather, they create an environment in the uterus and tubes that is unsuitable for pregnancy. The effectiveness rate is highest if ovulation is blocked consistently. When this happens, the woman tends to stop having her period or has prolonged time between menstrual bleedings. The minipill is generally less effective than the

CONTRAINDICATIONS FOR ORAL CONTRACEPTIVES

Absolute Contraindications	Strong Relative Contraindications	Other Considerations that Contraindicate
Thrombophlebitis or thromboembolic disorder (current or history)	Severe headaches that are vascular or migraines in nature, particularly when they start after initiation of oral contraceptives	Diabetes
Cerebrovascular accident (current or history)	Hypertension with resting diastolic blood pressure of 90 mm Hg or greater, or a resting systolic blood pressure of 140 mm Hg or greater on three or more separate occasions, or an accurate measurement of 110 mm Hg diastolic or more on a single occasion	Sickle cell disease
Coronary heart disease (current or history)	Acute phase of mononucleosis	Active gallbladder disease
Known or suspected breast cancer (current or history)	Elective major surgery requiring immobilization in the next four weeks	Congenital hyperbilirubinemia
Known or suspected estrogen-dependent neoplasia (current or history)	Long leg cast or major injury to lower leg	Over 50 years old
Benign or malignant liver tumor (current or history)	Over 40 years old, accompanied by a second risk factor for the development of cardiovascular disease such as diabetes or hypertension	Completion of term pregnancy within the past two weeks
Known impaired liver function	Over 35 years old and currently a smoker of 15 or more cigarettes a day	Weight gain of 10 or more pounds while on the pill in the past
Pregnancy	Any abnormal, undiagnosed bleeding	Cardiac or renal disease
Cholestasis during a pregnancy		Inability to follow instructions and comply with daily pill taking
		Lactation
		Family history of hyperlipidemia or heart disease causing myocardial infarction in a mother or sister before age 50

Figure 17–10 *Contraindications for the use of combined oral contraceptives*

combined pill, with its effectiveness rate ranging from 97% to 99% for perfect users. In lactating women, the effectiveness is higher, and the progestin does not alter the quantity of milk as the combined birth control pill does.

Progestin-only pills are desirable for women who want to use an oral contraceptive but have relative contraindications to combined pills. Women who have side effects from the estrogen component of the combined pills,

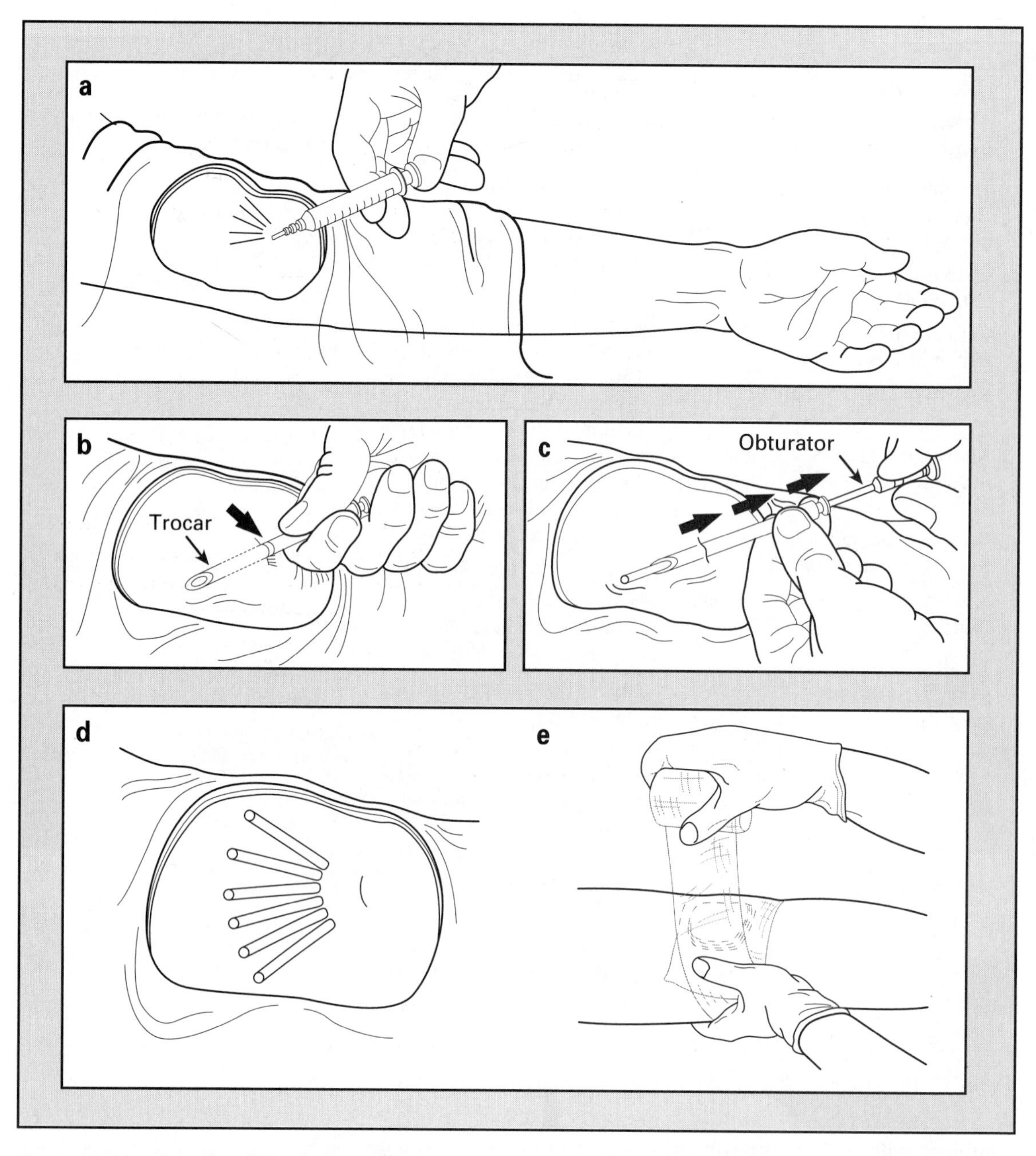

Figure 17–11 *Insertion of Norplant® capsules. (a) A local anesthetic is injected in a fan-shaped area on the inside of the upper arm. (b) A trocar, a metal tube into which a rod (obturator) fits, is inserted under the skin up to a special mark. (c) The first Norplant capsule is loaded and pushed out by the obturator, which is then withdrawn, leaving the trocar in place. (d) The same process is repeated until the remaining five implants are inserted in a fan shape. (e) The trocar is removed, and the incision is closed with a bandage.*

such as headaches or hypertension, may not be bothered by the minipill. Lactating women who desire hormonal contraception can safely use the progestin-only pill. The same absolute contraindications as for the combined pills apply to the minipill.

DEPO-PROVERA INJECTIONS (THE SHOT)

Injectable progestins have been used effectively in some countries as a method of birth control. The most commonly used injectable progestin is **Depo-Provera (DMPA)**. Its action is similar to progestin-only contraceptives. The effectiveness rate is about 99%. The FDA approved this method of birth control in the United States in October 1992. DMPA, 150 mg, is injected intramuscularly every three months. Because it is a long-acting injectable, DMPA is not related to sexual intercourse and offers privacy to the user. It eventually stops the menstrual period, thereby being beneficial to women who have problems with their periods.

Because some women prefer regular menstrual periods as assurance that they are not pregnant, the cycle irregularities for some users can be a disadvantage. The return of fertility may be delayed for 6–12 months after the use of DMPA. Some women find the injection itself a disadvantage. Animal studies also suggest that if a pregnancy were to occur while using DMPA, it may affect the fetus.

This method may be desirable for women who do not want more children but also do not want sterilization. Women who develop estrogen-related complications with combined oral contraceptives, such as high blood pressure, headaches, leg pain, or hyperlipidemia may be good candidates for the shot. Women who smoke or are over 40 may also benefit from this method.

STERILIZATION

After a couple have had their desired number of children, some couples request **sterilization**. This method is a surgical procedure that makes further conception impossible. Tubal occlusion, or **bilateral tubal ligation** is the blocking off of the fallopian tubes. The ovum, instead of passing into the uterus, disintegrates and is absorbed by the body. Special "temporary" tubal plugs are being developed, but as yet there is no guarantee that the procedure can be reversed and it must be viewed as a permanent form of birth control. The surgical procedure is performed under anesthesia and requires a brief period of recovery.

The sterilization procedure for men is called a bilateral vasectomy. A **vasectomy** is the cutting of the vas deferens to keep sperm from being ejaculated and reaching the ovum. This procedure does not interfere with erection or ejaculation. The ejaculate is simply missing the sperm. Vasectomy is simpler and less expensive than a tubal ligation. It also has less risk; it is a simple procedure performed in a doctor's office under a local anesthetic. Little recovery time is required, and sexual activity can be resumed in a week. It is wise, however, to advise additional birth control until the first semen count, done six weeks after the vasectomy, is found to be free of sperm. As with tubal ligation, procedures are being developed to reverse the vasectomy, but at this time, the vasectomy needs to be considered a permanent, irreversible method of contraception.

ABORTION

An abortion is not simply a medical procedure. It is an emotional and personal issue for many. Although there is much controversy surrounding abortion, each health-care provider must find his or her own "comfort zone" to discuss all the options with the pregnant woman. It is our belief that every woman is entitled to accurate information to make a decision regarding her own health and pregnancy.

Before 1970, legal abortions were not available in the United States. In 1973, abortions became legal through the U.S. Supreme Court decisions on two cases — *Roe v. Wade* and *Doe v. Bolton*. In these decisions it was stated:

1. In the first trimester of pregnancy, an abortion decision is the right of the woman and her physician.
2. In the second trimester, the state may regulate abortion procedures in ways that are reasonably related to a woman's health.
3. For pregnancy subsequent to viability, the state may, if it chooses, regulate and even outlaw abortion, except when necessary, according to appropriate medical judgment, for the preservation of the life or health of the pregnant woman.

On July 3, 1989, the Supreme Court ruled that states could place restrictions interfering with provision of abortion services to include such possibilities as waiting periods, informed consent requirements, parental or spousal notification, and hospitalization requirements. Over the next several years, confrontations from both sides of the abortion issue are likely to occur at the state legislative level.

The decision-making process regarding abortion begins when the woman learns she is pregnant. Women should be encouraged to always be aware of when their last menstrual period began. There is an increased risk if a woman chooses to terminate her pregnancy after the first two months.

All pregnancy-counseling staff should provide a supportive, nonjudgmental setting to explore feelings, options, and provide information and referrals. In some federally funded clinics, abortion counseling may not be allowed. The counselor or nurse needs to also be aware of his or her own feelings in each case. Personal ambivalence may affect one's ability to deliver quality care to the patient.

The goal of an abortion is to remove the products of conception. First-trimester abortions are performed within the first 13 weeks of pregnancy. A second-trimester abortion involves removing the pregnancy from 14 to 24 weeks of gestation. Surgical methods are the most common in the United States. They include **vacuum curettage** (most widely used procedure); **dilation and curettage (D&C)**; and **dilation and evacuation (D&E)**, which is the procedure done between 13 and 16 weeks gestation.

RU-486 is a drug being tested for various treatments. It is a progesterone antagonist that will effectively produce an abortion in 85% of women when given orally within three weeks of the expected onset of the missed period. The earlier it is used, the more effective it is in producing an abortion. The FDA has not approved its use in the United States. RU-486 is also being tested as a possible effective drug against various types of cancer.

A woman's fertility is usually unaffected by an abortion. In fact, a woman can become pregnant immediately after an abortion and therefore should be careful to use some form of birth control as soon as she resumes sexual activity. Learning about and using effective birth control methods are basic to preventing the future need for abortion. It is the health-care provider's responsibility to be sure the woman has all the information she needs to protect herself against unwanted pregnancies.

Figure 17–12 outlines the major methods of contraception and related concerns.

CONTRACEPTION METHODS AND CONCERNS

Method	Risks	Side Effects	Noncontraceptive Benefits
Oral contraceptives	Cardiovascular complications such as stroke, blood clots, high blood pressure, and heart attacks with the higher-dose combined oral contraceptive	Possible nausea, headaches, dizziness, spotting, weight gain, breast tenderness, chloasma, cramping	Protects against PID, decreases risk of ovarian and endometrial cancer, decreases menstrual blood loss and dysmenorrhea (cramps), decreases benign breast disease, regulates irregular menses, protects bone density, decreases risk of atherosclerosis, lessens the risk of rheumatoid arthritis, decreases uterine fibroids, and decreases ovarian cysts
IUD	Pelvic inflammatory disease, uterine perforation, anemia	Menstrual cramping, spotting, increased bleeding	None known except progestin-releasing IUD, which may decrease menstrual pain and blood loss
Condoms	None known	Decreased sensation, allergy to latex, less spontaneity in lovemaking	Protects against sexually transmitted disease, including AIDS; delays premature ejaculation
Norplant implants	Infection at implant site	Menstrual changes, weight gain, headaches	May protect against PID, may decrease menstrual cramps, and blood loss
DMPA	None definitely proven	Menstrual changes, weight gain, headaches	May protect against PID, lactation not disturbed, may protect against ovarian and endometrial cancer
Sterilization	Infection	Pain at surgical site, psychological reaction with subsequent regret	None known
Abstinence	None known	Psychological reactions	Prevents infections including AIDS
Abortion	Infection, pain, perforation, psychological trauma	Cramping	None known
Barriers (diaphragm, caps, sponges)	Mechanical irritation, vaginal infections, toxic shock syndrome	Pelvic pressure, cervical erosion, vaginal discharges if left in too long	Protects to some degree against sexually transmitted diseases

Figure 17–12 *Major methods of contraception and some related concerns*

REVIEW QUESTIONS

A. Multiple choice. Select the best answer.

1. The use of the combined oral contraceptives is absolutely contraindicated in women who have
   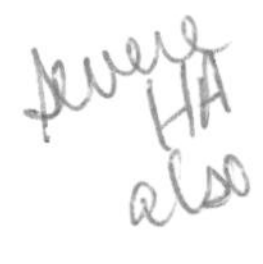
   a. thrombophlebitis and known impaired liver function
   b. menstrual irregularities and dysmenorrhea
   c. never borne children
   d. a family history of diabetes or heart disease

2. Side effects of the IUD include all of the following *except*
   a. increased dysmenorrhea
   b. increased bleeding and discharge
   c. nausea, headaches
   d. increased risk of pelvic infections

3. Spermicidal substances act by
   a. providing a mechanical barrier and destroying sperm
   b. altering the pH balance within the vagina
   c. suppressing ovulation
   d. stimulating growth of the vaginal lining

4. The Norplant system is a contraceptive method that
   a. gives 5 years of uninterrupted birth control and is highly effective
   b. needs to be surgically implanted and removed
   c. will cause irregularity in the menstrual cycle
   d. all of the above

5. Depo-Provera (DMPA), or "the shot"
   a. will usually stop a woman's period after 6 months of use and affects the return of fertility for 6–12 months after the medication is stopped
   b. is not an FDA-approved and effective method of contraception
   c. offers unpredictable contraception, at best
   d. causes breast cancer if used too long

6. The sterilization procedure for the male is
   a. condoms
   b. vasectomy
   c. spermicide
   d. all of the above

7. The possible side effects of a diaphragm include
   a. thromboembolic disease
   b. pelvic infections
   c. irritation from spermicide
   d. none

8. The effectiveness of the ovulation method depends on
   a. regular menstrual cycles
   b. observing and understanding vaginal secretions and temperature changes
   c. ovulating regularly
   d. using additional contraceptive methods

9. The cervical cap differs from the diaphragm by all of the following *except*
   a. the cap may be left in place 48 hours and remain effective without additional use of spermicide
   b. the cap covers the cervix as an airtight seal
   c. it offers greater contraceptive effectiveness
   d. extra spermicide does not need to be added if coitus occurs more than once in an 8-hour period

10. The minipill differs from the combined oral contraceptive by
    a. inhibiting ovulation
    b. being more effective
    c. offering a progestin-only effect on the body
    d. having fewer side effects

SUGGESTED ACTIVITIES

- Make a chart of the impact that the patient characteristics listed below may have on the choice of use of an oral contraceptive, the Norplant system, a diaphragm or cervical cap, natural family planning, condoms, and sterilization. Include aspects such as effectiveness rate and side effects.
  - Sexual activity pattern and habits
  - Reproductive life span
  - Age
  - Access to medical care
  - Ability to pay for contraception
  - Medical history
  - Health issues
- Define what is meant by fertility awareness. Demonstrate the ability to instruct a patient on fertility awareness.
- Discuss the issues surrounding abortion, and role play a counseling session with a woman requesting an abortion.

BIBLIOGRAPHY

Grimes, D. A. "Which Patients May Benefit from Alternative Contraceptive Methods?" *Contraceptive Report* 1(4):7–11, 1990.

Hatcher, R. *Contraceptive Technology 1991–1992*, 14th ed. New York: Irvington Publishers, 1991.

Heller, D. "The Emotional Issues of Abortion." *OB/GYN* 7:50–52, May, 1982.

CHAPTER

18

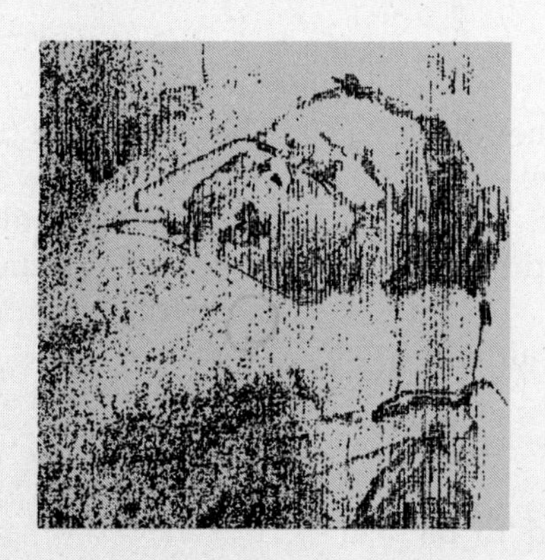

Characteristics and Care of the Neonate

OBJECTIVES

AFTER STUDYING THIS CHAPTER, THE STUDENT SHOULD BE ABLE TO:

- DIFFERENTIATE BETWEEN THE CHARACTERISTICS OF A FULL-TERM NEWBORN AND A PREMATURE INFANT.
- LIST NORMAL REFLEXES OF THE NEWBORN.
- DESCRIBE THE BRAZELTON NEONATAL BEHAVIORAL ASSESSMENT SCALE.
- IDENTIFY STANDARD NURSING CARE FOR A FULL-TERM AND A PREMATURE INFANT.
- LIST THE HOME-CARE INSTRUCTIONS FOR THE NEWBORN.

Key Terms

FONTANEL
CEPHALOCAUDAL DISPROPORTION
LANUGO
MILIA
JAUNDICE
VERNIX CASEOSA
MORO REFLEX
GALANT REACTION
TONIC NECK REFLEX
PRIMARY STANDING
AUTOMATIC WALKING
GRASP REFLEX
SUCKING REFLEX
ROOTING REFLEX
PLACING REACTION
PROTECTIVE REFLEX
PHENOTYPICAL
GENOTYPICAL
NEONATAL BEHAVIORAL ASSESSMENT SCALE (NBAS)
CONSOLABILITY
PHENYLKETONURIA (PKU)
PREMATURE INFANT
INCUBATOR
GAVAGE FEEDING
CIRCUMCISION

Although every baby is a unique individual, averages and the range of normality should be remembered so that a baby who deviates too far from the so-called normal may receive medical care. Understanding "normal" is important for nurses in evaluating the newborn.

Physical Appearance and Activities

The newborn looks surprisingly complete in contrast to its size. The hands, for example, resemble those of an adult with fingerprints, fingernails, and creases on the palms. The nurse soon learns that the newborn is a person in his own right and must be treated accordingly. The most important year in a baby's life is the first nine months in utero and the first three months after birth. During pregnancy all the baby's needs were supplied by the mother's body. After birth, it is necessary to protect and nourish the baby as an independent individual.

The weight of normal newborns varies, but about two-thirds of all full-term infants weigh from 6 to 8½ lb (2,700 to 3,850 g). During the first few days after birth the infant tends to lose about 6–10 oz (217 g–311 g) or 5%–10% of the birth weight. The length of the normal newborn varies also. The normal range is from 19 to 21½ in. (47.5 to 53.75 cm), Figure 18–1.

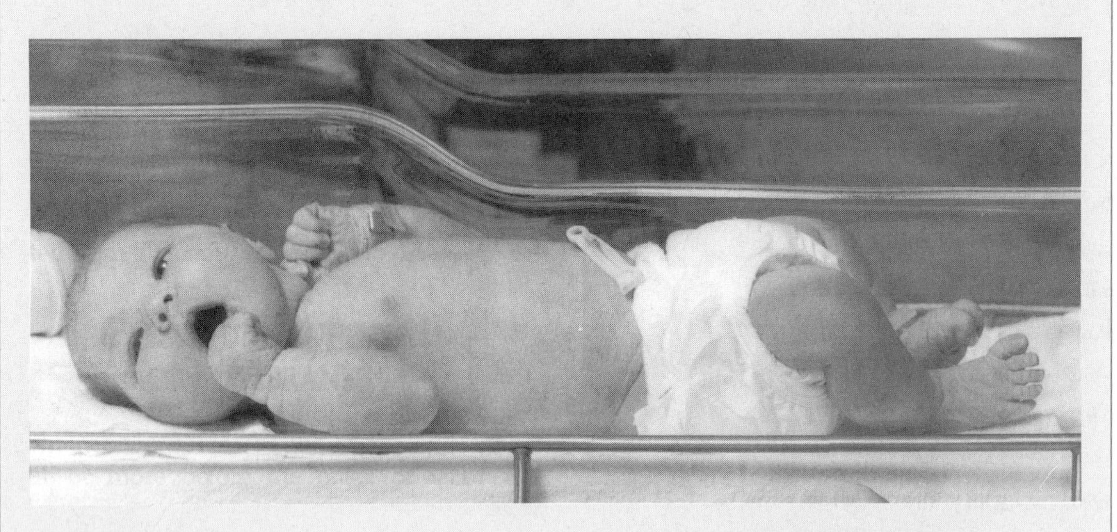

Figure 18–1 *What a healthy newborn baby looks like (Courtesy* Baby Talk Magazine, *Lew Merriam, photographer)*

The feet look more complete than they are. X-ray would show only one real bone at the heel. Other bones are now cartilage. Skin often loose and wrinkly.

Genitals of both sexes will seem large (especially scrotum) in comparison with the scale of, for example, the hands to adult size.

The trunk may startle you in some normal detail: short neck, small sloping shoulders, swollen breasts, large rounded abdomen, umbilical stump (future navel), slender, narrow pelvis and hips.

The skin is thin and dry. You may see veins through it. Fair skin may be rosy-red temporarily. Downy hair is not unusual. Some **vernix caseosa** (white, prenatal skin covering) remains.

Eyes appear dark blue, have a blank, staring expression. You may catch one or both turning or turned to crossed or wall-eyed position. Lids, characteristically, puffy.

Head usually strikes you as being too big for the body. It may be temporarily out of shape—lopsided or elongated—due to pressure before or during birth.

The legs are most often seen drawn up against the abdomen in prebirth position. Extended legs measure shorter than you'd expect compared with the arms. The knees stay slightly bent and legs are more or less bowed.

Weight unless well above the average of 6 or 7 lb will not prepare you for how really tiny newborn is. Top to toe measure: anywhere between 18 and 21 in.

A deep flush spreads over the entire body if baby cries hard. Veins on head swell and throb. You will notice no tears, as ducts do not function as yet.

The hands, if you open them out flat from their characteristic fist position, have: finely lined palms, tissue-paper thin nails, dry, loose-fitting skin and deep bracelet creases at wrist.

The face will disappoint you unless you expect to see: pudgy cheeks, a broad flat nose with mere hint of a bridge, receding chin, undersized lower jaw.

On the skull you will see or feel the two most obvious soft spots or **fontanels**. One is above the brow, the other close to crown of head in back.

The temperature of the newborn, though unstable, is usually about 37.5°C (99.5°F). The infant has an unstable heat-regulating system, and his body temperature is influenced by the environmental temperature, Figure 18–2. If the room is cold, so is his body. If he is covered with too many blankets, his body temperature rises. If the temperature about him is regulated, the newborn's temperature will return to normal.

The pulse rate is rapid, around 120–150 beats per minute. It is also irregular. If the infant is startled or cries, his pulse rate not only increases, but also becomes more irregular.

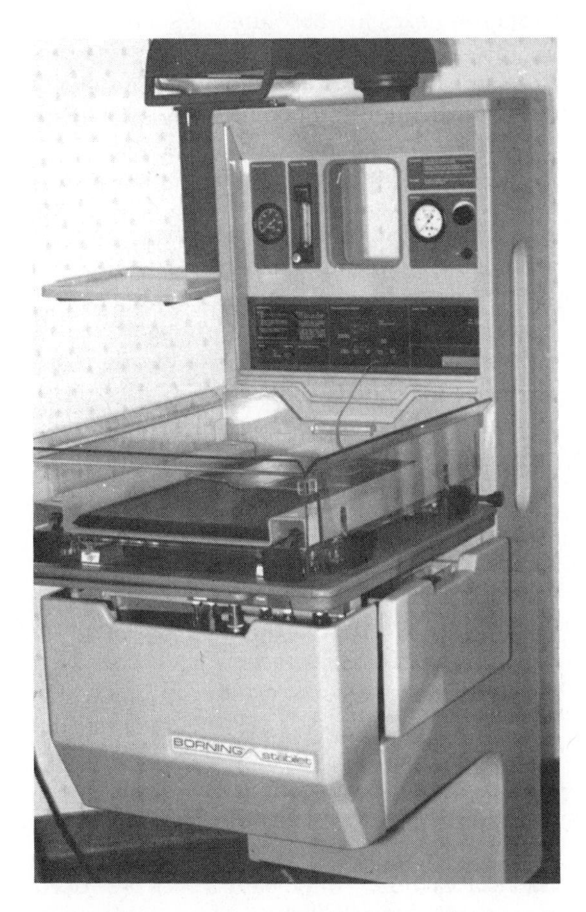

Figure 18–2 *Care center supports neonatal assessments, monitoring hookups, and maintains infant body temperature. (Courtesy Hill-Rom Corp.)*

The respiratory rate varies from 35 to 50 per minute. It is also irregular in depth and rhythm. Like the pulse rate, it is readily altered by internal or external stimuli.

The blood pressure is low. It is difficult to determine accurately and may vary with the size of the cuff used. The blood pressure is usually about 80/46.

The head seems too large for the body. The bones in the head have not grown together, and **fontanels** (soft spots) can be felt, Figure 18–3. The anterior fontanel is located above the brow, and the posterior fontanel is at the crown near the back of the head. The anterior fontanel closes within 18 months; the posterior fontanel takes 2 to 6 months to close. The circumference of the neonate's head is usually about 1 to 2 in. larger than the circumference of the chest. This rule of measurement is referred to as the law of **cephalocaudal disproportion**.

The skin is dark pink and soft. It is covered with **lanugo** (downy fine hair distributed

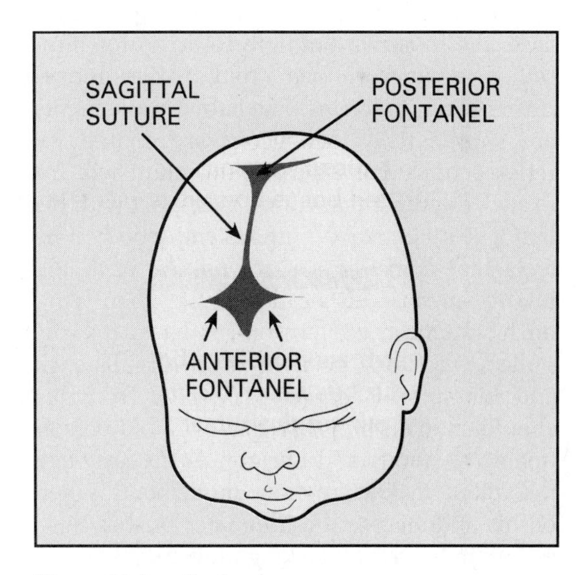

Figure 18–3 *Fontanels*

over the body). **Milia**, a condition in which tiny white pimples occur, particularly on the nose and chin, may be present. These spots are caused by obstructed sweat and oil glands. The skin may be **jaundiced** (yellow-tinged) but this color gradually disappears by the end of the first week. The skin may be covered with **vernix caseosa** (a cheeselike substance that protects the skin of the fetus), although the skin itself is thin and dry. Veins may be seen through it; when the baby cries, a deep flush spreads over the entire body. Babies of pigmented heritage can be evaluated for 0_2 by looking at mucous membranes (gums). Skin on the hands and feet is loose and wrinkled.

The breasts in both male and female neonates may be swollen because of maternal hormones they were exposed to before birth. Some babies even leak drops of milk from the breast nipples. This condition disappears without treatment. A slight milky or bloody vaginal discharge may be seen in female infants.

The muscles are weak, and the infant is unable to control them. The movements of the newborn are random and uncoordinated. He wiggles and stretches. His back and head must be supported when he is picked up, for he lacks the muscular strength to do so for himself. The newborn has rapid, varied movements in all directions. The baby's movements are simple reflex actions or are caused by reflex actions. For example, an infant will try to suck anything that comes in contact with his lips. The infant reacts with his entire body if he feels that something is wrong. At birth the infant can raise his head slightly when lying on his stomach but not on his back. If he is pulled to a sitting position, his head falls back and his spine is curved in a bow from his shoulders to his hips, like that of an old person unable to sit or stand upright. At an early age the infant makes crawling movements when on his abdomen and a little later pushes himself up in his crib by kicking movements.

The birth cry serves the two purposes of supplying the blood with sufficient oxygen and inflating the unexpanded lungs. Later, the newborn cries to express discomfort. If his discomfort is relieved when he cries, crying soon becomes a reflex action. It is the infant's method of expressing that he is hungry, wet, wants to be held, is in pain, or needs exercise. The newborn may sleep 15–20 hours each day. He is usually awakened by hunger.

REFLEXES

Certain reflexes are absolutely essential to the life of the infant because they protect him. Rooting, sucking, and swallowing are reflexes that enable the infant to obtain nourishment. Other reflexes help the newborn to relieve irritation or avoid unpleasant stimuli. Reflexes reflect the development of the newborn's nervous system. Some reflexes may also serve as the groundwork on which the baby begins the complicated business of learning to control his body, Figure 18–4.

Moro, or Startle, Reflex. After birth, when the baby reaches out and does not find a point of contact, he may have a feeling of falling into space. This sensation produces a reaction known as the Moro reflex. The **Moro reflex**, also known as the startle reflex, is a defensive response of newborns. The infant tenses, throws his arms out in an embracing motion and cries loudly. This reaction can occur when the infant is asleep or awake. By the fourth month, the baby is less easily startled and the response is less marked. By the sixth month the reflex disappears completely except in circumstances of extreme fright.

Galant Reaction. If the baby's back is stroked on one side while the baby is lying on his stomach, the whole trunk curves toward that side.

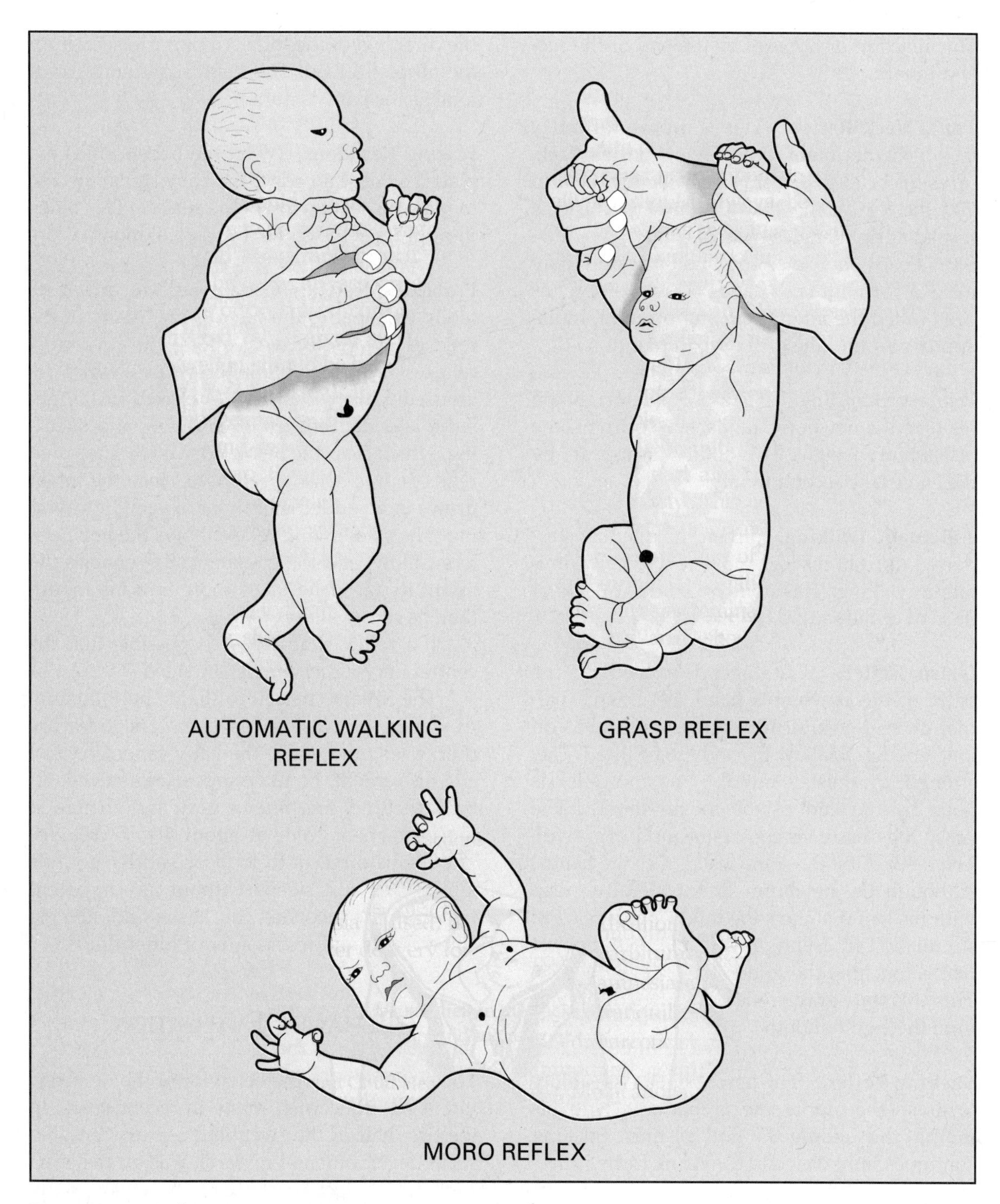

Figure 18–4 Reflexes

This reaction disappears by the end of the second month.

Tonic Neck Reflex. This is a postural reflex in which the infant, when lying on his back, turns his head to one side and extends the arm and the leg on the side to which the head is turned at right angles from his body. The newborn flexes the other leg and arm and may make a fist with both hands. This position has been called the infant's fencing position. It disappears around the fifth to sixth month.

Primary Standing. If supported upright on his feet, the newborn stands, supporting some of his body weight. This ability disappears by the end of the second month.

Automatic Walking. When the infant is supported upright his legs move reciprocally, imitating walking. This ability also disappears at the end of the second month.

Grasp Reflex. If a finger is placed on the palm of the newborn's hand, he grasps (palmar grasp reflex) firmly enough and holds on long enough to allow his body to be lifted. This strength diminishes rapidly, and the reflex is gone by the end of the fourth month. The grasp then becomes conscious and purposeful. The feet exhibit the same reaction as the hands. Although the newborn cannot literally grasp with his feet (Plantar), the infant's toes react to stimulation by trying to get hold of the object that is touching the sole of the foot or the toes. This (plantar) grasp reflex does not disappear until the eighth month.

Sucking Reflex. The newborn has the ability to grasp the nipple and areola area with his mouth, thus aiding the flow of milk. Sucking continues until the child can drink from a cup.

Rooting Reflex. The baby reacts to being touched on the cheek by turning his head in the direction of the touch in order to search for the nipple to feed. This reflex continues for as long as the baby is nursing.

Placing Reaction. When the baby's shins are placed against an edge, the baby steps upward to place his feet on top of the surface. This reflex disappears at the end of the second month.

Protective Reflex. Certain reflexes are absolutely essential to the infant's life; many of the reflexes are protective. Among the protective reflexes are the blinking reflex, which is aroused when the infant is subjected to a bright light, and the reflexes of coughing and sneezing, which clear the respiratory tract. The yawn reflex is, in a sense, protective, since the infant draws in an added supply of oxygen by yawning. The swallowing reflex allows the newborn to swallow, and the gagging reflex enables the infant to gag if he takes more into his mouth than he can swallow.

If a reflex is absent, it is possible that the central nervous system is damaged.

The infant reacts to light by blinking, frowning, or closing his eyes. The eyes are unfocused, and, since the baby cannot control eye movement, he may appear cross-eyed. At birth the eyes are blue or gray and change to the permanent color at about 3 to 6 months. The neonate reacts to loud or sudden sounds and wakes and sleeps without any apparent pattern. The neonate can taste and accepts sweet fluids and resists sour or bitter fluids.

BEHAVIOR EVALUATION

The evaluation of the behavior of the newborn infant has concerned many in recent years. In the first half of the twentieth century, emphasis in developmental research was on the environment's effect in shaping the child. Many researchers now feel that the individuality of the infant may be a powerful influence in shaping the relationship the infant has with his caregivers. For this reason, behavior should be evaluated as early as possible. By three months, a great deal of important interaction has already occurred, and the future patterns may already be set.

THE NEONATAL BEHAVIORAL ASSESSMENT SCALE

The behavior of the neonate is not the result of genetics alone. The intrauterine environment contributes to physiological and psychological development. The fetus in utero is influenced by such things as nutrition, infection, hormones, and drugs. Evidence is rapidly accumulating to substantiate the fact that the behavior of the newborn is **phenotypical** at birth, not **genotypical**; that is, it is a combination of heredity and environment rather than heredity alone.

Dr. T. Berry Brazelton developed an assessment scale for the propose of "obtaining more exact knowledge of the developing neurological functions as early as possible and the relationship of obstetrical complications to neurological abnormalities in later life." Designed with the help of many researchers and colleagues over a span of 20 years, the resultant psychological scale assesses the infant's capabilities that may be relevant to his social relationships. Abnormal signs that are present in the early days or weeks may disappear to be followed by the appearance of abnormal functions months or years later. Documentation of the wide span of behaviors available to the neonate may reveal some predispositions to personality development. Although the Apgar scores of the infant's responsiveness immediately after delivery have proven to have a moderate predictive value for the future outcome of the infant's central nervous system, there is a need for clinical evaluation that reflects the neonate's future social development.

New parents need guidelines for helping them evaluate the unfamiliar and unexpected situations that may arise in the course of caring for a newborn. They need reassurance that "normal" includes a variety of behaviors. This reassurance helps first-time parents to relax and enjoy caring for their baby. The nurse is in a unique position to help parents focus in on their newborn's special personality. One way to help parents understand their baby's uniqueness is to teach aspects of the **neonatal behavioral assessment scale (NBAS)**. The scale contains 27 characteristics of newborns grouped into four categories: irritability, social responsiveness, activity level and physical responsiveness, and response to stress. Every newborn scores differently. The baby's responses can reveal ways of approaching his care.

IRRITABILITY

Of the four categories of behavior on the scale, *irritability* focuses on behaviors that frequently distress new parents. Parents of the irritable, fussy baby feel helpless; their attempts to calm and console their baby are ineffective. Using scale items in this category can help determine whether the parents have a quiet calm baby, a fairly well-organized baby who gets upset only occasionally, or a very irritable baby who by nature spends a lot of time crying. The evaluation cannot assess parents' skill at consoling their baby, but it can demonstrate what personality traits the baby brings to the situation. The point is to show parents that a baby's unique behavior and responses to irritation are derived from his personality, not from their abilities as parents.

Items on the scale that determine how quickly a baby gets used to a light or a noise help evaluate how the infant controls his or her own behavior. A flashlight is shone briefly in a baby's eyes 10 times or a bell is rung 4 times. Many babies are startled by these activities at first. Then they gradually stop all eye and body movement as if they were unaware that anything is happening in their environment. Other babies seem to have no response to the bell or light at first and then are subsequently startled by it. The second type of baby may need a little assistance to help maintain calm — for example, a pat on the back for reassurance. Still other babies seem unable to tune out stimuli; in response to it, they get more and more upset. These babies need a lot of assistance from parents to calm down. It may be advisable for these babies to live in a quiet home where extra environmental stimuli are kept to a minimum.

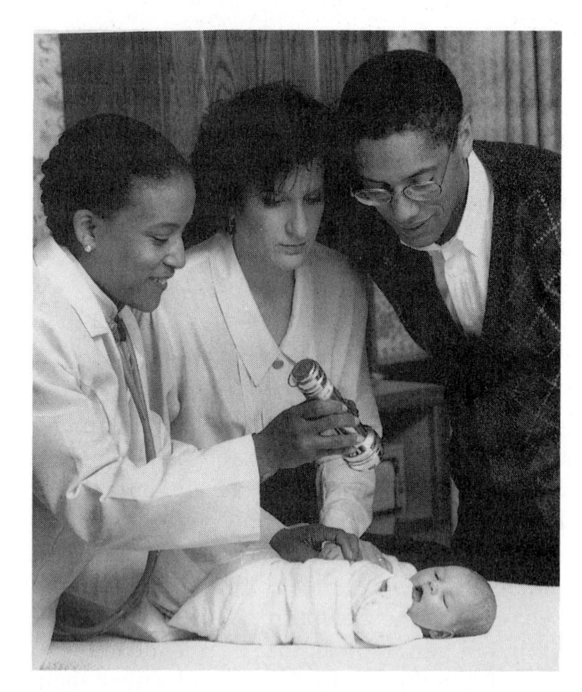

Figure 18–5 *Baby's responses are unique*

SOCIAL RESPONSIVENESS

One of the most satisfying aspects of a relationship with a baby is *social responsiveness*, Figure 18–5. The Brazelton scale gives parents a good idea of how easily they can get a social response from their baby, how long the baby sustains the response, and whether the baby prefers auditory or visual interactions with people and things.

When a shiny object, such as a ball, is moved in front of the baby's face slowly or a rattle is shaken out of sight, the baby may or may not follow the ball with his eyes or turn toward the rattle. A minimum response is for the baby to become still and alert. Sometimes parents have difficulty sustaining a response, or they stop trying. Parents can be taught to move the object more slowly and return it to the baby's line of vision, or to repeat the rattle sound. These exercises increase the opportunity for exchanges between parents and infant; they reveal how long a baby can sustain social interaction. They also increase the parents' insight into their baby's unique personality.

Consolability, another aspect of social responsiveness, is a measure of the infant's ability to calm down after fussiness. Babies quiet themselves by sucking on a fist or finger or by looking at or listening to something interesting. Consolability is particularly interesting to parents and can be assessed with the parents watching. Parents watch the crying baby for 10 seconds and slowly introduce a small amount of consolation such as talking soothingly. If this attempt is ineffective, parents can try gentle restraints, such as laying a hand on the baby's trunk or holding one or both arms. The next step is holding the baby, then rocking, then swaddling, or giving the infant a pacifier. These methods give parents a selection of strategies to quiet a baby who is fussy for no apparent reason. Some babies can calm themselves when they are fussing, but need help to stop crying. The benefit to parents is the discovery that consolability is not related to the effectiveness of their intervention, but rather to some internal process that the baby cannot yet control.

ACTIVITY LEVEL AND PHYSICAL RESPONSIVENESS

Activity level and physical responsiveness can be observed; these aspects will help parents learn whether they have an active, alert or a passive, quiet baby. Parents learn that their baby is unique and cannot be changed or molded to conform to expectations. Using information from the scale, parents may learn that their baby may be happier in a large crib rather than a small cradle. Some babies prefer to be carried facing outward and to be visually stimulated instead of being carried on a shoulder.

RESPONSE TO STRESS

The final category is *response to stress*. This category includes physical changes such as startles, tremors of the chin and limbs, and changes in skin color. Some infants rarely are startled; others are startled for no apparent reason. If the baby is easily startled and demonstrates frequent changes in skin color, parents can expect that he needs some restraint. Many parents do not know that babies normally have tremors; they mistakenly interpret them as shivers caused by cold.

The capabilities shown on the NBAS can give parents some idea of how a newborn contends with a new environment. In this way, nurses can teach parents and help influence the postnatal period. Even when the results are no longer valid, learning to observe and understand their child is a valuable parenting skill.

CARE IN THE NURSERY

In many hospitals, infants remain with their mothers 24 hours a day. Evaluation of the newborn is performed in the mother's room. In some hospitals, newborns are taken to the nursery for evaluation. The baby's temperature is taken either rectally or axillary and recorded and he is weighed and measured. Silver nitrate, erythromycin ointment, or tetracycline ointment is placed in the newborn's eyes within the first hour after birth to prevent gonococcal infection, which can cause blindness. Erythromycin is the only drug that also combats chlamydia, an infection that can also cause blindness in newborns. All of these medications may temporarily blur the baby's vision, so parents may request that the treatment be delayed for up to an hour so that they may have eye contact with their newborn. The passage of meconium and urine is recorded. The cord clamp is checked, and the baby is dressed in a shirt, diaper, and receiving blanket. The infant is placed in the Trendelenburg position in the bassinet with his head lower than his body. This position allows mucus to drain out of the nose and mouth. The crib card, in the appropriate color, is filled out and placed on the baby's bassinet. The cord clamp may be removed after 24 hours if the cord has dried.

Within a few hours after birth, the pediatrician gives the baby a complete physical examination. The examination includes the (1) head for fontanels; (2) mouth for lingual frenum (fold attaching underside of tongue to gum), precocious dentition (early eruption of teeth), cleft palate, and cleft lip; (3) heart; (4) lungs; (5) abdomen; (6) extremities; (7) genitals; and (8) anus.

The pediatrician may order an injection of vitamin K be given to the newborn. In adults, normal bacteria within the intestines help produce vitamin K. The newborn's intestines are sterile at birth and cannot contribute to the production of vitamin K needed for blood clotting.

A PKU (phenylketonuria) test is performed before the baby is discharged from the nursery. If the mother and baby are discharged from the hospital early, the mother should be instructed to return to the hospital nursery, or to her baby's physician's office for the PKU test. If taken before any source of protein has been ingested and absorbed by the baby, this test is invalid. **Phenylketonuria** results from a congenital defect in phenylalanine metabolism. It occurs in about 1 in every 10,000 births. The abnormal accumulation of phenylalanine prevents normal brain development. The diagnosis is made by a simple urine test for phenylketone bodies or blood tests for phenylalanine or both. If this condition is detected early, damage can be prevented by a special diet for the newborn (see Chapter 20).

The nurse closely observes the infant for the following and notes the results of the observation on the infant's chart.

- color: pallor (lack of color), cyanosis (bluish discoloration of the skin), jaundice (yellowish discoloration of skin)
- respirations, apical pulse
- presence of excess mucus
- condition of the cord
- passage of urine and meconium

The baby's temperature is recorded every four hours unless the doctor orders a more frequent check.

The doctor or hospital policy determines the kind of bath care the newborn receives. Usually the newborn is given a sponge bath with water and a bacteriostatic agent until the cord has fallen off. During the bath the nurse observes the infant for irritation to the eyes, skin, and umbilical cord. The nurse weighs the infant and takes his rectal or axillary temperature after the bath.

Unless contraindicated by the condition of the mother or baby, the infant is fed by the mother in her room, on demand (when he is hungry). Before taking the baby from the nursery bassinet, the nurse checks the bassinet card and Identabands. Identification of the mother and child is checked again in the mother's room. Also, if the baby is bottle feeding, the formula is checked to be sure it is the one prescribed for this particular child before the baby is taken to the mother's room for feeding. Feeding time is an excellent time for the nurse to instruct the mother in how to take care of her new baby and to answer any questions. If breast fed, the baby may be weighed before and after nursing.

CARE OF THE PREMATURE INFANT

If the baby is born three or more weeks before the calculated date of birth (less than 37 weeks gestation), it is said to be **premature** or preterm. Also, if the weight is less than 2,500 g (5½ lb) the newborn is designated premature. Weight is used to determine which babies require special care, see Figure 18–6. The behavior and appearance of the infant are also considered in reaching the diagnosis of prematurity.

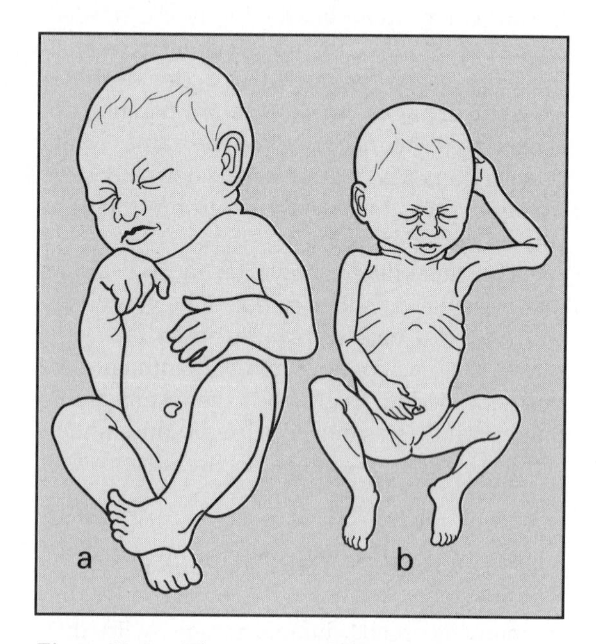

Figure 18–6 *The premature infant usually weighs under 2,500 g (5½ lb). Because he has no fat, the baby has thin arms and legs, thin cheeks and chin, a large head and large abdomen. The skin is loose and wrinkled, and the baby looks old and anxious. (a) Full-term baby. (b) Premature baby.*

Although only 7% to 10% of all live births are premature, prematurity is the most frequent cause of death in infants. Premature birth may be caused by abnormal conditions in the mother, multiple pregnancy, or induced labor. The premature infant appears listless and inactive, weighs less than 5½ lb (<2,500 g) and is less than 18 in. (45 cm) long. The fontanels are large, and the sutures (lines of closure) are quite prominent. The cry is feeble, and the sucking reflex is poor or absent. Features are sharp and angular; the skin is wrinkled because of the absence of subcutaneous fat. The skin is dull red and covered with lanugo. Respirations are shallow and irregular. Body temperature is unstable and subnormal, frequently between 34° and 36°C. (94° and 96°F). Since the blood vessels are frail, hemorrhage into the brain may occur. Many premature infants are unable to swallow and therefore require a great deal of care. An estimation of gestational age may be performed quickly in the delivery room or nursery by evaluating the infant's development by looking at the sole creases, size of the breast nodule, scalp hair, earlobe, and posture.

The survival of the premature infant depends on the skill, patience, judgment, and devotion of those giving nursing care. The basic principles to be observed in caring for the premature infant include:

- maintenance of body temperature
- protection from infection
- maintenance of airway and adequate oxygen intake
- conservation of infant's energy
- adequate fluid and calorie intake

Incubators are used to maintain the infant's body heat and to isolate the infant from sources of infection. Incubators can be regulated to control heat and humidity and to administer oxygen. Some incubators such as the Isolette have hand holes in each side, which enable the nurse to care for the infant without removing the infant from the incubator, Figure 18–7.

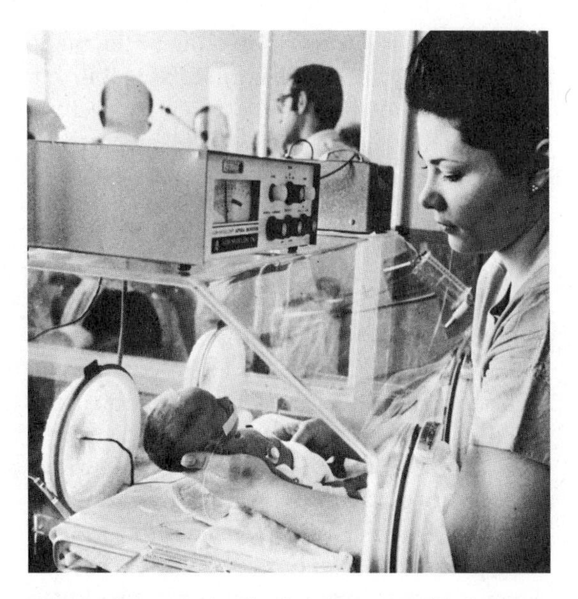

Figure 18–7 *Caring for the premature infant in the Air-Shields® Isolette® infant incubator (Courtesy Air-Shields, Inc.)*

The infant is placed in the incubator with the head of the bed lowered four to six inches to allow the mucus and secretions to drain from the throat. Suctioning equipment and oxygen should be available in case they are needed. Infants who remain in an incubator with an oxygen concentration greater than 40% for a prolonged period may develop blindness. Therefore, precautions must be taken to check the oxygen level frequently with an oxygen analyzer.

All babies weighing less than 2,500 g (5½ lb), those with cyanosis, babies having difficulty regulating body temperature, and infants who have respiratory difficulty require incubator care. In the incubator, the baby wears only a diaper; babies not in incubators are dressed in shirts and diapers and wrapped in blankets. Many babies may also wear stretchy cotton caps to prevent loss of heat from the head.

The temperature of the infant is taken every two to three hours until it has stabilized. Initially, the temperature is taken by rectum, but in smaller infants it may be taken by axilla every three hours until the weight of 2,500 g (5½ lb) is reached. As with the heavier infant, the temperature is then taken only twice a day after it has stabilized. The color, respiratory rhythm, and ease of breathing must be carefully checked at frequent intervals.

Babies weighing 1,500 g (3,165 oz) or more who can suck and swallow are fed in the usual manner with a bottle and soft nipple. Usually a 5% sugar solution is offered for four feedings on the second day of life. On the third day the baby is fed an individually calculated formula. Since premature infants are susceptible to deficiency diseases, vitamins and iron are given after the seventh day.

The infant who has no sucking or swallowing reflexes may have to be fed by **gavage** (tube feeding) or medicine dropper. The frequency and manner of feedings as well as the type and quantity of formula are prescribed by the physician.

To conserve the baby's energy, handling is kept to a minimum. The baby is left in bed for his bath, feedings, and examinations until weight increases to about 2,000 g (4 lb 7 oz). Weighing is done only twice a week unless the premature infant is in an incubator where trapeze-type scales can be used. If this is the case, the weight can be taken daily and the formula requirements calculated every 24 to 48 hours.

All personnel working in the premature nursery must be free of respiratory infections to protect the premature infant from infection. Routine checkups are given, and the use of masks may be ordered. In addition, personnel are required to wear special uniforms, scrub their hands carefully, and wear gowns when handling the premature infant.

CIRCUMCISION

Circumcision is a common minor operation in which the foreskin (prepuce) of the penis of the male baby is removed to facilitate cleaning and to prevent infection. There is no medical or legal reason for routine circumcision of the newborn; it is a matter of parental choice. Both the Jewish and Moslem people still practice circumcision as a religious rite. But for most, circumcision is a traditional choice passed from father to son. Circumcision is much less common in England, Canada, and Australia than in the United States. It is rarely performed in Asia, northern Europe, and Central and South America.

Some facts the nurse may present for consideration are:

- It is a brief procedure.
- The newborn experiences some pain because anesthetic is not used.
- Complications are rare.
- Possible complications include bleeding and irritation of the head of the penis from the friction of wet diapers, followed by pain on urination and scarring of urinary outlet.
- There is a fee.
- There is no evidence that circumcision prevents cancer of the penis or the prostate in the male or cancer of the cervix in the female partner.
- There is no evidence that circumcision or noncircumcision affects sexual performance.

There are several procedures for performing the circumcision. The method applied is decided by the attending physician. All circumcisions follow a similar procedure, Figure 18–8.

- The surgical area is cleaned.
- The foreskin is removed after a special

instrument or plastic ring is applied. There is minimal bleeding and it is easily controlled.

- Ointment and gauze may be placed over the cut to protect it from rubbing against the diaper.

The wound usually heals in two or three days. The penis is gently cleansed with a moist cotton ball at bath time. There is usually no need for additional care.

CARE OF THE INFANT AT HOME

Most new mothers are concerned about the proper skin care of the baby and the correct procedure for sterilizing the formula. These techniques may be demonstrated in the nursery before the mother and baby are discharged. This is an excellent time for the nurse to educate and support the new mother and offer outside resources for further questions or problems should they arise after discharge.

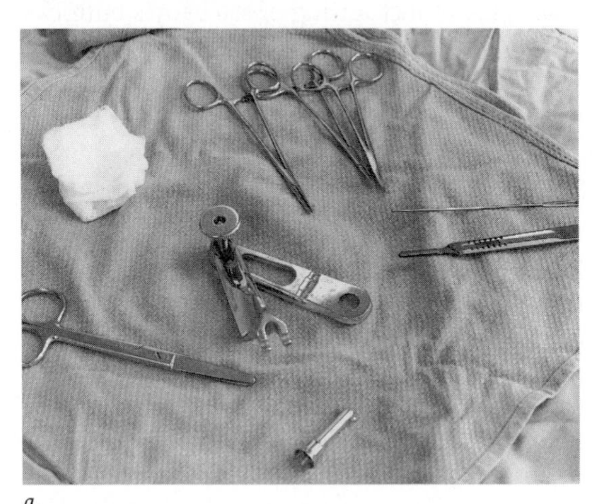

a.

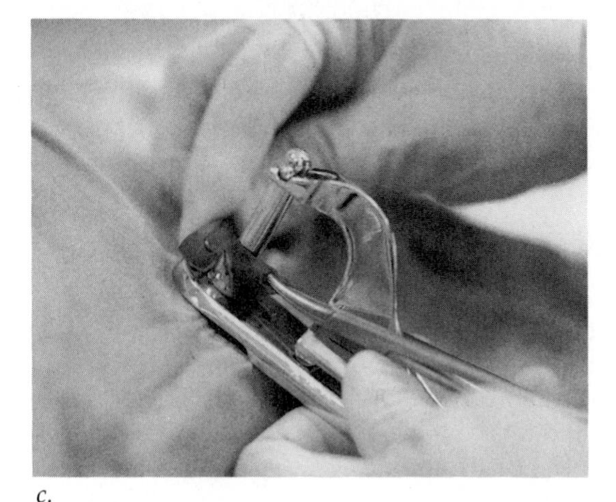

c.

b.

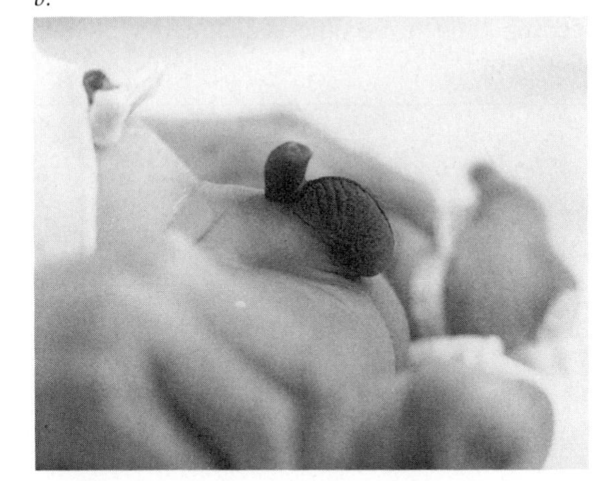

d.

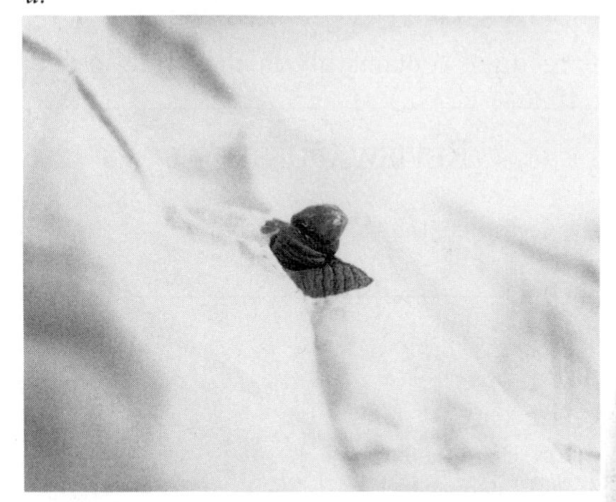

Figure 18–8 *(a) Equipment for circumcision. (b) Draped uncircumcised penis. (c) Circumcision in process. (d) The foreskin has been removed.*

BATHING THE BABY

A bath is given to the newborn with any mild castile soap, but it is recommended that a soap with cumulative antibacterial action be used. A small portable plastic tub may be used to bathe the baby. Placing a wash cloth on the inside bottom of the tub helps to prevent the baby from slipping during a tub bath. A specially designed sponge can also be obtained to offer support to the infant during the bath. The tub should be set down in a convenient place that is secure and free from slippage; a rubber bath mat may be used under the tub. The infant should be provided comfort while being bathed, and the bath experience should contribute to a loving parent-child relationship.

CARE OF THE UMBILICUS

The umbilicus should be washed off four times daily with ordinary rubbing alcohol until four days after the cord drops off. Some bleeding is common when the cord comes off. A large amount of blood or pus should be reported to the pediatrician.

DIAPER CARE

Since urine contains alkali, the urine-soaked diaper is also alkaline. Improper washing of cloth diapers does not remove all of the alkali that accumulates. Irritation to the skin can be prevented by removing the alkali with a final rinse of a vinegar and water solution. The diapers are first rinsed in cold water, then washed with a mild soap such as Ivory or pure castile soap before the solution (1 tablespoon of white vinegar to 1 quart of water) is used to remove the alkali. Many new parents use disposable diapers and discard them after they have been soiled. Careful cleansing of the baby's buttocks and genitals after each diaper change, along with the use of alkali-free diapers, prevents uncomfortable diaper rash.

TENDER LOVING CARE

Both the nurse and the mother should realize that the newborn infant reacts to the emotions of those who take care of him. The infant needs to be cuddled and loved just as he needs food, shelter, and rest. Understanding that the newborn reacts emotionally to people and situations is one reason that infants are fed on demand rather than on a rigid schedule. The mother should take advantage of bathing and feeding time to become acquainted with her new baby.

REVIEW QUESTIONS

A. Complete the following chart.

	Full-Term Newborn	**Premature Infant**
Size		
Cry		
Body shape		
Reflexes		
Skin tone		
Skin coating		

B. Multiple choice. Select the best answer.

1. When the newborn is admitted to the nursery, he is
   a. given a tub bath
   b. placed in the Trendelenburg position and weighed and measured
   c. given 2 oz of fluid
   d. administered the NBAS

2. Standard nursing care for the premature infant includes
   a. placement in an incubator with frequent checks of color and respiration
   b. minimal handling of the infant
   c. supplementary vitamins and iron
   d. all of the above

3. Some facts a nurse may present to parents regarding circumcision include the following *except*
   a. it is a brief procedure
   b. the newborn will not experience pain
   c. there is no evidence that circumcision prevents cancer
   d. complications are rare

4. A newborn is considered premature if he weighs less than
   a. 3,000 g
   b. 2,500 g
   c. 2,000 g
   d. 4,000 g

5. When a baby's back is stroked on one side while the baby is lying on his stomach, the whole trunk curves toward that side. This reaction is called
   a. tonic neck reflex
   b. Moro reflex
   c. placing reaction
   d. Galant reaction

6. The rooting reflex is present for
   a. the first six months
   b. the first two months
   c. as long as the baby is nursing
   d. the first year

7. The anterior fontanel usually closes by
   a. 6 months
   b. 12 months
   c. 24 months
   d. 18 months

8. Frequently the pediatrician orders the newborn be given an injection of vitamin K. Vitamin K aids in
   a. blood clotting
   b. preventing jaundice
   c. preventing the formation of phenylalanine
   d. iron absorption

SUGGESTED ACTIVITIES

- Describe the ways a premature infant differs from a full-term infant and how nursing care would differ.
- Describe the ways the nurse can use the Brazelton neonatal behavioral assessment scale to help the parents recognize the uniqueness of their newborn.
- List all the newborn reflexes, their function, and when each reflex is likely to disappear.

BIBLIOGRAPHY

Brazelton, T. Berry, W. B. Parker, and B. Zuckerman. "Importance of Behavioral Assessment of the Neonate." *Current Problems in Pediatrics* 7(2):1–82, December, 1976.

Cook, N., and P. Periz. "Brazelton Scale." *Childbirth Educator* 4(4):31–35, 1985.

Lesner, P. *Pediatric Nursing*, 2nd ed. Albany, NY: Delmar Publishers, 1985.

OGN Nursing Practice Resource, "Physical Assessment of the Neonate." *NAACOG*, October, 1986.

Plante, D., and B. Stiles. "Expanding the Nurse's Role through Formal Assessment of the Neonate." *JOGNN* 13(1):25–29, January-February, 1984.

Simkin, P., Whalley, J., and A. Keppler. *Pregnancy, Childbirth and the Newborn*. Deephaven, MN: Meadowbrook Books, 1991.

CHAPTER

19

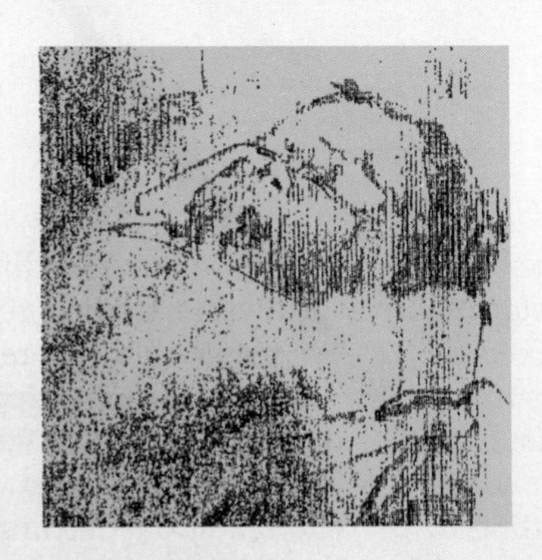

Feeding the Newborn

OBJECTIVES

AFTER STUDYING THIS CHAPTER, THE STUDENT SHOULD BE ABLE TO:

- DISCUSS THE PHYSIOLOGY OF BREAST FEEDING.
- LIST COMMON BREAST-FEEDING PROBLEMS AND NURSING INTERVENTIONS.
- UNDERSTAND THE DIFFERENCES BETWEEN BREAST FEEDING AND BOTTLE FEEDING.
- STATE THE PURPOSE OF GAVAGE FEEDING.

KEY TERMS

DEMAND FEEDING
PROLACTIN
COLOSTRUM
ALVEOLI
LET-DOWN REFLEX
HINDMILK
FOREMILK
MASTITIS
WEANING
GAVAGE FEEDING
LACT-AID

Successful infant feeding requires cooperation between the mother and her baby, starting with the initial feeding experience. Feeding time should be a pleasant and pleasurable period for both mother and infant. Maternal feelings are readily transmitted to the baby and largely determine the emotional setting in which feeding takes place. If a mother is tense, anxious, irritable, or easily upset, she is likely to experience difficulty in the feeding relationship. If she establishes a comfortable, satisfying feeding practice, this will contribute to the infant's emotional well-being. Figure 19–1 presents ways to promote breast feeding.

The emptying time of the infant's stomach may vary from 1 to 4 or more hours. Therefore, there may be considerable differences in the desire for food at different times of the day. Ideally the feeding schedule should be based on reasonable self-regulation by the infant. This approach is called **demand feeding**. Most healthy infants will want from 8 to 18 feedings in a 24-hour period. The majority will take enough at one feeding to satisfy them for one to three hours. Smaller babies, with more rapid gastric emptying, will want milk more frequently than larger birth weight babies. Babies do not necessarily eat on a regular schedule. Sometimes they will nurse four or five times in five to six hours and then sleep for a long stretch of time. It is important to encourage frequent daytime feedings if the baby sleeps for long periods during the night to ensure adequate nourishment.

PROMOTION OF BREAST FEEDING

1. Primary-care settings for women of childbearing age should have:
   - a supportive milieu for lactation
   - educational opportunities (including availability of literature, personal counseling, and information about community resources) for learning about lactation and its advantages
   - ready response to requests for further information
   - continuity allowing for the exposure to and development over time of a positive attitude regarding lactation on the part of the recipient of care.
2. Prenatal-care settings should have:
   - a specific assessment at the first prenatal visit of the physical capability and emotional predisposition to lactation. This assessment should include the potential role of the father of the child as well as other significant family members. An educational program about the advantages of and ways of preparing for lactation should continue throughout the pregnancy.
   - resource personnel — such as nutritionists, dietitians, social workers, public health nurses, La Leche League members, childbirth education groups — for assistance in preparing for lactation
   - availability and utilization of culturally suitable patient-education materials

Figure 19–1 (*From* Report of the Surgeon General's Workshop on Breastfeeding and Lactation, *presented by U.S. Department of Health and Human Services, 1984)*

PROMOTION OF BREAST FEEDING

- an established mechanism for a predelivery visit to the newborn care provider to ensure initiation and maintenance of lactation
- a means of communicating to the in-hospital team the infant feeding plans developed during the prenatal course.

3. In-hospital settings should have:
   - a policy to determine the patient's infant-feeding plan on admission or during labor
   - a family-centered orientation to childbirth including the minimum use of intrapartum medications and anesthesia
   - a medical and nursing staff informed about and supportive of ways to facilitate the initiation and continuation of breast feeding (including early mother-infant contact and ready access by the mother to her baby throughout the hospital stay)
   - the availability of individualized counseling and education by a specially trained breast-feeding coordinator to facilitate lactation for those planning to breast feed and to counsel those who have not yet decided about their method of infant feeding
   - ongoing in-service education about lactation and ways to support it. This program should be conducted by the breast-feeding coordinator for all relevant hospital staff.
   - proper space and equipment for breast feeding in the postpartum and neonatal units. Attention should be given to the particular needs of women breast feeding babies with special problems.
   - the elimination of hospital practices/policies which have the effect of inhibiting the lactation process, e.g., rules separating mother and baby
   - the elimination of standing orders that inhibit lactation, e.g., lactation suppressants, fixed feeding schedules, maternal medications
   - discharge planning which includes referral to community agencies to aid in the continuing support of the lactating mother. This referral is especially important for patients discharged early.
   - a policy to limit the distribution of packages of free formula at discharge only to those mothers who are not lactating
   - the development of policies to support lactation throughout the hospital units (e.g., medicine, surgery, pediatrics, emergency room, etc.)
   - the provision of continued lactation support for those infants who must remain in the hospital after the mother's discharge.

4. Postpartum ambulatory settings should have:
   - a capacity for telephone assistance to mothers experiencing problems with breast feeding
   - a policy for telephone follow-up 1–3 days after discharge
   - a plan for an early follow-up visit (within first week after discharge)
   - the availability of lactation counseling as a means of preventing or solving lactation problems
   - access to lay support resources for the mother
   - the presence of a supportive attitude by all staff
   - a policy to encourage bringing the infant to postpartum appointments
   - the availability of public/community-health nurse referral for those having problems with lactation
   - a mechanism for the smooth transition to pediatric care of the infant, including good communication between obstetric and pediatric care providers.

Figure 19–1 *continued*

At around 3 weeks, 6 weeks, and again at 3 months and 6 months, the baby may suddenly change his eating schedule to more frequent intervals. The baby may be fretful, irritable, and more sensitive to stimuli. He is probably experiencing a growth spurt and is stimulating the breasts to produce more milk to meet his increasing needs.

It is important to establish that the infant may cry for reasons other than hunger and that he need not be fed every time he cries. Other reasons for an infant's distress may include: too much clothing; soiled, wet, or uncomfortable diapers and clothing; colic; swallowed air; uncomfortably hot or cold environment; and illness. Some babies will cry for additional attention. Babies who stop crying when they are picked up or held do not usually need food. The habit of offering frequent, small feedings to pacify all crying should not be encouraged.

The postpartum period is often a time of great anxiety and insecurity for the new mother. She may feel temporarily overwhelmed by the responsibilities of motherhood. It is important that the nurse in the hospital setting be comforting and supportive while the mother finds and develops confidence in her maternal abilities.

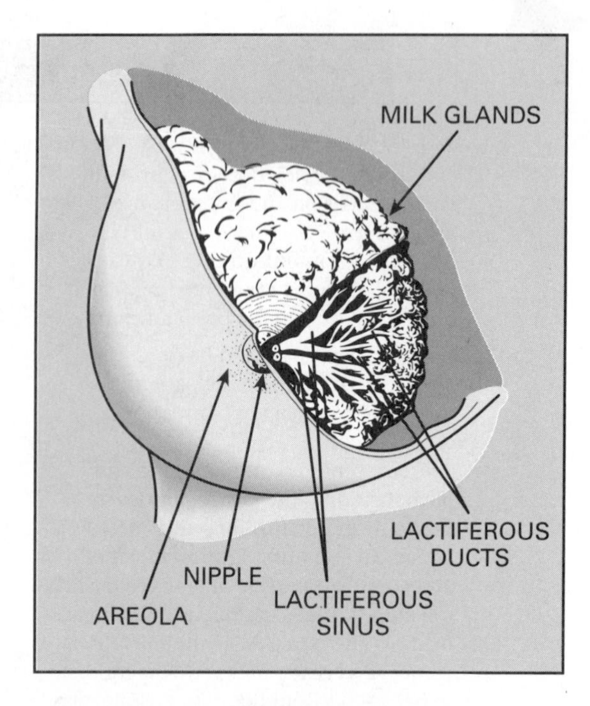

Figure 19–2 *Schematic drawing of the female breast*

BREAST FEEDING

Although milk is present in the breasts from the fifth or sixth month of pregnancy, high levels of hormones (progesterone and estrogen) prevent the milk from being released during the gestation period. At delivery, the levels of these hormones suddenly drop. This action triggers the production of large amounts of prolactin by the pituitary gland. The hormone **prolactin** is responsible for stimulating the mammary glands to produce milk.

During pregnancy and the first few days after delivery (before the milk is secreted) the breasts release colostrum. **Colostrum** is a thin, yellowish fluid composed chiefly of white blood cells and serum from the mother's blood. It is rich in antibodies, salt, protein, and fat. Colostrum also has a laxative effect and helps the newborn to expel the thick meconium in the neonate's intestinal tract.

About the third day after delivery, the breasts become warm, tender, and engorged with blood and lymph. The **alveoli** are lobules in the breast that contain milk-producing cells. They begin to function as a result of the prolactin, and a bluish-white milk replaces colostrum.

The success of giving an adequate supply of milk depends on the **let-down reflex**, a release of milk from the alveoli. As the infant sucks, the posterior pituitary releases oxytocin into the mother's system, causing the alveoli to contract. The milk flows into the main sinuses under the nipple and is released from the ducts in the nipple and areola of the breast. Although breast feeding is a natural function, a positive and confident attitude is all-important to its success. The mother must be calm and relaxed while nursing or the let-down reflex will be inhibited. Fear, pain, or other stresses release adrenalin through the body, causing blood vessels to constrict; constricted blood vessels prevent the hormone oxytocin from reaching the alveoli. (Oxytocin release may cause afterpains for a few minutes after nursing begins.) The nursing mother may either sit or lie on her side in a comfortable position while nursing. The baby can be stimulated to take the nipple and areola into his mouth by tickling the lip with the nipple. Proper positioning of the baby is essential to successful breast feeding, Figure 19–3. The arm supporting the baby should be under the baby's buttocks. The infant should be elevated to the height of the breast and then turned completely to face the mother, with abdomens touching. The other hand should support the breast with the thumb above and index finger below and behind the areola, compressing it to make the nipple thrust out. The milk reservoirs are directly behind the nipple, and they must be compressed by the baby's gums in order to release the milk. The mother should be sure the baby's nasal passage is not obstructed by breast tissue so that the baby can breathe easily while nursing. The nose, however, can be touching the breast without causing obstruction. To break suction when feeding is finished, the mother places her finger at the corner of the infant's mouth before removing the baby from the breast. The baby should not be pulled away from one breast so that he can nurse from the other. He will probably nurse at least 10 to 15 minutes. When the baby takes a rest, the mother can alternate breasts.

Both breasts should be offered at each feeding, as emptying the breasts stimulates milk production and prevents engorgement. The length of time the infant nurses varies widely from feeding to feeding and from infant to infant. Once a woman's milk supply is well established, a baby probably gets most of the milk from a breast in the first 10 minutes. A woman may want to allow the infant this amount of time on the first breast and let the baby nurse on the second breast as long as desired. Infants continue to derive pleasure from the sucking and contact with their mothers long after their hunger has been satisfied. Twenty to forty minutes overall is a good guideline if a mother wants to be sure her baby is getting enough milk.

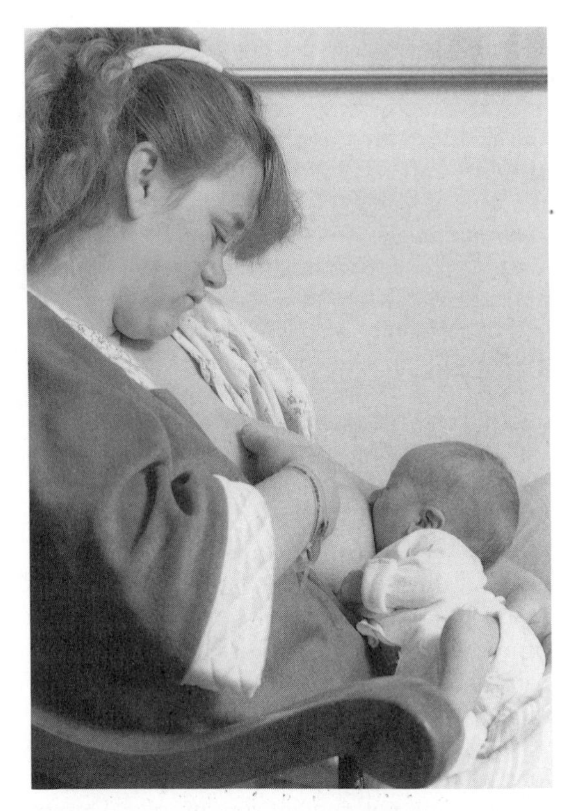

Figure 19–3 *Proper positioning adds to the success of breast feeding.*

There are numerous ways to know if the baby is getting enough milk. A baby who feeds well every two hours or so for 20 to 40 minutes with occasional shorter or longer periods between feedings will have 6 to 8 wet diapers a day. Some babies will have a loose stool with each feeding or three or more stools a day for the first month of life. The baby's elimination patterns and level of contentment after being fed are good indications that the baby is receiving adequate nourishment. An expected weight gain monitored by the pediatrician is another way to evaluate adequate intake.

Occasionally, a baby will prefer one breast, perhaps because the baby is more comfortable on that side or because the milk flows more readily. The mother may try feeding first on the side the baby likes best so that the milk flows readily from the other breast when the baby uses it. She also can feed the baby at the second breast without changing the baby's position (by just moving the baby over). The mother may have to express the milk by hand from the nonpreferred breast for a while. The baby should begin to accept both breasts if the mother keeps trying.

It is advisable to allow the baby to nurse as long as he wishes. Limiting feeding time, even initially, will not prevent sore nipples. During the first feedings after birth, the let-down reflex may not occur for three to five minutes after feeding begins. Researchers have found that limiting the amount of time the infant is at the breast does not affect the incidence of nipple soreness. The most critical factor in nipple soreness is how the baby latches on to the nipple. If the baby's mouth is properly positioned, soreness is rarely a serious problem. Restrictive schedules can delay milk coming in as a result of decreased nipple stimulation. Also, short feedings can prolong the engorgement period. Prolonged engorgement increases the likelihood of nipple trauma, if the baby has trouble latching on to overfull breasts. Once the milk-producing cells have begun to function, sucking and regular emptying of ducts in both breasts keep them producing milk for months or even years. The amount of milk produced is on a supply-and-demand system. The lactating cells of the alveoli replenish and produce the amount of milk the baby is demanding as it sucks and empties the ducts. To ensure an adequate supply of milk and to prevent the possibility of engorgement, the mother should empty both breasts regularly. The last breast offered at a feeding should be the first breast given at the next feeding. The milk in the second breast is a mixture of hindmilk and foremilk and is of much higher caloric value than the milk in the first. **Hindmilk** is stored in the alveoli and milk-producing cells of the breast. **Foremilk** is stored under the nipple and is not as rich in fats and calories.

Burping releases the air that may have been swallowed during the feeding. The baby should be burped frequently if on the breast, or burped every half-ounce if on the bottle. Otherwise, the baby will be uncomfortable and may burp spontaneously, regurgitating the entire feeding. Two methods of burping are shown in Figure 19–4.

A mother may be uncertain about whether to wake her baby to feed him. If it has been longer than four hours since the last feeding or her breasts are full and uncomfortable, it is perfectly all right to wake the baby. Some mothers wake their babies to feed if they are trying to establish a more regular feeding schedule, especially if there is a pattern of long naps during the day and frequent feedings at night.

The gastric emptying time of infants fed breast milk is often faster than that of formula-fed babies and ranges from one to four hours, so frequent feedings of breast-fed infants are warranted. The breast-feeding mother ideally uses the demand or unrestricted feeding schedule, offering her breast whenever her baby seems hungry, regardless of how long it has been since the last feeding. Frequent demand feeding is important to establish and maintain a woman's milk supply.

Milk contains large amounts of water. Therefore, it is not necessary to give young infants additional water to drink. There is no harm in giving babies an occasional bottle of cooled boiled water to drink for comfort, particularly if they are crying between feedings, but it should not be given regularly. It should be noted, however, that offering a bottle or pacifier in the early weeks may cause nipple confusion and the baby may not nurse as well.

The nursing mother's diet has a direct effect on the quantity and quality of her milk and, therefore, should be closely supervised. An increase to two to three quarts of fluid a day is also recommended. The amount of food and number of calories needed each day depend on a variety of factors. If a woman is active and has a large baby who nurses frequently, she may need to consume more calories to maintain her weight. If a woman is less active or is supplementing with formula, she may not need extra calories. It is best to eat a diet similar to that recommended during pregnancy and let weight be the guide for calorie intake. The nursing mother should be counseled about taking any medication, as some drugs cross into the milk supply. For example, some laxatives taken by the mother can produce loose stools in the baby. Certain foods also have a tendency to enter the milk supply;

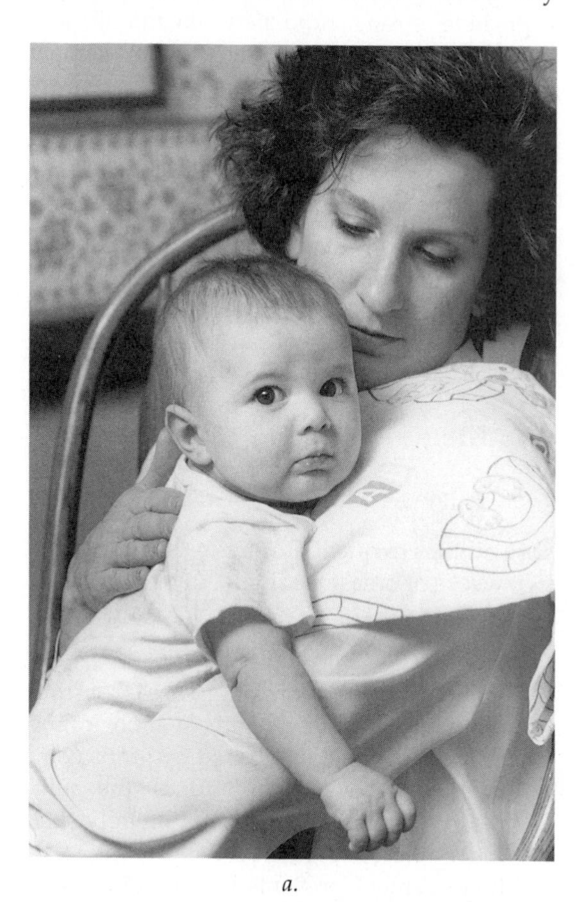

a.

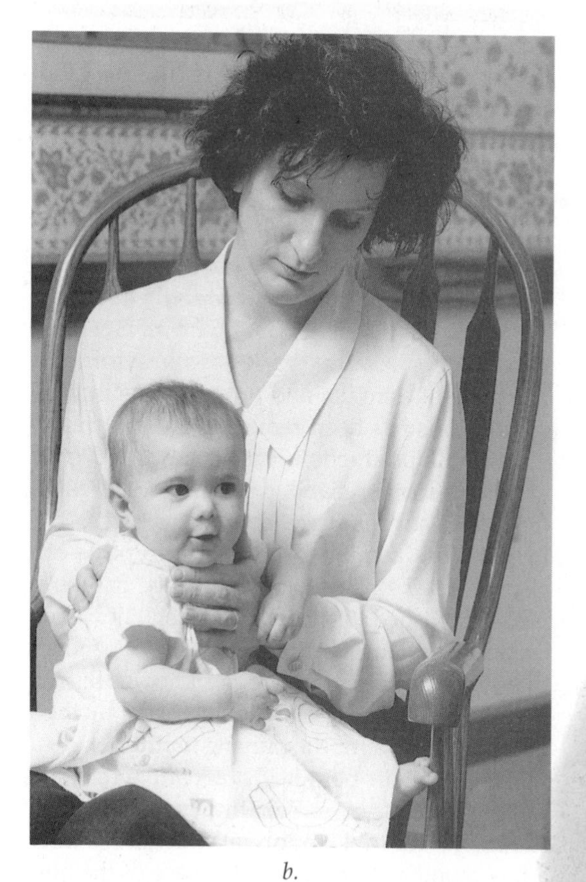

b.

Figure 19–4 *Burping a baby. (a) Hold baby so her chin rests against covered shoulder. Gently stroke her back. (b) Hold baby upright, leaning slightly forward. Support her head and chest with one hand and stroke her back with the other hand.*

heavily spiced foods, eggs, cola, chocolate, caffeine, citrus fruits, broccoli, cabbage, and tomatoes can adversely affect some babies. Occasionally, milk and milk products consumed by the mother may cause an adverse reaction in the infant. Eliminating these foods and gradually reintroducing them back into the mother's diet will tell her what foods may adversely affect her baby.

Some drugs can cause breast-feeding problems too. Vitamin B_6, when taken in doses over the daily FDA recommended amount of 2.1 mg, can inhibit lactation in sensitive women. The alcohol content in breast milk is approximately equal to the concentration of alcohol in the blood. Too much alcohol can inhibit the let-down reflex and reduce the hindmilk rich in calories. Heavy smoking will reduce milk production and vitamin C concentration in milk and may produce colic and diarrhea in the infant. Smoking near the baby will increase the risk of pneumonia and bronchitis in the baby. Cocaine use during lactation will affect the baby at least as profoundly as it does the adult. It is also associated with an increased incidence of sudden infant death syndrome. The level of estrogen and progesterone in birth control pills has been reduced so that it rarely affects milk production. The progestin-only pill or minipill is a reliable contraceptive method that does not influence the milk supply. The lowest dose combined oral contraceptive can also be used once the milk supply has been well established. Concern still exists, however, because the long-term effects these hormones may have on the infant are not known. Barrier methods are still the most widely used method of contraception for the nursing mother.

If a woman becomes pregnant while still breast feeding, she can continue to breast feed the baby. Her milk supply may diminish after a few months of pregnancy because of the hormones produced during gestation. The quality of milk, however, is not diminished, and a pregnancy does not mean that a mother must wean her infant. It is possible to continue breast feeding during pregnancy right through to delivery and relactation. It does place additional emotional and physical demands on the mother. Especially demanding are the nutritional requirements of pregnancy and lactation together. For example, a woman would need 800 mg of calcium above her maintenance needs, as well as additional quantities of other essential nutrients to continue to breast feed while she is pregnant.

Breast feeding can be a positive, rewarding experience for both mother and baby. The closeness, both physical and emotional, begins a positive, strong bond between mother and baby. Good instruction and encouragement from the nurse in the beginning can help make breast feeding a successful experience. In addition, mother's milk is allergen-free, the right temperature, and always available. If the nurse can assist the new mother through any breast-feeding problems she may encounter early in her experience, the mother will more likely choose to breast feed for an extended period of time with a high sense of satisfaction.

BREAST-FEEDING PROBLEMS

SORE NIPPLES

Sore nipples frequently occur in the first one to two weeks of breast feeding.

Causes:

- Infant is not properly put to breast; latches on to nipple instead of areola at beginning of feeding. Milk is obtained by gums compressing; the tongue strokes the milk reservoirs; the baby does not literally suck the nipple, see Figure 19–5.
- Engorgement prevents infant from grasping areola because of breast fullness caused by infrequent feedings or restricted nursing time.

- No variation in feeding positions; gums and tongue pressures are not distributed around entire nipple and areola surface.
- Slow let-down reflex; the infant nurses vigorously in an attempt to get milk.
- Frequent use of plastic-lined disposable breast pads; they retain moisture and delay the healing process.
- Improper technique in removing infant from breast; the suction is not broken; skin is stretched and traumatized as the infant tries to maintain a hold.
- Short, flat nipple; difficult for infant to latch on to breast, especially if engorgement is present.

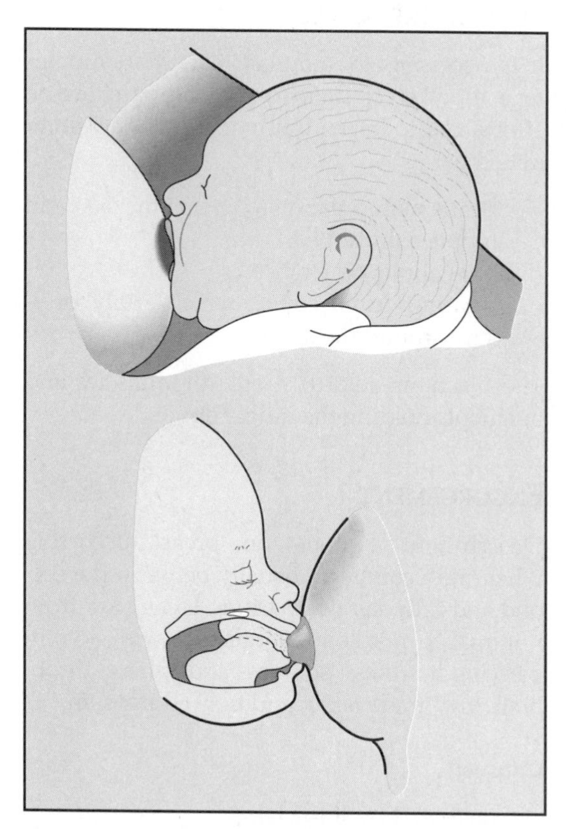

Figure 19–5 *Proper position of infant's mouth on breast (Courtesy Ross Laboratories)*

Fallacy: Limiting the time at the breast is the best way to prevent sore nipple.

Fact: The converse is true. Many women do not get an adequate let-down in a short period of time; the infant may nurse more vigorously, pull away, and make more frequent latching-on efforts. Limiting sucking time and slow let-down can aggravate engorgement, which further contributes to sore nipples.

Description: Amount of soreness may vary from slight to erosions and scabbing. Ongoing assessment should guide management.

Nursing Intervention:

- Facilitate proper latching-on techniques by guiding the mother in shaping the nipple and waiting until the baby's mouth is open enough to take hold of the areola. This technique decreases unproductive pressure and friction on the nipple.
- Assist mother to relax and thus enhance a quicker let-down. Infants can more quickly receive available milk and will satisfy hunger in less nursing time.
- Break suction before removing baby from breast by inserting little finger into corner of the mouth and between gums or by pulling down on the infant's chin. Breaking suction will decrease trauma to the nipple.
- Nurse more often but for shorter time periods if the nipple tissue is damaged and sore. Ten minutes each breast every 1 to 2 hours is better for nipple integrity and milk production than 30 minutes of each breast every 3 to 4 hours. This schedule will be less traumatic to nipples and more effective stimulation for milk production.
- Air-dry nipples after each feeding for 15 to 20 minutes; leave bra flaps down between feedings when possible. Use breast shields

without plastic liners. Exposure to air hastens healing; gentle friction with clothing will hasten toughening.

- Apply a small ice pack to the sore area for five minutes before feeding to provide some pain relief as the baby latches on.
- Rotate nursing positions (after mother has comfortably mastered one position); may want to practice at nonfeeding times. Using different positions will distribute pressure points around the entire areolar and nipple surfaces.
- Determine where the sore spots are to select the best alternative feeding position. Think of the areola as a clock face; if sore spots are at 2 and 8, select a position that will put the tongue and gum pressure at 10 and 4.
- Offer the least sore nipple first. The least affected breast is better able to handle vigorous sucking activity that occurs at the start of a feeding.
- Decrease sucking time on very sore nipples for a day (10 minutes or less); complete breast emptying by hand or pump expression. Efforts to promote healing by preventing milk stasis and to encourage milk production may have to be balanced.
- When the baby has finished with active, vigorous sucking activity, remove the infant from the breast. The infant should not be allowed to meet all emotional sucking needs when nipples are sore.
- Apply warm, moistened tea bags to nipple, before air drying, for approximately 10 to 15 minutes. (Use real tea, not herbal varieties.) Tannic acid has been found to help toughen nipples and promote healing.
- Heat-lamp treatment; have mother position herself approximately 16 to 20 in. away from an exposed 60-watt bulb for about 10 minutes. May need one to three treatments a day. Heat promotes healing, increases blood supply, brings oxygen, and carries away dead cells.
- Last-ditch measure; discontinue breast feeding for a day. Hand or pump express and give milk in a bottle. (Use a cylinder pump or electric pump — avoid the "bicycle-horn" pump.) Use this extreme measure only for bad cases of fissuring, erosion, large scab formation, and extreme pain.
- Have mother check infant's mouth for white patches that will not rub off. Infants may have a thrush infection, which can infect mother's skin, causing soreness. It can also cause sharp, deep nipple pain that continues between feedings. Consult with physician if patches are present; mother and infant both need treatment.

FLAT, SHORT NIPPLES

It is necessary to stimulate flat, short nipples to a more erect state to facilitate latching-on efforts and to lessen trauma. Nipples are stimulated by:

- gentle manipulation to stretch the skin and nipple, Figure 19–6
- brief application of ice
- wearing "milk cups," which apply pressure around the areola

These actions help to stretch the muscles and ligaments holding the nipple down.

ENGORGEMENT

Description: Fullness in breast occurring when milk comes in, usually between the second and fifth day postpartum. It can vary from minimal to marked enlargement with accompanying hardness, soreness and aching, throbbing, low-grade fever, and tight, shiny skin.

Causes:

- increased fluid in breast
- increased vascular and lymph supply
- increased interstitial fluid

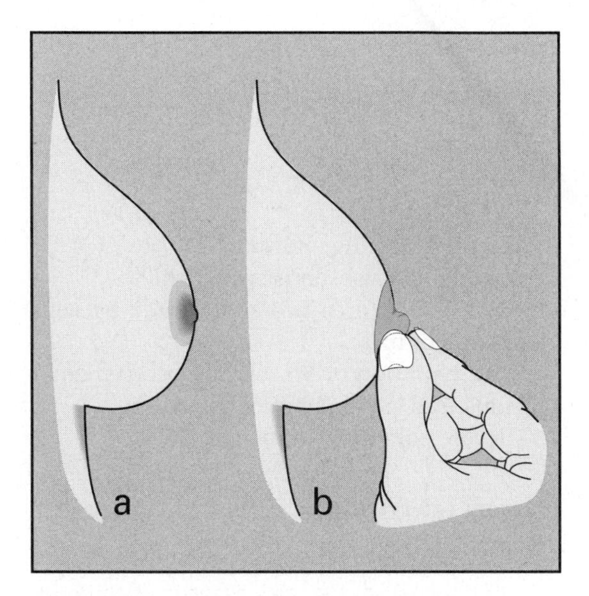

Figure 19–6 (a) Retracted nipple. (b) Prepare for breast feeding by exercising.

- increased pressure from newly produced milk

Nursing Intervention:

- Make sure that the mother knows that the acute phase of this problem will last 24 to 48 hours. Knowing that the problem is short-term is helpful to mothers. Engorgement dissipates as the milk supply and the baby's demand come into balance.
- The main goal in management is to prevent or minimize the degree of engorgement to spare the mother any unnecessary discomfort, to decrease the risk of plugged ducts, mastitis, and sore nipples, and to facilitate the infant's latching-on efforts.
- Management guidelines include shorter, more frequent nursing sessions around the clock as fullness begins to develop. Feeding approximately every 2 to 3 hours during the day and every 3 to 4 hours at night is suggested. Frequent emptying helps to prevent the breasts from becoming overfull. Night feedings are important.

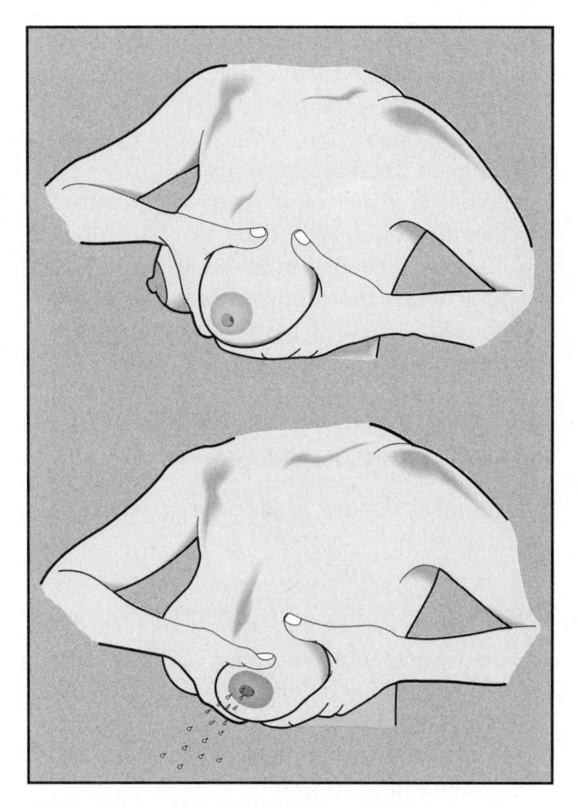

Figure 19–7 Massage the breast with downward strokes to manually express milk.

- Advise the mother to take a warm shower, or apply warm, wet towels to breast before nursing. Warmth may stimulate a spontaneous let-down reflex with a subsequent reduction in breast tension.
- Have the mother gently hand express milk to soften the areola before nursing, with or without warm, moist compresses, Figure 19–7. The infant is better able to latch on to the areola if it is softer and shapeable and there will be less trauma to the nipples. Also, sore nipples can inhibit a let-down, resulting in incomplete emptying, which aggravates engorgement.
- Ice packs may be applied after and between feedings. Cold will cause vasoconstriction and decrease breast tension.

- A properly fitted bra is advisable. It will offer support to overfull, heavy breasts. The bra must be big enough so as not to cause constriction, which could lead to plugged ducts and mastitis.
- Avoid the use of glucose water supplements. These will decrease the infant's hunger or interest in frequent nursing at a time when the mother needs the infant's emptying help. It may also interfere with the infant's imprinting on the breast.

PLUGGED DUCTS IN BREASTS

Symptoms: Tender and/or red areas on breast.

Causes:

- Inadequate milk emptying; stasis of milk
- Going too long between feedings
- Wearing a bra that is too tight; a tight bra causes pressure points or constriction of portions of the breast

Nursing Intervention:

- Advise mother to feel for full or tender areas in the breast by using a circular motion. Follow with gentle stroking action in the direction of the nipple. Early identification and management of plugged ducts will decrease the possibility of developing mastitis. To encourage milk flow, unplug involved ducts.
- Apply a warm, wet towel or small hot-water bottle to area. Warmth will enhance let-down reflex and emptying efforts. Increased circulation will aid in removal of dead cells and destruction of bacteria.
- Changing feeding positions will enhance emptying in affected areas by rotating the compression forces in the infant's tongue and gums.
- Nurse frequently.

MASTITIS

Mastitis is a generalized soft-tissue infection of the breast.

Symptoms:

- Flu-like feeling, fever (101° to 104°F), aching, malaise, nausea, and chills
- Red, tender area not as localized as with plugged duct
- Large portion of breast may be erythematous, and streaking may be present
- Severe pain may occur

Nursing Intervention:

- Consult with the physician when the above symptoms are present. Antibiotic therapy is indicated. Neglect can lead to formation of necrosis and breast abscesses.
- Advise the mother to continue nursing on the affected side; increase frequency of feeding to twice the number of usual feedings. Breast milk offers immunological help to infant to deal with the involved organism; high acid content of the stomach will assist in destruction of the offending organism.
- Allowing for pain threshold, suggest that the affected breast be offered first to maximize emptying with the infant's most vigorous sucking efforts. A mild analgesic 30 minutes before nursing may be helpful.
- Advise mother to apply hot, wet compresses, followed by massage and hand expression. Warmth will increase circulation to the breast, resulting in more oxygen, increasing white blood cell and enzyme activity to destroy bacteria and dead cells.
- An alternative approach is to use ice packs for 20 minutes or more. Pain may be lessened with initial vasoconstriction, decreasing tension in the affected area. Prolonged application of ice will cause vasodilation with the same benefit as heat therapy.

- Bed rest and increased fluids are advised to facilitate the body's healing efforts.
- Alternate feeding positions to facilitate emptying of all portions of the breast.
- Nurse the infant more frequently. Frequent emptying prevents further or recurrent milk stasis.
- Remove caked secretions on the nipple by soaking before nursing. Removing caked secretions will enhance nipple-duct patency, and soaking will soften scabs, allowing milk to flow more easily through softened covering.

INADEQUATE MILK SUPPLY

Description: When the infant fails to gain weight with breast feeding, or seems fussy, frustrated, and hungry after an adequate period of time at the breast, an inadequate milk supply may be the cause.

Nursing Intervention:

- Offer both breasts at every feeding. Adequate emptying of both breasts at each feeding will encourage increased milk production.
- Avoid supplementing or holding baby off. Because the breasts function on a supply-and-demand basis, the more the infant demands, the more the breasts will be stimulated to produce.
- Allow the baby to nurse as long as he is interested. Prolonged sucking, as long as the nipples are not becoming sore or irritated, will encourage increased milk production.
- Recognize growth spurts with increased need to nurse. These usually occur at around 3 weeks, 6 weeks, 3 months, and 6 months.
- Drink sufficient liquid (6–8 glasses daily); eat a good diet. Good nutrition is essential for an adequate milk supply.
- Get plenty of rest and avoid exhaustion. Extreme exhaustion will affect the let-down reflex as well as the quantity of milk produced.
- Recognize that the breasts, even while breast feeding, eventually return to a more normal size.
- Breast feed 10–12 times a day in the early weeks. Increased stimulation of the breasts will help to build milk supply.
- Learn proper technique for hand expression or use of the breast pump. Expressing milk will help keep the milk supply adequate if, for some reason, the infant cannot nurse well.

FUSSY BABY

Description: If the infant seems fussy for no apparent reason, it should not be assumed that the baby is not getting an adequate amount to eat. There are numerous reasons for a fussy baby.

Nursing Intervention:

- Help the parents to understand the various reasons for infant crying.
- Be aware that most babies normally have a fussy period (common time 1–11 P.M.). Hold and rock the baby. It is fine to offer the breast to sooth the infant as long as the nipples are not too sore.
- Understand infant's need for closeness and contact. Baby carriers are helpful.
- Be aware that breast-fed babies nurse more often than bottle-fed babies.
- Observe for possible illness in baby.
- Baby can sense if mother is overworked or underrested.
- Demand feeding works best. Because breast milk is easily digested, baby may need more frequent nursing.
- Evaluate mother's diet and eliminate possible allergens or foods that may produce gas (chocolate, cabbage, possibly cow's milk).

- Parent's emotional stress or crisis may affect baby's mood.
- Hold the baby frequently; offer various forms of stimulation.
- Decrease coffee and cola intake to decrease caffeine stimulation.
- Avoid bathing the baby while he is fussy.
- Burp the baby frequently during feeding to avoid gas pain.
- Allow the baby to nurse as long as swallowing is heard.
- Baby may be fussy during menstrual period. With total breast feeding, menses usually does not resume before four months. Milk production may be lessened due to hormones.

CESAREAN DELIVERY

Breast feeding is just as desirable after a cesarean delivery as after any other delivery. If the mother has had a general anesthetic, or if her hospital is one that routinely places all babies born by cesarean delivery in a special-care nursery for 12 to 24 hours, she may need to wait until the baby's second day of life to begin breast feeding. Although intravenous fluids and other equipment may decrease the mother's mobility, the baby can be put to the breast with the help of the nurse. Postoperative medication should not pose a problem. Even if the mother must wait two or three days, she can start and maintain her milk supply by expressing milk or by using a breast pump. Her breast milk can even be collected and fed to the baby by the nursing staff, if necessary.

The contractions of the uterus caused by the baby's nursing does not harm the mother's incision. With the help of a nurse, the mother can experiment to find the most comfortable position in which to feed her baby.

To protect the incision from the weight and wiggling of the baby, the mother can feed while sitting, positioning the baby on a pillow placed on her lap. Or put the baby, supported by pillows, in a football hold at the mother's side. Or the mother can lie on her side to nurse her baby, see Figure 19–8.

WHEN NOT TO BREAST FEED

There are situations when breast feeding is not recommended or possible. If the mother has had extensive breast reduction surgery in which the areola was removed, or if circulation to the breast was impaired or the duct system within the breast was altered by the surgery, she may not be able to successfully nurse. If the mother has hepatitis, untreated tuberculosis, a herpes sore on her areola or HIV infection, breast feeding is contraindicated. If the mother is receiving significant amounts of certain drugs (for example, chemotherapeutic drugs for cancer) or uses cocaine, she should not nurse. If the baby has galactosemia, a condition where the baby is unable to digest the sugar in milk, an alternative feeding program is necessary. If the mother feels uncomfortable, resentful, or unhappy about breast feeding, or if she has to be separated from her infant for days or weeks at a time, she should never be made to feel she has failed as a mother.

WEANING

Weaning means transferring a baby from dependence on mother's milk to dependence on another form of nourishment. A mother can wean her breast-fed infant whenever she wants. Some mothers want to breast feed for a few weeks, others for more than a year. However long a baby is breast fed, the most important thing to remember about weaning is that it should be done gradually, if possible, for both the mother's and the infant's sake. Generally, replacing one breast feeding at a time with a

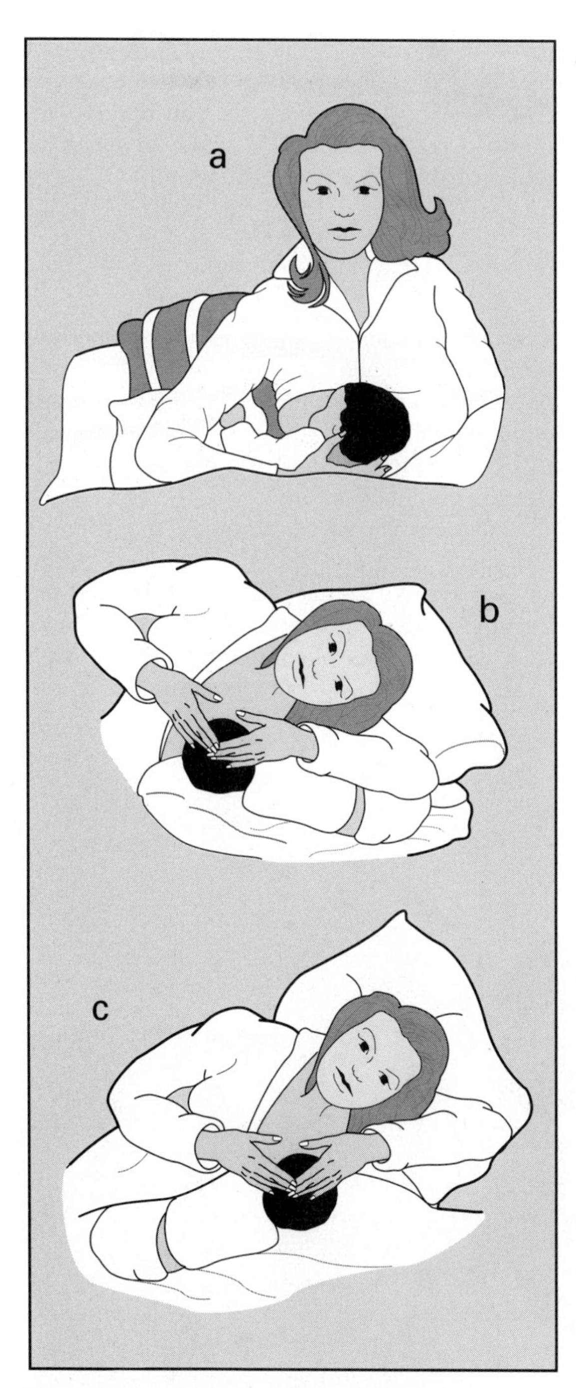

Figure 19–8 *Positions for breast feeding after a cesarean section. (a) Sitting. (b) Football position. (c) Lying on side.*

substitute feeding is a good way to wean. When the infant is used to one substitute feeding, a second substitute feeding can be given after a few days. This process continues until the baby is no longer feeding at the breast.

BOTTLE FEEDING

Both the nursing mother and the nonnursing mother should learn the techniques of bottle feeding. Supplementary bottles may be ordered by the pediatrician if the infant's need is greater than the mother's supply of milk. The nursing mother may want to give her baby an occasional bottle when her schedule does not allow her to breast feed.

On discharge from the hospital, the mother is given a set of instructions dealing with the formula. These instructions tell her the type of formula to use and how to prepare it. Formulas are available in ready-to-feed preparations, canned liquid concentrates, and powdered form. The baby may also be given specific prepackaged commercial formula preparations on the advice of the doctor. Whole, 2%, 1%, skim, or goat's milk are not considered good choices for an infant under one year old.

Care should be taken that the hole in the nipple is the proper size and that the nipple is full of milk to prevent the baby from swallowing air. The hole in the nipple is the right size if the formula drips out when the bottle is held upside down. If the milk comes out in a stream, the nipple hole is too big; if the milk drips too slowly or not at all, the baby will swallow too much air, tire, and not get enough at his feeding. The infant should be held in a semireclining position during bottle feeding. If his head is too low, the milk may pool back in his throat around his eustachian tubes (which extend from the back of the throat to the ears). This pooling could cause an infection in the middle ear. The mother should be encouraged to sometimes hold her baby with her right arm and sometimes with her left arm. Alternating will promote normal eye muscle development. The infant should be burped after completing about 1 to 2 oz of formula when he is little and about half-way through the feeding as he matures. The infant may not take in the same amount of formula at every feeding. The baby should not be coaxed to empty the bottle at each feeding if he seems satisfied with less. Encourage the mother to make feeding time a special time and never prop the bottle and leave the baby during a feeding. After feeding, the baby should be placed on his stomach or on his right side. The newborn baby is able to raise his head, so the mother should not be afraid that the baby might smother when lying on the stomach. If the baby is placed on the right side, the milk passes into the stomach, since the stomach contour is to the right, thereby lessening the chance of aspiration. One or two ounces of water twice daily should be given in addition to the formula. During hot weather, 2 or 3 oz of water could be given twice daily. If the baby is constipated, an increase in the amount of water given daily will probably remedy the situation.

GAVAGE FEEDINGS

Gavage feeding is a method of providing nourishment when the infant is unable to suck or swallow or when he becomes too fatigued or has difficulty breathing while nipple feeding. Gavage feeding also is a means of administering oral medications.

A tube is placed through the infant's mouth or nose into the stomach, see Figure 19–9. A syringe is attached to the tube, and the formula or feeding is poured into the syringe. In a careful, controlled manner, the feeding is allowed to flow from the syringe into the

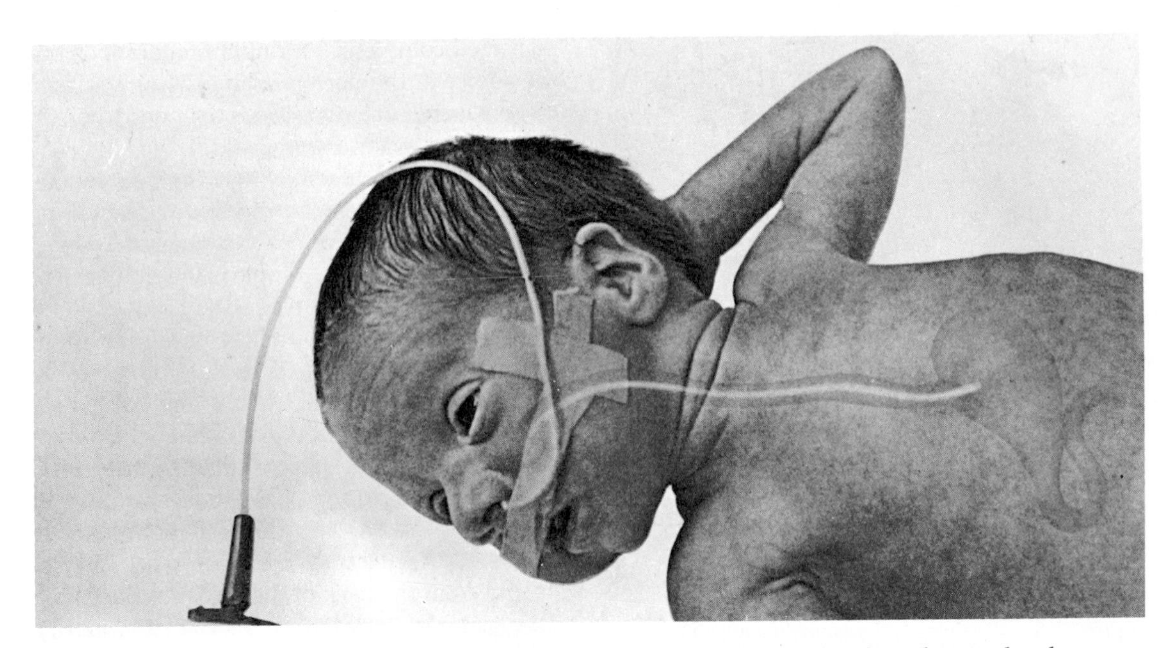

Figure 19–9 *Plastic indwelling catheter inserted through nose will remain in place 3–4 days when taped as shown. (Courtesy Ross Laboratories)*

infant's stomach. Care must be taken to ensure that the tube is actually in the infant's stomach. Also, the nurse should be sure that no air is forced into the infant's stomach.

Intermittent gavage feeding is often preferred to indwelling gavage feedings. An indwelling tube may coil, knot, perforate the stomach and cause nasal airway obstruction, ulceration, irritation to the mucous membrane and nosebleed. If intermittent intubation is not well tolerated and an indwelling tube is used, the catheter should be size #3.5 or #5, taped securely to the skin and flushed with 1–2 mL of sterile water after every use. The catheter should be changed every 24 to 72 hours. No studies have been done to determine long-term effects of indwelling nasogastric tubes. Alternate nares should be used when the tube is changed, and constant alertness to complications is stressed. When passing either an intermittent or indwelling catheter for feeding, observe the infant for bradycardia and apnea. Gavage feedings are usually increased in volume by 1-mL increments every other feeding, depending on the amount of residual obtained before administering the feeding and the tolerance of the infant.

SPECIAL FEEDING PROBLEMS

When the baby is matured enough to be fed by his mother, special feeding problems can still exist. Premature, small gestational age babies can require supplementation. These babies do not suck long enough or strongly enough to stimulate an adequate milk supply. They do not obtain enough calories and fluid without overtiring themselves. Mothers should be encouraged to express milk for supplementary use because of the benefits of breast milk and the need to stimulate continued milk production. The use of a **Lact-Aid** or similar device is also recommended, Figure 19–10. The formula-filled Lact-Aid is attached to the nursing bra or neck cord between the breasts and is positioned so that the formula cannot siphon out. The baby suckles the tip of the nursing tube and the nipple of the breast at the same time. As the infant nurses, formula is drawn from the bottom of the bag by the extension tube as well as from the breast. The Lact-Aid has an opening designed to provide the best rate of flow, slower than milk flows from the breast, but fast enough to keep from overtiring the infant.

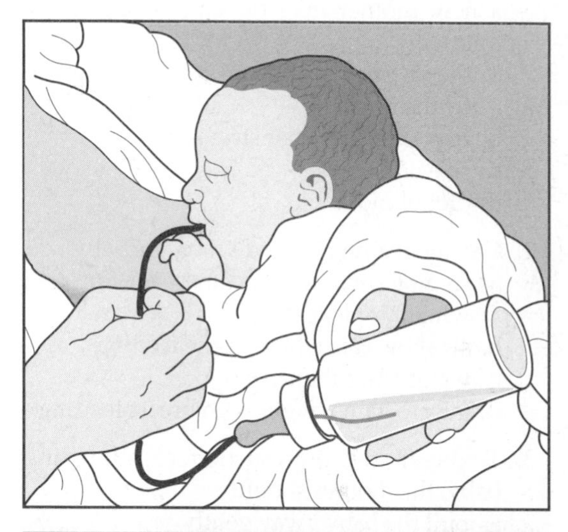

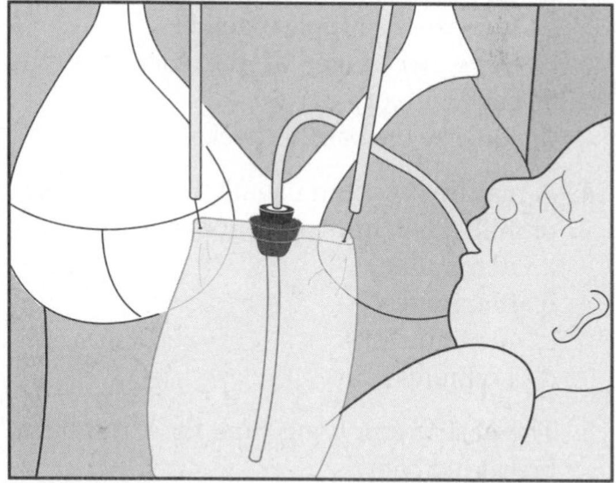

Figure 19–10 *Use of devices such as the Lact-Aid help build up the milk supply while providing adequate nutrition for the infant.*

When the infant is put to the breast, the flow of formula from the Lact-Aid rewards his nursing efforts. This reward provides a pleasant incentive for the baby to continue nursing, which in turn provides the breasts with suckling stimulation to build up the milk supply. Spoon, dropper, or an orthodontically correct nipple could also be used. With the Lact-Aid, the breast receives additional stimulation for milk production and as a result the infant is not overfatigued in efforts to receive required caloric intake.

REVIEW QUESTIONS

A. Multiple choice. Select the best answer.

1. The success or failure of breast feeding by a new mother may depend on all of the following *except*
   a. the instruction and encouragement given by the nurse
   b. fear, pain, or other stresses
   c. size of breasts
   d. diet of mother

2. Gavage feeding is used when the baby
   a. cannot suck and becomes too fatigued when nipple feeding
   b. swallows air while nipple feeding
   c. weighs less than 5½ lb
   d. fails to gain weight with breast feeding

3. To break the oral suction of a nursing baby, the mother should
   a. pull the baby away gently
   b. squeeze the nipple together
   c. place her finger at the corner of the baby's mouth
   d. squeeze the baby's cheeks

4. A mature baby can usually empty a breast of milk when nursing in about
   a. 20 minutes
   b. 10 minutes
   c. 40 minutes
   d. 3 minutes

5. The gastric emptying time for a full-term, breast-fed baby is
   a. 1 to2 hours
   b. 2 to 3 hours
   c. 1 to 4 hours
   d. usually more than 4 hours

6. For successful breast feeding to occur, the mother needs
   a. a comfortable, relaxed environment
   b. adequate fluids and a good diet
   c. correct positioning of the baby
   d. all of the above

7. Milk production is triggered by the hormone
   a. progesterone
   b. estrogen
   c. prolactin
   d. oxytocin

8. Colostrum is composed of all of the following *except*
   a. antibodies
   b. white blood cells and serum
   c. salt, protein, and fat
   d. milk products

9. Nipple soreness is caused by all of the following *except*
   a. engorgement
   b. nursing for 10 minutes on the first day
   c. slow let-down reflex
   d. improper latching on to the nipple

10. Symptoms of mastitis include
    a. inadequate milk supply
    b. flu-like symptoms and breast pain
    c. hard, full breasts
    d. sore nipples

SUGGESTED ACTIVITIES

- State how breast milk is formed.
- Discuss the advantages and disadvantages of breast feeding versus bottle feeding.
- List four common problems frequently encountered in breast feeding. Describe the technique to avoid or alleviate the problem.
- Demonstrate how to use the Lact-Aid; explain how to gavage feed an infant.
- Describe how to wean an infant with the least amount of discomfort.
- List reasons why a baby can be fussy besides hunger.

BIBLIOGRAPHY

Blair-Storr, G. "Prevention of Nipple Tenderness and Breast Engorgement in the Postpartal Period." *JOGNN* 17(3):203–209, May-June, 1988.

Dusdieker, L. B., B. M. Booth, B. F. Seals, and E. E. Ekow. "Investigation of a Model for the Initiation of Breastfeeding in Primigravida Women." *Social Science and Medicine* 20(7):695–703, 1985.

Helsing, E., and T. S. King. *Breast Feeding in Practice.* New York: Oxford University Press, 1982.

Kelly, M. "Will Mothers Breast-Feed Longer If Health Visitors Give Them More Support?" *Health Visitor* 56(11):407–409, 1983.

Lawrence, R. A. *Breast Feeding: A Guide for the Medical Profession,* 3rd ed. St. Louis, MO: C. V. Mosby, 1989.

Olds, S. W., and M. S. Eiger. *Maternal-Newborn.* Reading, MA: Addison-Wesley, 1984.

Simkin, P., Whalley, J., and A. Keppler. *Pregnancy, Childbirth and the Newborn.* Deephaven, MN: Meadowbrook Books, 1991.

Weibley, T. T., Adamson, M., Clinkscales, N., Curran, J., and R. Bramson. "Gavage Tube Insertion in the Premature Infant." *MCN* 12:24–27, January-February, 1987.

Worthington-Roberts, B. S., and S. R. Williams. *Nutrition in Pregnancy and Lactation*, 4th ed. St. Louis, MO: Times Mirror-Mosby, 1989.

CHAPTER

20

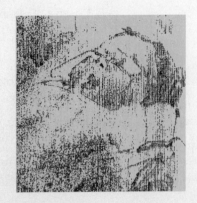

Disorders of the Neonate

Objectives

After studying this chapter, the student should be able to:

- Name three causes for asphyxia neonatorum.
- Describe the signs of respiratory distress.
- Identify principles to follow when treating a newborn with breathing difficulty.
- State one disorder of the newborn for each of the eight body systems.
- State the cause and treatment for specific disorders of the newborn.

Key Terms

congenital	narcosis
asphyxia neonatorum	respiratory distress syndrome (RDS)
anoxia	surfactant deficiency
cerebral injury	cyanosis

DYSPNEA
CONTINUOUS POSITIVE AIRWAY PRESSURE (CPAP)
CHEST RETRACTION
SILVERMAN-ANDERSON INDEX
PHYSIOLOGICAL JAUNDICE
BILIRUBIN
PHOTOTHERAPY
ERYTHROBLASTOSIS FETALIS
RHOGAM
ABO INCOMPATIBILITY
CLEFT LIP
CLEFT PALATE
THRUSH
PYLORIC STENOSIS
UMBILICAL HERNIA
IMPERFORATE ANUS
SPINA BIFIDA OCCULTA
MENINGOCELE
MENINGOMYELOCELE
DOWN SYNDROME
HYDROCEPHALUS
TORTICOLLIS
ERB'S PALSY
TALIPES
GYNECOMASTIA
NEONATAL HYPOGLYCEMIA
GLYCOGEN
PHENYLKETONURIA (PKU)
EXSTROPHY OF THE BLADDER
PSEUDOHERMAPHRODITISM
HERMAPHRODITISM
HYPOSPADIAS
EPISPADIAS
NEVI
MILIARIA RUBRA
CAPUT SUCCEDANEUM
CEPHALOHEMATOMA
IMPETIGO

Becoming a parent is a major event, a turning point in life, particularly for parents of a newborn with a disorder. Some parents can cope and adjust to the situation with increased maturity; others react with distress, which leaves them emotionally drained. It is the responsibility of the health care team to understand the psychodynamics that are taking place in both the parents and themselves. Only then can the situation be dealt with constructively and therapeutically.

ATTITUDES OF THE STAFF

The delivery of an infant with a disorder is difficult for the entire health care team. The mother may sense their frustration and misinterpret it as hostility. She may feel sadness rather than the anticipated feeling of joy. All of this distress comes at a time when the mother may be physically and emotionally exhausted. The importance of the nurse's presence should never be underestimated. The mother needs to feel that someone understands. By simply holding the mother's hand or encouraging her to express her feelings, the nurse renders tremendous emotional support.

Realistic reassurance should be given to the mother and father. The parents need to feel that the child is accepted and treated like any other newborn and that hospital personnel will give any assistance possible. The nurse can help by cuddling the newborn and calling the infant by name. Also, the nurse can encourage the parents to talk about their feelings openly. The hospital staff should be careful not to offer the mother helpful platitudes such as "you can always have other children" or "don't feel so bad." This attitude simply conveys a lack of understanding and empathy.

ETIOLOGY AND TREATMENT

Observation of the newborn is one of the nurse's most important duties both in the delivery room and in the nursery. Serious threats to the baby's health may be averted. Early treatment of congenital anomalies and diseases may be initiated when an alert nurse reports unusual signs and symptoms. These observations alert the physician or supervising nurse to the fact that a condition may exist for which medical attention is necessary.

Disorders of the newborn are acquired during development in the uterus **(congenital)**, during the birth process, or as a result of medical conditions. Disorders may affect any one of the following body systems or may overlap and involve more than one system:

- respiratory system
- circulatory system
- digestive system
- nervous system
- musculoskeletal system
- endocrine/metabolic system
- genitourinary system
- integumentary system

A few of the more commonly seen birth disorders of neonates are discussed in this chapter.

RESPIRATORY SYSTEM OF THE NEWBORN

The newborn's respirations are normally slightly irregular. They may vary from 40 to 60 per minute. If respirations have not begun within 30 seconds after birth, the condition may be called **asphyxia neonatorum** (imperfect breathing in the newborn). Failure of the infant to breathe spontaneously is usually due to one or a combination of three causes:

- deprivation of oxygen **(anoxia)**
- damage to brain tissue **(cerebral injury)**
- unconscious state caused by drugs **(narcosis)**

Anoxia. Any interference with the function of the placenta or the umbilical cord, which supplies oxygen to the baby, puts the baby in great danger of anoxia. A prolapsed cord, nuchal cord, premature separation of the placenta (placenta abruptio), or extremely severe uterine contraction could all produce intrauterine asphyxia. The child may literally suffocate while in the uterus because of the lack of oxygen.

Cerebral Injury. Cerebral injury is a common cause of apnea at birth when the delivery is particularly difficult. There may be brain hemorrhage that damages the respiratory center; other vital centers may also be injured. A disproportion between the size of the baby's head and the mother's pelvis can cause compression of the skull severe enough to cause damage to the brain.

Narcosis. A state of narcosis (unconsciousness) may be produced in the baby by analgesic and anesthetic drugs given to the mother during labor. Although the respirations may be sluggish at first, the infant usually does quite well when the effects of the medication have worn off.

RESPIRATORY DISTRESS SYNDROME

Respiratory distress syndrome (RDS) (formerly called hyaline membrane disease) often occurs from minutes to several hours after birth. The reason why RDS occurs is unknown but it is thought to be due to a **surfactant deficiency** in the infant's system. The lack of this phospholipid inhibits the complete expansion of the alveoli in the lungs. As a result, the lungs lose their elasticity.

The main symptoms of RDS are **cyanosis** (bluish tinge to nails, lips, and skin) and **dyspnea** (difficult breathing). The disorder is found more frequently in premature infants and those born by cesarean section than in full-term or vaginal birth babies. Observation and recording of respiratory signs and symptoms are important. Treatment consists of placing the infant in an incubator to meet the need for oxygen and maintenance of high humidity. **Continuous positive airway pressure (CPAP)** can be given to assist in ventilation. Antibiotics are often given along with intravenous feedings.

SIGNS OF RESPIRATORY DISTRESS

The nurse should be alert to the following signs of respiratory distress, which may be evident at birth or may develop several days later:

- nasal flaring
- excessive mucus
- increase in rate of respirations accompanied by regular rhythm
- **chest retraction** upon inspiration (see-saw type of respirations)
- expiratory grunt or feeble cry
- cyanosis, except for hands and feet

Normally, the newborn is slightly blue at the moment of birth because its lungs have not yet expanded. The skin becomes rosy pink as soon as breathing begins. The development of pallor and cyanosis should be reported immediately because they are signs of respiratory or circulatory difficulty.

There are five main principles to follow when treating a baby who does not breathe spontaneously at birth.

- gentleness
- warmth
- removal of mucus
- positioning
- artificial respiration

Often the baby is in a state of shock and gentleness is essential in all procedures. Physical stimulation should be limited to rubbing the back or flicking the soles of the feet. The temperature of the room may also aggravate the state of shock, so the baby must be kept warm. Excessive mucus should be reported immediately and emergency measures taken if necessary. Mucus may be removed with a suction catheter or with a bulb syringe. The baby should be placed in the Trendelenburg position with the head turned to one side. If the baby does not respond to these measures within 90 seconds after delivery, oxygen must be administered, and possibly external cardiac massage. Once the baby begins to breathe on his own, continued close observation is vital. See the procedure for resuscitation of the newborn given later in this chapter, on page 383.

SILVERMAN-ANDERSON INDEX

The **Silverman-Anderson Index** is designed to provide a continuous evaluation of the infant's respiratory status, Figure 20–1. Values are assigned to five criteria: chest lag, intercostal retraction, xiphoid retraction, nares dilatation,

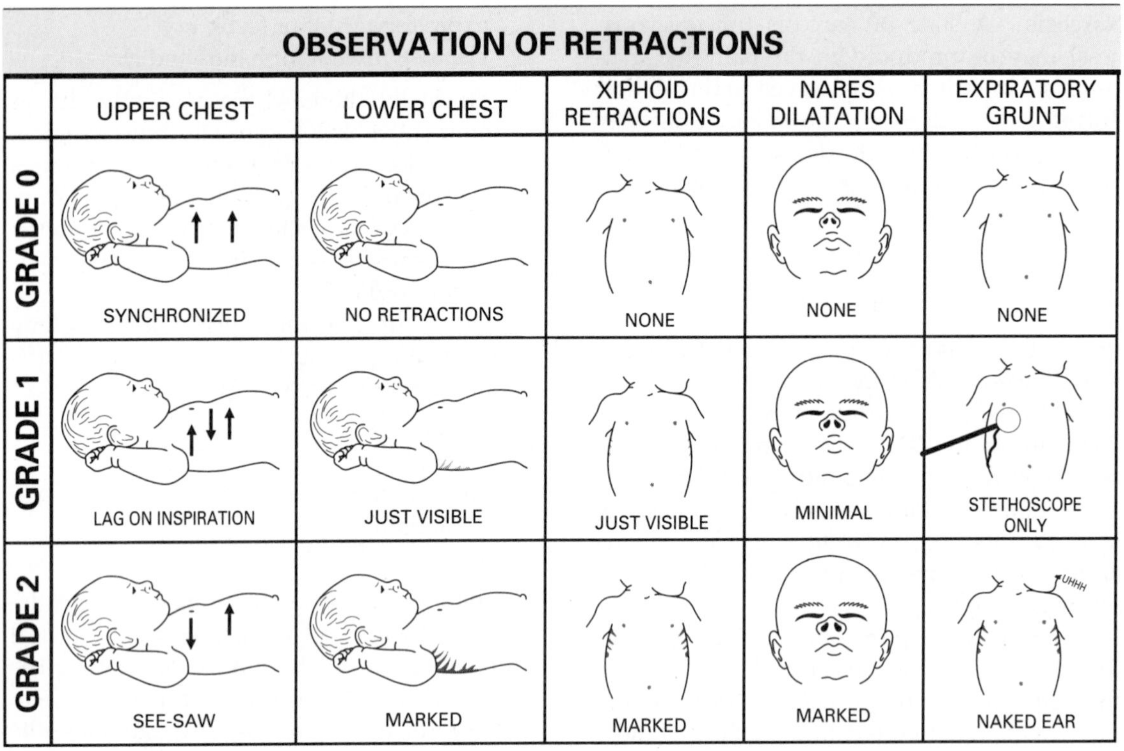

OBSERVATION OF RETRACTIONS

	UPPER CHEST	LOWER CHEST	XIPHOID RETRACTIONS	NARES DILATATION	EXPIRATORY GRUNT
GRADE 0	SYNCHRONIZED	NO RETRACTIONS	NONE	NONE	NONE
GRADE 1	LAG ON INSPIRATION	JUST VISIBLE	JUST VISIBLE	MINIMAL	STETHOSCOPE ONLY
GRADE 2	SEE-SAW	MARKED	MARKED	MARKED	NAKED EAR

Figure 20–1 *The Silverman-Anderson Index for the evaluation of respiratory status*

and expiratory grunt. A score of zero indicates no respiratory distress; a score of 10 indicates severe respiratory distress.

CIRCULATORY SYSTEM OF THE NEWBORN

The heart, blood vessels, lymph vessels and lymph nodes make up the circulatory system. Blood is pumped to all body tissues. The circulating blood carries oxygen, nutrients, and chemicals to the cells of the body and takes away waste materials from the cells.

JAUNDICE

As the circulatory system adapts to extrauterine life, many newborns develop mild jaundice. This normal characteristic, which appears in up to 50% of full-term infants and 80% of premature newborns, is called **physiological jaundice**. It is caused by the liver's failure to cope with the breakdown of red blood cells no longer needed by the newborn. This liver failure causes increased amounts of **bilirubin** (a product of red blood cell destruction) to appear in the bloodstream, thus causing a yellowish tint to the skin. This type of jaundice becomes apparent between the third and fifth day of life and subsides around the eighth day; it has little medical significance. Jaundice can and frequently does occur in breast-fed babies because of a compound present in some mothers' milk that inhibits the breakdown of bilirubin. If the bilirubin level is too high, the mother may be asked to interrupt her breast feeding for 24 to 48 hours and pump her breasts to maintain her milk supply. Breast feeding can then be tried again and the bilirubin level monitored. The mother should always be assured that there is nothing wrong with her breast milk.

Jaundice that appears before the third day of life should be promptly reported to the physician. Jaundice at this time could indicate the presence of a hemolytic disease such as erythroblastosis fetalis or ABO incompatibility.

A blood test to determine the level of bilirubin is made to assess the degree of jaundice in the infant. The pediatrician may order **phototherapy** (the exposure of the infant to fluorescent blue light). The baby is placed unclothed under the light, which helps to remove the yellow or jaundice from the skin by helping the body break down the bilirubin more efficiently. The nurse must protect the baby's eyes with a cover of soft bandage. The baby's body temperature should be monitored carefully, and the infant should receive extra fluids. A newer form of phototherapy utilizes a plastic body wrap and fiberoptic lights. The baby does not need eye patches and may be fed and held without interrupting treatment.

ERYTHROBLASTOSIS FETALIS

The Rh factor caused by an Rh-negative woman giving birth to an Rh-positive baby may cause a disease technically known as **erythroblastosis fetalis**, Figure 20–2. In this condition the baby's red blood cells are destroyed by Rh antibodies. Antibodies are proteins that are made as a response to foreign antigens. When Rh-positive red blood cells enter the bloodstream of an Rh-negative person, the recipient may produce Rh antibodies capable of destroying Rh-positive cells. Some of the Rh-positive red blood cells of the fetus may spill into the woman's bloodstream during a pregnancy and even more frequently at the time of spontaneous or induced abortion or delivery. The Rh-negative woman may then develop antibodies against the fetus's Rh-positive red blood cells. Rh antibodies produced by the mother can destroy the red blood cells of the fetus in the uterus. Destruction of the fetus's red blood cells is indicated by increased levels of bilirubin in the baby's blood. Erythroblastosis fetalis is characterized by anemia, jaundice, enlargement of the liver and spleen, and generalized edema of the newborn. If the anemia is severe enough, brain damage, heart failure, or death can occur.

The treatment of this disorder consists of giving the infant frequent transfusions of Rh-negative blood during the first weeks of life. Phototherapy is a simple and safe method of treating mild hemolytic disease and greatly reduces the need for exchange transfusions. It is relatively ineffective, however, when serum bilirubin rises rapidly in severe cases. Phototherapy is also helpful for infants with low birth weight, respiratory distress, acidosis, and sepsis.

A specific gamma globulin, **RhoGAM**, has made erythroblastosis fetalis rare. RhoGAM is a specially prepared gamma globulin that contains a concentration of Rh antibodies. These antibodies suppress the Rh-negative mother's immune response to the foreign Rh-positive red blood cells that may enter her bloodstream. RhoGAM provides virtually complete protection by preventing the woman from producing her own permanent Rh antibodies. It is administered intramuscularly within three days after delivery of an Rh-positive infant. It has been shown that administration of RhoGAM between 28 and 32 weeks of pregnancy, as well as after delivery, further decreases the risk of antibody production. RhoGAM should also be administered to the woman who has had a miscarriage or abortion after 12 weeks of pregnancy, even though the Rh type of the fetus cannot be confirmed. MICRhoGAM is a reduced dose of RhoGAM and is administered to the Rh-negative woman if she aborts within the first 12 weeks of pregnancy.

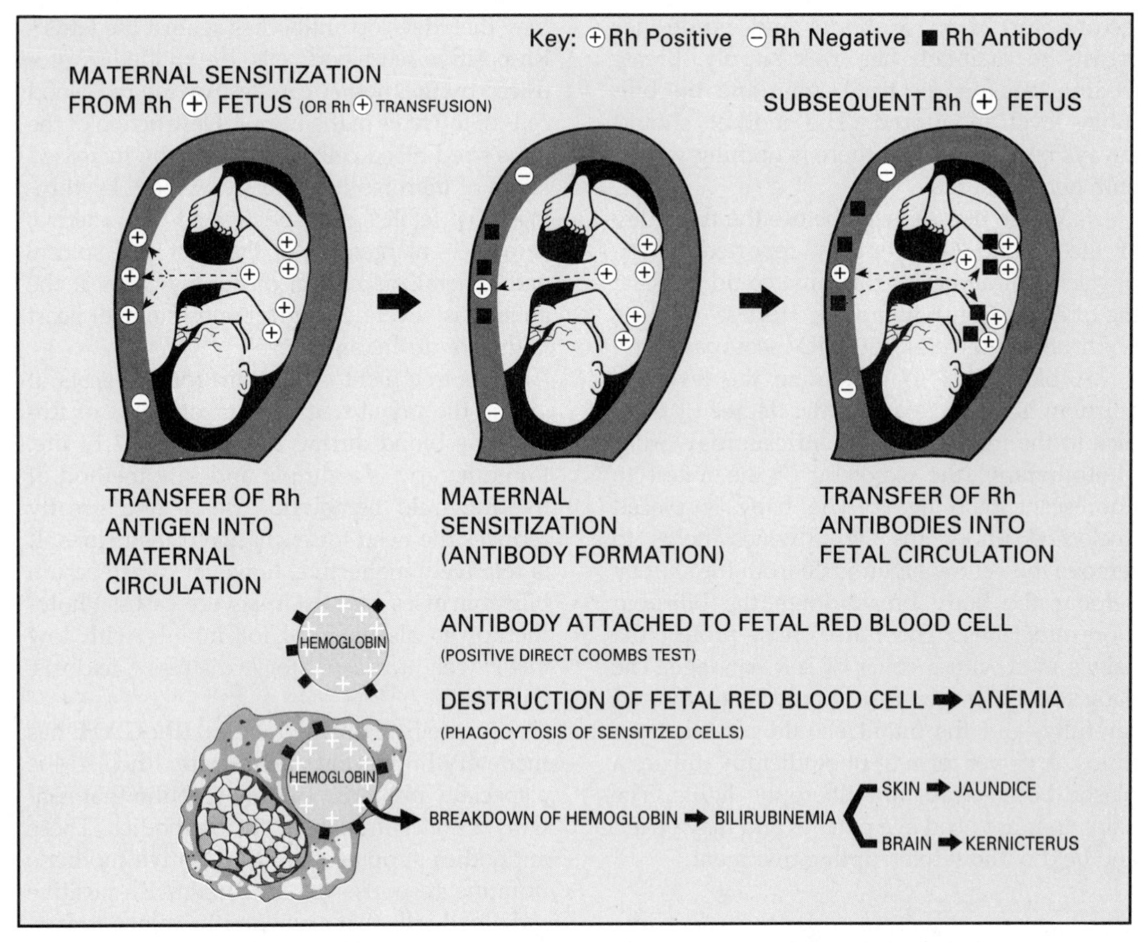

Figure 20–2 *Erythroblastosis fetalis (Adapted from Nursing Education Aid, No. 9, Ross Laboratories)*

ABO INCOMPATIBILITY

In **ABO incompatibility**, the etiologic process is much the same as in Rh incompatibility. The difficulty is caused by the presence of the naturally occurring antigen of the blood group A or B factors. Hemolytic disease due to A or B incompatibility is not usually anticipated unless there is a history of this problem among previous children in the family. The disease of the newborn is usually mild and may even pass unnoticed. It should be treated, however, if signs are well developed:

- mild jaundice during the first 36 hours of life
- enlargement of the liver and spleen
- central nervous system complications (rare)
- varying degrees of anemia or erthroblastosis

The treatment consists of phototherapy or an exchange transfusion using group O blood of appropriate Rh type if the infant's serum bilirubin level approaches 20 mg per 100 mL. The majority of affected infants need no treatment but should be watched carefully with special attention to respirations, pulse, temperature, and increasing lethargy. The nurse should also watch for and report any increased jaundice, pigmentation of urine, edema, cyanosis, convulsions, and any changes of the vital signs.

DIGESTIVE SYSTEM OF THE NEWBORN

The digestive system is made up of all the organs of the body that are involved in taking food and converting it into substances that the body can use and discarding those elements that are considered waste. The digestive system includes the mouth, teeth, pharynx, and the alimentary or gastrointestinal tract (esophagus, stomach, intestines, and other organs such as the liver, gallbladder, and pancreas).

CLEFT LIP AND CLEFT PALATE

A **cleft lip** is a vertical cleft or split in the upper lip, Figure 20–3. It is also known as harelip. A **cleft palate** is a fissure in the roof of the mouth and nasal cavities.

Feeding is usually the most immediate problem. It is best accomplished by placing the infant in an upright position and directing the flow of milk against the side of the mouth. This method decreases the amount of air swallowed. The baby should be bubbled or burped at frequent intervals. A variety of nipples may be tried, including regular nipples with enlarged holes. Cleft palate nipples are also available. Breast feeding may be tried as well.

Cleft lip and cleft palate can occur separately or together. Both conditions result from failure of the soft or bony tissues or both of the upper jaw and palate to unite during the 8th to 12th weeks of gestation. Surgical repair is the usual course of action. Depending on the severity, the plan of treatment may be immediate or it may be delayed until the second year of life. The parents often require a great deal of support, as this disorder can be quite disfiguring. Repair is generally successful; it is helpful if the parents know and understand this fact.

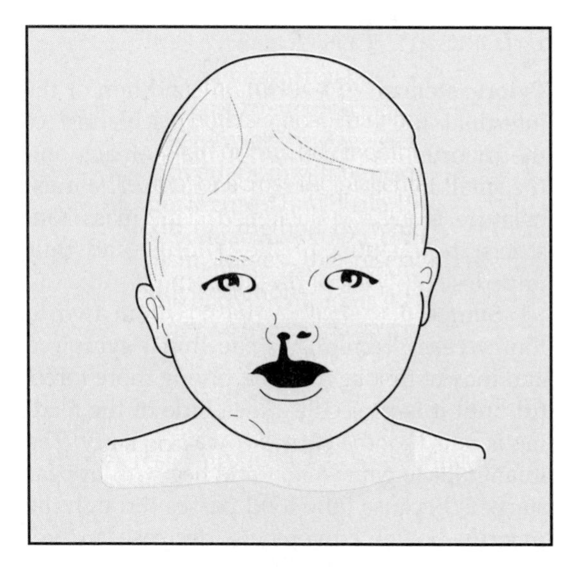

Figure 20–3 *A complete cleft lip*

THRUSH

Thrush, or oral candidiasis is an infection caused by the fungus *Candida (Monilia) albicans*, which is generally found in the vagina of the mother. Spores grow on the delicate tissue of the infant's mouth. An infant can be infected by improperly cleaned nipples or breast of the mother.

Thrush appears as pearly white, elevated lesions resembling milk curds. It is usually found on the tongue margin, inside the lips and cheeks, and on the hard palate. Prognosis with treatment is good, and recovery usually takes place in three to four days. Nystatin or aqueous gentian violet (1% solution) or 1:1,000 aqueous solution of Zephiran may be used in treating thrush.

PYLORIC STENOSIS

Pyloric stenosis is a common condition of the intestinal tract. The circular musculature of the pylorus (the junction of the stomach and the small intestine) increases in size. The musculature is greatly thickened. This mass constricts the opening of the pylorus, and thus impedes emptying of the stomach.

Symptoms usually appear within two to four weeks. Vomiting is the initial symptom and may at first be mild, becoming more forceful until it is projectile. Since little of the feeding is retained, the baby is always hungry. The infant fails to gain weight and begins to appear starved. Because little food passes through the pylorus bowel movements decrease in frequency and amount.

The signs of pyloric stenosis are dehydration, poor skin turgor, and an olive-shaped mass that can be felt in the right upper quadrant of the abdomen. Surgical intervention is usually necessary. If surgery is performed early enough, the prognosis is excellent.

UMBILICAL HERNIA

A hernia is a protrusion of part of an organ through the wall of the cavity in which it is normally contained. An **umbilical hernia** is caused by a weakness or incomplete closure of the umbilical ring, allowing a portion of the small intestine or omentum to protrude. Omentum is a double fold of peritoneum attached to the stomach that connects it to the abdominal viscera. The hernia is indicated by a soft swelling at the site of the umbilicus. The swelling may disappear when pressure is applied and reappear again when pressure is removed or when the baby cries. The condition often disappears by itself when the abdominal muscles become strengthened, usually when the child learns to stand or walk. It can also be repaired surgically after the first year of life.

COLIC AND DIARRHEA

Colic is most common during the first three to four months and is characterized by intestinal cramping due to accumulation of excessive gas. The infant may pass gas from the anus or belch it up from the stomach. The infant draws up his knees and cries loudly in pain. The exact cause of colic is unknown but it is felt that predisposing causes are excessive swallowing of air, too much excitement, too rapid feeding, or a tense mother who communicates this tenseness to the infant.

The treatment is to bubble or burp the infant frequently, holding him upright to get rid of the air in the intestinal tract. Letting the baby suck on a pacifier, breast, or finger, walking and rocking him, swaddling him, or holding him by lying him on the arm while he is facing outward may also help comfort the colicky baby. Colic is not a serious condition, and infants usually gain weight despite the periods of pain.

Diarrhea is a symptom of a variety of conditions that can be mild or severe, Figure 20–4. Faulty preparation of formula, overfeeding, an unbalanced diet (excessive sugar), and spoiled food may all cause diarrhea. A diagnosis is made from history and clinical evaluations. Weight loss and dehydration may follow. Treatment is usually a reduction in formula feedings in order to put less stress on the gastrointestinal tract. Fluid (5% glucose in saline solution) is increased and given orally every three to four hours until the diarrhea subsides. Diarrhea can be a serious problem. The mother should be encouraged to report continued episodes of diarrhea to the baby's physician.

IMPERFORATE ANUS

In the eighth week of embryonic life, a membrane that separates the rectum from the anus is usually absorbed, leaving a continuous canal whose outlet is the anus. If this membrane is

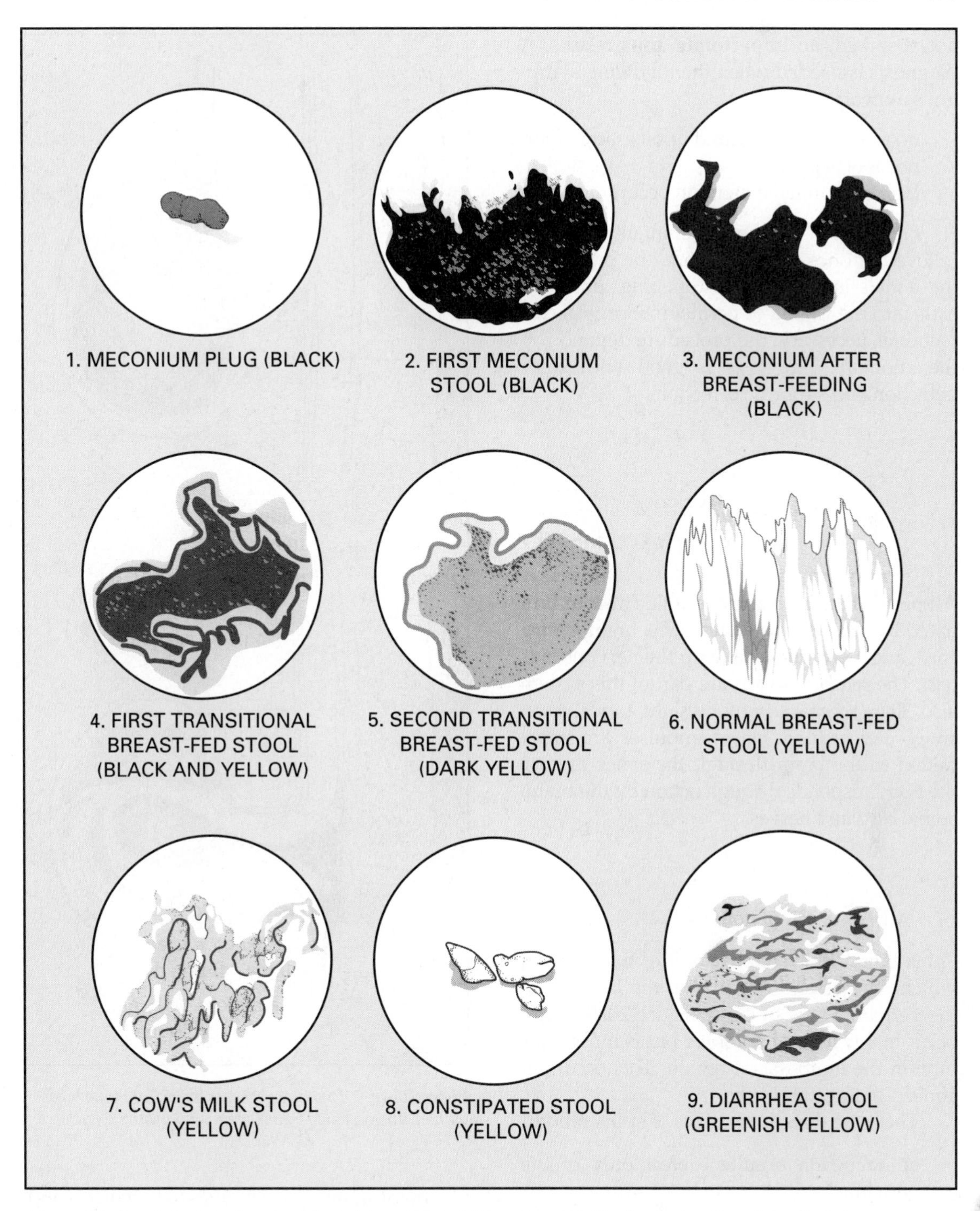

Figure 20–4 *Infant stool cycle (Adapted from Clinical Education Aid, No. 3, courtesy Ross Laboratories)*

not absorbed, an **imperforate anus** results. A diagnosis is needed when the following symptoms appear:

- no anal opening is found upon examination
- no stool is passed
- later abdominal distention occurs

Obstruction in the male infant must be relieved at once for stool cannot be passed. In the female infant a fistula (opening) probably exits into the vagina or perineum. Surgical correction is necessary; the procedure depends on the anomaly. Prognosis is good with early detection and surgical correction.

NERVOUS SYSTEM OF THE NEWBORN

All parts of the body are controlled and coordinated by the nervous system. The brain, spinal cord, and the nerves make up the nervous system. The sensory organs are part of this system also. They receive stimuli by sight, touch, taste, smell, and hearing. When impulses are transmitted to the brain through the sense organs, the body responds through action by the brain, spinal cord and nerves.

SPINA BIFIDA

Spina bifida is a malformation of the spine in which the posterior portion of the laminae of the vertebrae fails to close, Figure 20–5. It can occur in any area of the spine but is most common in the lumbosacral region. This occurs in about 1 out of 1000 births.

There are three basic types of spina bifida.

spina bifida occulta (defect only of the vertebrae)

meningocele (meninges protrude through the opening of the spinal cavity)

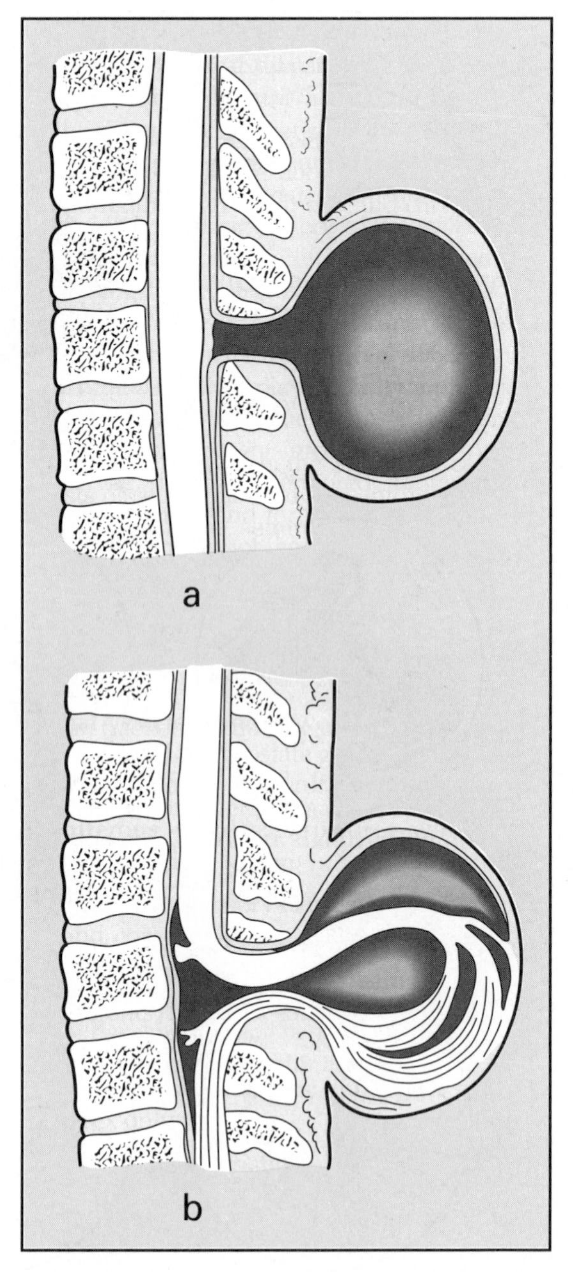

Figure 20–5 *Two types of spina bifida. (a) Spina bifida with meningocele. (b) Spina bifida with meningomyelocele.*

meningomyelocele (spinal cord and meninges protrude through the defect in the bony rings of the spinal canal)

With spina bifida occulta, there is no need for treatment unless neurological symptoms show involvement of the spinal cord. Surgical correction is necessary with meningocele, but prognosis is excellent. There is generally no evidence of weakness in the legs or lack of sphincter control.

With meningomyelocele, there may be anything from minimal weakness to a flaccid paralysis of the legs and absence of sensation in the feet. With surgical correction the neurological deficit can be improved. Therapy may further improve function as the nervous system matures.

Nursing care in meningocele and meningomyelocele is mainly of a protective nature until surgery:

- Protect the bladder from infection by frequent emptying. Emptying is done by applying firm, gentle pressure starting at the umbilical area and progressing downward.
- Protect the protruding sac from pressure.
- Protect the sac from dangers of infection from urine and feces.
- Protect the feet from deformity when the infant is placed on his abdomen. Ankles should be supported with foam rubber pads so that the toes do not rest on the bed.

Good general nursing care is vital for these babies as well as a caring attitude. Special consideration should also be given to the parents to help them understand this disorder.

The alpha fetoprotein screen, which is performed between the 15th and 20th weeks of gestation from maternal serum, will often indicate the presence of this neural tube defect. An ultrasound will confirm the diagnosis by actually visualizing the defect. Early detection gives the parents a choice. They can continue with the pregnancy, knowing their newborn will need special attention at birth and may have permanent disabilities, or they can decide to terminate the pregnancy within the legal time restrictions. In either case, nursing support is needed to help a family understand the nature of a neural tube defect and all the possible outcomes.

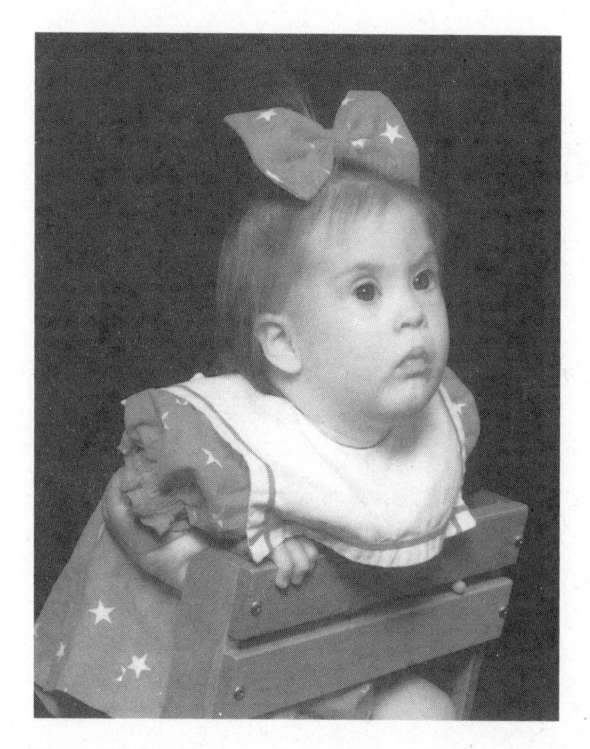

Figure 20–6 *Down syndrome child*

DOWN SYNDROME

Down Syndrome is a congenital disorder that is characterized by irreparable brain and body damage, Figure 20–6. The true cause of this disorder is unknown. However, an abnormal chromosome count has been found to be present in the body cells of children afflicted with the disease, Figure 20–7. Mental retardation is sometimes severe. Deformities are most often noticed in the skull and eyes. The eyes are set close together and slanted, the nose is flat, and the tongue is large and usually protrudes from an open mouth. The head is small; the hands short and thick. Some of these children die early in life because of infection, which their bodies cannot handle.

DOWN SYNDROME AND MATERNAL AGE

Maternal Age	Frequency of Down Syndrome
30	1 in 885 births
31	1 in 826 births
32	1 in 725 births
33	1 in 592 births
34	1 in 465 births
35	1 in 365 births
36	1 in 287 births
37	1 in 225 births
38	1 in 176 births
39	1 in 139 births
40	1 in 109 births
41	1 in 85 births
42	1 in 67 births
43	1 in 53 births
44	1 in 41 births
45	1 in 32 births
46	1 in 25 births
47	1 in 20 births
48	1 in 16 births
49	1 in 12 births

Figure 20–7 *Risk of giving birth to a Down syndrome infant by maternal age*

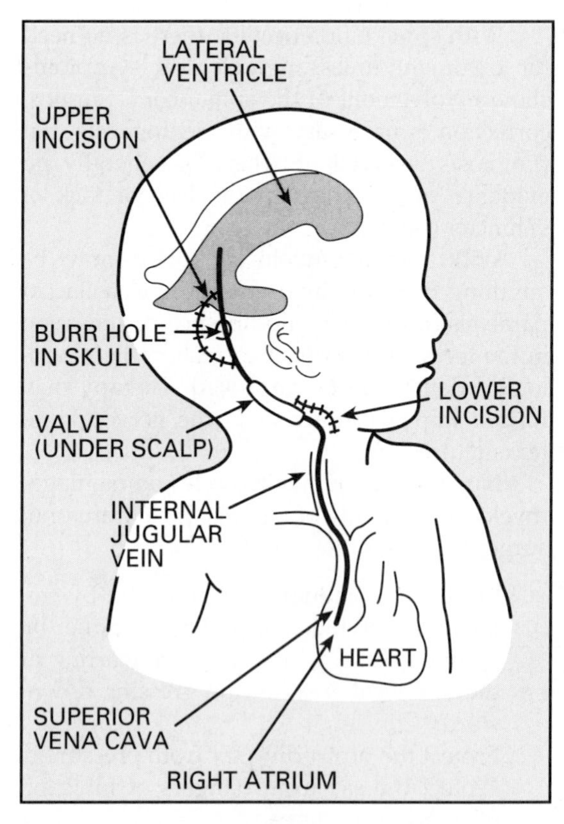

Figure 20–8 *A ventriculoatrial shunt drains spinal fluid in a child with hydrocephalus.*

HYDROCEPHALUS

Hydrocephalus is due to inadequate absorption of cerebrospinal fluid and an increase of fluid under some degree of pressure within the intracranial cavity, Figure 20–8.

The accumulation of fluid in the ventricles generally enlarges the infant's skull since the bones are not yet closed and will yield to pressure. Treatment should begin as soon as symptoms appear and before damage to the brain results. Several shunting procedures are now in use. Prognosis depends on the promptness of treatment and the operation performed.

FACIAL PARALYSIS

Pressure of the forceps on the facial nerve may cause a temporary paralysis of the muscles on one side of the face. The mouth may be drawn to the other side; this lopsidedness is most noticeable when the baby cries. The condition usually disappears in a few days or even a few hours. The parents need assurance that this is a temporary condition. During initial feedings, sucking may be difficult for the infant. The mother needs support and patience in feeding her baby.

MUSCULOSKELETAL SYSTEM OF THE NEWBORN

The bones provide support and protection. Skeletal muscles are attached to the bones. Body movements are due to the action of these muscles. Some disorders of the newborn affect this system.

TORTICOLLIS

Torticollis is a condition caused by the abnormal shortening of the sterocleidomastoid muscle. The neck is tilted to one side. Exercise or traction may be prescribed.

ERB'S PALSY

An infant with **Erb's palsy** may suffer partial paralysis of the arm due to injury to the brachial plexus. The infant cannot raise his arm. Usually this injury is not permanent if it is caused by the delivery process.

FRACTURES

Fractures may occur during delivery. The bones usually affected are the clavicle (collarbone), the humerus (upper arm), or femur (thigh bone). The clavicle usually heals without treatment. Long bones need to be splinted, but these fractures usually heal quickly.

TALIPES

Talipes (clubfoot) may involve one or both feet. The foot may turn inward, outward, downward, or upward, Figure 20–9. Sometimes simple exercises, foot braces, special shoes, or casts may be used successfully. In other instances, surgery may be necessary.

CONGENITAL DISLOCATED HIP

Congenital dislocated hip is believed to be due to lack of embryonic development of the joint. The etiology, however, is not clear. Most commonly, the dislocation occurs when the head of the femur does not lie entirely within the shallow acetabulum (socket of the pelvis). An observable sign is limitation in abduction of the hips (away from the body). Normally, when an infant is lying on his back with knees and hips flexed, the hip joint permits the femur to be abducted until the knee almost touches the table at a 90-degree angle. With dislocation, abduction on the affected side is limited to not more than 45 degrees. Also, the leg on the affected side is shorter than the other leg, and there is a prominence of the soft tissue of the gluteal folds. Treatment should be started as soon as a diagnosis is made. The objective of treatment is to place the head of the femur within the acetabulum and to enlarge and deepen the socket by constant pressure. Ultimately, the dislocation is corrected.

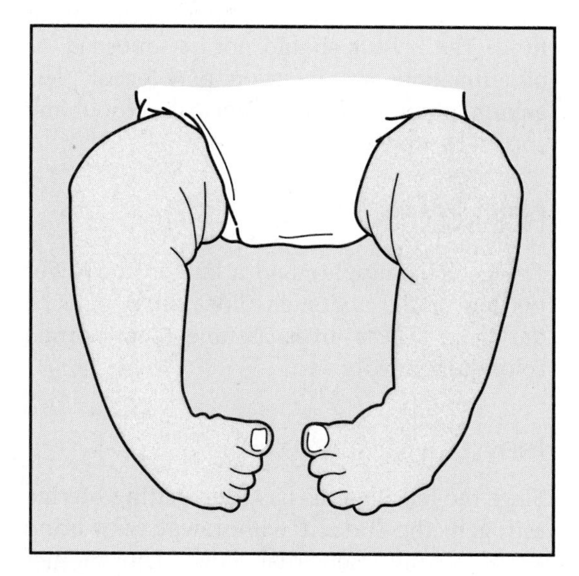

Figure 20–9 *Anterior view of bilateral talipes (clubfoot)*

ENDOCRINE/METABOLIC SYSTEM OF THE NEWBORN

Hormonal interactions take place while the fetus is in utero. Not only does the fetus have its own endocrine system but it is also receiving hormones produced by the mother. The placenta also secretes hormones. The mother secretes large amounts of estrogen during pregnancy. Endocrine disturbances of the mother such as diabetes and hyperthyroidism may affect the newborn's hormonal balance. The result may be a child with hypertrophy of the Islands of Langerhans (from diabetic mothers) or congenital exophthalmic goiter (from mothers with hyperthyroidism). Other disorders of the newborn due to maternal hormones are less severe and usually are of a temporary nature.

GYNECOMASTIA

Gynecomastia may affect both male and female infants. The breasts of the newborn enlarge and sometimes secrete tiny amounts of fluid. The breasts should not be squeezed, as inflammation and infection may occur. The enlarged breasts return to normal without any special treatment.

PIGMENTATION

The genitals, nipples, and a line on the lower portion of the abdomen (linea alba) may be darkened. These areas assume their normal color quite rapidly.

INFANTILE MENSTRUATION

Since the female fetus has been getting uterine estrogen, the sudden withdrawal may bring about a tiny menstrual flow. The mother should be reassured and told that it is no cause for concern. Usually it ceases in a day or two. (*Caution:* If blood loss is considerable, hemorrhagic disease may be present.)

NEONATAL HYPOTHERMIA

Neonatal hypothermia is a problem more commonly seen in the small for gestational age (SGA) baby. It can be a serious metabolic problem. Babies usually produce heat primarily by nonshivering thermogenesis. That is, they metabolize brown fat, which is concentrated in the neck, between the scapula, and behind the sternum, along the vertebral column, and around the kidneys and adrenal glands. These fat stores often are depleted in the SGA infant. Therefore, heat production is impaired. The temperature of full-term babies can also drop rapidly immediately after birth. If the naked newborn is exposed to the usually cool delivery room, this chilling may produce shivering and increased oxygen requirements. The infant's temperature is unstable, responding to slight stimuli with considerable fluctuations. Monitoring temperature and assuring an adequately warm environment are essential to the baby's health.

NEONATAL HYPERTHERMIA

Neonatal hyperthermia can occur when the newborn is bundled up against an outside low temperature that does not exist in his immediate indoor environment. The low sweating capacity of the newborn infant is a contributing factor. The body temperature is often as high as 106°F (41°C), the skin is hot and dry, and the infant appears flushed and apathetic. This stage may be followed by stupor, grayish pallor, coma, and convulsions. This condition can be prevented by providing clothing suitable for the temperature of the immediate environment. If infection or illness is the cause of hyperthermia, the causative agent must be treated appropriately. Immersion of the baby in tepid water usually suffices to bring the temperature back to normal levels. Attention to possible fluid and electrolyte disturbance is essential.

NEONATAL HYPOGLYCEMIA

Neonatal hypoglycemia is an insufficiency of glucose in the newborn. The fetus derives glucose directly from maternal blood by a process of diffusion through the placenta. **Glycogen** is the stored source of glucose. It is stored in the placenta as an additional source of fetal glucose. At 20 to 24 weeks' gestation, the fetal liver becomes the major storage site for glycogen. The fetal heart and skeletal muscles are also storage sites and are essential sources of energy. A defective heart or skeletal muscles lessen the infant's ability to withstand asphyxia. A direct relationship exists between the quantity of glucose stored at birth and the capacity to survive.

At birth, glycogen stored in the liver is normally twice the amount of adult concentrations. Glycogen stored in the heart is 10 times as great; skeletal muscle stores are three to five times as great.

Increased energy is needed for breathing, temperature regulation, and muscle activity at birth. This increased energy output causes a sharp decline in glycogen stores. A low supply of glycogen is a serious threat to the infant. Blood sugar concentration reflects the release of glucose from the liver and the use of glucose by tissues. Use of glucose by tissues is abnormally increased by the metabolic response to cold stress, acidosis, and hypoxia (lack of sufficient oxygen in inspired air). Signs associated with low blood sugar include:

- apnea
- rapid and irregular respirations
- tachypnea
- tremors
- jitters and twitches
- convulsions
- lethargy
- coma
- abrupt pallor, cyanosis, gray shock
- sweating
- upward rolling of the eyes
- weak cry; high-pitched cry
- refusal to feed
- inability to regulate temperature

These signs should subside within five minutes if intravenous glucose is administered. If the signs do not subside, they are due to a cause other than hypoglycemia.

Normal blood sugar concentrations range from 30 to 125 mg per 100 mL in full-term infants weighing over 2,500 g (5½ lb) and from 20 to 100 mg per 100 mL in infants weighing less than 2,500 g. Untreated hypoglycemia in the infant may cause death.

PHENYLKETONURIA

Normally the liver produces an enzyme that acts on an amino acid called phenylalanine; the enzyme changes it to tyrosine. **Phenylketonuria (PKU)** is a metabolic disease caused by failure of the body to oxidize phenylalanine because of the missing or inadequate enzyme. Since the amino acid isn't broken down, it builds up in the blood and tissues causing damage to the brain. If left untreated, mental retardation usually results from phenylketonuria.

Treatment consists of early detection and dietary management restricting phenylalanine intake. Since phenylalanine makes up 5% of the protein factor in all foods, a low-phenylalanine diet is a very restricted one. PKU disorders can be diagnosed from both blood and urine tests. Blood tests are done routinely on newborns in the hospital nursery about the third day of life. Urine tests are done about the second week. Retardation can be prevented with early detection and prompt treatment. Best results are obtained if treatment is started by the third week of life.

GENITOURINARY SYSTEM OF THE NEWBORN

The kidneys, ureters, bladder and urethra make up the urinary system. The external sex organs and related inner structures which are concerned with the production of new individuals make up the reproductive system. The genitourinary system is related to both reproduction and urination.

MALFORMATION OF THE URINARY TRACT

It is important to record the time, description, and kind of urine flow of every newborn. Although little urine is voided in the first two days, ample water should be given to handle the needs for hydration and excretion of wastes. Malformations may lead to death if they are obstructive and renal failure occurs. Abnormalities of the ureters, double kidneys, and double pelves on one or both kidneys cause no harm in themselves but may lead to renal infection and problems of the urinary tract.

EXSTROPHY OF THE BLADDER

Exstrophy of the bladder is a condition in which the interior of the bladder lies completely exposed through an abdominal opening. Infection takes place often but can usually be treated by the use of antibiotics. Surgery must be done to remedy this disorder. There is always the danger of kidney damage resulting from inadequate drainage and infection.

PSEUDOHERMAPHRODITISM

A newborn who has the external sex organs of one sex and the gonads of the other sex is said to be intersexual. The condition is called **pseudohermaphroditism**. Female pseudohermaphrodites have female internal organs, but the enlarged clitoris and fused labia of the external organs resemble a penis and scrotum. The male pseudohermaphrodite has testes, but they are usually in the abdomen. The external genitals may be feminine. There are no ovaries.

HERMAPHRODITISM

An infant who has the gonads and genitals of both sexes is a hermaphrodite. This condition, **hermaphroditism**, is rare. Treatment consists of removing the gonads of one sex.

UNDESCENDED TESTICLE

Sometimes the testes fail to descend into the scrotum. Usually only one testicle has not descended. If the testicle descends spontaneously, it usually does so during the first year. Otherwise, surgery is indicated.

HYPOSPADIAS

In the condition called **hypospadias** the urethra terminates on the under side of the penis. Since the child will not be able to direct his urinary stream, he will be subject to embarrassment and ridicule if the situation is not corrected. Less common is the condition called **epispadias**; the urethra opens on the upper surface of the penis. This condition is sometimes associated with exstrophy of the bladder. Both are correctable by surgery.

INTEGUMENTARY SYSTEM OF THE NEWBORN

The integumentary, or skin, system includes the epidermis and its appendages: hair, nails, sweat glands, oil glands, and the corium layer, which is sometimes referred to as the true skin. The newborn may have skin disorders that range from a mild irritation to more severe infection.

PROCEDURE

Resuscitation of the Newborn

Purpose:

The purpose of resuscitation is to establish or reestablish regular breathing patterns in the infant, see Figure 20–10.

1. Establish an open airway by wiping or suctioning the mouth of any mucus.
2. Tilt the infant's head back slightly by placing your hand at the base of the infant's neck. The breathing passages may be obstructed if the head is too far back.
3. Place your mouth over the infant's nose and mouth to establish an airtight seal.
4. Gently blow air from your cheeks into the infant's nose and mouth at the rate of about three puffs per second. The infant's chest should rise and fall after each breath. If it does not, reposition the infant's head so that his tongue is not resting on the back of his throat or resuction to establish a clear airway.
5. After each puff of air, raise your mouth and turn your head to the side. This allows air to escape back out of the infant's lungs and gives you a chance to take a breath.
6. Continue artificial breathing until proper medical equipment can help ventilation.
7. Observe for signs that the infant is breathing on his own.

Equipment:

- Radiant heat source
- Bulb syringe or DeLee mucus trap
- Oxygen tank and liter gauge
- Oxygen tubing

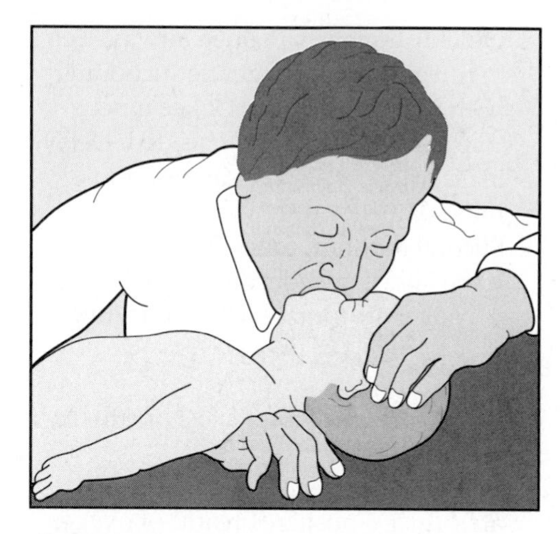

Figure 20–10 *Resuscitation of the newborn*

- Infant oxygen mask
- Pen-Lon valve bag
- Ambu bag
- Wall suction tubing
- Suction catheters #8 and #6.5
- Bottle of sterile water
- Laryngoscope with two blades
- Portex blue-line endotracheal tubes #3.0, #3.5, #2.5
- Stylette
- Clean scissors
- Connector adaptor
- Closed system bag with water manometer
- Stethoscope

Precautions:

1. Keep the baby warm. Keeping the baby warm minimizes oxygen demands while resuscitation is in progress. The infant's temperature should be maintained at 36.5°C. (98° to 98.6°F) axilla.

PROCEDURE

Resuscitation of the Newborn *continued*

2. Quickly establish an open airway. Ten to fifteen seconds of gentle suctioning with a bulb syringe or DeLee mucus trap is all that is usually needed. Delay in clearing the airway can result in brain damage.
3. Suction the oropharynx before the nose. If the nose is suctioned first, the infant may aspirate mucus or amniotic fluid.

Procedure:

1. Briefly flick the infant's feet or rub his back gently.
2. If breathing does not begin immediately, give 5 positive breaths of oxygen-enriched air by mask.
3. Maintain the first 5 inspirations for 4 to 5 seconds at a water pressure of 30 cm on the manometer. Use this high pressure for the first few breaths only to clear excess fetal lung liquid and to open collapsed alveoli.
4. Check for chest movement and breath sounds.
5. If breathing does not start, suction and/or intubate.
6. If breathing begins, heart rate, color, and tone should improve immediately.
7. If breathing does not start, continue bag breathing at a rate of 40 per minute with water pressures that do not exceed 20 to 25 cm.
8. Check the infant's apical pulse.
9. If the apical pulse is below 100 beats per minute and falling in spite of assisted ventilation, initiate cardiac massage.
10. To give cardiac massage, place one hand under the baby's back.
11. With the tips of the index and middle fingers of the other hand, depress the midsternum about ½ to ¾ in.
12. Gently but forcibly do this at a rate of 80 to 100 compressions per minute (a little more than once per second). Do not push too hard, to prevent injury to the infant.
13. Ventilate once after every 5 compressions. Do not interrupt the compressions while ventilating, but avoid compressing the chest and giving breath at the same time.

If the Apgar score is less than 6 at 3 to 5 minutes of age, the infant may need to be transferred to the intensive care unit. Resuscitation must continue during transport to the unit.

NEVI

Nevi (birth marks) are local anatomic alterations of the cellular or vascular components of the skin. They are usually present at birth. Generally, these lesions are minor defects, but on occasion they are so extensive that they cause cosmetic or functional problems. Removal of birth marks depends on their type, severity, and location. Many will fade on their own in time.

MILIARIA RUBRA

Miliaria rubra is another name for prickly heat or heat rash. The sweat pores are blocked, so the sweat seeps into the epidermis or dermis. Overdressing the baby should be avoided. Light powdering of the skin with cornstarch may be helpful.

CHAFING

The skin in folds may become quite inflamed because of friction caused by the rubbing together of the skin areas. Chafing can be prevented by keeping the area dry and clean. Creases such as those in the neck, groin, and buttocks require good hygiene.

CAPUT SUCCEDANEUM

The soft tissues of the scalp may become swollen as a result of the delivery. The condition is called **caput succedaneum**. Fluid collects under the scalp on top of the skull. After a few days, the fluid is absorbed.

CEPHALHEMATOMA

Cephalhematoma differs from caput succedaneum in that the fluid is bloody and collects under the covering layer of the skull bone and is located within the bone structure. Although it is disfiguring, the condition requires no treatment. The fluid is absorbed in a few days.

IMPETIGO

Impetigo is a serious skin infection caused by staphylococcal organisms. Lesions appear on the body; when ruptured, they spread to other areas. It is a contagious skin disorder; the condition can spread quickly unless strict isolation of the infant is carried out. An antibacterial soap, usually hexachlorophene, is used. Ointments and systemic penicillin may be ordered by the physician.

INCIDENCE OF BIRTH ANOMALIES

The majority of babies born are perfectly formed, mature, healthy babies. A small percent, however, are born with a disease or defect. With modern technology and advanced medical science, many diseases and deformities that once caused death can now be cured or greatly lessened.

REVIEW QUESTIONS

A. Multiple choice. Select the best answer.

1. A metabolic disease caused by failure of the body to oxidize a certain amino acid is
   a. erythroblastosis fetalis
   b. hyaline membrane disease
   c. narcosis
   d. phenylketonuria

2. Jaundice that appears before the third day of life
   a. has little medical significance
   b. is called physiological jaundice
   c. may indicate a hemolytic disease
   d. is to be expected in all infants

3. The color of the normal newborn at the moment of birth is
   a. rosy pink
   b. slightly blue
   c. pale white
   d. slightly yellow

4. Temporary paralysis of the muscles on one side of the face can be caused by
   a. pressure of forceps on the facial nerve
   b. severe uterine contractions
   c. analgesic drugs given the mother during labor
   d. disproportion of the baby's head size and mother's pelvis

5. Mental retardation can be caused by
   a. phenylketonuria
   b. narcosis
   c. thrush
   d. pyloric stenosis

6. Meningomyelocele is a condition in which
   a. a vertebra is defective
   b. the meninges protrude through the opening of the spinal cavity
   c. the spinal cord and meninges protrude through the defect in the bony rings of the spinal canal
   d. the posterior portion of the laminae of the vertebrae fails to close

7. Erb's palsy is defined as
   a. an abnormal shortening of the sternocleidomastoid muscle
   b. partial paralysis of the arm due to injury to the brachial plexus
   c. temporary paralysis of the muscle on one side of the face
   d. one or both feet may turn inward, outward, downward, or upward

8. A condition which can affect both male and female infants where the breasts enlarge and sometimes secrete tiny amounts of fluid is known as
   a. congenital exophthalmic goiter
   b. linea alba
   c. pseudohermaphroditism
   d. gynecomastia

9. The principles to follow when treating a baby who does not breathe spontaneously at birth are
   a. gentleness and proper positioning
   b. artificial respiration
   c. removal of mucus
   d. all of the above

10. Intrauterine asphyxia could be caused by all of the following *except*
    a. prolapsed cord
    b. placenta abruptio
    c. omentum
    d. extremely severe uterine contractions

B. Match the term in column II to the correct description in column I.

Column I	Column II
1. unconscious state caused by drugs	a. anoxia
2. deprivation of oxygen	b. asphyxia neonatorum
3. fissure in the roof of the mouth	c. bilirubin
4. product of red blood cell destruction	d. cleft palate
5. exposure to fluorescent blue light	e. dyspnea
6. vertical split in upper lip	f. harelip
7. an amino acid	g. hyaline membrane disease
8. imperfect breathing in the newborn	h. narcosis
9. Respiratory distress syndrome	i. phenylalanine
10. difficult breathing	j. phototherapy

C. Briefly answer the following questions.

1. List five signs of respiratory distress.
2. What is the treatment for erythroblastosis fetalis?

SUGGESTED ACTIVITIES

- Discuss the possible causes of birth defects. Draw on your personal experiences and talk about emotions involved.
- Write a report on how you think you would react when assisting in the birth of a severely deformed infant. Determine ways to overcome any negative feelings you may have.
- With another classmate, role play a nurse presenting a baby with a birth defect to the mother for the first time. Be prepared to offer acceptance and encouragement. Encourage the "mother" to talk about her feelings. Exchange roles and play the mother while another student plays the nurse.
- Research the causes for mental retardation. Present a paper or talk on one of the causes.
- Contact community resources for information about prenatal clinics. Make arrangements to attend one and discuss your observations with the class.

BIBLIOGRAPHY

Lesner, P. *Pediatric Nursing*, 2nd ed. Albany, NY: Delmar Publishers, 1985.

Smith, C. A. *A Critically Ill Child*, 3rd ed. Philadelphia: W. B. Saunders, 1985.

UNIT

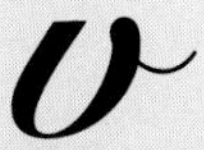

Growth and Development

CHAPTER

21

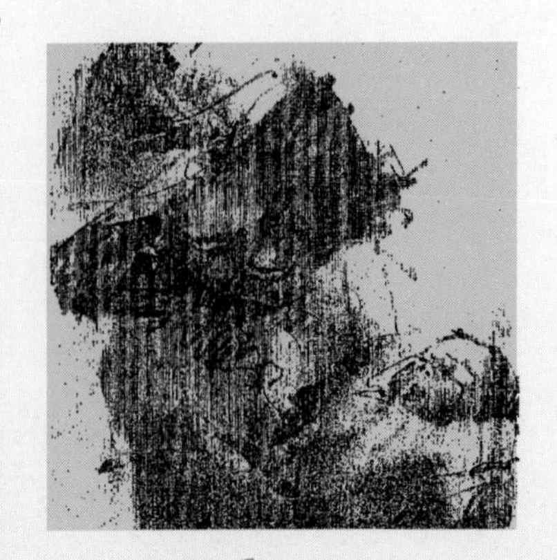

Principles of Growth and Development

Objectives

After studying this chapter, the student should be able to:

- Discuss principles of growth and development.
- Distinguish between cephalocaudal growth and proximodistal growth.
- Identify the variations in growth rate that occur as children mature.
- Describe the differences in growth rates for various parts of the body.
- Identify two factors that influence growth and development and give an example of each.

Key Terms

GROWTH
DEVELOPMENT
CEPHALOCAUDAL
PROXIMODISTAL
DIFFERENTIATION
INTEGRATION

Growth is the continuous and complex process in which the body and its parts increase in size. It can be evaluated numerically; for example, height, weight, arm length, leg length, and head circumference can be measured using numbers. **Development** is the qualitative, continuous process in which the child's level of functioning and progression of skills become more complex. For example, children babble before they use words and use two- or three-word phrases before they speak in sentences.

Several principles that govern how growth and development proceed are listed in Figure 21–1. This chapter discusses these principles and provides an overview of general patterns in growth and development. More detailed information on physical growth, cognitive development, and developmental milestones is provided in Chapters 22 and 23.

Patterns of Development

Directional Patterns

Growth and development proceed in a cephalocaudal and a proximodistal direction, Figure

Principles of Growth and Development

- Growth and development proceed in a cephalocaudal and proximodistal direction and follow an orderly, sequential pattern.
- The pace of growth and development varies, and different parts of the body grow and develop at different rates.
- Behavior becomes more versatile as development proceeds.
- Differentiation of skills occurs with maturation and practice.
- Development involves the ability to move from simple to more complex tasks.
- Growth and development are influenced by such factors as heredity and environment. Development cannot proceed without appropriate stimulation.

Figure 21–1

21–2. **Cephalocaudal** refers to the process in which maturation begins at the head and moves downward to the toes. For instance, infants are able to lift their heads before they can lift their chests, and they have control of their hands before they have control of their feet. **Proximodistal** refers to the process in which development proceeds from the center of the body outward toward the extremities. Again, infants control their shoulder movements before their hand movements, grasp objects with their whole hand before using their fingers, and gaze at items before they can reach out and grasp them.

Predictable Patterns

Throughout childhood and adolescence, other definite patterns in motor, physical, cognitive, and psychosocial growth and development can also be observed. Although the time and rate at which growth and development occur

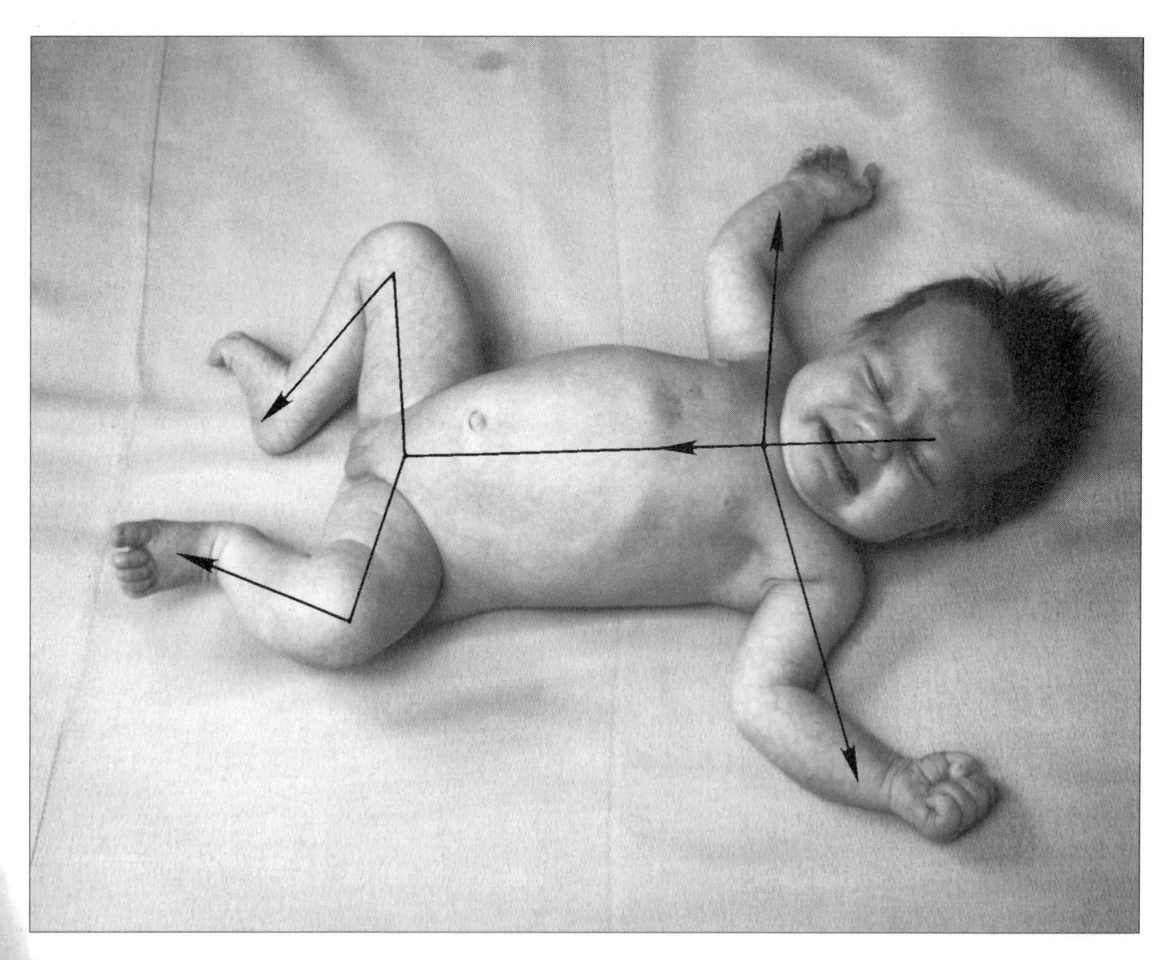

Figure 21–2 *Growth and development proceed in a cephalocaudal and a proximodistal direction.*

may vary from child to child, growth and development are predictable and follow an orderly sequence. Children achieve milestones in motor development at different ages but within an expected time frame. Although one child may walk at 10 months of age and another at 12 months, both children achieve this milestone at the expected point in their development. Furthermore, the sequence of motor development is consistent; children always sit before they stand and stand before they walk.

Cognitive development also proceeds in an orderly and sequential pattern. For example, 2-year-olds use one word to describe several objects; thus, the word *ball* describes both apple and ball. Five-year-olds, on the other hand, use words that accurately represent the objects; an apple is called an apple and a ball is called a ball. In addition, children progress from literal interpretation of words to more complex associations in a predictable sequence (Erikson 1963).

DEVELOPMENTAL PACE

Although growth and development are orderly and sequential, the pace of these processes varies throughout childhood and adolescence. In the fetus and infant, the rate of growth is very rapid. After the age of 12 months, however, growth slows and progresses at a steady pace. The growth rate again increases dramatically during adolescence. The pace of maturation for different body systems also varies. For example, the cardiovascular system matures earlier than the respiratory system. In addition, when one area is developing, development of another area seems to slow down. Thus, while children are learning to walk they concentrate on this activity, and their speech development slows.

Rates of growth and development of the parts of the body also differ. Infants' heads are large compared with the rest of their bodies; their arms and legs are relatively short. The feet and legs of toddlers and preschoolers grow more rapidly than the trunks of the body. This disproportion makes toddlers clumsy, and contributes to the number of falls they experience.

DIFFERENTIATION

Children progress from general and simple responses to more specific and complex responses as they mature. This process is termed **differentiation**. Differentiation can be seen in language development. In infancy, children only cry and babble, but by adolescence they can express complex thoughts and feelings (Gottlieb 1983). The same is true of gross motor skills. For example, 2-year-olds can jump in place, and 7-year-olds can jump rope. Differentiation also takes place throughout psychosocial development as children progress from concrete thinking to abstract thinking (Erikson 1963). Differentiation is influenced by maturation and practice. Thus, children are not able to ride a bicycle until their muscles are developmentally ready and until they have had the opportunity to learn how to ride the bicycle and practice the necessary skills.

INTEGRATION OF SKILLS

As they mature, children are able to combine simple movements or skills to achieve complex tasks (Dacey and Travers 1991). This pattern, referred to as **integration**, is seen in the progression from the simple movements of crawling to the more complex movements of walking, running, and hopping. Children learn to play catch long before they combine the skills of throwing, catching, fielding, and batting in the game of baseball. Integration is also demonstrated in cognitive development. For instance, children progress from performing simple addition and subtraction to using these abilities in the more complex calculations of higher mathematics.

FACTORS INFLUENCING GROWTH AND DEVELOPMENT

Growth and development are influenced by many interacting factors such as heredity and environment.

INFLUENCE OF HEREDITY (GENETIC FACTORS)

Genetic factors influence the child's physical characteristics, such as bone structure and height and weight. Intellectual potential and personality type are also determined by inheritance. The sex of the child, which is randomly determined at conception, affects growth patterns and how others behave toward the child.

Certain physical or mental defects that affect the child's development may be inherited. For example, muscular dystrophy (of which there is more than one kind) is a chronic, hereditary, degenerative muscle disease that affects muscle development. Children with Duchenne muscular dystrophy, the most common and severe form of the disease, usually develop noticeable muscle weakness by the third year of life. Eventually they are confined to a wheelchair.

INFLUENCE OF ENVIRONMENT

Although a child is born with certain potential features and capacities, interaction with the environment influences how and to what extent this potential is realized. If children are well nourished, growth is stimulated. If, however, children are malnourished, growth is retarded (Tanner 1978).

A stimulating environment is also important to fostering growth and development. The period of infancy and each developmental stage thereafter require stimulation by parents and caregivers. Parents can provide auditory and visual stimulation to their infants by simply talking to them while maintaining eye contact. Physical contact between parents and their young children is also important. Simple toys such as balls and wooden blocks encourage development and early exploration of the environment. Involvement in appropriate activities promotes and enhances growth and development.

Social, economic, and educational factors are part of the cultural environment that affects growth and development. Children learn how to act in certain situations by observing the people around them. Behavior that is acceptable in some families may be considered improper in other families from different ethnic backgrounds.

NURSING CARE RELATED TO PRINCIPLES OF GROWTH AND DEVELOPMENT

- Knowledge of the principles of growth and development is an important aspect of the care that nurses provide to children and adolescents.
- Nurses should anticipate the needs of parents in fostering optimal growth and development in their children.
- Nurses should act as advocates for children and adolescents so that people who work with children (teachers, coaches, and others) understand what the child is capable of accomplishing at various developmental stages.

REVIEW QUESTIONS

A. Multiple choice. Select the best answer.

1. Which of the following is most true about growth?
   a. It can be measured numerically.
   b. It refers to changes in behavior as well as size.
   c. It proceeds most rapidly in school-age children.
   d. It proceeds mainly in the limbs of newborns and infants.

2. Being able to sit before being able to stand is an example of
   a. cephalocaudal development
   b. proximodistal development
   c. growth
   d. stimulation

3. Growth and development proceed
   a. from the feet to the head
   b. at a constant rate through infancy and childhood
   c. in predictable sequences
   d. without outside stimulation

4. Which of the following variations in the rate of growth and development would you most expect?
   a. rapid growth in the preschool years
   b. rapid growth in the school-age years
   c. rapid growth in adolescence
   d. steady growth in infancy

5. Which of the following are you most apt to see?
   a. toddlers with head and body well proportioned
   b. well-coordinated toddlers
   c. preschoolers that seem to be all legs
   d. infants with head and body well proportioned

6. Which of the following is true of differentiation?
   a. It is not a progression from general to increasingly specific responses in a given area of ability.
   b. It does not apply to psychosocial development.
   c. It is unaffected by practice.
   d. It increases as muscles develop.

7. Integration has occurred in which of the following examples?
   a. being able to use a fork to help cut food after learning to hold the fork
   b. being able to sit on a bicycle before being able to ride it
   c. being able to hold a bat before being able to swing it
   d. being able to hold knitting needles before being able to knit

8. Which of the following is not an example of environmental influences on growth and development?
   a. diet
   b. culturally defined ways of training children
   c. an inherited hip defect
   d. parental expectations

B. Match the term in column I to the correct definition in column II.

Column I	Column II
1. integration	a. head-to-toe direction
2. growth	b. from center to extremity
3. proximodistal	c. an increase in size
4. differentiation	d. increase in level of functioning
5. development	e. combining simple movements or skills to achieve complex tasks
6. cephalocaudal	f. general responses becoming more specific

SUGGESTED ACTIVITIES

- List three examples of each of the following:
  - the impact of the environment on growth and development
  - the impact of heredity on growth and development
- Prepare a teaching poster to demonstrate how parents or other caregivers can stimulate some aspect of childhood development.
- List three examples of:
  - cephalocaudal development
  - proximodistal development
- Interview the parent of one child to do a case history of growth and development for a period of a child's life.
- Work individually or in teams to find three examples of each of the following developmental concepts:
  - differentiation
  - integration

BIBLIOGRAPHY

Dacey, J., and J. Travers. *Human Development across the Lifespan*. Dubuque, IA: Wm. C. Brown Publishers, 1991.

Erikson, E. H. *Childhood and Society*, 2nd ed. New York: W. W. Norton, 1963.

Gottlieb, G. The psychobiological approach to developmental issues. In P. Mussen, ed. *Handbook of Child Psychology*, 4th ed. New York: Wiley, 1983.

Tanner, J. M. *Foetus into Man: Physical Growth from Conception to Maturity*. Cambridge, MA: Harvard University Press, 1978.

CHAPTER

22

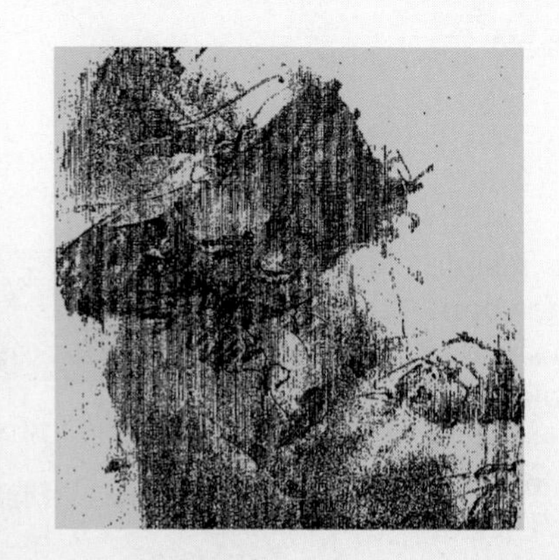

Physical Growth

Objectives

AFTER STUDYING THIS CHAPTER, THE STUDENT SHOULD BE ABLE TO:

- IDENTIFY THE MOST RAPID PERIOD OF GROWTH OCCURRING DURING THE LIFESPAN.
- DESCRIBE THE CHANGES IN HEIGHT AND WEIGHT THAT OCCUR DURING INFANCY, TODDLERHOOD, AND THE PRESCHOOL YEARS.
- DESCRIBE THE CHANGES THAT OCCUR IN THE SCHOOL-AGE YEARS AND DURING ADOLESCENCE.
- IDENTIFY THE AVERAGE AGE OF SKELETAL MATURITY IN BOYS AND GIRLS.
- DESCRIBE THE PROCESS OF PRIMARY (DECIDUOUS) AND SECONDARY (PERMANENT) TOOTH ACQUISITION.

Key Terms

INFANCY
TODDLERHOOD
PRESCHOOL
SCHOOL AGE
ADOLESCENCE
PREPUBERTAL GROWTH SPURT
ADOLESCENT GROWTH SPURT
SEXUAL MATURITY
PRIMARY (DECIDUOUS) TEETH
SECONDARY (PERMANENT) TEETH

Physical growth is one of the most visible changes of childhood. The tiny newborn becomes a strong and sturdy toddler, a slender schoolchild, and finally a gangly adolescent. Parents and relatives are often astonished at the rapid changes that occur during infancy, early childhood, and adolescence. "I can't believe how big you've gotten," is a common refrain during this period.

This chapter describes patterns of height and weight gain, skeletal growth, and tooth eruption from infancy through adolescence. Growth patterns during this period can be summarized as follows:

Infancy: A period of very rapid growth and development occurring between birth and 1 year of age

Toddlerhood: A period of slower growth occurring between 1 and 3 years of age

Preschool: A period in which physical growth slows and stabilizes occurring between 3 and 6 years of age

School Age: A period of slow, steady growth occurring between 6 and 12 years of age

Adolescence: A period of increased physical growth and development, characterized by the development of primary and secondary sex characteristics, occurring between the ages of 12 and 19 years

Cross-sectional growth charts are used to plot a child's growth from infancy through adolescence. These charts provide a statistical definition of what is considered normal by comparing the child with others of similar age and sex. Normal variations in growth may reflect ethnic or individual genetic differences in both potential for growth and timing of growth spurts (Rudolph 1991). Chapter 28 provides a detailed discussion of the techniques for measuring physical growth; refer to the appendixes at the back of this textbook for pediatric growth charts.

PHYSICAL GROWTH DURING INFANCY

Age	Physical Size
1–6 months	Birth weight is regained by 10th–14th day; gains 1.5 pounds per month until 5 months. Birth weight doubles by 6 months. Grows 1 inch per month during the first 6 months.
6–12 months	Birth weight triples by 12 months. Birth length increases 50% by the end of the first year.

Figure 22–1

PHYSICAL GROWTH

In the first year, physical growth is faster than it will be in any other period of the lifespan. The newborn baby gains weight and length rapidly, maturing into a stronger and more active infant and toddler. Physical growth continues more slowly between toddlerhood and the school-age years, until another rapid growth spurt occurs at puberty.

INFANCY AND TODDLERHOOD

By the age of 6 months, the average infant has doubled his or her birth weight, attaining a weight of about 15 pounds. By one year, birth weight has tripled, to about 22 pounds. The infant's height increases during this period by about 10 to 12 inches, with the average 1-year-old attaining a height of about 30 inches, Figure 22–1.

This period of rapid growth decreases during the second and third years. The average child gains about 5 to 6 pounds and grows approximately 3½ to 5 inches by the second birthday. During the third year, the increase is less, about 3 to 5 pounds and 2 to 2½ inches, Figure 22–2.

As the child grows, body proportions change as well. The head, which is disproportionately large in the newborn baby and toddler, becomes smaller in proportion to the rest of the body until the individual reaches his or her full adult height, Figure 22–3. Most children also become leaner in this period. Thus, by age 3, the characteristically potbellied toddler has become a slender preschooler.

PHYSICAL GROWTH DURING TODDLERHOOD

Age	Physical Size
1–2 years	Gains ½ pound or more per month. Grows 3½–5 inches during this year.
2–3 years	Gains 3–5 pounds per year. Grows 2–2½ inches per year.

Figure 22–2

PRESCHOOL AND SCHOOL-AGE YEARS

During the preschool (3–6) and school-age (6–12) years, the average child goes through a period of slow but steady growth, Figure 22–4. As the young child grows, body weight and

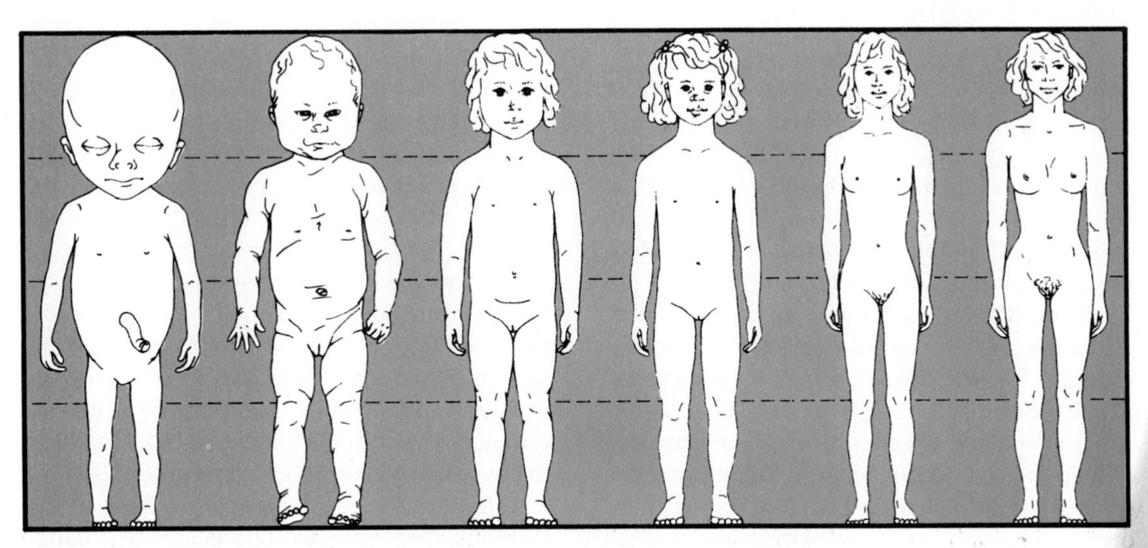

Figure 22–3 *Changes in body proportions through adolescence and young adulthood*

PHYSICAL GROWTH DURING PRESCHOOL AND SCHOOL-AGE YEARS

Age	Physical Size
3–6 years (preschool)	Gains 3–5 pounds per year. Grows 1½–2½ inches per year. Birth length doubles by 4 years.
6–12 years (school-age)	Gains 3–5 pounds per year. Grows 1½–2½ inches per year.

Figure 22–4

shape change as well. The legs are the fastest-growing part of the body during childhood. Fat tissue increases slowly until approximately age 7, when the **prepubertal growth spurt** begins. This phase precedes the true growth spurt of adolescence.

PUBERTY AND ADOLESCENCE

The trunk and legs continue to become proportionately longer during adolescence. Puberty is characterized by a rapid growth spurt, which generally begins in girls between the ages of 9½ and 14½ (usually at about age 10) and in boys between the ages of 10½ and 16 (usually at about age 12 or 13). This period of accelerated growth typically lasts about 2 years.

In both sexes, the **adolescent growth spurt** affects practically all skeletal and muscular growth. During this period, the adolescent gains almost half of his or her final adult weight, and the skeleton and organ systems double in size. These changes are more pronounced in boys than in girls and follow their own timetables. Thus, parts of the body may be out of proportion for a time. The familiar awkwardness that characterizes the teenage years is a result of this unbalanced, rapid growth. During adolescence, boys also develop broader shoulders and greater muscle mass than girls, and girls develop a wider pelvis in preparation for childbearing. Growth in height is virtually complete by age 18, Figure 22–5.

PHYSICAL GROWTH DURING ADOLESCENCE

Age	Physical Size
12–18 years	Weight gain peaks during growth spurts and accounts for over 40% of the ideal body weight. During growth spurt, girls gain approximately 20–25 pounds; boys approximately 15–20 pounds. Girls grow approximately 5–6 inches and boys 4½–5 inches. This secondary growth spurt accounts for approximately 25% of final adult height.

Figure 22–5

Soon after the growth spurt ends, the adolescent reaches **sexual maturity**. Under the influence of the hypothalamus, pituitary, and gonadal hormones, the reproductive organs double in size during adolescence and mature to adult function. The principal sign of sexual maturity in girls is menstruation. The principal sign of sexual maturity in boys is the presence of sperm in the urine. Like that of the adolescent growth spurt, the timing of sexual maturity in boys and girls varies greatly, Figure 22–6.

Refer to the appendixes at the back of this textbook for growth charts from infancy through adolescence.

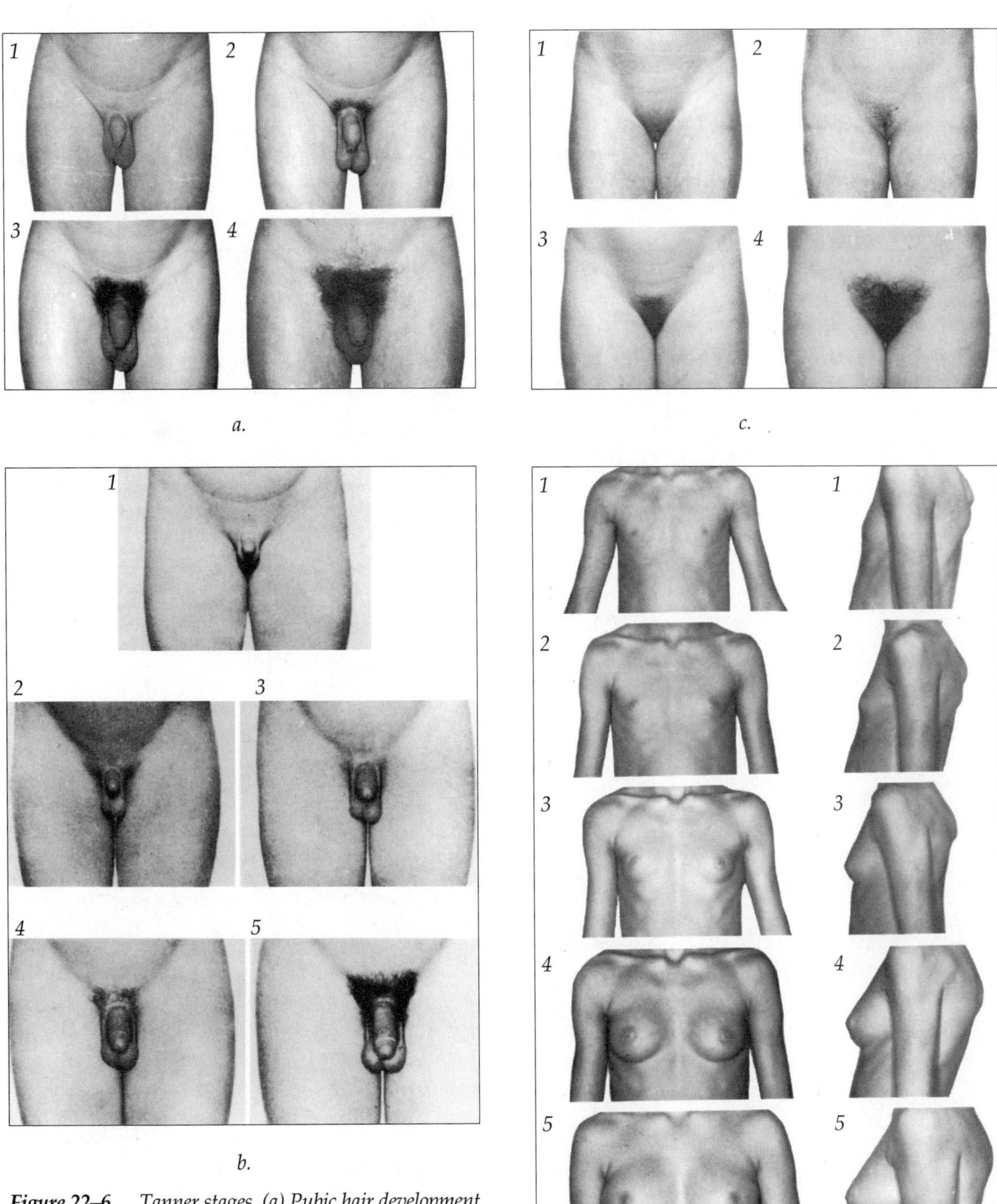

Figure 22–6 *Tanner stages. (a) Pubic hair development in males. (b) Penis and testes/scrotum development in males. (c) Pubic hair development in females. (d) Breast development in females. (From J. M. Tanner.* Growth at Adolescence, *2nd ed. Blackwell Scientific, 1962.)*

SKELETAL DEVELOPMENT

Changes in body proportion as the child grows from infancy to adulthood are related to the pattern of skeletal growth.

Skeletal growth is considered complete when the growth plates of the long bones of the arms and legs have completely fused. Completion of skeletal growth occurs, on average, in boys at 17½ years and in girls at 15½ years.

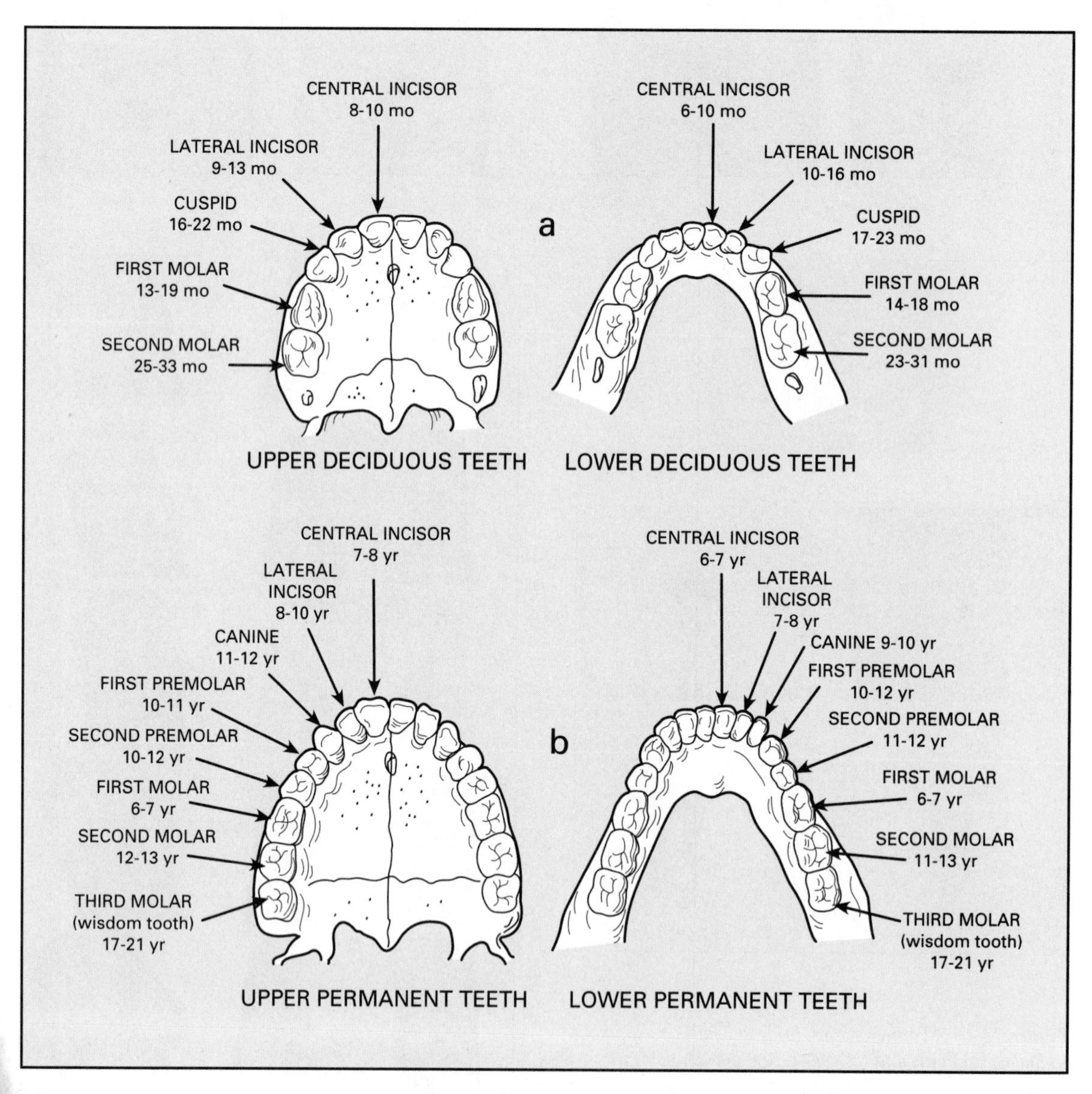

Figure 22–7 *Tooth development. (a) Primary (deciduous) teeth. (b) Secondary (permanent) teeth. (From G. L. Smith, P. E. Davis, and J. T. Dennerll.* Medical Terminology: A Programmed Text, *6th ed., Delmar Publishers, 1991.)*

Minor skeletal growth continues until approximately age 30, as additional bone is deposited to the upper and lower surfaces of the vertebrae. But this additional bone deposition accounts for only a 3- to 5-mm increase in height.

TOOTH DEVELOPMENT

PRIMARY (DECIDUOUS) TEETH

In most infants, the first tooth erupts between the ages of 5 and 9 months. By 1 year, 6 to 8 teeth usually are present. By the time a toddler reaches 33 months, approximately 20 **primary (deciduous) teeth** will have been acquired in a characteristic pattern, Figure 22–7a.

SECONDARY (PERMANENT) TEETH

The first **secondary (permanent) teeth** emerge at about 6 years, and the child continues to shed and replace teeth throughout childhood and early adulthood, see Figure 22–7b. The timing of the shedding of primary teeth and that of the eruption of secondary teeth vary widely among children.

REVIEW QUESTIONS

A. Multiple choice. Select the best answer.

1. The most rapid rate of growth during the lifespan occurs
   a. in the first year
   b. during adolescence
   c. between 3 and 6 years of age
   d. between 6 and 12 years of age

2. Which of the following is most true of first-year growth?
   a. Weight at the age of 6 months is about triple the birth weight.
   b. Birth weight triples by the end of the first year.
   c. Infant height doubles by the age of 6 months.
   d. Infant height at the end of the first year is about 40 inches.

3. You are likely to observe which of the following changes in body proportions as the child grows?
   a. The head of the toddler is well proportioned relative to the body.
   b. The legs of the growing child will be longer relative to the rest of the body than in infancy.
   c. The potbelly of the school-age child will flatten as adolescence approaches.
   d. The trunk of the adolescent looks smaller relative to the limbs than that of the school-age child.

4. After the age of 2, the number of pounds gained each year
   a. will increase until the age of 18
   b. will remain constant until the adolescent growth spurt
   c. will be about 10
   d. will be about 6
5. Which statement is true? Height increases
   a. about ½ inch per month during the first 6 months
   b. 2 to 2½ inches per year for the toddler
   c. are smaller each year from ages 3 to 12
   d. 5 to 6 inches per year for girls during the adolescent growth spurt
6. Which of the following statements is true of the adolescent growth spurt?
   a. The adolescent gains almost half of his or her final adult weight.
   b. It lasts approximately 4 years.
   c. It usually occurs between the ages of 10 and 12 years in boys.
   d. Organs triple in size.
7. Sexual maturity
   a. occurs immediately before the adolescent growth spurt
   b. occurs soon after the adolescent growth spurt ends
   c. is characterized primarily by the growth of breasts in girls
   d. is characterized primarily by the voice change in boys
8. Which of the following best describes skeletal growth?
   a. Skeletal growth is considered complete when the growth plates of the arms and legs have completely fused.
   b. The long bones of the arms and legs fuse during the school-age years.
   c. Minor skeletal growth continues throughout adult life.
   d. All skeletal growth stops after adolescence.
9. Tooth development shows which of the following patterns?
   a. The first tooth erupts between 2 and 4 months.
   b. The shedding and replacement of natural teeth continue throughout life.
   c. Before the toddler is 2 years old, 20 primary (deciduous) teeth will erupt.
   d. The first permanent teeth emerge at about 6 years of age.
10. Which of the following best describes the growth patterns of boys and girls?
    a. Growth patterns are similar during infancy and childhood.
    b. Growth patterns are markedly different in the preschool years.
    c. The rate of skeletal development differs throughout early childhood.
    d. Teeth erupt at different times in boys and girls.

SUGGESTED ACTIVITIES

- List the physical changes that you expect to occur in:
  - infancy
  - toddlerhood
  - preschool years
  - school-age years
  - adolescence
- Make color-coded charts to help you remember and compare changes in height and weight for each stage.
- Observe a growing infant, child, or adolescent for the changes discussed in this chapter. List the changes that you observe.

BIBLIOGRAPHY

Behrman, R. E. and V. C. Vaughn. *Nelson's Textbook of Pediatrics*, 13th ed. Philadelphia: W. B. Saunders, 1987.

Papalia, D. E. and S. W. Olds. *A Child's World: Infancy through Adolescence*, 6th ed. New York: McGraw-Hill, 1993.

Rudolph, A. M. *Rudolph's Pediatrics*, 19th ed. Norwalk, CT: Appleton & Lange, 1991.

Seidel, H. M., J. W. Ball, J. E. Dains, and G. W. Benedict. *Mosby's Guide to Physical Examination*, 2nd ed. St. Louis, MO: Mosby-Year Book, 1991.

Tanner, J. M. *Foetus into Man: Physical Growth from Conception to Maturity*. Cambridge, MA: Harvard University Press, 1978.

Wong, D. L. *Whaley & Wong's Essentials of Pediatric Nursing*, 4th ed. St. Louis, MO: Mosby-Year Book, 1993.

CHAPTER

23

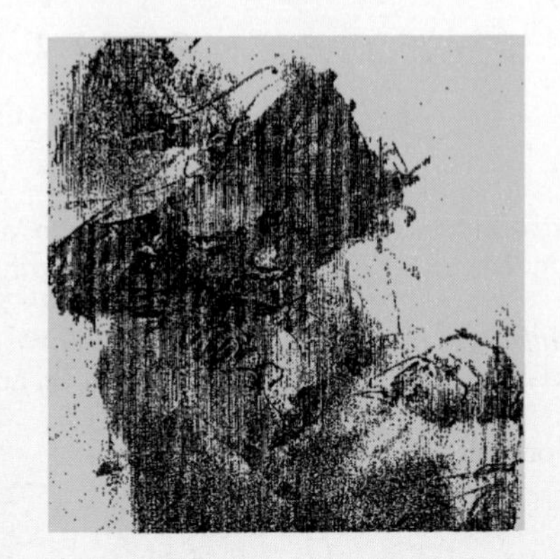

Developmental Stages

Objectives

After studying this chapter, the student should be able to:

- Identify and describe the stages of Freud's theory of psychosexual development.
- Identify and describe the stages of Erikson's theory of psychosocial development.
- Identify and describe the stages of Piaget's theory of cognitive development.
- Identify and describe the stages of Kohlberg's theory of moral development.
- Describe physical characteristics of children at various stages of development.
- Identify fine motor ability at various stages of development.
- Identify gross motor ability at various stages of development.
- Identify language skills at various stages of development.
- Identify sensory ability at various stages of development.

Key Terms

- PERSONALITY
- TEMPERAMENT
- ID
- EGO
- SUPEREGO
- PSYCHOSEXUAL DEVELOPMENT
- PSYCHOSOCIAL DEVELOPMENT
- COGNITIVE DEVELOPMENT
- MORAL DEVELOPMENT
- DENVER II DEVELOPMENTAL SCREENING TEST
- GROSS MOTOR SKILLS
- FINE MOTOR SKILLS
- ANTICIPATORY GUIDANCE

Infants and children act on their environment and in turn are stimulated by the responses they help to bring about. Through this interaction, motor, cognitive, language, and social skills are developed. This chapter introduces several theories of child development and identifies behaviors and skills that are characteristic of children at various stages of development. This information provides a useful guide for nurses who care for pediatric patients of various ages.

The following developmental stages are used in this chapter and throughout the text:

Infant: Birth through 1 year
Toddler: 1 through 3 years
Preschool Child: 3 through 6 years
School-Age Child: 6 through 12 years
Adolescent: 12 through 19 years

Personality and Temperament

Each child is a unique individual whose personality and temperament influence how the child deals with others and with the environment. **Personality** is the pattern of characteristic thoughts, feelings, and behaviors that distinguishes one person from another (Phares 1991). **Temperament** refers to a person's style of approaching other people and situations (Thomas and Chess, 1977). Early in life, children display identifiable differences in temperament. For example, parents of a new baby girl may tell the nurse, "She's such a fussy baby; she cries all the time. Our older child was so different; she was such an easy baby, laughing and smiling constantly." A child's temperament usually remains consistent as the child grows older.

THEORIES OF DEVELOPMENT

Many theorists have examined the process of child development. Among the most well known are Freud, Erikson, Piaget, and Kohlberg. These theorists identified stages of development common to all children as they mature. But because each child develops individually, he or she also demonstrates unique differences in achievement of developmental milestones.

FREUD'S THEORY OF PSYCHOSEXUAL DEVELOPMENT

According to Sigmund Freud, the personality consists of three aspects: the id, ego, and superego. The **id** represents one's desires. It is present at birth and seeks immediate gratification under the pleasure principle. The pleasure principle is the attempt to gratify needs immediately. The **ego** represents reason or common sense. The goal of the ego is to find a way to gratify the id. The **superego** represents one's conscience. It incorporates socially approved "shoulds" and "should nots" into the person's own value system.

Freud's theory of **psychosexual development** focuses on the shift of gratification from one body zone to another as the child matures. According to Freud, the developing child passes through five stages: *oral*, *anal*, *phallic*, *latent*, and *genital*, Figure 23–1.

ERIKSON'S THEORY OF PSYCHOSOCIAL DEVELOPMENT

Erik Erikson's theory of **psychosocial development** stresses societal and cultural influences on the ego at eight stages of the lifespan (Erikson 1963). Only the first five stages are related to childhood, Figure 23–2. Erikson identifies a conflict or problem — that is, a particular challenge — that must be resolved during critical periods of personality development in order for a healthy personality to develop.

PIAGET'S THEORY OF COGNITIVE DEVELOPMENT

Cognitive (or intellectual) **development** encompasses a wide variety of mental abilities, including learning, language, memory, reasoning, and thinking. Jean Piaget proposed that changes in children's thought processes result in a growing ability to acquire and use knowledge about their world (Piaget 1969). If the child is given nurturing experiences, his or her ability to think will unfold and mature naturally.

Piaget identified several stages and substages of cognitive development. The principal stages are the *sensorimotor stage*, from birth to 2 years; the *preoperational stage*, from 2 to 7 years; the *concrete operational thought stage*, from 7 to 11 years; and the *formal operational thought stage*, from 11 years through adulthood (Piaget 1969). Figure 23–3 summarizes the changes that occur during each stage.

KOHLBERG'S THEORY OF MORAL DEVELOPMENT

Lawrence Kohlberg's focus is on the aspect of cognitive development that deals with moral reasoning. He identifies three levels of **moral development**: preconventional, conventional, and postconventional (Kohlberg 1975). In the *preconventional stage* (4–7 years), the young child's decisions are based on the desire to please others and avoid punishment. In the *conventional stage* (7–11 years), conscience or an internal set of standards becomes increasingly important. In the *postconventional stage* (12 years and older), the child uses internalized ethical standards in making decisions. The person

FREUD'S STAGES OF PSYCHOSEXUAL DEVELOPMENT

Stage	Age	Description
Oral	Birth–1 year	Infant gains pleasure through the mouth, with sucking and eating the primary desires.
Anal	1–3 years	Pleasure is centered in the anal area, with control over excretion a primary force in behavior.
Phallic	3–6 years	Sexual energy becomes centered in the genitalia. During this stage the child shifts his or her identification from the parent of the same sex to the parent of the opposite sex.
Latent	6–12 years	Sexual energy is at rest. Children focus on skills and traits learned earlier. Energy is directed at learning and play.
Genital	12 years–adulthood	Focus is on mature sexual function and developing relationships with others.

Figure 23–1

who achieves this level is able to evaluate different moral approaches and make decisions on the basis of personal ethical standards.

Although Kohlberg provides age guidelines for the attainment of these stages, he emphasizes that they are approximate and that many individuals never reach the postconventional stage of moral development.

DEVELOPMENTAL SCREENING

The **Denver II Developmental Screening Test** is given to children between 1 month and 6 years of age in order to assess normal development and identify potential developmental delays, Figure 23–4 (pages 412–413). The test assesses four areas: gross motor skills, fine motor skills, personal and social development, and language development.

Gross motor skills demonstrate the child's ability to control the large muscle groups of the body. Examples of gross motor skills are rolling over, crawling, and throwing a ball. **Fine motor skills** demonstrate the child's ability to coordinate the small muscle groups. Examples of fine motor skills are grasping an object, holding a crayon, and playing a musical instrument.

Development is difficult to assess because all children demonstrate individual variations in behavior and in their acquisition of skills.

ERIKSON'S STAGES OF PSYCHOSOCIAL DEVELOPMENT

Stage	Age	Description
Trust versus mistrust	Birth–1 year	The infant must develop trust in the people who provide care. Caregivers encourage this trust when they provide food, cleanliness, touch, warmth, comfort, and freedom from pain. From this basic sense of trust develops a sense of trust in the world, other people, and oneself, and feelings of faith and optimism. If these needs are not met, the infant will mistrust others.
Autonomy versus shame and doubt	1–3 years	The toddler demonstrates a sense of autonomy or independence through control over his or her body and environment and by saying "no" when asked to do something. From this sense of autonomy, the child develops self-control and willpower. Children who are consistently criticized for expressions of independence or for lack of control will develop a sense of shame about themselves and will doubt their abilities.
Initiative versus guilt	3–6 years	The child explores the world, tries out new activities, and considers new ideas. This period of exploration creates a child who is involved and busy, with a sense of purpose and direction. Conversely, consistent criticism during this period will lead to feelings of guilt and lack of purpose.
Industry versus inferiority	6–12 years	Characterized by involvement in many interests and activities. The older child takes pride in his or her accomplishments at school, home, and in the community and learns to compete and cooperate with others. The child who is free to exercise skill and intelligence in the completion of activities develops a sense of competence. A sense of inferiority can develop if the child cannot accomplish what is expected.
Identity versus role confusion	12–18 years	Characterized by examination and redefinition of the self or identity. The adolescent questions the self, family, peers, and the community. Successful completion of this stage results in devotion and fidelity, the ability to maintain allegiance to others and to values and ideologies that are accepted during this period. Conversely, the adolescent who is unable to establish a meaningful definition of self will experience role confusion later in life.

Figure 23–2

PIAGET'S STAGES OF COGNITIVE DEVELOPMENT

Stage	Age	Description
Sensorimotor	Birth–2 years	The child learns about the world through input from the senses and by motor activity. During this period, the child begins to link cause with effect and to recognize object permanence (i.e., that an object continues to exist even when it cannot be seen). Language provides the child with a tool for understanding the world.
Preoperational	2–7 years	The child now thinks by using words as symbols, but logic is not well developed.
Concrete operational thought	7–11 years	The child develops a more accurate understanding of cause and effect, and reasons well if concrete objects are used.
Formal operational thought	11 years–adulthood	Mature intellectual thought is attained. The adolescent can reason abstractly and consider different alternatives or outcomes.

Figure 23–3

Overall Denver II test results are analyzed, and the child is classified as normal, suspect, or untestable. When results are not normal, retesting and referral should occur.

ANTICIPATORY GUIDANCE

Anticipatory guidance is an important form of teaching that provides parents with information to help them understand their children's behavior and improve their parenting skills. Anticipatory guidance about the range of normal behaviors characteristic of a particular developmental stage can increase parents' confidence in their parenting abilities by reinforcing that their expectations for their child are typical. Parents can benefit from information about the following topics:

- normal growth and development
- safety
- stimulation
- nutrition and feeding practices
- bathing
- immunizations
- sexual curiosity
- toilet training
- exercise
- vocational guidance (adolescents)
- common health problems

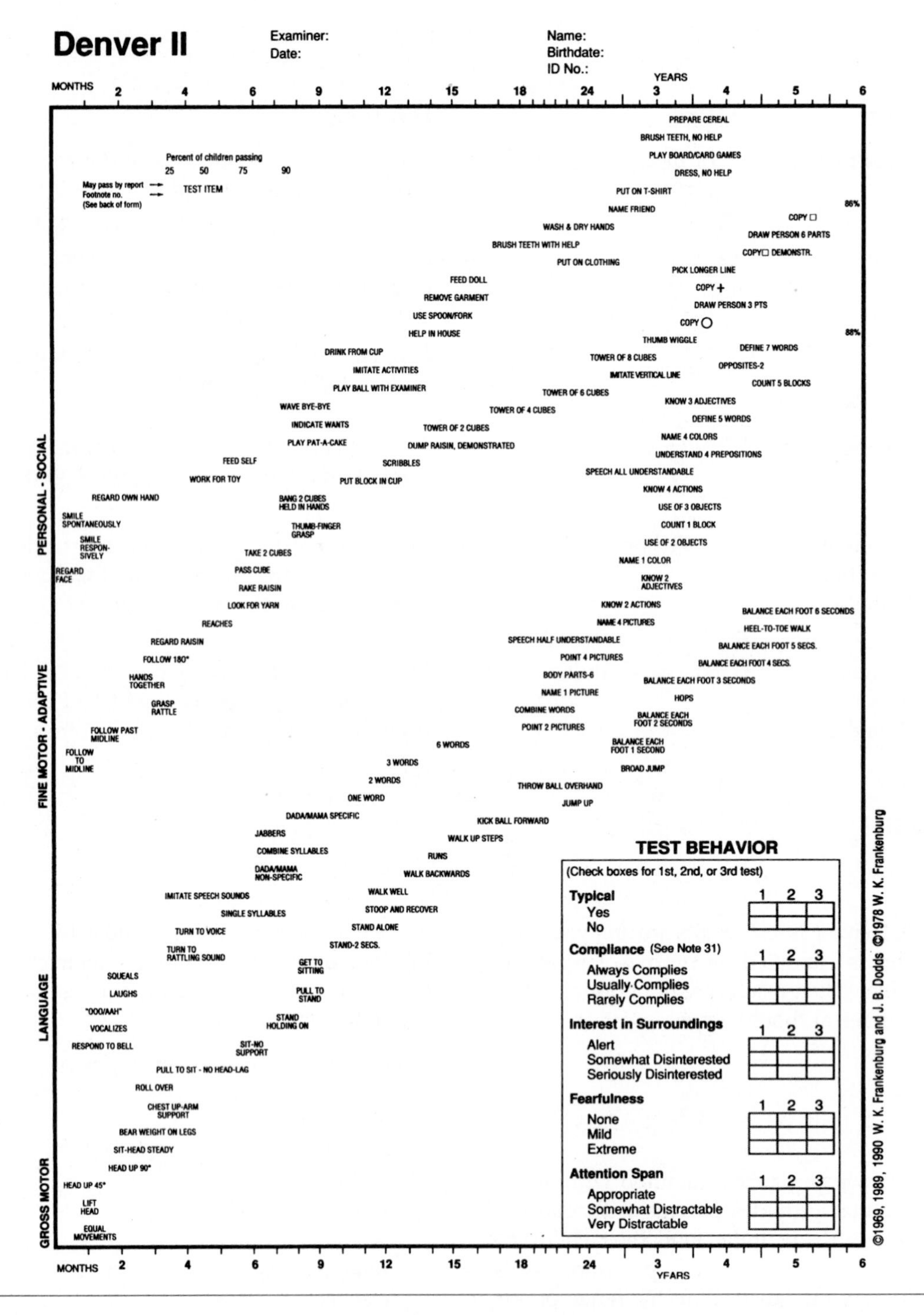

Figure 23–4 *Denver II — Revision and Restandardization of the Denver Developmental Screening Test. (From W. K. Frankenberg and J. B. Dodds, 1990)*

DIRECTIONS FOR ADMINISTRATION

1. Try to get child to smile by smiling, talking or waving. Do not touch him/her.
2. Child must stare at hand several seconds.
3. Parent may help guide toothbrush and put toothpaste on brush.
4. Child does not have to be able to tie shoes or button/zip in the back.
5. Move yarn slowly in an arc from one side to the other, about 8" above child's face.
6. Pass if child grasps rattle when it is touched to the backs or tips of fingers.
7. Pass if child tries to see where yarn went. Yarn should be dropped quickly from sight from tester's hand without arm movement.
8. Child must transfer cube from hand to hand without help of body, mouth, or table.
9. Pass if child picks up raisin with any part of thumb and finger.
10. Line can vary only 30 degrees or less from tester's line.
11. Make a fist with thumb pointing upward and wiggle only the thumb. Pass if child imitates and does not move any fingers other than the thumb.

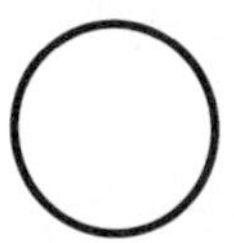

12. Pass any enclosed form. Fail continuous round motions.

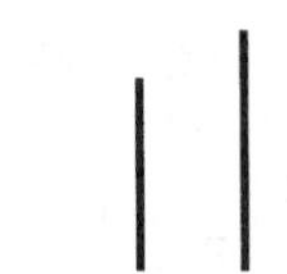

13. Which line is longer? (Not bigger.) Turn paper upside down and repeat. (pass 3 of 3 or 5 of 6)

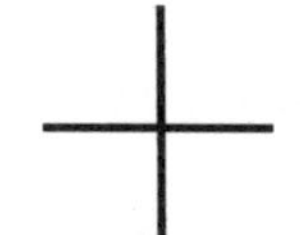

14. Pass any lines crossing near midpoint.

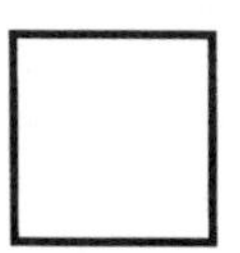

15. Have child copy first. If failed, demonstrate.

When giving items 12, 14, and 15, do not name the forms. Do not demonstrate 12 and 14.

16. When scoring, each pair (2 arms, 2 legs, etc.) counts as one part.
17. Place one cube in cup and shake gently near child's ear, but out of sight. Repeat for other ear.
18. Point to picture and have child name it. (No credit is given for sounds only.)
    If less than 4 pictures are named correctly, have child point to picture as each is named by tester.

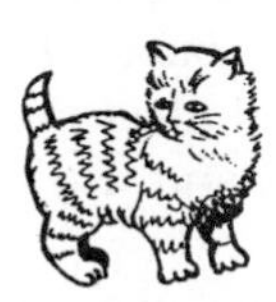
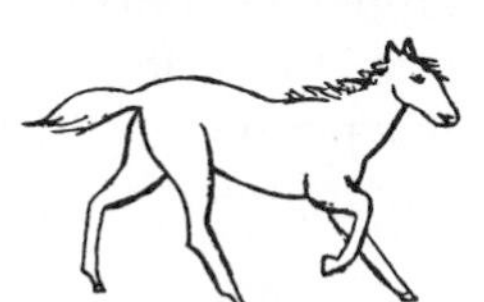
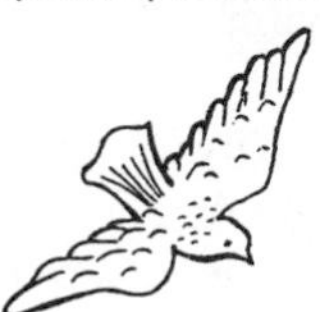
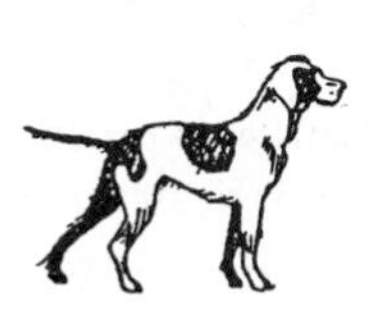
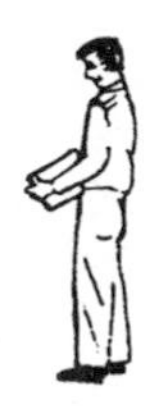

19. Using doll, tell child: Show me the nose, eyes, ears, mouth, hands, feet, tummy, hair. Pass 6 of 8.
20. Using pictures, ask child: Which one flies?... says meow?... talks?... barks?... gallops? Pass 2 of 5, 4 of 5.
21. Ask child: What do you do when you are cold?... tired?... hungry? Pass 2 of 3, 3 of 3.
22. Ask child: What do you do with a cup? What is a chair used for? What is a pencil used for?
    Action words must be included in answers.
23. Pass if child correctly places <u>and</u> says how many blocks are on paper. (1, 5).
24. Tell child: Put block **on** table; **under** table; **in front of** me, **behind** me. Pass 4 of 4.
    (Do not help child by pointing, moving head or eyes.)
25. Ask child: What is a ball?... lake?... desk?... house?... banana?... curtain?... fence?... ceiling? Pass if defined in terms of use, shape, what it is made of, or general category (such as banana is fruit, not just yellow). Pass 5 of 8, 7 of 8.
26. Ask child: If a horse is big, a mouse is __? If fire is hot, ice is __? If the sun shines during the day, the moon shines during the __? Pass 2 of 3.
27. Child may use wall or rail only, not person. May not crawl.
28. Child must throw ball overhand 3 feet to within arm's reach of tester.
29. Child must perform standing broad jump over width of test sheet (8 1/2 inches).
30. Tell child to walk forward, → heel within 1 inch of toe. Tester may demonstrate.
    Child must walk 4 consecutive steps.
31. In the second year, half of normal children are non-compliant.

OBSERVATIONS:

Figure 23–4 *continued*

Infant (Birth through 1 Year)

General Characteristics

Physical growth and development occur more rapidly during infancy than at any other period of life. During the first year, the infant triples his or her birth weight and by the year's end begins to walk and communicate with others.

Motor, Language, and Sensory Development

Over the course of the first year, the infant develops greater motor control, following a cephalocaudal and proximodistal pattern of development (see Chapter 21). The infant participates actively in learning through the senses and through motor activities, progressing from reflexive behaviors such as sucking and grasping to purposeful activities, such as the manipulation of objects.

Communication skills also progress rapidly during this period. Within the first few weeks of life, two-way interaction is occurring between the infant and parents or caregivers. The infant expresses comfort by cooing, cuddling, and eye contact. Discomfort is displayed by kicking the legs, arching the back, and vigorous crying. By the end of the first year, the infant has refined these communication skills and is able to speak several words.

Changes in motor, language, and sensory development during infancy are summarized in Figure 23–5.

Toddler (1 through 3 Years)

General Characteristics

The term *toddler* aptly describes children from 1 to 3 years old, who toddle from side to side as they walk, holding out their arms for balance. The ability to walk increases the toddler's independence from parents. For this reason, the toddler period has been called the first adolescence. An infant only months before, the toddler now demonstrates increasing autonomy and negativism, responding with an emphatic "No!" to parents' instructions.

Motor, Language, and Sensory Development

During the toddler period, motor skills continue to develop. The eyes now work well together, and hearing is well developed. Sometime between the end of the second and third years, toddlers learn bowel and bladder control.

The rapid growth of language skills during this period emphasizes the importance of communication with toddlers. The 12- to 15-month-old child may use four to six words in addition to "mama" and "dada." By the end of this period, the 3-year-old has a vocabulary of more than 500 words and uses short sentences.

Changes in motor, language, and sensory development during toddlerhood are summarized in Figure 23–5.

Preschool Child (3 through 6 Years)

General Characteristics

The preschool years are characterized by increasing initiative and independence. Preschoolers have mastered many gross motor and some fine motor skills, and they can communicate both verbally and nonverbally. During the preschool period, these skills are refined, and children learn the social skills that will prepare them to function in the school environment.

DEVELOPMENTAL STAGE — INFANCY

Age	Gross Motor	Fine Motor	Language	Sensory
Birth–1 month	• Assumes tonic neck posture • When prone lifts and turns head	• Holds hands in fist • Draws arms and legs to body 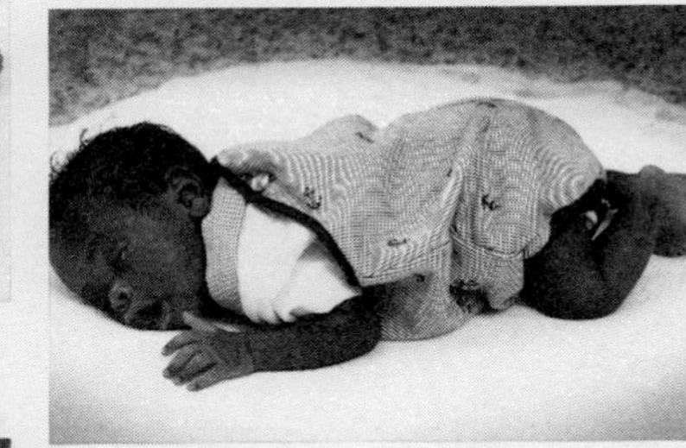 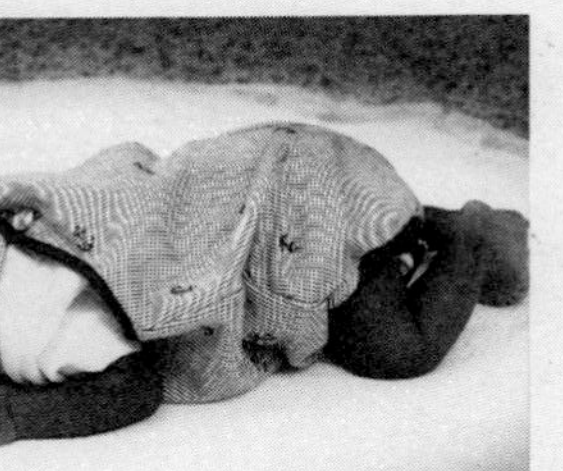	• Cries	• Comforts with holding and touch • Looks at faces • Follows objects when in line of vision • Alert to high-pitched voices • Smiles
2–4 months	• Can raise head and shoulders when prone to 45°–90°; supports self on forearms • Rolls from back to side 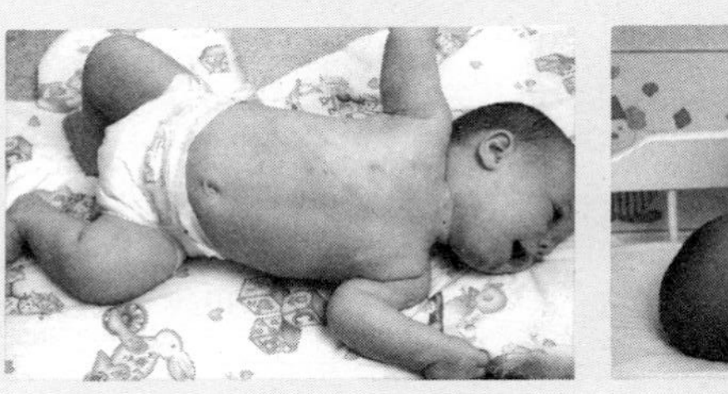	• Hands mostly open • Looks at and plays with fingers • Grasps and tries to reach objects 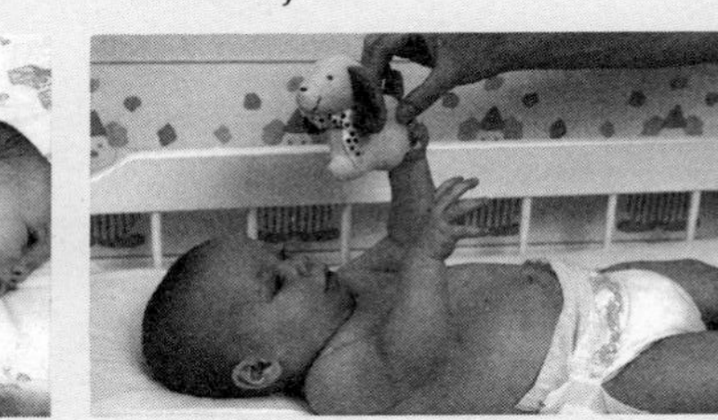 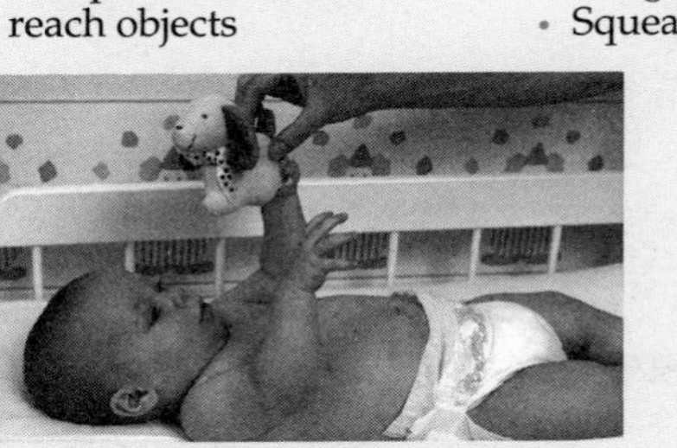	• Vocalizes when talked to; coos, babbles • Laughs aloud • Squeals	• Smiles • Follows objects 180 degrees • Turns head when hears voices or sounds

Figure 23–5 *Stages of development; infancy through adolescence (Developed by Barbara Ellen Norwitz, BSN, RN, PNP)*

DEVELOPMENTAL STAGE — INFANCY

Age	Gross Motor	Fine Motor	Language	Sensory
4–6 months	• Turns from stomach to back and then back to stomach • When pulled to sitting almost no head lag	• Can hold feet and put in mouth • Can hold bottle	• Squeals	• Watches a falling object • Responds to sounds
	• By 6 months can sit on floor with hands forward for support	• Can grasp rattle and other small objects • Puts objects in mouth		

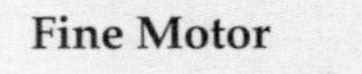

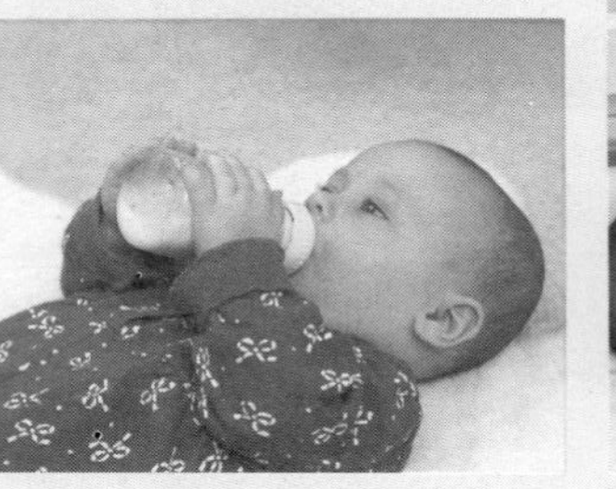

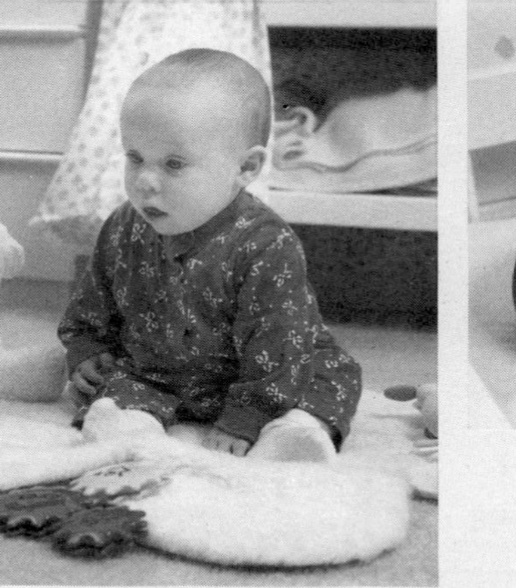

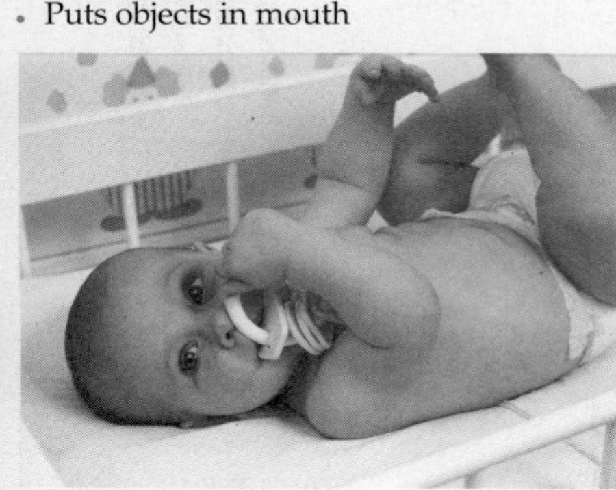

Figure 23–5 *continued*

DEVELOPMENTAL STAGE — INFANCY

Age	Gross Motor	Fine Motor	Language	Sensory
6–8 months	• Puts full weight on legs when held in standing position • Can sit without support • Bounces when held in a standing position	• Transfers objects from one hand to the other • Can feed self a cookie • Can bang two objects together	• Babbles vowel like-sounds, ooh or aah • Imitation of speech sounds, (mama, dada) beginning • Laughs aloud	• Responds by looking and smiling • Recognizes own name

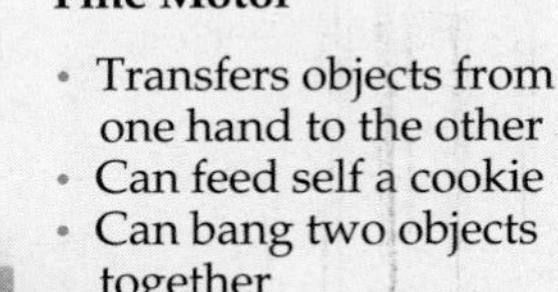
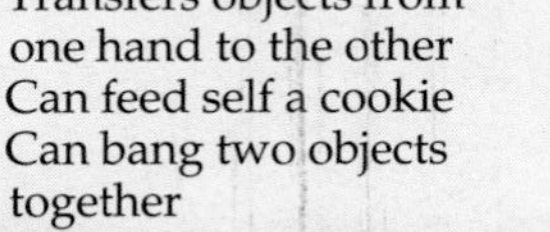
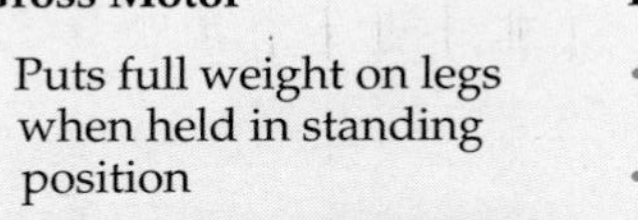
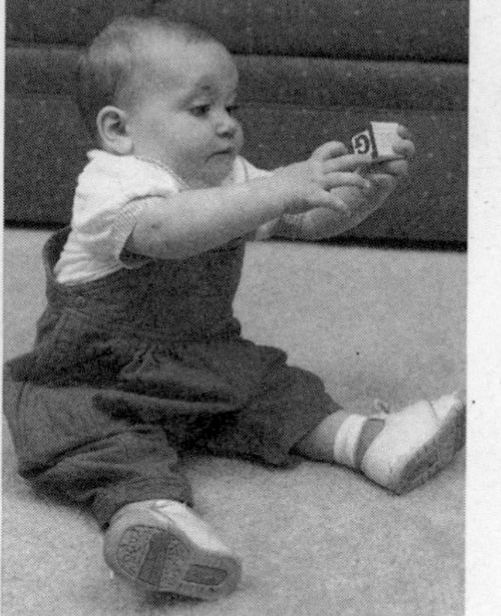
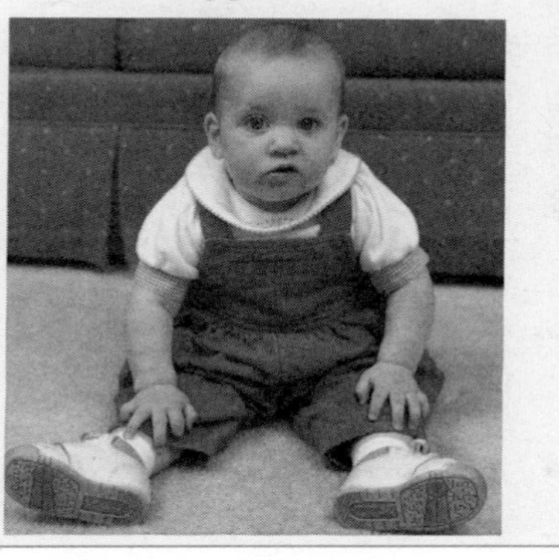

Figure 23–5 *continued*

DEVELOPMENTAL STAGE — INFANCY

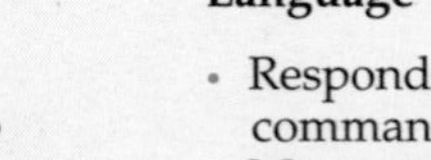

Age	Gross Motor	Fine Motor	Language	Sensory
8–10 months	• Crawls on all fours or uses arms to pull body along floor	• Beginning to use thumb-finger grasp • Dominant hand use • Has good hand-mouth coordination	• Responds to verbal commands • May say one word in addition to "mama" and "dada"	• Recognizes sounds

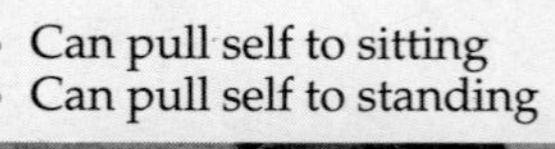

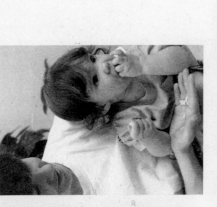

• Can pull self to sitting
• Can pull self to standing

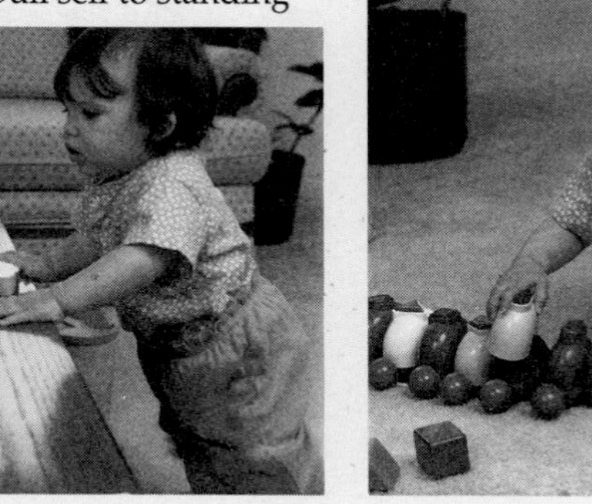

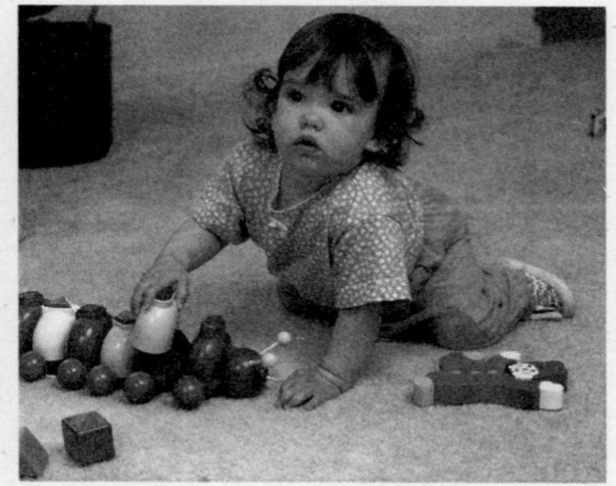

Figure 23–5 *continued*

DEVELOPMENTAL STAGE — INFANCY

Age

10–12 months

Gross Motor

- Can sit down from standing
- Walks around room holding onto objects
- Can stand alone

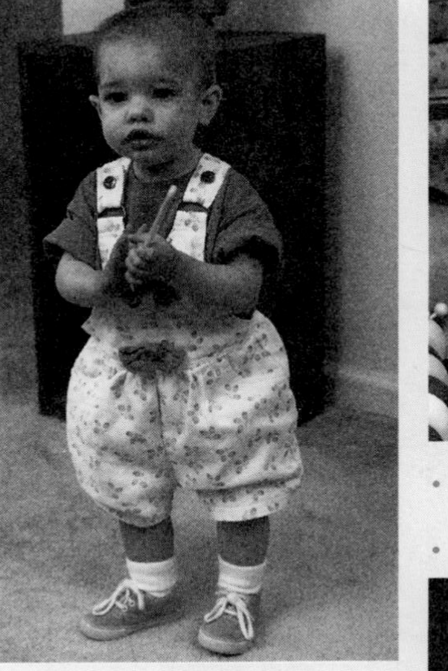

Fine Motor

- Picks up and drops objects
- Can put small objects into toys or containers through holes

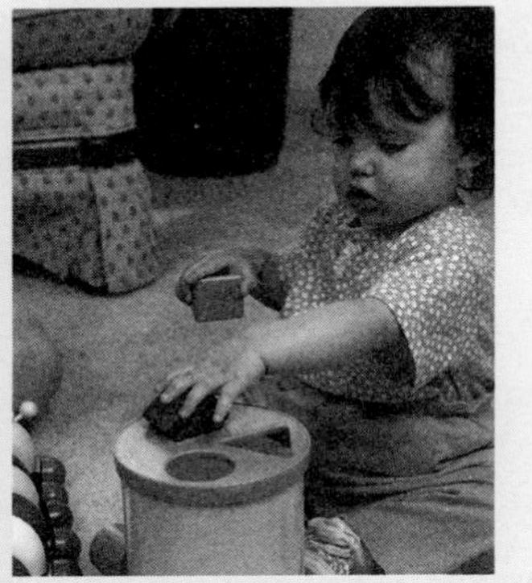

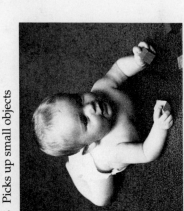

- Turns many pages in a book at one time
- Picks up small objects

Language

- Understands "no" and other simple commands
- Learns 1–2 other words
- Imitates speech sounds
- Speaks gibberish

Sensory

- Follows fast-moving objects
- Indicates wants
- Likes to play imitative games such as patty cake and peek-a-boo

Figure 23–5 *continued*

DEVELOPMENTAL STAGE — TODDLERHOOD

Age	Gross Motor	Fine Motor	Language	Sensory
12–15 months	• Can walk alone well • Can crawl up stairs	• Can feed self with cup and spoon • Puts raisins into a bottle • May hold crayon or pencil and scribble • Builds a tower of two cubes	• Says four to six words	• Binocular vision developed

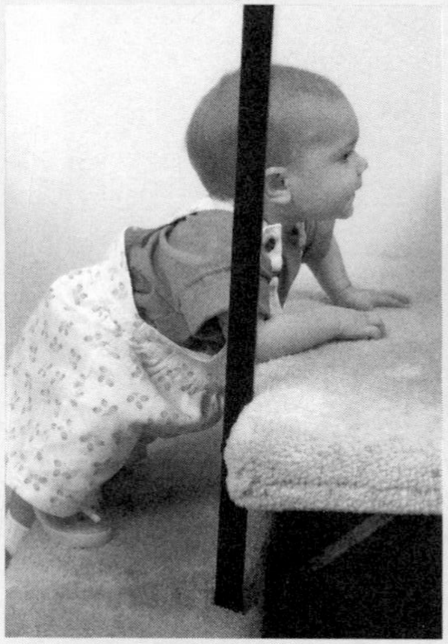

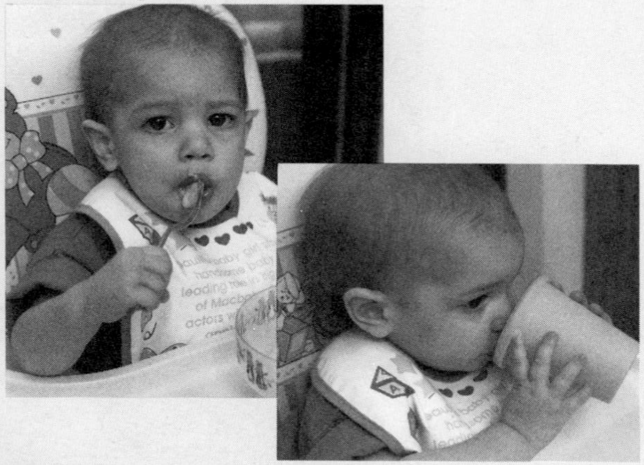

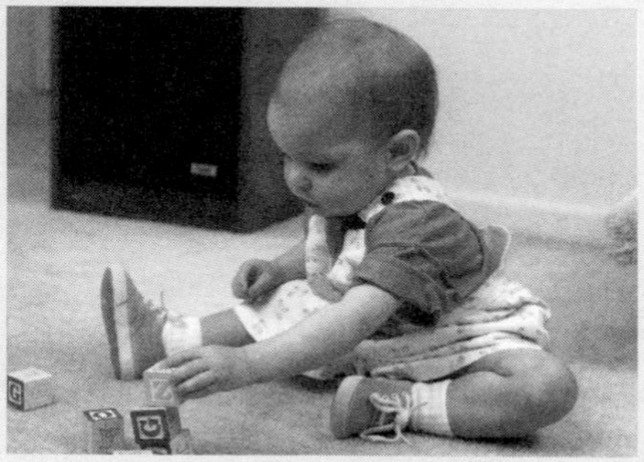

Figure 23–5 *continued*

DEVELOPMENTAL STAGE — TODDLERHOOD

Age	Gross Motor	Fine Motor	Language	Sensory
18 months	• Runs, falling often • Can jump in place • Can walk up stairs holding on • Plays with push and pull toys	• Can build a tower of 3–4 cubes • Can use a spoon	• Says 10 or more words • Points to objects or body parts when asked	• Visual acuity 20/40

Figure 23–5 *continued*

DEVELOPMENTAL STAGE — TODDLERHOOD

Age	Gross Motor	Fine Motor	Language	Sensory
24 months	• Can walk up and down stairs • Can kick a ball • Can ride a tricycle	• Can draw a circle • Tries to dress self	• Talks a lot • Approximately 300-word vocabulary • Understands commands • Knows first name, refers to self • Verbalizes toilet needs	
30 months	• Throws a ball • Jumps with both feet • Can stand on one foot for a few minutes	• Can build a tower of 8 blocks • Can use crayons • Learning to use scissors	• Knows first and last name • Knows the name of 1 color • Can sing • Expresses needs • Uses pronouns appropriately	

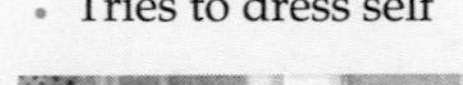

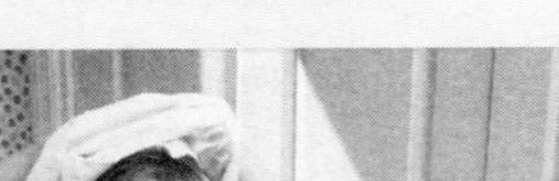

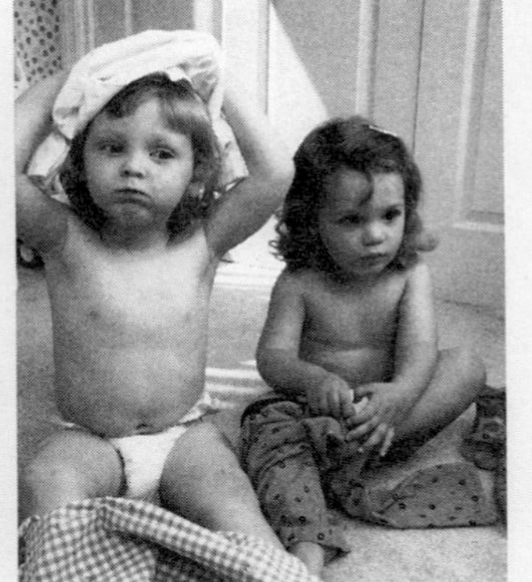

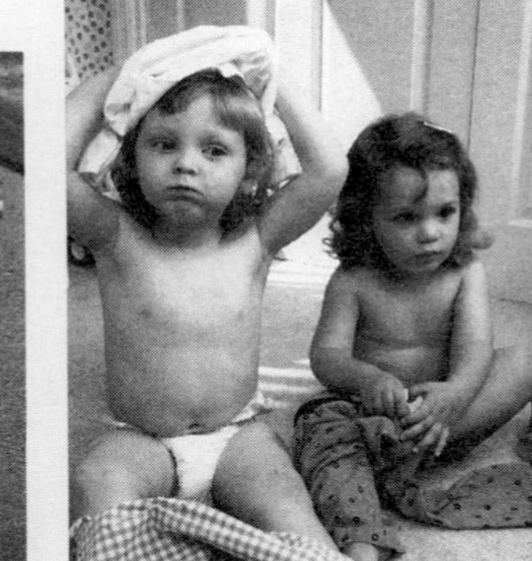

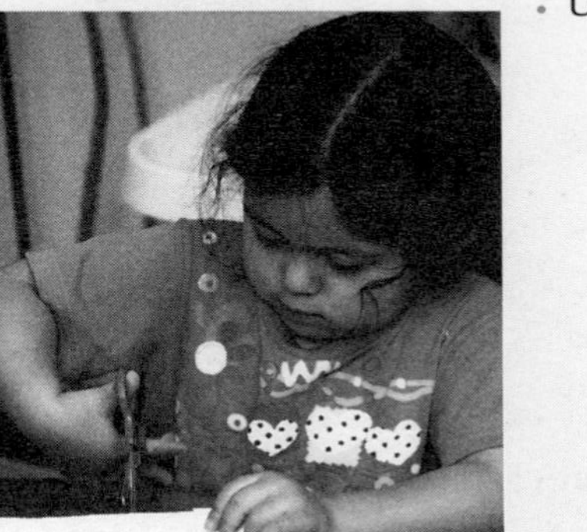

Figure 23–5 *continued*

DEVELOPMENTAL STAGE — PRESCHOOL AGE

Age	Gross Motor	Fine Motor	Language	Sensory
3–6 years	• Can ride a bike with training wheels • Can throw a ball overhand • Skips and hops on one foot • Can climb well • Can jump rope	• Can draw a six-part person • Can use a scissors • Can draw circle, square or cross • Likes art projects, likes to paste and string beads • Can button • Learns to tie and buckle shoes • Can brush teeth	• Language skills are well developed with the child able to understand and speak clearly • Vocabulary grows to over 2,000 words • Talks endlessly and asks questions	• Visual acuity well-developed • Focused on learning letters and numbers

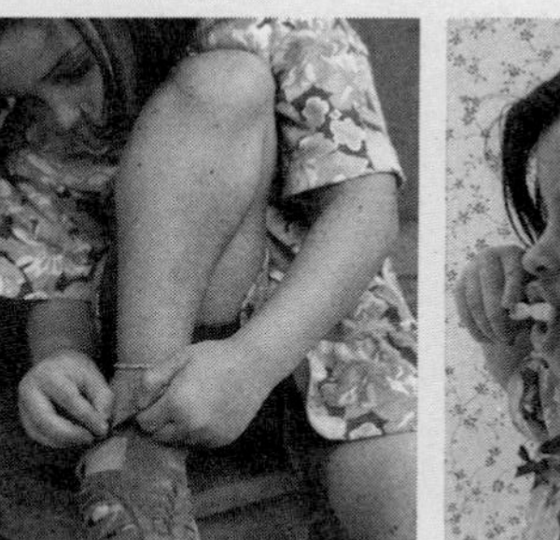
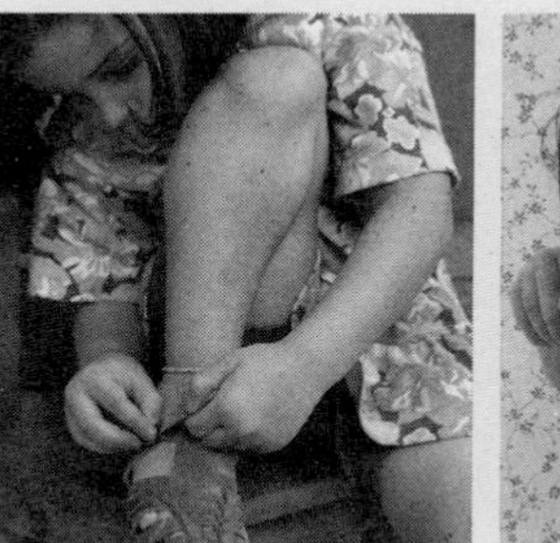
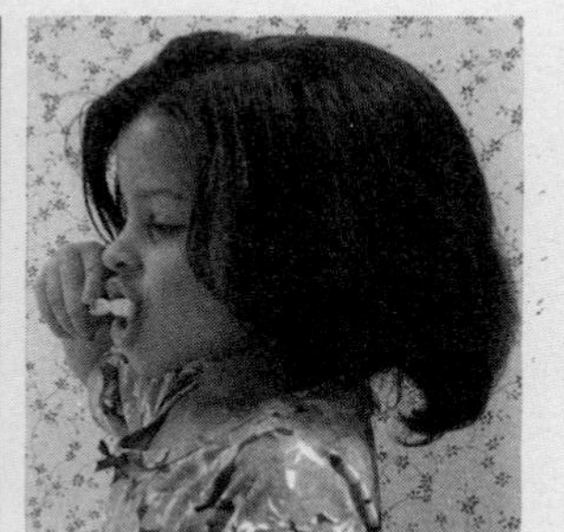

Figure 23–5 *continued*

Developmental Stage — Preschool Age

Age	Gross Motor	Fine Motor	Language	Sensory
6–12 years	• Can use rollerblades or ice skates • Able to ride two-wheeler • Plays baseball	• Can put models together • Likes crafts • Enjoys board games, plays cards	• Vocabulary increases • Language abilities continue to develop	• Reading • Able to concentrate on activities for longer periods

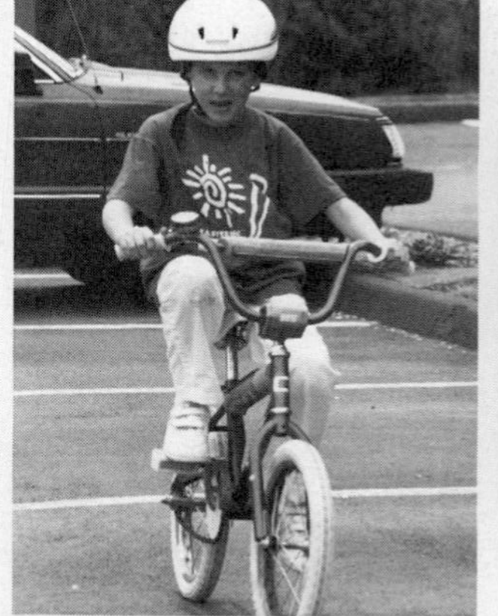

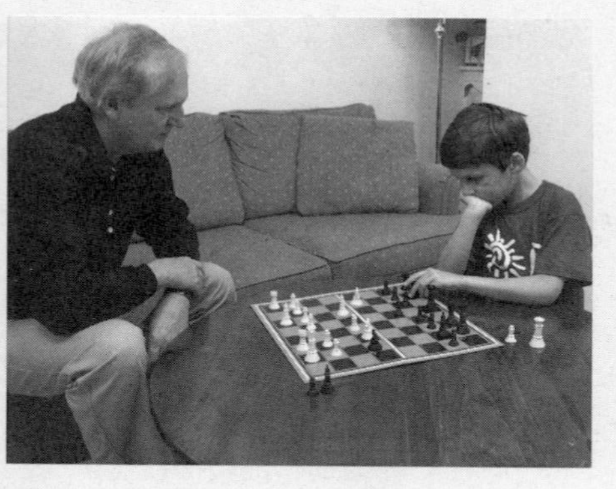

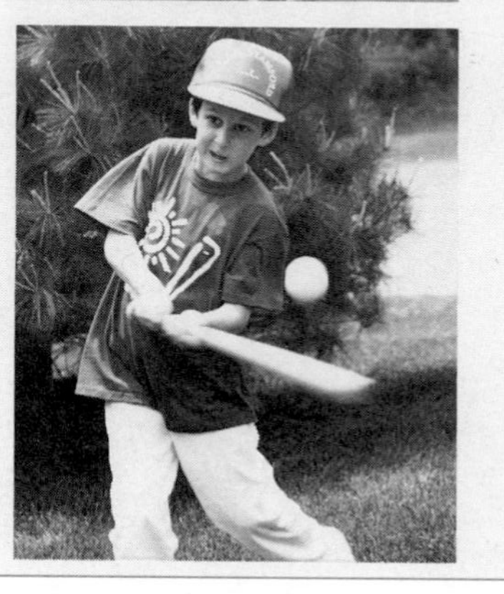

Figure 23–5 *continued*

DEVELOPMENTAL STAGE — ADOLESCENCE

Age	Gross Motor	Fine Motor	Language	Sensory
12–19 years	• Muscles continue to develop • At times awkward, with some lack of coordination	• Well-developed skills	• Vocabulary fully developed	• Development complete

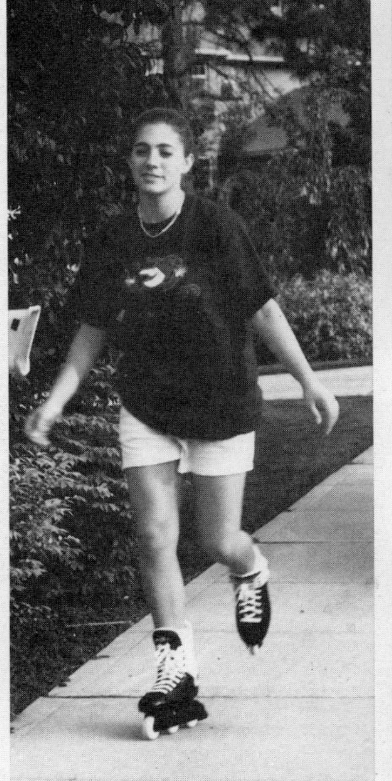

Figure 23–5 *continued*

MOTOR, LANGUAGE, AND SENSORY DEVELOPMENT

Most preschool children display more precisely controlled movements than they demonstrated as toddlers. The ability to participate successfully in games and other physical activities enhances preschoolers' self-esteem. Interaction with others during play, in turn, encourages the growth of social skills.

Language skills continue to expand during the preschool years. The preschooler has a vocabulary of more than 2,000 words and uses complete sentences of several words. Although many words are used, the preschooler's grasp of their meaning is usually quite literal. For example, children may interpret a statement such as "you're going to cough your head off" to mean that their head is going to fall off.

Figure 23–5 summarizes changes in motor, language, and sensory development during the preschool years.

SCHOOL-AGE CHILD (6 THROUGH 12 YEARS)

GENERAL CHARACTERISTICS

Interactions with peers, growth of intellectual skills, and continued refinement of fine motor and gross motor skills characterize children in the school-age period. Activities such as playing an instrument or helping with chores help the school-age child to develop a sense of self-worth.

MOTOR, LANGUAGE, AND SENSORY DEVELOPMENT

School-age children have the fine motor skills necessary to color, draw, write, and play a musical instrument or board game, and they have the physical and social skills needed for team sports and group activities. Vocabulary continues to increase, and the child's reading and writing skills expand rapidly. Children in this period also learn to apply rules for interacting with people outside their families.

Refer to Figure 23–5 for a summary of changes in motor, language, and sensory development during the school-age years.

ADOLESCENT (12 THROUGH 19 YEARS)

GENERAL CHARACTERISTICS

Adolescence is generally thought of as a time of transition into adulthood. Adolescents are trying to establish an identity of their own by experimenting with adult roles and behaviors.

MOTOR, LANGUAGE, AND SOCIAL DEVELOPMENT

Although some awkwardness and lack of coordination may accompany the adolescent growth spurt, increased dexterity, strength, and endurance are characteristic of the teenage years. Language skills are well developed. The adolescent increasingly demonstrates independence from parents, establishing close ties with peers. These relationships form the basis of an adult identity. Traditional values that were accepted during childhood are often questioned. But the adolescent must also develop the emotional maturity and motivation to make wise choices. Encouragement from family and significant others and practice in dealing with difficult decisions can help adolescents to become less impulsive and self-centered when solving problems.

Refer to Figure 23–5 for a summary of changes in motor, language, and sensory development during adolescence.

NURSING CARE RELATED TO DEVELOPMENTAL STAGES

- When caring for or teaching pediatric patients, always keep in mind the age and developmental stage of the child.
- Review with parents realistic expectations for their child's stage of development, and caution them not to expect skills that are beyond the developmental level of their child.
- Provide infants with touch, comfort, and security.
- Anticipate the infant's need to suck by providing a pacifier.
- Anticipate the preschool child's concerns about sexuality by providing privacy and clear explanations about any procedures involving the genital area.
- When speaking to preschoolers, remember that they interpret your words literally.
- Allow children to manipulate medical equipment safely in order to see for themselves how it works.
- Anticipate the adolescent's focus on relationships by asking about friends and family.
- Provide adolescents with information and allow them, when possible, to choose among alternative treatments.

REVIEW QUESTIONS

A. Multiple choice. Select the best answer.

1. The theory of cognitive (intellectual) development was proposed by
   a. Freud
   b. Piaget
   c. Erikson
   d. Kohlberg
2. The final stage of development in Freud's theory is
   a. oral
   b. anal
   c. phallic
   d. genital
3. According to Erikson, a child between the ages of 3 and 6 years is in the stage of
   a. trust versus mistrust
   b. autonomy versus shame and doubt
   c. initiative versus guilt
   d. identity versus industry
4. The final stage of cognitive development according to Piaget is
   a. formal operational thought
   b. sensorimotor
   c. concrete operational thought
   d. preoperational
5. The highest stage of moral development according to Kohlberg is the
   a. conventional
   b. preconventional
   c. postconventional
   d. nonconventional

6. Which of the following statements is true according to Kohlberg's theory?
   a. The young child's moral decisions are based on the desire to please others or to avoid being punished.
   b. The young child earns approval by following rules.
   c. The school-age child begins to internalize ethical standards for forming his or her own decisions and weighing the value of differing moral approaches.
   d. Most people reach the postconventional stage before age 20.

7. Erikson's theory holds that
   a. trust develops first in children between 3 and 6 years of age
   b. the toddler must learn to obey others
   c. the adolescent is mainly concerned with building a sense of competence
   d. a particular social or psychological challenge has to be met at each stage for a healthy personality to develop

8. Freud's stages focus on
   a. shifts in gratification from one body area to another as development unfolds
   b. how a child learns right from wrong
   c. how children think as they develop
   d. developmental tasks

9. The Denver II Developmental Screening Test assesses
   a. cognitive development
   b. intelligence quotient
   c. personal and social development
   d. sexual development

10. The infant stage of development is typically characterized by
    a. the infant's active participation in sensory and motor learning
    b. one-way interaction until the second week of life
    c. lack of purposeful activities
    d. a vocabulary of more than 100 words

11. During the toddler stage, you can observe
    a. the ability to coordinate games with other toddlers
    b. well-developed fine motor skills
    c. a precisely controlled gait
    d. the use of short sentences

12. The preschool child
    a. has mastered all fine motor skills
    b. cannot yet participate in games with other children
    c. uses complete sentences of several words
    d. has mastered few gross motor skills

13. When working with preschoolers, you ought to
    a. joke about their literal interpretation of words
    b. acknowledge concerns about sexuality by maintaining privacy and giving clear explanations about procedures involving the genital area
    c. avoid explaining procedures in order to lessen anxiety
    d. discourage parents from participating in care in order to promote independence

14. When dealing with adolescents, you will want to
    a. avoid focusing on the importance of relationships in their lives
    b. prevent them from making choices about their own care
    c. help them become less impulsive when solving problems
    d. encourage self-centeredness

SUGGESTED ACTIVITIES

- Interview a parent about his or her child's behavior patterns. Find two examples of each of the four theories discussed in this chapter.
- Try to write a history of your own development to see how many examples of developmental changes you can recall.
- Identify three personality patterns in yourself or someone you are close to.
- Visit a day-care center or early childhood learning center and observe children's skills and activities at various ages.
- Prepare an anticipatory guidance poster for teaching parents. You choose the age group and topic to be presented.
- List the five stages of development and three characteristics unique to each one.
- Compare several children of the same age in one of the following areas:
  - fine motor ability
  - gross motor ability
  - sensory ability
  - language skills

BIBLIOGRAPHY

Erikson, E. H. *Childhood and Society*, 2nd ed. New York: W. W. Norton, 1963.

Kohlberg, L. The cognitive-developmental approach to moral education. *Phi Delta Kappa* 56, (1975): 670–677.

Papalia, D. E., and S. W. Olds. *A Child's World: Infancy through Adolescence*, 6th ed. New York: McGraw-Hill, 1993.

Phares, E. J. *Introduction to Personality*, 3rd ed. Glenview, IL: Scott, Foresman, 1991.

Piaget, J. *The Theory of Stages in Cognitive Development.* New York: McGraw-Hill, 1969.

Thomas, A. and S. Chess. *Temperament and Development*. New York: Brunner/Mazel, 1977.

Thompson, J. M., and A. C. Bowers. *Health Assessment: An Illustrated Pocket Guide*, 3rd ed. St. Louis, MO: Mosby-Year Book, 1992.

Wong, D. L. *Whaley & Wong's Essentials of Pediatric Nursing*, 4th ed. St. Louis, MO: Mosby-Year Book, 1993.

UNIT

vi

Pediatric Health Promotion

CHAPTER

24

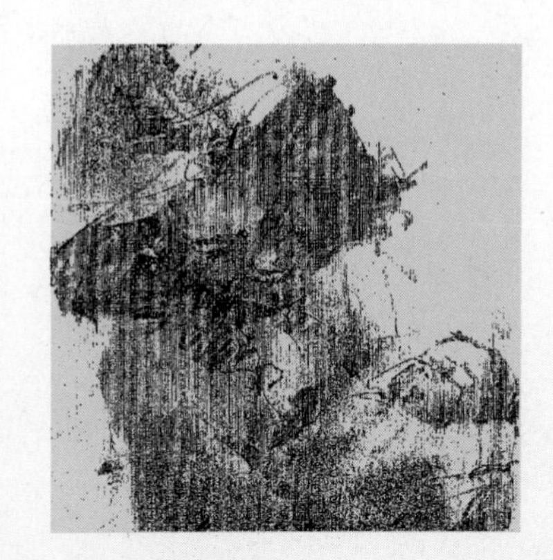

Basic Nutrition

Objectives

After studying this chapter, the student should be able to:

- List essential nutrients of a well-balanced diet and describe their functions.
- Identify several sources of each essential nutrient.
- Identify age-related nutritional needs of children.
- Explain characteristic eating patterns of children of different developmental stages.
- Provide nutritional teaching to assist parents in planning a healthy diet for children from infancy through adolescence.

Key Terms

nutrients
malnutrition
lactose
nonessential amino acids
essential amino acids
lipids
triglycerides
fatty acids
food pyramid
Recommended Dietary Allowances
ritualistic behavior

Nutrition is essential to the health and well-being of children. Adequate nutrition is especially important during periods of rapid growth and development, such as infancy and early childhood (Marotz et al. 1993). Life-long eating habits are formed in early childhood, and a healthy diet can lay the foundation for healthy eating habits in adulthood.

THE ROLE OF THE NURSE

Nurses are frequently involved in counseling children and families about diet and the importance of good nutrition. Nutritional counseling can be challenging as well as rewarding. It is important to emphasize positive eating habits that already exist in the child's diet. To be effective in counseling families and children, the nurse needs to be able to:

1. Recognize outward signs of good and poor nutrition.
2. Assess a family's nutritional intake.
3. Modify existing dietary habits to meet the goals of a prescribed treatment plan.
4. Plan meals that incorporate the child's food preferences, where possible.

Culture and religion influence the selection of food. Because there are many different cultural and religious groups in the United States, nurses must also have a knowledge of cultural food habits and preferences that affect diet, Figure 24–1.

ESSENTIAL NUTRIENTS AND THEIR FUNCTIONS

Five major **nutrients** are essential for proper body function: carbohydrates, protein, fats, minerals, and vitamins. Water, which is essential to life, is sometimes included in the category of essential nutrients. A daily intake of essential nutrients depends on eating a variety of foods in adequate amounts. Inadequate intake of essential nutrients results in **malnutrition**, Figure 24–2 (page 436).

CARBOHYDRATES

The primary function of carbohydrates is to meet the body's need for energy. Carbohydrates are the most readily available and easily converted source of energy for body metabolism. There are two categories of carbohydrates: simple and complex.

Simple carbohydrates include monosaccharides, such as glucose, fructose, and galactose, and disaccharides, such as sucrose (table sugar) and **lactose** (found in milk). Complex carbohydrates include starch and dietary fiber. The dietary fiber in carbohydrates passes through the intestinal tract unchanged because the body lacks the enzymes to digest it. There are many sources of carbohydrates, including grains and grain products, fruits, root vegetables, sugars, and syrups.

The nurse needs to use a sensible approach when teaching parents guidelines for a child's intake of sugar. Many "scare tactics" have been used to discourage sugar ingestion, leading some parents to give honey to infants and sugar substitutes to children. Parents should be warned that honey has been linked to cases of botulism in infants and that the long-term effects of many sugar substitutes are yet to be determined. A moderate approach to the intake of sugars in childhood is therefore advised.

A carbohydrate deficiency is manifested by weight loss, because protein and fat sources are being used for energy. Prolonged carbohydrate deficiency can lead to liver damage.

ETHNIC AND REGIONAL FOOD PATTERNS

Ethnic Group	Bread and Cereal	Eggs, Meat, Fish, Poultry	Dairy Products	Fruits and Vegetables	Seasonings and Fats
Italian	Northern Italy: Crusty white bread, cornmeal, and rice Southern Italy: Pasta	Beef, chicken, eggs, fish	Milk in coffee, cheese	Broccoli, zucchini, other squash, eggplant, artichokes, string beans, tomatoes, peppers, asparagus, fresh fruit	Olive oil, vinegar, salt, pepper, garlic
Puerto Rican	Rice, noodles, spaghetti, oatmeal, cornmeal	Dry salted codfish, meat, salt pork, sausage, chicken, beef	Coffee with hot milk	Starchy root vegetables, green bananas, plantain, legumes, tomatoes, green pepper, onion, pineapple, papaya, citrus fruits	Lard, herbs, oil, vinegar
Near Eastern	Bulgur (wheat)	Lamb, mutton, chicken, fish, eggs	Fermented milk, sour cream, yogurt, cheese	Nuts, grape leaves	Sheep's butter, olive oil
Greek	Plain wheat bread	Lamb, pork, poultry, eggs, organ meats	Yogurt, cheese, butter	Onions, fresh fruit, tomatoes, legumes	Olive oil, parsley, lemon, vinegar

Figure 24–1 *(Compiled from Mahan, L. K. and M. Arlin.* Krause's Food, Nutrition, and Diet Therapy, *8th ed. Philadelphia: W. B. Saunders, 1992).*

ETHNIC AND REGIONAL FOOD PATTERNS

Ethnic Group	Bread and Cereal	Eggs, Meat, Fish, Poultry	Dairy Products	Fruits and Vegetables	Seasonings and Fats
Mexican	Lime-treated corn	Little meat (ground beef or pork), poultry, fish	Cheese, evaporated milk as beverage for infants	Pinto beans, tomatoes, potatoes, onions, lettuce	Chili pepper, salt, garlic
Chinese	Rice, wheat, millet, corn, noodles	Little meat and no beef, fish (including raw fish), eggs of hen, duck, and pigeon	Water buffalo milk occasionally, soybean milk, cheese	Soybeans, soybean sprouts, bamboo sprouts, soy curd cooked in lime water, radish leaves, legumes, vegetables, fruits	Sesame seeds, ginger, almonds, soy sauce
American Black	Hot breads, cookies, pastries, cakes, cereals, white rice	Chicken, salt, pork, ham, bacon, sausage	Milk and milk products	Kale, mustard, turnip greens, cabbage, hominy grits, sweet potatoes	Molasses
Jewish	Noodles, crusty white seed rolls, rye bread, pumpernickel bread	Kosher meat (from forequarters and organs from beef, lamb, veal), milk not eaten at same meal, fish	Milk and milk products	Vegetables — usually cooked with meat (kosher), fruits	

Figure 24–1 *continued*

SIGNS OF HEALTH AND MALNUTRITION

	Normal/Healthy	**Malnourished**
Hair	Shiny and firm in scalp	Dull, brittle, dry and loose
Eyes	Clear pink membranes; adjust easily to darkness	Pale membranes, spots, redness; adjust slowly to darkness
Skin	Smooth, hydrated skin	Pale, sallow, ashen, scaly, and cracked skin
Tongue	Red, bumpy, rough	Smooth, sore, purplish, swollen
Nails	Smooth and pink	Spoon-shaped, brittle, ridged
Behavior	Alert and attentive	Irritable and inattentive, apathetic or hyperactive

Figure 24–2 *(Adapted from E. Whitney and S. Rolfes.* Understanding Nutrition. *Minneapolis/St. Paul: West Publishing, 1993).*

Excess ingestion of simple carbohydrates can result in obesity and dental caries.

It is now recommended that approximately 55% to 60% of daily caloric intake be in the form of carbohydrates, with no more than 10% of these in the form of simple sugars (Marotz et al. 1993).

PROTEIN

The primary function of protein is to promote cellular and tissue growth and repair. Protein is used as an energy source only when other sources (carbohydrates and fats) are lacking. Proteins are made up of hundreds of individual units called amino acids. **Nonessential amino acids** can be manufactured by the body. **Essential amino acids** cannot be manufactured and must be provided in food.

Proteins are classified as complete or incomplete depending on whether they supply all of the essential amino acids needed by the body in adequate amounts. Complete proteins are generally found in animal sources such as meat, fish, poultry, and dairy products, which also tend to be high in fat and cholesterol. Plant sources, such as nuts, seeds, vegetables, and legumes, individually supply incomplete proteins. These sources, however, can be combined to provide the equivalent of a complete protein.

The child who lacks protein appears weak and apathetic, with edema and muscle wasting. The child's skin may appear patchy and scaly, and the hair dull and colorless.

FATS

Fats are stored in the body and serve an important role in the diet as a reserve of energy. Too much fat, however, can be harmful. Fats, oils, and fatlike substances called sterols are classified as **lipids**. Chemically, fats are made up of **triglycerides**, which consist of three fatty acids combined with glycerol.

Fatty acids are classified as saturated or unsaturated. All animal products — including milk, butter, egg yolks, and red meat — contain some amounts of saturated fat. Polyunsaturated or monounsaturated fat is found in vegetable fats and oils (with the exception of coconut oil and palm oil). Saturated fats have been linked with high levels of cholesterol and low-density lipoproteins (LDLs) and with an incidence of hypertension in children.

When excess kilocalories are ingested, they are turned into fat and stored for later use. Fat functions to maintain body temperature, cushion vital organs, and facilitate the absorption of the fat-soluble vitamins (A, D, E, and K). It is also the source of one of the essential amino acids, linoleic acid. Excess ingestion of fat, however, can lead to obesity and atherosclerosis.

It is now recommended that no more than 30% of daily calories come from fat.

MINERALS

Minerals help to regulate body functions and build body tissue. Calcium, phosphorus, potassium, and sodium are four minerals that are essential to proper body functioning. Milk products, meats, whole grains, legumes, and green leafy vegetables are good sources of many minerals. A well-balanced diet supplies necessary quantities of these and other minerals, such as iron, iodine, magnesium, and zinc.

Children need calcium and phosphorus for normal bone and tooth development. Fluoride is an important mineral that makes teeth harder and more resistant to decay. Fluoride supplementation of drinking water and the use of fluoride-containing toothpastes is therefore recommended during childhood to help prevent dental caries (Marotz et al. 1993). Iron supplements are usually recommended for infants after the age of 6 months to prevent deficiency (see later discussion). Other mineral supplements are usually unnecessary for children who consume a variety of foods.

VITAMINS

Vitamins are essential for the regulation of normal body functions. For example, vitamins regulate energy metabolism, cellular reproduction and growth, bone growth, neuromuscular activities, and blood formation (Marotz et al. 1993). Vitamins are classified as either fat-soluble or water-soluble.

The fat-soluble vitamins are A, D, E, and K. These vitamins are stored in the body, mainly in the liver. Vitamin A helps the eyes to accommodate to dim light and also maintains the skin and mucous membranes. Vitamin D aids in the formation of bones and teeth. Food sources high in vitamins A and D include yellow fruits and vegetables and green leafy vegetables. Other sources include fish liver oil, animal liver, and sunlight.

Water-soluble vitamins are the B-complex vitamins and vitamin C. Once the body has absorbed a maximum concentration of these vitamins, the excess is excreted in the urine. Because water-soluble vitamins are not stored in the body, children need a daily intake of these vitamins to maintain health.

The B-complex vitamins include thiamin, riboflavin, niacin, B_{12}, folacin, pantothenic acid, and biotin. These vitamins aid in energy metabolism. Wheat germ, whole grains, legumes, organ meats, and eggs are good sources of B-complex vitamins. Deficiencies of these vitamins can result in symptoms of anorexia, muscle weakness, anemia, diarrhea, nausea, irritability, or depression.

Vitamin C, also known as ascorbic acid, has a significant role in the formation of collagen. It also functions in the metabolism of amino acids, the absorption of iron, and the synthesis of collagen. Vitamin C is found in citrus fruits (such as oranges, strawberries, and grapefruit) and dark green leafy vegetables. A deficiency of vitamin C can result in easy bruising, scurvy, sore mouth and gums, and joint tenderness due to disruption of cartilage.

GUIDELINES FOR NUTRITIONAL INTAKE DURING CHILDHOOD

Growth rate, body size, and physical activity influence a child's nutritional requirements. Several guidelines are available to help in planning nutritionally sound diets for children from infancy through adolescence.

Most nutritional recommendations until 1992 were based on the four basic food groups (milk and milk products, meat and meat alternatives, fruits and vegetables, and bread and cereal). In 1992, however, the U.S. Department of Agriculture (USDA) published a new guide for daily food planning, the **food pyramid**, Figure 24–3. This revised planning guide encourages limited intake of fats, increased intake of fiber (fruits, vegetables), and increased intake of carbohydrates (grains and grain products).

The U.S. **Recommended Dietary Allowances**

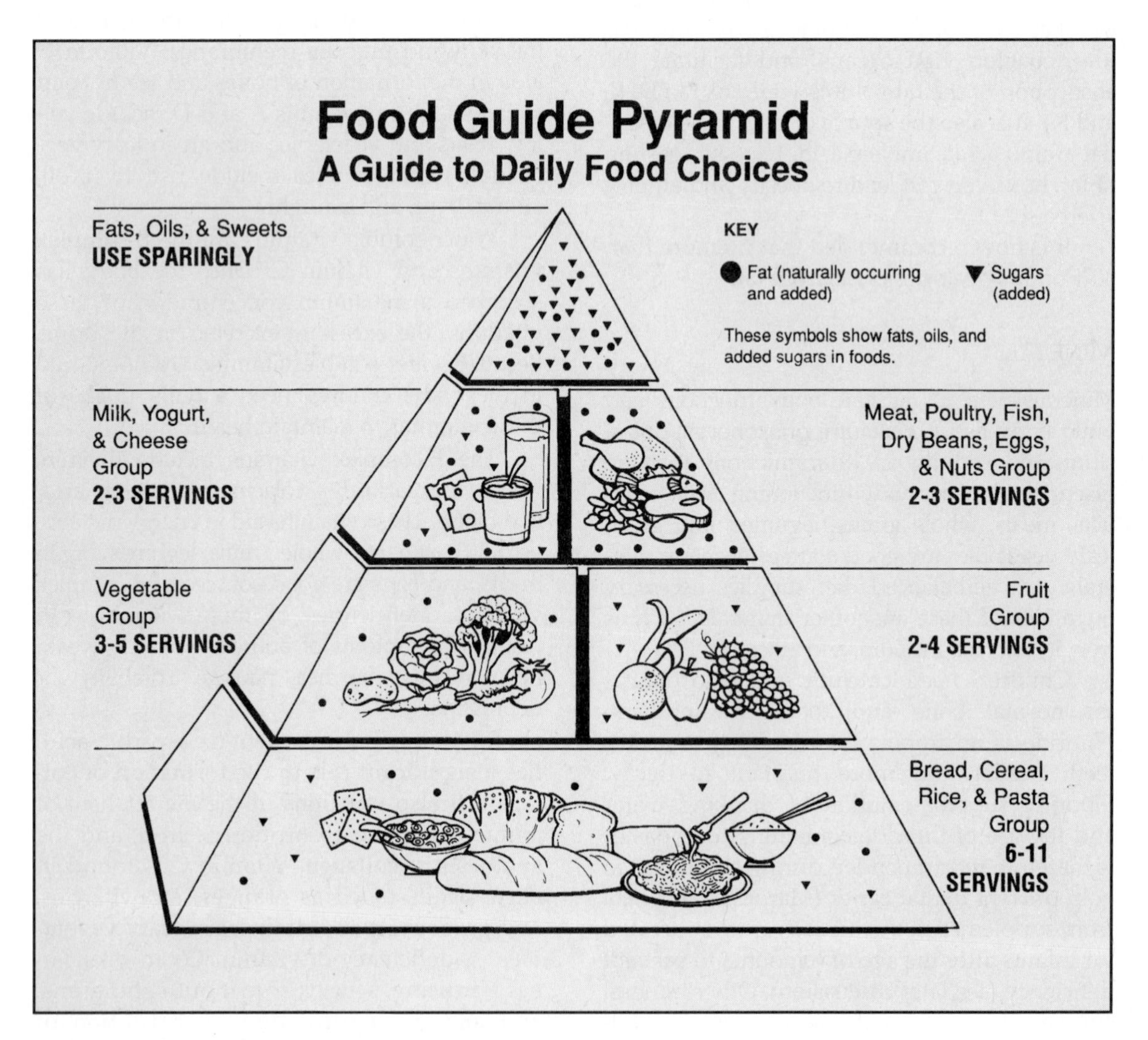

Figure 24–3 (Courtesy of the U.S. Department of Agriculture)

(RDAs), developed and updated periodically by the Food and Nutrition Board of the National Academy of Sciences, is a guide to intake of essential nutrients from infancy through adulthood, Figure 24-4. The committee on Nutrition of the American Academy of Pediatrics has also published several guidelines related to infant feeding, composition of formulas, and recommended dietary intake for children.

INFANT

During the first year of life, breast milk or infant formula is the infant's major source of food. Breast milk has certain advantages over formula. Breast milk contains easily digested protein and carbohydrate (in the form of lactose), fat (including linoleic acid), and minerals and vitamins. It is less likely to cause food allergies and also contains maternal antibodies, which help protect the infant from infection in the first months of life. Cow's milk or soy-based formulas closely parallel the nutritional content of breast milk. Cow's milk alone, however, is insufficient as a source of food for infants (American Academy of Pediatrics 1983). It lacks sufficient quantities of vitamin C and iron, contains excess sodium and less-digestible forms of protein, is higher in fat, and contains less sugar than breast milk.

The addition of solid foods in pureed form to the infant's diet is not recommended for the first 4 to 6 months of life (American Academy of Pediatrics 1984). Although the infant's stomach and intestines are able to digest the components of breast milk and formula, they cannot digest the starches found in many other foods. By the time an infant is 4 to 6 months of age, he or she is producing enzymes capable of digesting complex carbohydrates and proteins.

Neonatal iron stores are exhausted between 4 and 6 months of age, and this deficit becomes a significant factor when considering the infant's diet. Iron recommendations for infants are 10 mg per day by 6 months of age. An iron supplement or iron-fortified cereal is usually recommended after the age of 6 months to decrease the risk of iron deficiency and associated developmental delays.

New foods should be introduced one at a time at intervals of about one week in order to observe for symptoms of allergy or sensitivity. Iron-fortified rice cereal is usually the first solid food introduced, followed by pureed fruits, vegetables, and meats. Rice cereal, pears, yellow vegetables, and lamb usually are introduced first because they are the least likely to cause reactions. Another factor influencing introduction of foods is the need to select foods high in vitamin C to enhance iron absorption.

By 12 months of age, the normal infant has tripled his or her birth weight and is nearing a three-meal-per-day pattern. Explain to parents that experimentation with foods and feeding is a normal part of the infant's growth and development. Allow the older infant to begin self-feeding at 7 to 8 months of age.

Nursing Considerations. Teach parents the following points about the infant's diet and nutritional intake:

- Breast milk or formula provides a complete diet for the infant during the first 6 months of life.
- Self-feeding should be encouraged when the infant reaches about 7 months of age.
- Solids in pureed form may be added one at a time to the infant's diet after the age of 4 months.
- When new foods are introduced, observe for signs of food allergy or sensitivity (vomiting, diarrhea, abdominal pain, hives, and eczema).
- Because iron stores normally will be low after 6 months, iron-fortified food or iron supplementation may be required.
- Never prop bottles or allow the infant to take a bottle to bed. Juice, sweetened water, and formula can pool in the infant's mouth, causing tooth decay (nursing bottle-mouth syndrome). A propped bottle may cause choking and aspiration.

TODDLER

After the age of 1 year, the rapid growth and development of infancy begins to slow and the toddler's body begins to change proportions (see Chapter 23). The toddler's nutritional needs are directly related to these physical changes.

During this period, the child's appetite and the need for calories decrease. Adequate protein intake is necessary, however, to main-

RECOMMENDED DIETARY ALLOWANCES

Recommended dietary allowances[a] designed for the maintenance of good nutrition of practically all healthy people in the United States

Category	Age (years) or condition	Weight[b] (kg)	Weight[b] (lb)	Height[b] (cm)	Height[b] (in)	Protein (g)	Fat-soluble vitamins: Vitamin A (μg RE)[c]	Vitamin D (μg)[d]	Vitamin E (mg/α-TE)[e]	Vitamin K (μg)
Infants	0.0–0.5	6	13	60	24	13	375	7.5	3	5
	0.5–1.0	9	20	71	28	14	375	10	4	10
Children	1–3	13	29	90	35	16	400	10	6	15
	4–6	20	44	112	44	24	500	10	7	20
	7–10	28	62	132	52	28	700	10	7	30
Males	11–14	45	99	157	62	45	1000	10	10	45
	15–18	66	145	176	69	59	1000	10	10	65
	19–24	72	160	177	70	58	1000	10	10	70
	25–50	79	174	176	70	63	1000	5	10	80
	51+	77	170	173	68	63	1000	5	10	80
Females	11–14	46	101	157	62	46	800	10	8	45
	15–18	55	120	163	64	44	800	10	8	55
	19–24	58	128	164	65	46	800	10	8	60
	25–50	63	138	163	64	50	800	5	8	65
	51+	65	143	160	63	50	800	5	8	65
Pregnant						60	800	10	10	65
Lactating	1st 6 months					65	1300	10	12	65
	2nd 6 months					62	1200	10	11	65

From Food and Nutrition Board, National Research Council: *Recommended dietary allowances*, ed 10, Washington, DC, 1989. National Academy of Sciences.

[a]The allowances, expressed as average daily intakes over time, are intended to provide for individual variations among most normal persons as they live in the United States under usual environmental stresses. Diets should be based on a variety of common foods in order to provide other nutrients for which human requirements have been less well defined.

[b]Weights and heights of reference adults are actual medians for the U.S. population of the designated age, as reported by National Health and Nutrition Examination Survey (NHANES) II. The median weights and heights of those under 19 years of age were taken from Hamill PV and others: Physical growth: National Center for Health Statistics percentiles. *Am J Clin Nutr* 32:607–629, 1979. The use of these figures does not imply that the height-to-weight ratios are ideal.

Figure 24–4 *(Reprinted with permission from* Recommended Dietary Allowances, *10th ed. Copyright 1989 by The National Academy of Sciences. Courtesy of the National Academy Press, Washington, D.C.)*

tain optimal growth. Milk is an excellent source of protein for children, and from 16 to 24 ounces of milk per day is recommended. No more than 24 ounces is desirable, however, as milk contains little iron and excess intake can result in inadequate intake of other foods containing this mineral. Toddlers from 1 to 3 years of age remain at high risk for iron-deficiency anemia because of the rapid growth and depletion of iron stores during infancy

Water-soluble vitamins							Minerals						
Vitamin C (mg)	Thiamin (mg)	Riboflavin (mg)	Niacin (mg NE)[f]	Vitamin B_6 (mg)	Folate (μg)	Vitamin B_{12} (μg)	Calcium (mg)	Phosphorus (mg)	Magnesium (mg)	Iron (mg)	Zinc (mg)	Iodine (μg)	Selenium (μg)
30	0.3	0.4	5	0.3	25	0.3	400	300	40	6	5	40	10
35	0.4	0.5	6	0.6	35	0.5	600	500	60	10	5	50	15
40	0.7	0.8	9	1.0	50	0.7	800	800	80	10	10	70	20
45	0.9	1.1	12	1.1	75	1.0	800	800	120	10	10	90	20
45	1.0	1.2	13	1.4	100	1.4	800	800	170	10	10	120	30
50	1.3	1.5	17	1.7	150	2.0	1200	1200	270	12	15	150	40
60	1.5	1.8	20	2.0	200	2.0	1200	1200	400	12	15	150	50
60	1.5	1.7	19	2.0	200	2.0	1200	1200	350	10	15	150	70
60	1.5	1.7	19	2.0	200	2.0	800	800	350	10	15	150	70
60	1.2	1.4	15	2.0	200	2.0	800	800	350	10	15	150	70
50	1.1	1.3	15	1.4	150	2.0	1200	1200	280	15	12	150	45
60	1.1	1.3	15	1.5	180	2.0	1200	1200	300	15	12	150	50
60	1.1	1.3	15	1.6	180	2.0	1200	1200	280	15	12	150	55
60	1.1	1.3	15	1.6	180	2.0	800	800	280	15	12	150	55
60	1.0	1.2	13	1.6	180	2.0	800	800	280	10	12	150	55
70	1.5	1.6	17	2.2	400	2.2	1200	1200	320	30	15	175	65
95	1.6	1.8	20	2.1	280	2.6	1200	1200	355	15	19	200	75
90	1.6	1.7	20	2.1	260	2.6	1200	1200	340	15	16	200	75

[c]Retinol equivalent. 1 retinol equivalent = 1 mg retinol or 6 mg b-carotene.

[d]As cholecalciferol. 10 μg cholecalciferol = 400 IU vitamin D.

[e]α-Tocopherol equivalents. 1 mg *d*-α-tocopherol = 1 α-TE.

[f]1 NE (niacin equivalent) is equal to 1 mg of niacin or 60 mg of dietary tryptophan.

(Mahan 1992). Thus, intake of foods rich in iron is advised.

Toddlers have fluctuating appetites with strong food likes and dislikes. Serving size is important. Toddlers tend to like colorful dishes with foods cut into bite-size pieces. **Ritualistic behavior** at mealtime is common. For example, toddlers like to use a special plate, fork, or spoon; they may want to eat one food first at each meal or follow a sequence in eating.

Nursing Considerations. Teach parents the following points about the toddler's diet, nutritional needs, and eating patterns:

- Limit milk to no more than 24 ounces per day.
- Toddlers can feed themselves and want to do so, Figure 24–5.
- Toddlers demonstrate definite food likes and dislikes. Be flexible but consistent in presenting food. Serve small portions.
- Toddlers are easily distracted during meals. Avoid interruptions.
- Insufficient iron intake during infancy can leave toddlers vulnerable to iron-deficiency anemia.

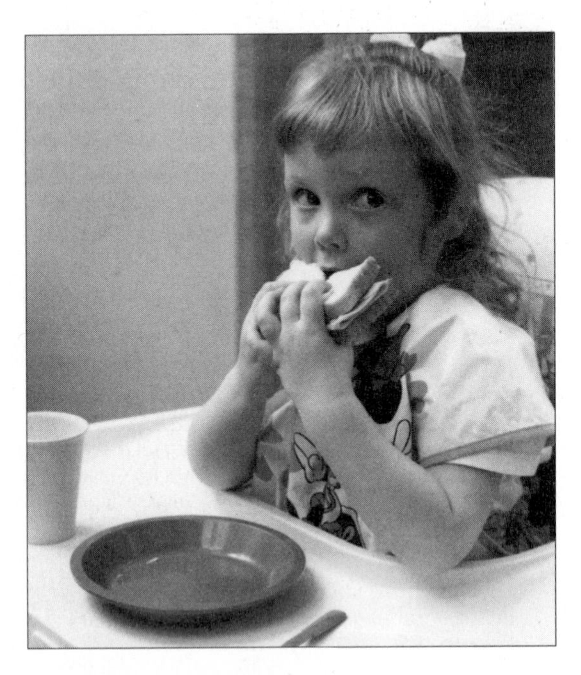

Figure 24–5 A toddler enjoys self-feeding and demonstrates definite food likes and dislikes.

PRESCHOOL CHILD

Nutritional requirements for preschool children are similar to those for toddlers. Caloric requirements continue to decrease slightly between 3 and 6 years of age. Fluid requirements also decrease slightly, and protein requirements remain much the same. Preschool children, like toddlers, have definite food likes and dislikes and occasionally display ritualistic behavior By 5 years of age, however, most preschoolers become more agreeable to trying new foods, especially if they are allowed to help in food preparation.

The quantity of food a preschooler eats is not as important as the quality. The American Academy of Pediatrics' Committee on Nutrition (1984) recommends a moderate intake of fat (30% to 40% of total energy-source intake), but cautions against extremes in dietary restrictions.

During the preschool· period children should be screened for nutritional deficiencies. A healthy diet during this period can lay the foundation for healthy eating patterns as an adult.

Nursing Considerations. Teach parents the following points about the preschool child's diet, nutritional needs, and eating patterns:

- The preschool child has definite food preferences.
- Preschool children are vulnerable to communicable diseases. Illness and fever increase metabolic rate, and therefore caloric needs.
- As ritualistic behavior diminishes, the preschooler becomes more flexible in eating habits.

SCHOOL-AGE CHILD

Because the young school-age child (age 6 to 7 years) chooses which foods to eat when at school or away from parental supervision, deficiencies in iron, vitamin A, and riboflavin are common during this period. Uneven growth patterns and lack of interest in eating contribute to the extreme fluctuations in the appetite of school-age children. In addition, peer pressure related to eating habits begins to appear.

Unless the diet of an 8- or 9-year-old child is well planned, it may be deficient in calcium, iron, and thiamin. Meats, legumes, and milk in sufficient quantities are needed to assure adequate amounts of these minerals and vitamins.

In the late school-age period (8 to 10 years) and in preadolescence (11 to 12 years), caloric requirements increase and nutritious snacks are required to meet dietary requirements. As the child reaches 11 to 12 years of age, protein requirements diminish. Growth of new bone and muscle slows; however, energy needs to maintain the child's additional tissue mass are high.

The manner in which food is offered to the school-age child is important. Encourage nutritious meals by presenting food in an appealing manner. Children can be encouraged to choose nutritious foods by labeling them "food to make us grow." Similarly, holiday foods such as dried fruit in Christmas stockings, peanuts in Easter baskets, and fresh fruit at Halloween promote good nutrition. One mother's approach exemplifies this philosophy: "When they were good I gave them a vegetable as a reward. Now they ask for vegetables and other nutritious snacks."

Nursing Considerations. Teach parents the following points about the school-age child's diet, nutritional needs, and eating patterns:

- During the school-age years, children's food choices begin to be influenced by peers, fads, and "junk food" advertising.
- School-age children are vulnerable to deficiencies in iron, calcium, and B-complex vitamins.
- The child's activities may interfere with mealtime routines and good eating habits.

ADOLESCENT

Caloric needs during adolescence are high because of the accelerated growth and development characteristic of this developmental stage. Individual variation is the single most significant feature of adolescent growth. Girls usually begin pubertal growth at about 10 years and complete their growth spurt by 16 years of age. Boys tend to start their pubertal growth two years later than girls (refer to Chapter 22).

Stress, fatigue, and peer pressure influence the adolescent's appetite and dietary intake. Most adolescent boys have a fairly adequate dietary intake because they eat massive quantities of food. This diet, however, is often high in fat. The diet of adolescent girls is often lacking in essential nutrients. Low-calorie diets and poor food choices contribute to nutrient deficiencies, particularly of calcium, protein, B vitamins, and iron. Eating disorders such as anorexia nervosa and bulimia nervosa often manifest during adolescence (refer to Chapter 44).

Although the adolescent's diet should be similar to the ideal diet recommended for adults, teenagers frequently model their eating patterns after adults who have poor diets. The nurse needs to understand the factors influencing adolescents' dietary intake when helping them plan meals. Creative approaches can help to promote a healthy diet. Teenagers who eat fast foods can be encouraged to eat pizza instead of high-salt, high-fat hamburgers and french fries from fast-food outlets, Figure 24–6.

Teenagers are concerned about their body image and a diet that enables them to maintain a healthy, physically fit body will be followed more readily than one that does not. Adolescents are also more likely to comply with a planned diet if they are involved in the decision-making process regarding food choices.

Nursing Considerations. Teach parents the following points regarding adolescent diet, nutritional needs, and eating patterns:

- The adolescent has an increased appetite and an increased need for calories.
- Requirements for calcium, iron, and protein are increased during adolescence.
- Diet during this period is greatly influenced by peer groups.
- Adolescents are vulnerable to eating disorders and food fads.

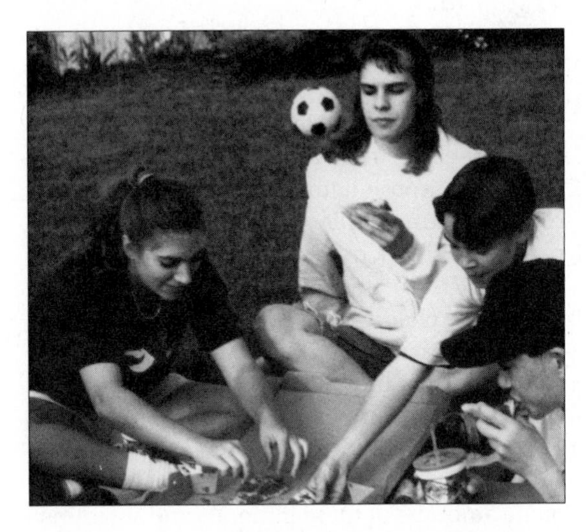

Figure 24–6 *Adolescents should be encouraged to eat healthy alternatives such as pizza, rather than high-fat, high-salt, low-nutrient fast foods.*

REVIEW QUESTIONS

A. Multiple choice. Select the best answer.

1. In counseling a mother whose 10-month-old infant is overweight, what advice should be given first?
   a. Recommend reducing the quantity of food given at each meal and allow one bottle feeding.
   b. Recommend the use of skim milk instead of whole milk in infant's formula.
   c. Ask the mother to keep a log of feedings and bring it to the clinic next week.
   d. Tell the mother that the baby needs to be more active.

2. Which of the following practices may help prevent the development of obesity?
   a. Encourage eating animal protein rather than plant protein.
   b. Avoid fats.
   c. Eat saturated fats, not polyunsaturated fats.
   d. Ingest caloric requirements for maintenance and growth.

3. Which of the following foods is the least likely to cause an infant to have an allergic reaction?
   a. apples
   b. green vegetables
   c. pears
   d. oatmeal

4. How does human milk differ from cow's milk? Human milk
   a. is more easily digested
   b. supplies more protein
   c. provides fewer calories
   d. contains less lactose

5. A 3-year-old boy is encouraged to drink a cup of orange juice to promote
   a. tissue regeneration
   b. iron absorption
   c. carbohydrate metabolism
   d. an acidic urine

6. Most normal infants who weigh 7 pounds (3.175 kg) at birth can be expected at 12 months of age to weigh
   a. 14 pounds (6.35 kg)
   b. 21 pounds (9.325 kg)
   c. 28 pounds (12.5 kg)
   d. 35 pounds (15.675 kg)
7. A mother at the well-baby clinic says she is worried because her 2-year-old daughter's appetite is decreasing. Which is the best response?
   a. Advise supplementing her meals with nutritious snacks several times a day.
   b. Suggest restricting her play activities until she eats all of the food at each meal.
   c. Emphasize that her caloric needs are lower now and her appetite reflects these reduced needs.
   d. Advise adding high-calorie foods to her diet to improve caloric intake.
8. The 6-year-old child who is at the expected developmental level will most likely have which of the following characteristic attitudes about food and eating?
   a. food likes and dislikes that fluctuate from day to day
   b. an eagerness to try new foods
   c. a dislike of fruits and vegetables
   d. a preference for familiar foods that are simply prepared
9. The infant should be weaned from only breast or bottle feeding to eating some solid foods at approximately 6 months of age because
   a. the infant should learn new tastes and textures
   b. extended breast and bottle feeding promote tooth decay
   c. the infant requires dietary fiber for proper growth and development
   d. the child's iron stores begin to diminish at 6 months of age
10. The adolescent's diet often lacks which of the following nutrients?
    a. carbohydrates and vitamin D
    b. fats and zinc
    c. proteins and iron
    d. fluids and calcium

SUGGESTED ACTIVITIES

- Identify four suggestions that you can give parents to encourage preschoolers to eat new or different foods. Be specific.
- Describe key differences in nutritional requirements and diet from infancy through adolescence.

BIBLIOGRAPHY

American Academy of Pediatrics, Committee on Nutrition. The use of whole cow's milk in infancy. *Pediatrics* (1993): 253–255.

American Academy of Pediatrics, Committee on Nutrition. Toward a prudent diet for children. *Pediatrics* 73 (1984): 876.

Anderson, J. B. The status of adolescent nutrition. *Nutrition Today* (March/April, 1991): 7–10.

Laquatra, I., and M. J. Gerlach. *Nutrition in Clinical Nursing*. Albany, NY: Delmar Publishers, 1990.

Mahan, L. K. and M. Arlin *Krause's Food, Nutrition and Diet Therapy*, 8th ed. Philadelphia: W. B. Saunders, 1992.

Marotz, L. R., M. Z. Cross, and J. M. Rush. *Health, Safety, and Nutrition for the Young Child*, 3rd ed. Albany, NY: Delmar Publishers, 1993.

Pipes, P., and C. Trahms. *Nutrition in Infancy and Childhood*, 5th ed. St. Louis, MO: Mosby-Year Book, 1993.

Whitney, E., and S. Rolfes. *Understanding Nutrition*. Minneapolis/St. Paul: West Publishing, 1993.

CHAPTER

25

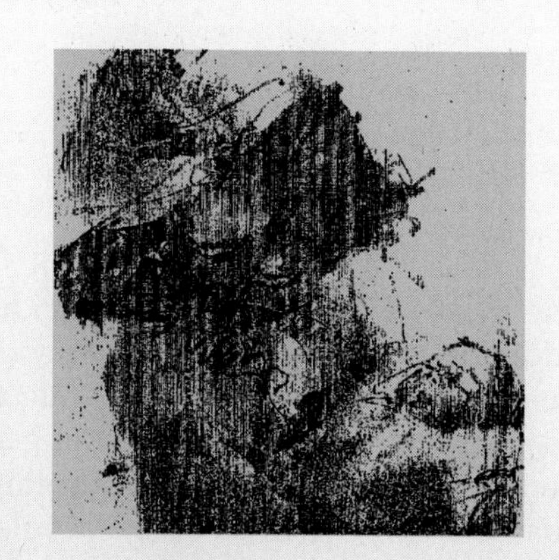

Immunizations

OBJECTIVES

AFTER STUDYING THIS CHAPTER, THE STUDENT SHOULD BE ABLE TO:

- DISTINGUISH BETWEEN PASSIVE AND ACTIVE IMMUNITY.
- DISCUSS THE RECOMMENDED IMMUNIZATION SCHEDULE FOR HEALTHY CHILDREN.
- DESCRIBE THE CURRENT ACTIVE IMMUNIZATIONS AVAILABLE TO CHILDREN AND POSSIBLE REACTIONS TO THESE IMMUNIZATIONS.
- DESCRIBE GENERAL CONCERNS AND NURSING RESPONSIBILITIES WHEN ADMINISTERING VACCINES TO CHILDREN.

KEY TERMS

IMMUNE RESPONSE

ACTIVE IMMUNITY

PASSIVE IMMUNITY

VACCINE

TOXOID

LIVE ATTENUATED VIRUS

KILLED INACTIVATED VIRUS

The routine immunization of children against specific infectious diseases is one of the most significant advances in health care worldwide. The occurrence of childhood diseases that were once considered major public health problems has been dramatically reduced because of the development of immunizing agents that prevent specific diseases.

In 1977 the U.S. Department of Health and Human Services initiated a childhood immunization program. Many children were immunized against childhood diseases because of this initiative and the enactment of laws by all 50 states requiring documentation of immunization as a condition of a child's enrollment into school.

Many children still remain underimmunized today, however. In some cities in the United States, as many as 50% of children under the age of 2 have not received the recommended immunizations. Nurses can be important advocates of childhood immunizations and should become familiar with the immunizations available to children, as well as the immune responses that these immunizations produce to specific childhood diseases.

THE IMMUNE RESPONSE

Immunity is a state in which an individual is resistant to a particular disease. Individuals become immune to specific diseases through exposure to the disease or vaccination against the disease. An **immune response** occurs when the body's lymphocytes are stimulated to produce antibodies that react with antigens (protein substances found on the surface of microorganisms). These disease-specific antibodies destroy or neutralize antigens and remain in the blood plasma to prevent reinfection by the specific infectious agent.

Active immunity (or humoral immunity) occurs when individuals form antibodies or antitoxins against specific antigens, either by exposure to the infectious agent or by introduction of the antigen. For example, a child develops active immunity to the measles virus when he or she develops the disease or is vaccinated against the virus. In each instance, the child responds to the measles antigen by forming antibodies against it. If the child is exposed to measles again, reinfection will not occur because active immunity against the disease has been developed.

Passive immunity occurs when an individual receives ready-made antibodies from a human or animal that has been actively immunized against the disease. An example of passive immunity is the transfer of antibodies from a mother to her fetus. A newborn baby who has received measles antibodies from his or her mother in utero will be immune from measles for as long as 6 months to 1 year of age. Passive immunity provides only temporary immunity because the recipient has not developed his or her own antibodies against the disease.

VACCINES

Active immunity is achieved through the introduction of a **vaccine**, an active immunizing agent that incorporates an infectious antigen. The vaccine can be given in the form of a **toxoid**, an agent that has been treated to destroy its toxic qualities; a **live attenuated virus**, a weakened virus; or a **killed inactivated virus**.

Vaccines stimulate the body to produce antitoxins or antibodies against the specific disease. Some immunizing agents provide lifetime protection against a disease, some provide partial protection, and some must be

VACCINATION SCHEDULE

2 mo	4 mo	6 mo	12 mo	15 mo	4–6 yr	11–12 yr	14–16 yr
DTP	DTP	DTP		DTP[a] or DTaP	DTP or DTaP		Td[b]
Polio	Polio			Polio[a]	Polio		
				MMR[c]		MMR[d]	
Hib[e]	Hib	Hib		Hib			
or							
Hib	Hib		Hib				

Birth	1–2 mo	4 mo	6–18 mo
HB	HB[f]		HB[f]
	HB[f]	HB[f]	HB[f]

Notes:
DTP = diphtheria-tetanus-pertussis vaccine
DTaP = acellular pertussis
Polio = live oral polio vaccine (OPV) drops or killed (inactivated) polio vaccine (IPV) shots
MMR = measles, mumps, and rubella vaccine
Hib = *Hemophilus influenzae* b conjugate vaccine
HB = hepatitis B vaccine
Td = diphtheria-tetanus adult

[a] Many experts recommend these vaccines at 18 months.
[b] Repeat every 10 years.
[c] In some areas, this dose of MMR vaccine may be given at 12 months.
[d] Unless second dose given previously.
[e] Hib vaccine is given in either a four-dose schedule or a three-dose schedule, depending on the type of vaccine used.
[f] HB vaccine can be given simultaneously with DTP, polio, MMR, and Hib conjugate vaccine.

Figure 25–1 *Recommended schedule of vaccinations for all children (From American Academy of Pediatrics,* Report of the Committee on Infectious Diseases, *22nd ed. 1991)*

readministered at intervals in the form of booster immunizations to maintain the antibodies at protective levels (American Academy of Pediatrics 1991).

RECOMMENDED IMMUNIZATION SCHEDULE

There are currently nine infectious diseases for which routine immunizations in childhood are recommended: diphtheria, tetanus, pertussis, infections caused by *Hemophilus influenzae*, polio, measles (rubeola), rubella (German measles), mumps, and hepatitis B.

The American Academy of Pediatrics' Committee on Infectious Diseases recommends that immunization for children begin at 2 months of age, with the exception of the hepatitis B vaccine, which can be given initially at birth (American Academy of Pediatrics 1991). Figure 25–1 gives the recommended schedule for active immunization of healthy infants and children.

DIPHTHERIA, TETANUS, AND PERTUSSIS VACCINES

Diphtheria-Tetanus-Pertussis. The diphtheria-tetanus-pertussis (DTP) immunization is usually given in one injection of combined diphtheria and tetanus toxoids, and a suspension of killed whole-cell pertussis organisms. For primary immunization of children, DTP is given in a series of four doses. The first three doses of 0.5 mL each are given intramuscularly at four- to eight-week intervals (usually at 2 months, 4 months, and 6 months of age). A booster dose of DTP is given to children one year after the third dose (usually at 18 months of age). At 4 to 6 years, or before entering school, children who have received the fourth dose of DTP at ages younger than 4 years should receive a fifth dose of DTP. An interruption in the recommended schedule does not affect immunity. It is not necessary to begin the series again if an immunization is delayed.

Forty to seventy percent of children will experience mild reactions following administration of the DTP immunization. These mild reactions include redness and tenderness at the injection site, fever, drowsiness, fretfulness, and loss of appetite. Rarely children have more severe reactions; these include fever of 40.5°C (104.9°F) or higher, persistent crying for three or more hours, unusual high-pitched crying, and convulsions. If a severe reaction occurs, further immunization with pertussis is contraindicated (DHHS 1991a). Other contraindications to administration of pertussis vaccine are listed in Figure 25–2.

DTaP. In December 1991, the U.S. Food and Drug Administration (FDA) licensed a new pertussis vaccine. Instead of being made from killed whole-cell pertussis organisms, the new vaccine is made of a few parts of the pertussis cell (Edwards et al. 1991). Combined with the diphtheria and tetanus vaccines (DTaP) for administration, it can be used as the fourth and fifth dose for children only if they have been immunized previously with at least three doses of the DTP vaccine (DHHS 1992).

Diphtheria-Tetanus Pediatric. Diphtheria-teta-

CONTRAINDICATIONS TO VACCINATIONS

Vaccine	Contraindications
Pertussis	Progressive neurologic disorder Any of the following reactions after receiving the vaccine: convulsion, persistent uncontrollable cry, fever of 104°F or more
Live attenuated polio (OPV)	Immunosuppressed children or children who share a household with individuals who are immunosuppressed (e.g., those with HIV infection or those receiving steroids, chemotherapy, or radiation therapy)
Measles, mumps, rubella	Egg sensitivity (vaccine contains egg antigens), which may lead to an anaphylactic reaction Anaphylactic reaction to neomycin

Figure 25–2

nus (DT) pediatric vaccine is administered instead of DPT to children for whom the pertussis vaccine is contraindicated. DT contains full amounts of the diphtheria and tetanus toxoids. This preparation is not given to children over the age of 7 because adverse reactions can occur from the administration of the full-strength diphtheria toxoid.

Diphtheria-Tetanus Adult. Diphtheria-tetanus (Td) adult vaccine is administered to children over the age of 7 and adults. It contains less diphtheria toxoid than the DPT or DT vaccines.

POLIOVIRUS VACCINES

There are two types of polio vaccine available in the United States: live oral poliovirus vaccine (OPV) and inactivated polio vaccine (IPV).

OPV. OPV is the vaccine of choice for immunizing children against the poliovirus in the United States. This vaccine is given orally at the same time that the DTP immunization is administered. The primary series of three doses is usually given at 2 months, 4 months, and 18 months of age. If the infant lives in an area at high risk for polio, an additional dose is recommended at 6 months of age. A booster dose of OPV is given at 4 to 6 years of age.

OPV is a live attenuated virus that is excreted in the stool for about a month after administration. It should not be given to children if they or their household contacts are immunosuppressed from such conditions as cancer, HIV infection, or because of radiation or drug therapy that would make it difficult for the body to fight infection (DHHS 1991b), see Figure 25–2. Very rarely OPV will cause vaccine-related paralysis.

IPV. IPV is a killed virus that is given subcutaneously. It is recommended for children in whom OPV is contraindicated (American Academy of Pediatrics 1991).

HEMOPHILUS INFLUENZAE TYPE B CONJUGATE

Hemophilus influenzae type b infection is a major cause of meningitis, epiglottitis, septic arthritis, and bacteremia in infants and children under the age of 5. Current recommendations require all children be immunized by intramuscular injection with *H. influenzae* type b conjugate (Hib) beginning at approximately 2 to 3 months of age in a three-dose series at two-month intervals. A fourth dose is recommended at 15 months of age. Hib may be given simultaneously with DTP, polio, and measles, mumps, rubella (MMR) immunizations. A different injection site and separate syringes should be used (American Academy of Pediatrics 1991). Recently the FDA approved a combined Hib and DTP vaccine.

Hib is a very safe vaccine. About 2% of children receiving the vaccine develop redness and soreness at the injection site and mild fever.

MEASLES, MUMPS, AND RUBELLA VACCINES

Measles, mumps, rubella (MMR) is a live attenuated vaccine that is usually administered in one subcutaneous injection at 15 months of age. It is recommended that a second immunization be given to children 11 to 12 years of age unless state law requires administration at 4 to 6 years.

Contraindications to the MMR vaccine are listed in Figure 25–2. Reactions may occur 5 to 12 days after administration of the measles, mumps, and rubella vaccines because they are live attenuated virus vaccines.

Measles. Measles (rubeola) is a serious disease that is easily prevented by the administration of the measles vaccine to all children. The vaccine is available in measles-only form (M), in combination with rubella (MR), and in combination with mumps and rubella (MMR). The initial measles immunization should be given at 15 months of age. If the vaccine is given earlier than 15 months, many children fail to become immune because of the presence of maternal antibodies to measles that were passed to the infant through the placenta during pregnancy. Any child vaccinated with MMR before 12 months of age should have a repeat vaccination at 15 months and a third dose at 11 to 12 years (Merenstein et al. 1991).

Because of the increase in measles cases in vaccinated children, a two-dose schedule for administration of MMR is recommended (*Vaccine Bulletin* 1993). Some experts recommend that the second dose be given before entry into school (at 4 to 6 years), while others recommend that the second dose be given before entry into middle school (at 11 to 12 years) (*MMWR* 1989a).

The measles vaccine may sometimes cause a rash and fever.

Mumps. The mumps vaccine is a live attenuated virus that is usually combined with measles and rubella vaccines (MMR) for administration.

Rarely after receiving the mumps vaccine, the child may develop swelling of the parotid glands.

Rubella (German Measles). Rubella is usually a mild infection in children. When a pregnant woman develops the disease, however, serious consequences may occur. Babies born to mothers who have had rubella in pregnancy may be blind, deaf, or have heart disease (*MMWR* 1989b). Rubella vaccine is administered in a single subcutaneous dose of 0.5 mL in combination with measles and mumps (MMR), with measles (MR), or alone.

The current recommendation is to vaccinate all children 12 months of age or older. The vaccine usually is given combined with the measles and mumps vaccines (MMR), starting at 15 months of age. In addition, all post-pubertal adolescent girls who are not known to be immune to rubella should be immunized (American Academy of Pediatrics 1991).

The rubella vaccine may cause swelling of the lymph glands or a rash. Mild pain or stiffness may also occur one to three weeks after vaccination with rubella.

HEPATITIS B VACCINE

Hepatitis B virus infection is a major health problem in the United States. Both adolescents and adults are at high risk. Currently the hepatitis B vaccine is not required for entry into school (*MMWR* 1991).

Hepatitis B (HB) vaccine is recommended in a series of three intramuscular doses. The first dose is administered within 24 hours of birth. The second and third doses are administered one to six months, respectively, after the first dose, see Figure 25–1. The third dose acts as a booster dose. If the vaccination series is interrupted after the first dose, the second dose should be administered as soon as possible. The second and third doses of HB should be separated by an interval of two months (*MMWR* 1991).

Few reactions have been reported with HB vaccination. Those reported include soreness and redness at the injection site.

GENERAL CONSIDERATIONS IN IMMUNIZATION

INFORMED CONSENT

The benefits and risks of the immunizations should be explained to parents before administering the vaccine. Religious beliefs may be a factor. For example, Christian Scientists may not permit their children to have immunizations.

Several documents developed by the Centers for Disease Control and Prevention (CDC) can be used for securing informed consent. These forms are frequently updated as new developments in immunization occur.

RECORD KEEPING

Standard immunization records have been developed for parents' use, Figure 25–3. The

Vaccine Administration Record

Patient Name ______________________

Birthdate ______________________

Record # ______________________

Clinic Name/Address

"I have been provided a copy, and have read or have had explained to me, information about the diseases and the vaccines listed below. I have had a chance to ask questions that were answered to my satisfaction. I believe I understand the benefits and risks of the vaccines cited, and ask that the vaccine(s) listed below be given to me or to the person named above (for whom I am authorized to make this request)."

Vaccine	Date Given m/d/y	Age	*Site	Vaccine Manufacturer	Vaccine Lot Number	**Handout Publ. Date	***Initials	Signature of Parent or Guardian
DTP 1								
DTP 2								
DTP 3								
DTP/DTaP4								
DTP/DTaP5								
DT								
DTP/Hib1								
DTP/Hib2								
DTP/Hib3								
DTP/Hib 4								
Td								
OPV/IPV 1								
OPV/IPV 2								
OPV/IPV 3								
OPV/IPV 4								
MMR 1								
MMR 2								
Hib 1								
Hib 2								
Hib 3								
Hib 4								
Hep B 1								
Hep B 2								
Hep B 3								

*** Initials — Signature of Vaccine Administrator

____

____

____

(Use reverse side if more signatures are needed)

*Site Given Legend

RA = Right Arm
LA = Left Arm
RT = Right Thigh
LT = Left Thigh
O = Oral

** If required by state law

American Academy of Pediatrics

HE0116

Figure 25–3 *(Used with permission of the American Academy of Pediatrics, Elk Grove Village, IL)* child's health record should contain the following information about immunizations:

1. date of immunization (day, month, year)
2. vaccine
3. manufacturer
4. batch or lot number
5. site and route of administration
6. name and title of person administering immunization

The National Childhood Vaccine Injury Act (*MMWR* 1988) requires that any adverse reactions to the vaccine be reported to the state health department, which notifies the CDC.

SCHEDULING

Vaccinations should be postponed if the child has a febrile illness. An upper respiratory infection without fever does not necessitate postponing the immunization. A lapse in the routine schedule does not interfere with the immune response, so it is unnecessary to reinitiate the series if such a lapse occurs. If the child's immunization status is unknown, he or she should be considered susceptible (Derschewitz 1988).

NURSING CONSIDERATIONS WHEN ADMINISTERING VACCINES

- Refer to the manufacturer's insert for the proper storage and route of administration for the vaccine.
- Obtain informed consent from parents before administering the vaccine.
- Minimize minor, local reactions to intramuscular injection (for example, DTP) by:
  - using a 1-inch long, 22-gauge, needle
  - injecting the vaccine into the anterolateral thigh muscle in children 18 months old or younger (the deltoid muscle can be used in older children)
- Use a ⅝-inch long, 25–gauge needle for subcutaneous injections.
- Give each vaccine at a separate site.
- Adequately restrain the child when administering the vaccine.
- Know that multiple vaccines may be given in a single visit without adverse effects.
- Accurately document the administration of immunizations for parents and on the child's health record.

REVIEW QUESTIONS

A. Multiple choice. Select the best answer.

1. Vaccines can be given in which of the following forms?
   a. toxoid
   b. live active virus
   c. topical
   d. live enhanced virus

2. Routine immunizations are not recommended for
   a. polio
   b. AIDS
   c. *Hemophilis influenzae*
   d. mumps

3. The American Academy of Pediatrics' Committee on Infectious Diseases recommends that immunization for healthy children should begin at
   a. 2 months of age
   b. 6 months of age
   c. 18 months of age
   d. 2 years of age

4. DTP immunizes against which of the following diseases?
   a. diphtheria, tetanus, polio
   b. diphtheria, toxoid, polio
   c. diphtheria, toxoid, pertussis
   d. diphtheria, tetanus, pertussis

5. Which of the following is true about reactions to DPT immunization?
   a. Approximately 20% of children will experience mild reactions.
   b. Mild reactions include redness at site, fever, drowsiness, fretfulness, loss of appetite.
   c. If a severe systemic reaction occurs, further immunization with pertussis is needed.
   d. Many children develop a high fever, with high-pitched crying and sometimes convulsions.

6. Measles, mumps, and rubella vaccines are usually given
   a. if the child has a neomycin or egg sensitivity
   b. before 12 months of age
   c. while maternal antibodies are still present
   d. initially at about 15 months of age

7. Reactions to the MMR vaccine do not include
   a. swelling of the parotid glands or lymph glands
   b. rash and fever
   c. encephalitis
   d. mild pain or stiffness

8. The child's health record must contain the following information about immunizations
   a. the day and hour of immunization
   b. a family history of communicable diseases
   c. immunizations of brothers and sisters
   d. the site and route of administration

9. Vaccinations should be postponed
   a. if the child has an upper respiratory infection with no fever
   b. if the child has a febrile illness
   c. if a lapse in the routine immunization schedule has occurred
   d. if a nurse cannot determine the child's immunization status

10. When administering vaccines, the nurse's responsibilities include
    a. administering vaccines over the religious objections of parents
    b. giving each vaccine at the same site
    c. limiting administration to one vaccine per visit
    d. giving each vaccine at a separate site

B. Match the terms in column I to the correct definition in column II.

Column I	Column II
1. immunity	a. an antigenic agent that has been treated to destroy its toxic qualities
2. toxoid	b. a weakened virus
3. vaccine	c. a state in which an individual is resistant to a specific disease
4. immune response	d. antibodies or antitoxins formed as a result of exposure to the infectious agent or antigen
5. passive immunity	e. lymphocyte production of antibodies that neutralize antigens
6. active immunity	f. an active immunizing agent incorporating an intact infectious antigen
7. live attenuated virus	g. transfusion with ready-made antibodies from another human or an animal

SUGGESTED ACTIVITIES

- Make a chart to teach parents when immunizations are given, what they protect against, and possible side effects or reactions.
- Make your own drug cards indicating the various forms of each vaccine, when indicated and contraindicated, and possible reactions.
- List examples of each of the terms included in the matching exercise, above.

BIBLIOGRAPHY

American Academy of Pediatrics. *Report of the Committee on Infectious Diseases*, 22nd ed. Elk Grove Village, IL: American Academy of Pediatrics, 1991.

Department of Health and Human Services (DHHS). *Diphtheria, Tetanus, Pertussis*. Atlanta, GA: Centers for Disease Control, October 15, 1991a.

Department of Health and Human Services (DHHS). *Polio*. Atlanta, GA: Centers for Disease Control, October 15, 1991b.

Department of Health and Human Services (DHHS). *DTaP*. Atlanta, GA: Centers for Disease Control, March 25, 1992.

Derschewitz, R. A. *Ambulatory Pediatrics*. Philadelphia: J. B. Lippincott, 1988.

Edwards, K. M., N. A. Halsey, T. Townsend, and D. T. Karson. Differences in antibody response to whole-cell pertussis vaccines. *Pediatrics* 88, no. 5 (1991): 1019–1023.

Merenstein, G., W. Kaplan, and A. Rosenberg. *Handbook of Pediatrics*. Norwalk, CT: Appleton & Lange, 1991.

MMWR. National Childhood Vaccine Injury Act: Requirements for permanent vaccination records and for reporting of selected events after vaccination. *MMWR* 37, no. 13, (1988): 197–200.

MMWR. Measles prevention: Recommendations of the Immunization Practices Advisory Committee. *MMWR* 38 (S-9) (1989a).

MMWR. Rubella vaccine during pregnancy — United States, 1971–1988. *MMWR* 38, no. 17 (1989b): 289–293.

MMWR. Hepatitis B virus: A comprehensive strategy for eliminating transmission in the United States through universal childhood immunization. *MMWR* 40 (RR 13) (November, 1991).

Vaccine Bulletin. Measles and herd immunity: The association of attack rates with immunization rates in preschool children. *Vaccine Bulletin* 61 (January, 1993).

CHAPTER

26

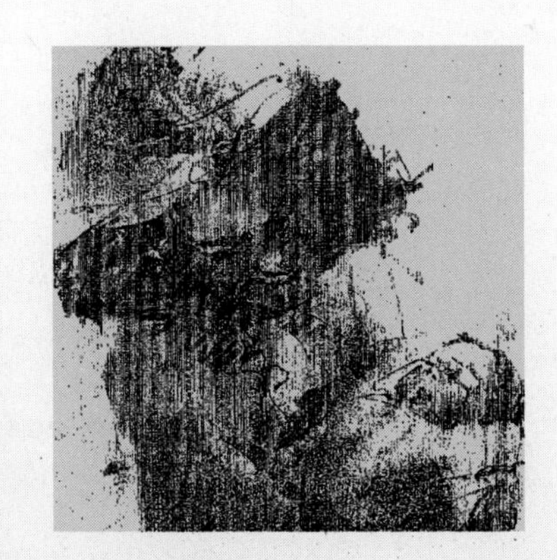

Child Safety

Objectives

After studying this chapter, the student should be able to:

- Identify the leading cause of death and permanent injury in children.
- Identify specific federal regulations designed to reduce the incidence of unintentional injury among children.
- Discuss measures for preventing unintentional injuries in children from infancy through adolescence.
- Identify poisons commonly found in the home.
- Define child abuse and differentiate among physical abuse, emotional abuse, sexual abuse, and neglect.
- Describe signs of physical abuse, sexual abuse, and neglect.
- Identify the ABCs of cardiopulmonary resuscitation.
- Describe variations for performing cardiopulmonary resuscitation on an infant or child victim.
- Describe variations for removing a foreign body obstruction in an infant or child victim.

Key Terms

- GASTRIC LAVAGE
- CHILD ABUSE
- PHYSICAL ABUSE
- EMOTIONAL ABUSE
- SEXUAL ABUSE
- NEGLECT
- CARDIOPULMONARY RESUSCITATION
- RESCUE BREATHING
- STRIDOR
- HEIMLICH MANEUVER

Infants and children depend on others to maintain a safe environment in which they can develop and grow. Providing a safe environment requires knowledge of behaviors that characterize children at different stages of their development. An essential part of the nurse's role involves educating parents about behaviors that place children at risk for unintentional injury or death.

Children who grow up in an abusive home environment are especially at risk for injury or death. Nurses must therefore be alert to the signs of physical or emotional abuse and ready to intervene promptly to protect the child from further harm.

Emergency measures are, at times, necessary to help children who have sustained injury. Nurses and other health care providers must be able to perform techniques for cardiopulmonary resuscitation and removal of an object causing airway obstruction. Nurses should encourage parents and others in the community to become familiar with these lifesaving techniques.

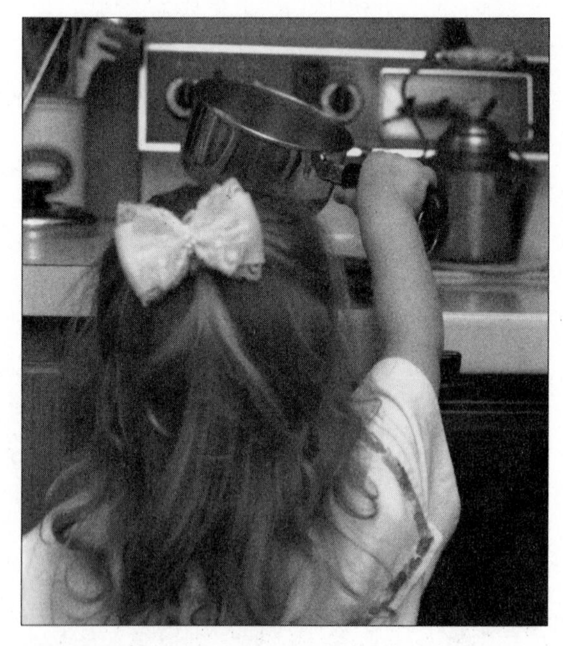

Figure 26–1 *Burns are a common cause of unintentional injury among toddlers, who can reach stove tops. Teach parents to place pots on back burners and turn pot handles toward the back of the stove, away from inquisitive hands.*

ACCIDENTS

Accidents kill and permanently injure more children than any disease and are the leading cause of death in childhood. Most accidents occur in or near the home. Statistics also indicate that certain injuries are more common among specific age groups. Burns, for example, are a common occurrence in children. Toddlers are especially at risk, Figure 26–1. For these reasons, a primary focus of nurses and other health care providers is educating parents about accident prevention through age-appropriate precautions, Figure 26–2.

ACCIDENT PREVENTION IN CHILDREN

Injury	Anticipatory Guidance
Falls	• Secure infant in infant seat. • Do not leave infant unattended on tables or beds. • Use gates to block doorways and stairs. • Move chairs and ladders away from counters and cabinets.
Burns	• Be sure bath water and foods are not too hot. • Use safety covers on electrical outlets. • Keep fireplace screens closed. • Do not leave barbecue grills unattended. • Turn pot handles toward back of stove.
Poisoning	• Lock cabinets that contain medicines and cleaning products. • Keep all house plants out of child's reach. • Keep syrup of ipecac in the home. • Have poison control center number by the telephone.
Motor vehicle, pedestrian, biking accidents	• Be sure that car seats have approved infant/toddler restraint systems. • Use seat belts at all times. • Do not leave small children unattended out of doors. • Keep small children in a fenced-in yard if possible. • Have children use bicycle helmets at all times. • Teach children bicycle safety. • Have teenagers take driver education classes before getting their driver's license. • Discuss the importance of not drinking and using drugs while driving.
Drowning	• Do not leave children unsupervised near water or on a boat. • Use life jackets approved for children. • Keep home swimming pools covered when not in use. • Remember that a child can drown in a bath tub or a bucket of water.
Firearms	• Keep guns unloaded, out of reach, and locked away.

Figure 26–2

The federal government and various private agencies have attempted to provide regulations for certain factors that influence some accidents. For example, regulations mandate the use of nonflammable fabric for children's sleepwear. Laws also require proper restraints for infants and small children while riding in automobiles, Figure 26–3. These restraints must meet standards set by the federal government.

The Child Protection and Toy Safety Act, passed in 1970, has helped to stop the distribution of unsafe toys. Nurses, however, should caution parents to inspect any toy purchased for small or loose parts that might cause injury.

NURSING CONSIDERATIONS REGARDING CHILD SAFETY

- Teach parents accident prevention techniques regarding falls, burns, choking.
- Emphasize to parents the importance of keeping household plants out of the reach of children and locking up medications and household toxins.
- Stress to parents the proper use of car seats.
- Suggest that parents buy toys that are developmentally appropriate for their child.

POISONING

Poisoning — by the ingestion, inhalation, absorption, or injection of a toxic substance requiring intervention — is the most common pediatric emergency. Over 2 million poisoning cases involving children are reported to poison control centers in the United States each year; 5,000 of these cases result in death (Budassi Sheehy 1990). Poisoning is a major cause of preventable death in children under 5 years of age, with a peak incidence in children between 2 and 3 years of age. Children in this age group are at greater risk for poisoning because of their characteristic behaviors that involve exploration and testing of the environment (Eichelberger et al. 1992), Figure 26–4.

More than 90% of poisonings occur in the home and are usually caused by common household products, Figure 26–5. Poisonous substances that are commonly ingested by young children are listed in Figure 26–6. The Poison Prevention Packaging Act of 1970 requires that child safety caps be put on all potentially toxic substances and drugs. These caps are not, in fact, "child-proof," but rather are designed to delay access to the substance by a child under 4 years of age.

In order to assess a situation and provide appropriate emergency instructions and care, the health care professional must obtain specific information from the parent or caregiver regarding the poison and the child's condition (Budassi Sheehy 1990), Figure 26–7. Because most substances are absorbed within two to four hours, it is important to act quickly.

Further absorption of a poison may be prevented by chemical removal, mechanical removal, or antidotes. Examples of each method are (1) syrup of ipecac, (2) gastric lavage, and (3) activated charcoal, respectively. The approach used will depend on the substance ingested.

Administer syrup of ipecac to stimulate vomiting. If a parent has syrup of ipecac at home, the recommended dose (Rosenstein and Fosarelli 1989) is

- *9 months:* 5 cc or 1 teaspoon (tsp)
- *9–12 months:* 10 cc or 2 tsp
- *1–12 years:* 15 cc or 1 tablespoon (Tbsp)
- *over 12 years:* 30 cc or 2 Tbsp

Ipecac usually takes effect in 15 to 20 minutes. Do not give ipecac if the child has ingested a

☐ **Do you have the instructions?**
Follow them and keep them with your seat for use as your child grows older.

☐ **Is your child facing the right way, for both weight and age?**
- If you use a seat made only for infants (a), **always** face it backward.
- A baby should ride facing the back of the car up to 20 pounds, and as close as possible to age one (b).
- A child over 20 pounds faces forward (c).

☐ **Is the auto safety belt in the right place, and pulled tight?**
- The belt must go in the correct, marked path to hold the seat in place.
- A convertible seat faces backward for an infant and forward for a toddler (b and c). It has two different belt paths, one for each direction.

☐ **Is the harness snug; does it stay on her shoulders?**
- Shoulder straps go in the lowest slots for babies riding backward, and in the top slots for children facing forward.
- The retainer clip at armpit level (c), holds harness straps on the shoulders.

☐ **Does your child use a booster seat if he is close to 40 pounds and has outgrown his convertible seat?**
- A booster seat helps the safety belt protect your child until she grows big enough to fit the belt alone.
- A booster seat with no shield is used only with a lap and shoulder belt (d). Use a booster with a shield (e) if you car has only lap belts.

☐ **Have you fixed your child's car seat if it has been recalled?**
Call the Auto Safety Hotline (1-800-424-9393) for a list of recalled seats that need repair.

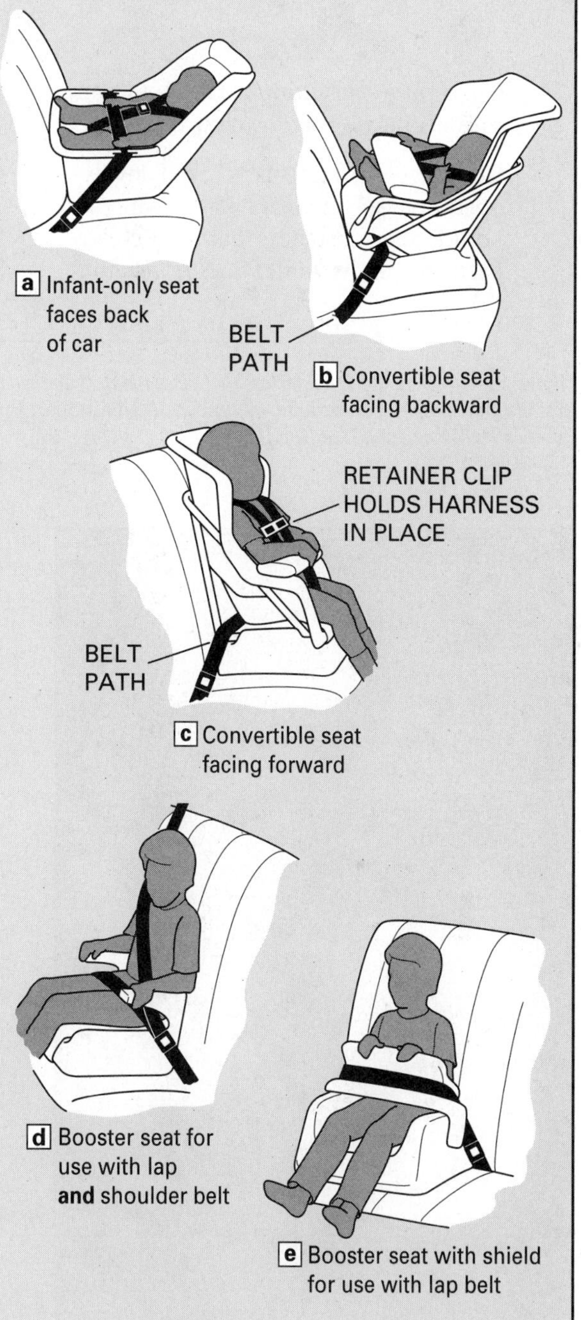

a Infant-only seat faces back of car

BELT PATH

b Convertible seat facing backward

RETAINER CLIP HOLDS HARNESS IN PLACE

BELT PATH

c Convertible seat facing forward

d Booster seat for use with lap **and** shoulder belt

e Booster seat with shield for use with lap belt

Figure 26–3 *Proper use of a car seat for infants and small children is key to preventing or reducing injury in motor vehicle crashes. (Reproduced with permission of the American Academy of Pediatrics, Elk Grove Village, IL)*

DEVELOPMENTAL FACTORS THAT INCREASE POISONING RISK

- Child puts everything in the mouth as a means of exploring the environment.
- Child's sense of taste is not well developed, so he or she will drink or eat many liquids and substances that older children and adults would find distasteful.
- Child is becoming more independent, mobile, and curious.
- Child is now able to open drawers, closets, and most containers.
- Child cannot read labels.

Figure 26–4 *Developmental factors that place toddlers and small children at risk for poisoning (From Eichelberger, Ball, Pratsch, and Runion,* Pediatric Emergencies: A Manual for Prehospital Care Providers, *1992. Adapted by permission of Prentice-Hall, Englewood Cliffs, NJ)*

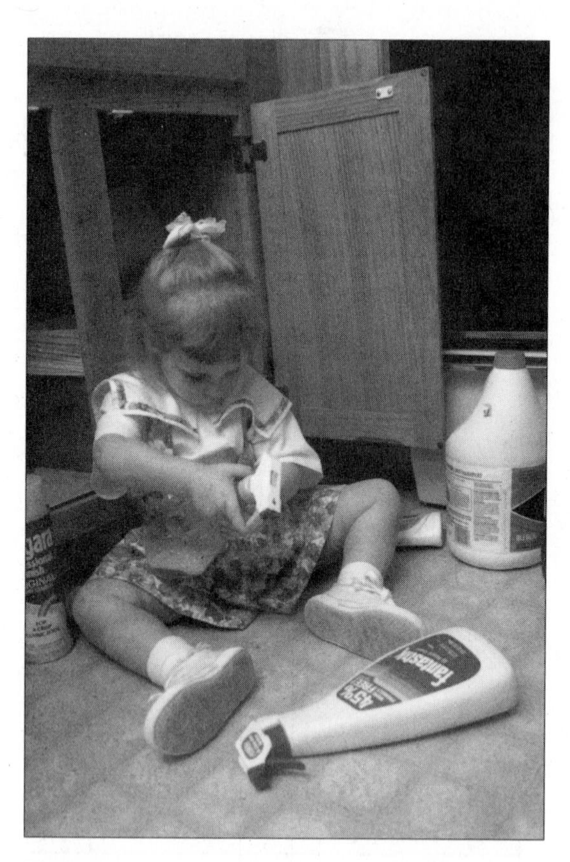

Figure 26–5 *Many substances found in the home present hazards to small children and should be kept in locked cabinets.*

caustic or hydrocarbon, is having a seizure, or is comatose. If there is no response to ipecac or vomiting is contraindicated, gastric lavage is ordered. **Gastric lavage** involves instilling large amounts of warm normal saline through a nasogastric tube into the child's stomach until the return is clear. Lavage is contraindicated for the ingestion of corrosives (lye, strong acids), strychnine, or hydrocarbons (kerosene, gasoline, paint thinner, cleaning fluid).

Ingestions are also treated with the administration of activated charcoal. Activated charcoal prevents absorption of the poison and promotes excretion from the body. There are no known contraindications or side effects. Charcoal has an ugly appearance and can be mixed with water, fruit juice, or syrup to make it easier for the child to drink. Charcoal can also be given by nasogastric or orogastric tube.

Ingestion of a poison may not, in fact, be accidental. Sometimes a child is abused by the administration of drugs. Often, the abuse continues while the child is in the hospital. Be suspicious if the child is less than 1 or more than 5 years of age; if more than one ingestion episode has occurred; if the clinical findings are inconsistent; and if risk factors for abuse are present (Rosenstein and Fosarelli 1989).

POISONOUS SUBSTANCES COMMONLY INGESTED BY CHILDREN

- Over-the-counter medications such as aspirin, acetaminophen, vitamins with iron, skin care preparations, and diaper care products
- Prescription drugs and sedatives
- House and garden plants, such as poinsettias, Boston ivy, elephant ear, ivy (leaves), mistletoe (berries), philodendron, daffodil (bulbs), azalea (foliage and flowers), and rhubarb (leaves)
- Household cleaners
- Petroleum products, such as heavy greases, oils, turpentine, furniture polish, gasoline, and lighter fluid
- Alcohol in alcoholic beverages, cold remedies, mouthwash, perfume, and alcohol-based paints and thinners
- Lead in lead-based paint, unglazed pottery, lead water pipes, and acid juices in leaded pottery

Figure 26–6 *(From Eichelberger, Ball, Pratsch, and Runion,* Pediatric Emergencies: A Manual for Prehospital Care Providers, *1992. Adapted by permission of Prentice-Hall, Englewood Cliffs, NJ)*

WHEN POISONING IS SUSPECTED

- What drug or product did the child take?
- How much did the child take?
- Is the child having any symptoms?
- Is the child having difficulty breathing?
- Has the child ever done this before?
- Tell parents or caregivers to transport the child to the nearest emergency department for evaluation and treatment if needed.
- Tell them to bring the product and product container — including empty containers — to the emergency department.
- Instruct them to save all emesis.

Figure 26–7 *Information to be obtained in suspected cases of pediatric poisoning (Adapted from Budassi Sheehy,* Mosby's Manual of Emergency Care, *3rd ed. Mosby-Year Book, St. Louis, 1990)*

NURSING CONSIDERATIONS REGARDING TOXIC SUBSTANCES

- Emphasize to parents the importance of keeping the poison control center number next to the telephone.
- Teach parents how to use syrup of ipecac, and stress the importance of keeping it in the home.
- Help parents express feelings of fear, anger, and guilt accompanying a child's unintentional injury or poisoning.

CHILD ABUSE

Child abuse — the intentional physical or emotional maltreatment or neglect of children — is a growing social problem. Physical abuse, physical neglect, emotional abuse, emotional neglect, verbal assault, or sexual assault are all forms of child abuse (Harris 1993).

In the United States, it is estimated that there are 50,000 to 70,000 child abuse cases each year (Budassi Sheehy 1990). After sudden infant death syndrome, child abuse is the leading cause of death in infants under 6 months of age (Eichelberger et al. 1992). Many children die each year as a result of child abuse injuries. The child should be removed from the abusive situation as soon as possible to prevent further injury.

It is the nurse's duty to report suspected cases of child abuse to the appropriate legal authorities. Every state has laws that protect children from abuse. Although coming to the realization that a child has been abused is difficult, it is a moral and legal responsibility to report such findings.

PSYCHOSOCIAL FACTORS CONTRIBUTING TO ABUSE

Abuse usually occurs because the abuser is having difficulty coping. Many factors can contribute to the abuse of a child, including economic stressors (poverty, unemployment, too many children), marital problems, single parenthood, inadequate or lack of support systems, and drug or alcohol abuse (Eichelberger et al. 1992). In addition, a child's personality, chronic illness, or physical disabilities can place him or her at high risk for abuse.

TYPES OF ABUSE

Physical Abuse. **Physical abuse** is defined as deliberate physical maltreatment that causes injury to the body. The injuries may be caused by beatings, burns, shaking, or throwing the child. Characteristic signs of physical abuse are listed in Figure 26–8.

Emotional Abuse. Any interaction over a period of time that causes a child unnecessary psychological pain is **emotional abuse**, including excessive demands, verbal harassment, excessive yelling, belittling, teasing, or rejection. Because the signs of emotional abuse are often subtle, this is one of the most difficult types of abuse to identify and prevent.

Sexual Abuse. **Sexual abuse** entails sexual contact between a child, 16 years of age or younger, and a person in a position of authority, no matter what the age, in which the child's participation was obtained through force, threats, bribes, or gifts. Sexual contact can include intercourse, masturbation, fondling, exhibitionism, sodomy, or prostitution (Eichelberger et al. 1992, Rosenstein and Fosarelli 1989).

Physical signs of sexual abuse include bruises on the genitals; a small tear or laceration of the vagina, penis, or anus; semen on the body; and discharge from the urethra, vagina, or penis.

Neglect. **Neglect** refers to the deliberate or unintentional lack of care for a child's basic needs that places the child's life or health in danger (Eichelberger et al. 1992). Neglect can include poor nutrition, inadequate medical care, lack of psychosocial support systems, or lack of education. The absence of daily care and abandonment of the child are also considered neglect.

NURSING CONSIDERATIONS REGARDING CHILD ABUSE

- Become familiar with state laws for the prevention of child abuse and neglect.
- Develop skills to recognize the signs of abuse in children.

SIGNS OF PHYSICAL ABUSE IN CHILDREN

- Small round burns or scars.
- Glove or stocking burns from immersion of the hands or feet in hot water. These burns have a characteristic lack of splash marks.
- Burns to buttocks, legs, and feet, often with creases behind the knees and lack of involvement of the upper thighs.
- Clearly defined burns showing the shape of the object used — for example, an iron, stove burner, oven rack, or radiator.
- Slap marks resembling the shape of a hand.
- Welts showing the shape of the object used — for example, a belt, buckle, hanger, electrical cord.
- Suspicious bruises in various stages of healing. Active children often have bruises over bony prominences such as the shins, hips, spine, lower arms, forehead, and under the chin. These are caused by falling and bumping into objects during play. Suspicious sites for bruises are on the upper arms, trunk, upper thighs, sides of the face, ears and neck, genitalia, and buttocks.
- Human bite marks indicating the pattern of teeth and size of an adult's mouth.

Figure 26–8 *(From Eichelberger, Ball, Pratsch, and Runion,* Pediatric Emergencies: A Manual for Prehospital Care Providers, *1992. Adapted by permission of Prentice-Hall, Englewood Cliffs, NJ)*

PEDIATRIC BASIC LIFE SUPPORT: THE ABCS OF CPR

CARDIOPULMONARY RESUSCITATION

Cardiopulmonary resuscitation (CPR) provides basic life support to a victim who, unable to breathe or pump sufficient blood through the body, would otherwise die. There are three basic skill groups known as the ABCs of CPR: *A*irway, *B*reathing, and *C*irculation.

Airway — Determine Responsiveness. The nurse must first determine whether the infant or child is conscious and breathing. To determine the level of responsiveness, tap the child and speak loudly. When the child is unconscious, the muscles in the mouth and throat relax, allowing the tongue to fall back into the throat and obstruct the airway. The airway should be opened immediately using the head tilt–chin lift maneuver, Figure 26–9a, b. If neck injury is suspected, the head tilt should be avoided and the airway opened using a jaw thrust, instead, keeping the cervical spine completely immobilized.

Breathing — Assessment. Once the airway is opened, check for breathing. Look for a rise and fall of the chest and abdomen, listen for exhaled air, and feel for exhaled air flow at the mouth. If no movement is observed, **rescue breathing** is begun, Figure 26–9c, d.

If the victim is an infant (under 1 year of age), place your mouth over the infant's nose and mouth, creating a seal. If the victim is a large infant or child (1–8 years of age), make a mouth-to-mouth seal, pinching the victim's nose tightly with your thumb and forefinger and maintaining the head tilt with your other hand. Provide two slow breaths to the victim, pausing in between to take a breath. If a mask

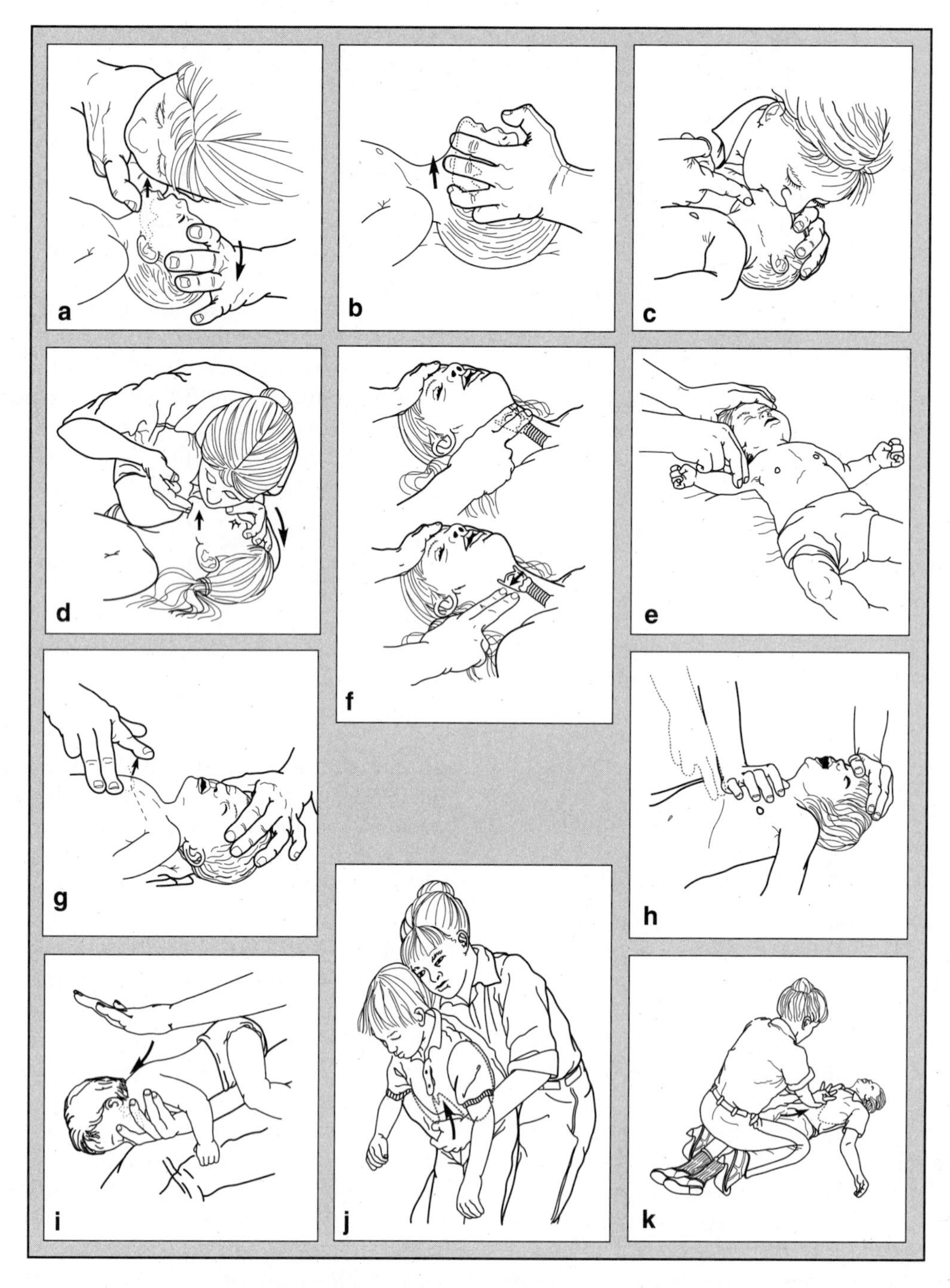

Figure 26–9 *Procedures for cardiopulmonary resuscitation (a–h) and removal of a foreign body obstruction (i–k) (From Emergency Cardiac Care Committee and Subcommittees, American Heart Association, 1992. Guidelines for cardiopulmonary resuscitation and emergency cardiac care. V. Pediatric basic life support.* Journal of the American Medical Association, *vol. 268, no. 16)*

with a one-way valve or other infection-control barrier is available, it should be used when performing rescue breathing.

If the chest does not rise after the initial breaths, airway obstruction may be the cause. Reposition the victim's head by performing the head tilt–chin lift or jaw thrust maneuver. If the chest still does not rise, the obstruction may be from a foreign body. Once the airway is opened and two rescue breaths have been provided, determine whether chest compression is needed.

Circulation — Assessment (Pulse Check). Assess the pulse in a large central artery. The short, chubby neck of children under 1 year of age makes rapid location of the carotid artery difficult, so palpation of the brachial artery is recommended, Figure 26–9e. In children over 1 year of age, the carotid artery on the side of the neck is used, Figure 26–9f.

If a pulse is present but the infant or child is not breathing, rescue breathing alone should be provided at a rate of 20 breaths per minute (once every 3 seconds) until spontaneous breathing resumes. If a pulse is not palpable, external chest compressions are begun.

Chest Compressions

Chest compressions must always be accompanied by ventilations. To achieve optimal compressions place the infant or child in a supine position on a hard, flat surface.

The area of compression for infants is the lower third of the sternum, Figure 26–9g. Landmarks and technique for chest compression in an infant are as follows:

1. Draw an imaginary line (intermammary line) between the nipples, over the breastbone.
2. Place your index finger on the sternum just below the intermammary line. Place your middle and ring fingers approximately a fingerwidth below the line where it intersects the sternum. Avoid compression of the xiphoid process.
3. Compress the chest ½ to 1 inch at the rate of at least 100 times per minute. Pause for ventilation.
4. At the end of each compression, pressure is released without removing the fingers from the surface of the chest.

Landmarks and technique for chest compression in a child are as follows:

1. Using the middle and index fingers of the hand nearer the victim's feet, trace the lower margin of the victim's rib cage, on the side of the chest next to you.
2. Using the middle finger, follow the margin of the rib cage to the notch where the ribs and sternum meet.
3. With the middle finger on this notch, place the index finger next to the middle finger.
4. Place the heel of the same hand next to the point where the index finger was located, with the long axis of the heel parallel to that of the sternum, Figure 26–9h. The fingers should be held up off the ribs while the heel of the hand remains in contact with the sternum.
5. Use your other hand to maintain the child's head position.
6. Compress the chest 1–1½ inches at the rate of 100 times per minute. Pause for ventilation.
7. Compressions should be smooth. Allow the chest to return to its resting position after each compression, but do not lift your hand off of the chest.

Coordination of Compressions and Rescue Breathing. External chest compressions must always be accompanied by rescue breathing. At the end of every five compressions, a pause of 1–1½ seconds should be allowed for a ventilation. The infant and small child should be reassessed after 20 cycles of compressions and ventilations (approximately 1 minute) and every few minutes thereafter for any sign of resumption of spontaneous breathing or pulses.

If you are alone, call for help after 1 minute of rescue support (20 breaths including chest compressions, if necessary). If the victim is small and no trauma is suspected, it may be possible to carry the child (supporting the head and neck carefully) to a telephone while CPR is provided so that you can call for help.

FOREIGN BODY AIRWAY OBSTRUCTION

The most common cause of respiratory distress in children is airway obstruction. Aspiration of a foreign body can result in airway obstruction and death. Foreign body aspiration is the second leading cause of unintentional injury deaths in infants between 1 month and 1 year of age and the fifth leading cause in children 1 to 4 years of age. Commonly aspirated foods include hot dogs, uncooked vegetables, peanuts, grapes, beans, candy, and seeds. The size, shape, and consistency of the object contribute to the severity of the symptoms.

The Infant. If an infant or child experiences the sudden onset of respiratory distress associated with coughing, gagging, or **stridor** (a high-pitched, noisy sound or wheezing), suspect foreign body aspiration. Relief of the obstruction should be attempted only if the cough is or becomes ineffective (loss of sound) or the child is having increasing respiratory difficulty, accompanied by stridor.

The Child: The Heimlich Maneuver. In children under 1 year of age, a combination of five back blows and five chest thrusts is used to try to remove the obstruction, Figure 26–9i. Back blows are delivered while the infant is supported in the prone position. Chest thrusts are delivered while the infant is supine. Remove the foreign body if it can be seen.

In older children, subdiaphragmatic abdominal thrusts are performed with the child either sitting, standing, or lying (**Heimlich maneuver**), Figure 26–9j, k.

When the child is conscious and is either standing or sitting, perform the following steps.

1. Stand behind the child with your arms directly under the child's axillae and encircling the child's chest.
2. Make a fist with one hand, placing the thumb side against the midline of the child's abdomen, slightly above the navel and below the tip of the xiphoid process.
3. Grasp the fist with the other hand and exert a series of up to five quick upward thrusts. Take care not to press on the xiphoid or the rib cage because of the potential for damage to internal organs.

When the child is unconscious and lying on the floor, perform these steps.

1. Place the child supine and kneel beside the child or straddle the child's hips.
2. Place the heel of one hand in the midline of the child's abdomen above the navel and below the rib cage and xiphoid process. Place the other hand on top of the fist.
3. Press both hands into the abdomen with a quick upward thrust. Each thrust is directed upward in the midline and should not be directed to either side of the abdomen.

Individual thrusts should continue until the foreign body is expelled or until five abdominal thrusts have been delivered. If the foreign body can be seen, remove it.

NURSING CONSIDERATIONS REGARDING CPR

- Promote classes in CPR for the general public.
- Encourage new parents to learn CPR and to recertify periodically to maintain these skills.

REVIEW QUESTIONS

A. Multiple choice. Select the best answer.

1. The most common pediatric emergency is
   a. child abuse
   b. poisoning
   c. burns
   d. drowning

2. The recommended dose of syrup of ipecac for a 3-year-old toddler is
   a. 5 cc (1 tsp)
   b. 10 cc (2 tsp)
   c. 15 cc (1 Tbsp)
   d. 30 cc (2 Tbsp)

3. Syrup of ipecac may be used
   a. to stimulate vomiting when some poisons have been ingested
   b. when the child is in a coma from poisoning
   c. to stop convulsions from poisoning
   d. as an antidote for caustics

4. Gastric lavage is indicated when
   a. a corrosive, such as lye or strong acid, has been ingested
   b. there is no response to ipecac or when vomiting is contraindicated
   c. strychnine poisoning occurs
   d. a child drinks a hydrocarbon such as kerosene

5. The incidence of child abuse in the United States each year is approximately
   a. 10,000–15,000 cases
   b. 20,000–30,000 cases
   c. 50,000–70,000 cases
   d. 100,000–150,000 cases

6. Which of the following is *not* a form of emotional abuse?
   a. intimidation
   b. rejection
   c. teasing
   d. starvation

7. Which of the following is *not* true of sexual abuse?
   a. Sexual contact is not limited to intercourse.
   b. Most of the signs of sexual abuse are easily spotted.
   c. Overt signs of sexual abuse include bruising on the genitals, lacerations of the vagina or anus, semen on the body, discharge from the vagina or penis.
   d. It involves a child, 16 years or younger, with another person in a position of authority.

8. The rate of chest compressions used when performing CPR on a 10-year-old child should be
   a. 60 times/minute
   b. 80 times/minute
   c. 100 times/minute
   d. 120 times/minute

9. When performing CPR on an unconscious child, one should not
   a. shake the child gently to determine the level of response
   b. open the airway manually using the head tilt–chin lift
   c. open the airway manually using the jaw thrust maneuver
   d. leave the neck unstabilized if a cervical spine injury is suspected

10. The most common cause of respiratory distress in children is
    a. cardiac arrest
    b. airway obstruction
    c. asthma
    d. child abuse

SUGGESTED ACTIVITIES

- Create a teaching tool to educate peers or parents about one of the following:
  - falls
  - poisoning
  - burns
  - vehicle/bicycle crashes
  - choking
  - drowning
  - firearms
  - assault
- Describe and demonstrate how the procedure for performing CPR on an infant differs from the procedure for a child.
- Describe and demonstrate how the procedure for removing a foreign body obstruction from an infant differs from the procedure for a child.
- Discuss how the nurse can help parents express feelings of fear, anger, and guilt when a child is injured or poisoned, and list three ways of providing emotional support.

BIBLIOGRAPHY

American Heart Association. *Healthcare Provider's Manual for Basic Life Support*. Dallas: American Heart Association, 1988.

Budassi Sheehy, S. *Mosby's Manual of Emergency Care*, 3rd ed. St. Louis, MO: Mosby-Year Book, 1990.

Eichelberger, M. R., J. W. Ball, G. S. Pratsch, and E. Runion. *Pediatric Emergencies: A Manual for Prehospital Care Providers*. Englewood Cliffs, NJ: Brady/Prentice-Hall, 1992.

Emergency Cardiac Care Committee and Subcommittees, American Heart Association. Guidelines for cardiopulmonary resuscitation and emergency cardiac care. V. Pediatric basic life support. *Journal of the American Medical Association* 268, no. 16 (1992): 2251–2261.

Harris, P. *A Child's Story: Recovering through Creativity*. St. Louis, MO: Cracom Corporation, 1993.

Jones, N. E. Prevention of childhood injuries: Motor vehicle injuries. *Pediatric Nursing* 18, no. 4 (1992): 380–382.

Kottmeier, P. K. The battered child. *Pediatric Annals* 16, no. 4 (April, 1987): 343–351.

Rosenstein, B. J., and P. D. Fosarelli. *Pediatric Pearls: The Handbook of Practical Pediatrics*. St. Louis, MO: Mosby-Year Book, 1989.

Seidel, J., et al. Presentation and evaluation of sexual misuse in the emergency department. *Pediatric Emergency Care* 2 (1986): 157–164.

Willens, J. S. Strengthen your life-support skills. *Nursing 93* 23, no. 4 (1993): 54–58.

Wong, D. L. *Whaley & Wong's Essentials of Pediatric Nursing*, 4th ed. St. Louis, MO: Mosby-Year Book, 1993.

UNIT

vii

Hospitalization

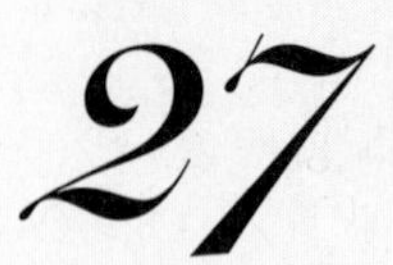

CHAPTER 27

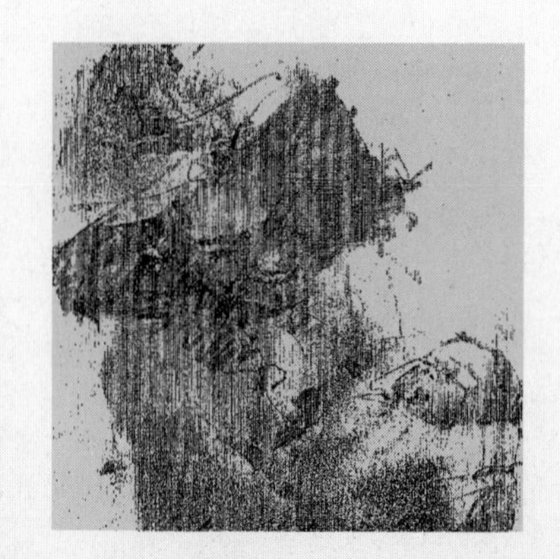

Preparing for Hospitalization

OBJECTIVES

AFTER STUDYING THIS CHAPTER, THE STUDENT SHOULD BE ABLE TO:

- DISCUSS THE ROLE OF THE NURSE IN PREPARING A CHILD AND FAMILY FOR HOSPITALIZATION.
- IDENTIFY THE TYPE OF INFORMATION NEEDED BY THE FAMILY OF THE HOSPITALIZED CHILD PRIOR TO ADMISSION.
- IDENTIFY INDICATORS OF STRESS AMONG SIBLINGS OF A HOSPITALIZED CHILD.
- IDENTIFY STRATEGIES THAT CAN BE USED TO PREPARE CHILDREN OF DIFFERENT AGES FOR HOSPITALIZATION.
- DISCUSS THE IMPORTANCE OF COMMUNICATION IN PREPARING CHILDREN OF DIFFERENT AGES FOR HOSPITALIZATION.

KEY TERMS

STRESSORS
RITUALS
DISBELIEF

Hospitalization of a child can be planned or unplanned. For most children, regardless of the reason for admission, hospitalization is a fearful bewildering experience (Faller 1988). Even with preparation, it places stress on the child and the family. Unfamiliar sounds, smells, routines, and strangers; confinement; separation from parents and siblings; and loss of control are only a few of the **stressors** with which a child must cope during hospitalization.

PREPARING THE FAMILY FOR HOSPITALIZATION

Adequate preparation of the family can influence the child's adjustment to hospitalization, Figure 27–1. The focus of this preparation is to minimize stress and avoid crisis. A planned hospitalization can be an organized effort to comfort both the family and the child. Planning can involve a hospital teaching program that encompasses preadmission activities, day of admission activities, and discharge planning. The trend in many pediatric acute care settings is to include the family in a significant way (Brown and Ritchie 1990).

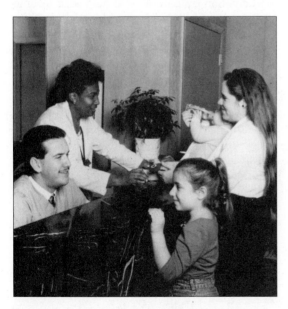

Figure 27–1 *Preadmission and day of admission activities can help prepare children and their families for the planned hospitalization. (From Keir, Wise, and Krebs,* Medical Assisting Administrative & Clinical Competencies, *3rd edition, Delmar Publishers Inc., 1993)*

FAMILY ASSESSMENT

The first step in preparing the family is assessing their level of knowledge. What do they know? What do they need to know? Good communication skills and interviewing techniques are essential because the seriousness of the child's illness affects family reactions.

In the assessment process, the nurse should allow for a free exchange of information. This approach helps to build a positive relationship in which parents are able to talk openly about concerns and fears. It also gives the nurse an opportunity to learn the family structure, ages of siblings, and support systems that may already be present. Note the socioeconomic level and cultural and spiritual affiliation of the family, as well as the interaction between parents. Illness of a child can place additional stressors on the parents' relationship and reduce their ability to cope.

Throughout the assessment phase, reinforce to parents that they are an integral part of the child's recovery. Parenting the child should not change, and preparation for discharge should begin on admission. Observe and assess the parents' reaction to the child's illness. If the child has been diagnosed with an illness such as leukemia or cystic fibrosis that has long-term effects, parents may have difficulty believing that this is actually happening to their child. This **disbelief** is often coupled with anger and guilt. Anger, which may be directed at themselves or at others, is common. Parents may look for reasons for the onset of illness in their own actions or perceived shortcomings. Feelings of guilt can surface when parents anticipate their helplessness when confronted by their child's illness and pain.

The importance of the assessment phase should not be minimized. Hospitals in which preadmission teaching or conferences take place provide the nurse with an opportunity for conducting a planned interview.

PREADMISSION TEACHING AND INTERVIEW

Dialogue should be geared toward the parents' level of understanding. Language barriers and cultural patterns need to be considered to make teaching effective.

Ideally both parents should participate in the teaching process. Sometimes, however, one parent is more accepting and ready to participate than the other.

The information presented to parents should be honest and accurate. It should include anticipated reactions of the child to hospitalization. Telling the child about hospitalization can be traumatic for parents. How much do they say? What do they say? The answers to these questions will depend on the child's age and developmental level and the seriousness of the illness. Allow time between sessions for parents to formulate questions and develop strategies to help the child learn about hospitalization. Several resources are available to parents to help them formulate their approach, Figure 27–2. Particularly effective are books that can be read to the child in preparation for hospitalization, Figure 27–3.

Parents should be encouraged to participate in the care of the child during hospitalization. Mutual participation is ideal but not always practical. Parents may need to take turns visiting the child, particularly if there are other children at home. Working parents may find it difficult to care for their hospitalized child, so planning for extended family members to participate may be appropriate. Adjusting a work schedule may take some planning. But participation by parents will help ease feelings of helplessness, loss of control, and loss of the parenting role (Petrillo and Sanger 1980).

Be aware that in some cultures, adults other than the child's parents may provide important support to the child and family. Among Mexican Americans, for example, a godparent may be an important participant in

RESOURCE BOOKS

Curious George Goes to the Hospital, M. Rey and H. A. Rey, Houghton Mifflin Company.

Doctors and Nurses: What Do They Do? C. Green, Harper & Row Junior Books.

The Hospital Book, J. Howe, Crown Publishers.

Richard Scarry's Nicky Goes to the Doctor, R. Scarry, A Golden Book.

Why Am I Going to the Hospital? C. Ciliotta and C. Livingston, Lyle Stuart.

Your Child Goes to the Hospital: A Book for Parents, H. Love et al., Charles C. Thomas.

Note: Most major bookstores will special order books if they are not available on the shelf.

Figure 27–2 *Resource books to help prepare children for hospitalization*

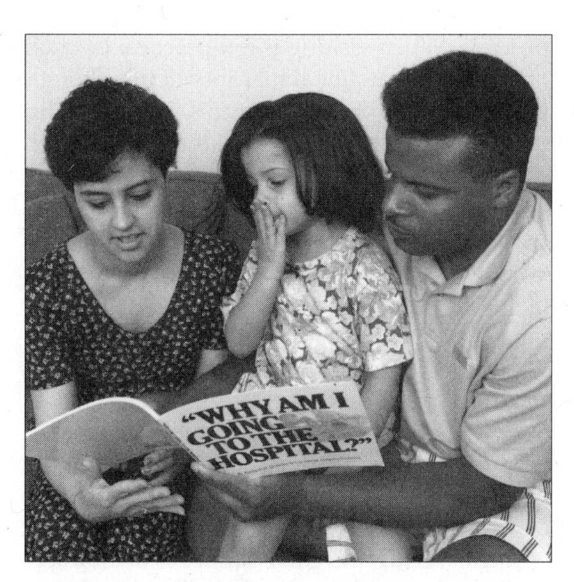

Figure 27–3 *Reading the child books that describe the hospital stay is one strategy that parents can use to prepare the child before admission.*

care of the hospitalized child. The presence of these support persons reduces the family's fear and anxiety and facilitates adjustment to the hospital setting (Giger and Davidhizar 1991). When extended family members or godparents will be present, it is important that they be identified to the staff.

Parents should be taught that the hospitalized child may exhibit uncharacteristic behaviors. That is, the child may be stubborn, overly quiet, sad, uncommunicative, or unruly. The child may cry without much provocation, and younger children, especially, may regress to behaviors such as bed wetting, thumb sucking, and use of the bottle or pacifier (Bolig and Weedle 1988). Hospitalization is particularly stressful for toddlers, who experience separation anxiety when parted from parents (see Chapter 29). Advising parents of these anticipated behavioral changes can help them cope when these behaviors occur.

During the preadmission interview, ask parents to describe the child's daily routine. Ask about the child's toileting habits and the words used for toileting. It is important to know if the child takes an afternoon nap or if there is a favorite afterschool activity or television program. These **rituals** can be comforting and provide for emotional stability. Encourage parents to bring the child's favorite toys, blankets, books, or other objects from home. Figure 27–4 lists age-appropriate toys and activities that can be provided for the hospitalized child. Rooming-in also should be encouraged where it is permitted. The focus of this strategy is to minimize separation and maintain the appearance of the child's basic routine (Brown and Ritchie 1990).

Parents should be prepared for anticipated tests and procedures before admission and informed about pertinent preoperative and postoperative care. Blood workups and x-rays are common preadmission procedures. Information about anesthesia can be discussed at this time.

SIBLINGS

One area of teaching that is often neglected is the impact of hospitalization on the siblings of the hospitalized child. Age-appropriate information should be shared with the siblings. Clear, concise, truthful answers are best. Often, siblings feel neglected and less loved because the attention is on the hospitalized child. The parents' role should include listening to siblings and allowing them time to express their feelings and concerns. Time should be taken to praise them and reinforce their need to be loved (Craft and Craft 1989). Siblings often wonder if they will get sick too. Magical thinking is common among preschool children and may lead siblings at this developmental stage to believe that their thoughts and deeds caused the hospitalized child's illness. Rivalry, which may have existed before hospitalization, also can be a source of guilt and shame.

Separation does nothing to foster family ties, so siblings are encouraged to visit when

ANTICIPATORY GUIDANCE

Age	Toys/Activities
Infant	Mobiles Cradle gyms Busy box Stuffed animals
Toddler	Stuffed animals Doctor's kit Dolls Picture books Simple puzzles
Preschool child	Balloons Puppets Crayons Toy hospital Books In-room television
School-age child	Playing cards Television Video games Transistor radio Books Simple games Cut outs Writing materials Art supplies Cuddly toys
Adolescent	Telephone Television Video games/movies Books Writing materials Art supplies Board games

Figure 27–4 *Anticipatory guidance: Age-appropriate toys and activities for hospitalized children*

possible. When visiting is not practical because of the age or emotional maturity of the siblings, they can send letters, pictures, photographs, cards, and even telephone the hospitalized child to maintain contact (Petrillo and Sanger 1980). Parents who are already having to cope with their own feelings and emotions have the added task of monitoring the support needed by the siblings.

PREPARING THE CHILD FOR HOSPITALIZATION

Preparation of the child for hospitalization is dependent on the child's age and stage of development. Telling the child about hospitalization, explaining procedures, and gaining cooperation are linked to the child's developmental readiness (Faller 1988). Timing of preparation is also age-dependent. Young children can be told about the planned hospitalization one to three days before admission, school-age children one week before admission, and adolescents as soon as the need for hospitalization is determined (Cowen 1993).

Theories of development proposed by Freud, Piaget, and Erikson provide a framework for anticipating responses of children at particular ages (refer to Chapter 23). Erikson's approach, based on psychosocial tasks or crises, is useful in developing age-appropriate approaches to children (Erikson 1963). Knowing what is normal can help nurses formulate the plan of care for children in stressful situations.

Using Erikson's theory as a framework, the following discussion provides both the family and nurse with information to meet the needs of the child before and during hospital admission.

INFANT

According to Erikson, psychosocial tasks in the first year center on trust versus mistrust. At this stage, the infant can signal needs by crying or contentment. The infant's sense of self is closely tied to the caregiver. Talking to the infant, holding, and cuddling can lessen the traumatic experience of hospitalization. Encourage parents to room in, hold, feed, play, and provide some level of stimulation to the infant during hospitalization to encourage normal development.

TODDLER

From 1 to 3 years, psychosocial tasks focus on autonomy versus shame and doubt. The toddler is aware of hospitalization, separation, and loss of control. Parents and caregivers should explain in simple terms what is happening and how it will help to make the child better.

PRESCHOOL CHILD

The preschool years, from 3 to 6 years, are characterized by the psychosocial tasks of initiative versus guilt. The preschool child responds verbally and has many questions. Particular care must be given to explain hospitalization and procedures. Fear of bodily mutilation is common in this age group. At this age, the child responds well to prehospitalization programs. Introduce the child to the environment, particularly the unit or room, to help reduce the fear of the unknown. Emphasize healing and helping when discussing the need for hospitalization and procedures.

SCHOOL-AGE CHILD

The school-age years, from 6 to 12, are characterized by the psychosocial tasks of industry versus inferiority. The school-age child needs to have positive reinforcement. Be sure the child understands that hospitalization is not a punishment for something he or she did wrong. Self-confidence can be fragile, and trust at this stage is paramount. Preparation can involve simple books, diagrams, videotapes, and the opportunity to handle equipment (Cowen 1993).

ADOLESCENT

Adolescence, the period between 12 and 18 years, is characterized by the psychosocial tasks of identity versus role diffusion. Adolescents have an increasing sense of self and are influenced by peer groups and leadership. Hospitalization is particularly stressful because the adolescent is viewed as separate from the group. Visits from peers should be encouraged. Adolescents understand simple to complex medical terms and can be provided with verbal explanations, books, and diagrams to explain planned procedures (Cowen 1993). Adolescents have the ability to make decisions and should be involved in planning for hospitalization and given options, when appropriate.

NURSING CONSIDERATIONS IN PREPARING CHILDREN FOR HOSPITALIZATION

- Understanding growth and development milestones can assist the nurse in teaching and caring for the hospitalized child.
- In an ideal situation, in which hospitalization is planned, preadmission preparation should help meet parents' need to provide support and participate in care, as well as their needs for information and reinforcement. Siblings should have an opportunity to participate, ask questions, and continue to participate within the family circle.
- For the child, developmentally appropriate preparation can reduce stressors such as separation anxiety, fear of the unknown, and loss of control. A less-stressful experience, in turn, aids in the healing process.

REVIEW QUESTIONS

A. Multiple choice. Select the best answer.

1. Interviewing the parent(s) is an integral part of the assessment process before the hospitalization of a child. Which of the following techniques is the best method to obtain information?
   a. Let parents direct the course of the interview.
   b. Give parents a checklist of questions.
   c. Talk to parents using open-ended questions.
   d. Quiz parents about how you can meet their needs.

2. The goal of the assessment process is to collect information and ultimately plan with the family a positive hospital experience. What would be the best first step?
   a. Use your interviewing skills to find out what the family knows about the child's hospitalization and illness.
   b. Be cordial and upbeat in your first meeting.
   c. Let parents take the inquiring role, since they know all about the child.
   d. Talk to only one parent at a time.

3. Preparing for the hospitalization of a child can create stress in the relationship of the parents. Even though it is best to talk to both parents, in which situation would you talk to only one?
   a. when one parent keeps interrupting your presentation with questions
   b. when one parent refuses to participate in the discussion
   c. when one parent keeps blaming the other for the child's problem
   d. when one parent cries all the time

4. Participating in care is important for parents because
   a. it allows the parents to remain occupied
   b. parents know how to take care of the child better than the staff
   c. it is comforting for the child to have familiar caregivers
   d. it allows parents to monitor the staff

5. Many hospitals have preadmission programs and perform tests on an out-patient basis. The reason for this approach to child care is to
   a. save money
   b. introduce the family and child to the hospital in an organized manner
   c. help the staff form a relationship with the family
   d. get all the information needed before hospitalization

6. The role of the nurse in preparing the family for hospitalization is to
   a. provide support information as reinforcement for parents
   b. make sure the parents will not give false information to the child
   c. keep the child from being anxious about hospitalization
   d. allow the parents and child to pick out the room

7. Which of the following measures can be used to promote family harmony during a child's hospitalization?
   a. Siblings should not be told the truth about the hospitalization so that they do not worry too much.
   b. Parents should encourage and plan for visits by the siblings.
   c. Parents should have a significant other take care of the children at home because their time is limited.
   d. Parents should maintain a happy disposition.

8. Preparation for hospitalization for a child between the ages of 1 and 3 should include
   a. limiting parents' time with the child, since the child cries when they leave
   b. encouraging parents to keep the child neat and clean
   c. holding, cuddling, and talking to the child
   d. keeping the child in his or her own room to avoid exposure to any other illness

9. For children between the ages of 6 and 12, the preparation for hospitalization should include
   a. a truthful explanation in language that is nonthreatening
   b. an explanation that omits all the hurtful parts
   c. an explanation in terms they will not really understand to keep them from being afraid
   d. an explanation that is given only by the nurse, since she understands most about the illness

10. When an adolescent is hospitalized, the best preparation includes
    a. having a regular time for school friends to visit
    b. having the adolescent participate in decision making
    c. having the adolescent view all the procedures in which he or she will be involved
    d. limiting parents' visits, since the parents really do not understand this child

---

SUGGESTED ACTIVITIES

- Contact your local hospital's public relations department and inquire about the programs that are conducted to prepare for the hospitalization of a child. Make arrangements to view audiovisual materials that may be available.
- Practice communication techniques by role playing with classmates. Have a fellow student pick a developmental stage and diagnosis; then prepare the student for hospitalization.
- Contact a childcare center and arrange to observe normal child interactions. Compare and contrast the behaviors you observe with those of a hospitalized child.
- Read several of the books on the resource list in Figure 27–2 and develop a book review for each so that you can recommend particular books with some knowledge of their content.

Bibliography

Bolig, R., and K. D. Weedle. Resiliency and hospitalization of children. *Child Health Care* 16, no. 4 (1988): 255–260.

Brown, J., and J. A. Ritchie. Nurses' perceptions of parent and nurse roles in caring for hospitalized children. *Child Health Care* 19, no. 1 (1990): 28–36.

Cowen, K. J. Hospital care for children. In D. Broadwell Jackson and R. B. Saunders, eds. *Child Health Nursing*. Philadelphia: J. B. Lippincott, 1993.

Craft, M. J., and J. L. Craft. Perceived changes in siblings of hospitalized children: A comparison of sibling and parent reports. *Child Health Care* 18, no. 1 (1989): 42–48.

Erikson, E. H. *Childhood and Society*, 2nd ed. New York: W. W. Norton, 1963.

Faller, H. S. A child's perception of the hospital. *American Journal of Maternal-Child Nursing* 13 (1988): 38.

Giger, J. N., and R. F. Davidhizar. *Transcultural Nursing: Assessment and Intervention*. St. Louis, MO: Mosby-Year Book, 1991.

Petrillo, M., and S. Sanger. *Emotional Care of Hospitalized Children*, 2nd ed. Philadelphia: J. B. Lippincott, 1980.

Pontious, S. L. Practical Piaget: Helping children understand. *American Journal of Nursing* 82 (1982): 114–117.

CHAPTER

28

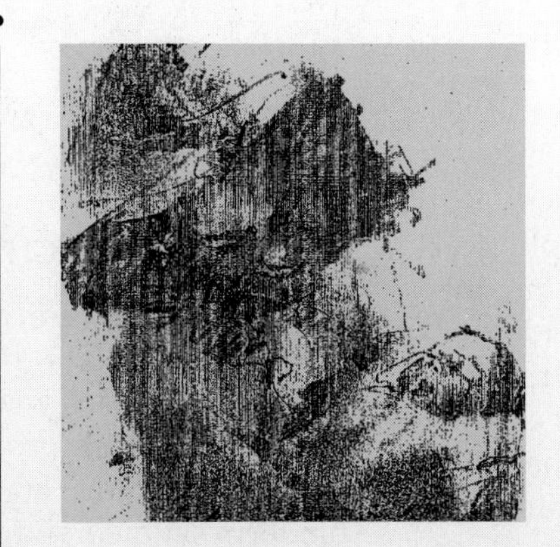

Assessment

Objectives

After studying this chapter, the student should be able to:

- Identify common methods for measuring a child's physical growth.
- Describe the various methods available for measuring weight and height in infants, children, and adolescents.
- Describe the various methods available for taking a child's temperature.
- Describe the recommended methods for taking a child's pulse.
- Define sinus arrhythmia and explain its significance to pediatric assessment.
- Describe methods for taking a child's blood pressure.
- Discuss nursing considerations in pediatric assessment.

Key Terms

Head circumference

Sinus arrhythmia

Apical pulse

Routine pediatric assessment includes physical measurements (height, weight, head circumference, and chest circumference) and vital sign assessment (temperature, pulse, respirations, and blood pressure). Physical measurements help the nurse to determine whether a child's growth is within the normal parameters for his or her age. These measurements, along with vital sign assessment, provide valuable information that contributes to assessment of overall health status.

MEASUREMENTS

Measurement of physical growth in children is a key element in assessment of health status. Indicators of physical growth include height (length), weight, head circumference, and chest circumference. Values are plotted on growth charts, and the child's measurements in percentiles are compared with those of the general population (see the appendixes at the back of this textbook).

HEIGHT AND WEIGHT

Various devices are available for measuring height and weight in children. Infants and small children are weighed on an infant platform scale, which provides a measurement in ounces and grams, Figure 28–1. The scale has a platform with curved sides in which the child may sit or lie. Weigh the infant or child in as few clothes as possible, removing the diaper and shoes or slippers. A small sheet, cloth diaper, or paper towel should be placed on the scale before weighing the infant or child, to avoid the transfer of microorganisms from bare skin.

Infant length can be measured using an infant measuring board, which consists of a rigid headboard and movable footboard, Figure 28–2. Place the measuring board on a table and position the infant on his or her back on the board, with the head touching the headboard. Move the footboard up until it touches the bottom of the infant's feet.

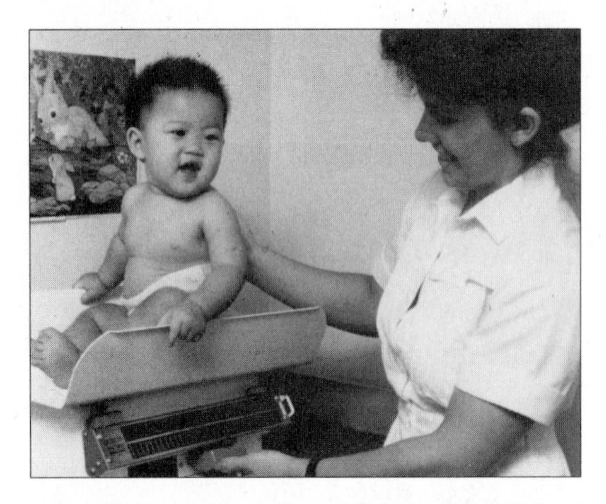

Figure 28–1 *Infant platform scale (From Keir, Wise, and Krebs,* Medical Assisting: Administrative and Clinical Competencies, *3rd ed. Delmar Publishers Inc., 1993)*

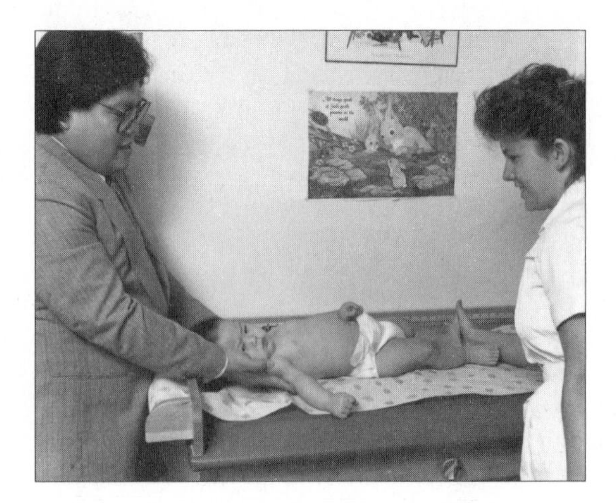

Figure 28–2 *Foot- and headboard for measuring the length of an infant (From Keir, Wise, and Krebs,* Medical Assisting: Administrative and Clinical Competencies, *3rd ed. Delmar Publishers Inc., 1993)*

An infant can also be measured on a pad by placing a pin into the pad or making a pencil mark at the top of the head and a second pin or mark at the heel of the extended leg. The length is the distance between the two pins. A tape measure can also be used.

A stature-measuring device may be used to measure height once the child is able to stand erect without support. The device consists of a movable headpiece attached to a rigid measuring bar and platform, Figure 28–3. A paper towel should be placed on the platform before use to avoid the potential transmission of microorganisms from bare feet.

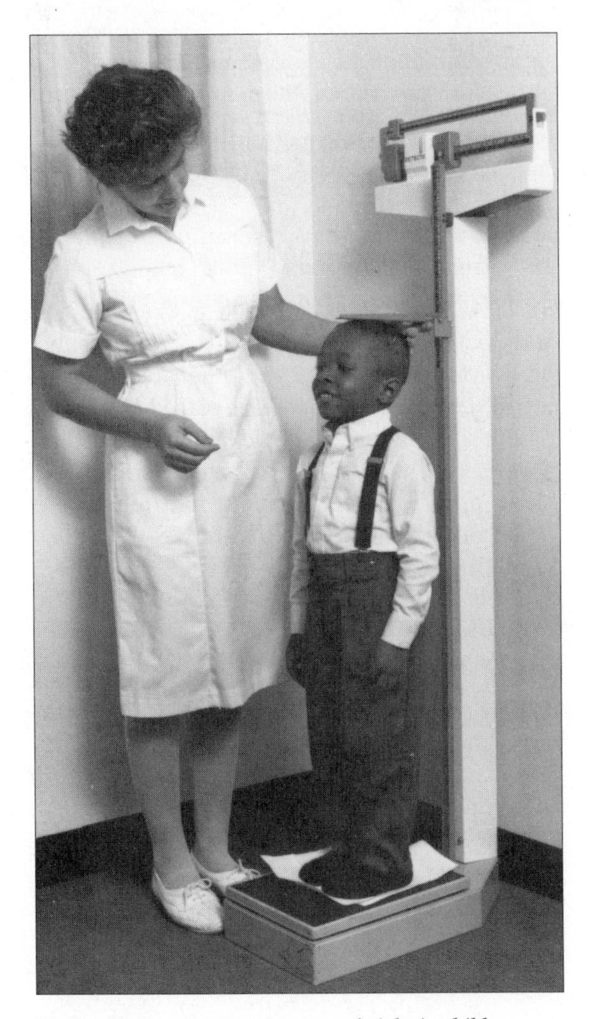

Figure 28–3 Device to measure height in children (From Keir, Wise, and Krebs, Medical Assisting: Administrative and Clinical Competencies, *3rd ed. Delmar Publishers Inc., 1993)*

HEAD CIRCUMFERENCE

Head circumference is usually measured in all children up to 3 years of age and in any child whose head size is questionable. Measure the head at its greatest circumference, slightly above the eyebrows and pinnae of the ears and around the occipital prominence at the back of the skull. Use a paper or metal tape, since a cloth tape may stretch and give a falsely small measurement, Figure 28–4. Generally head and chest circumference are equal at about 1 to 2 years of age.

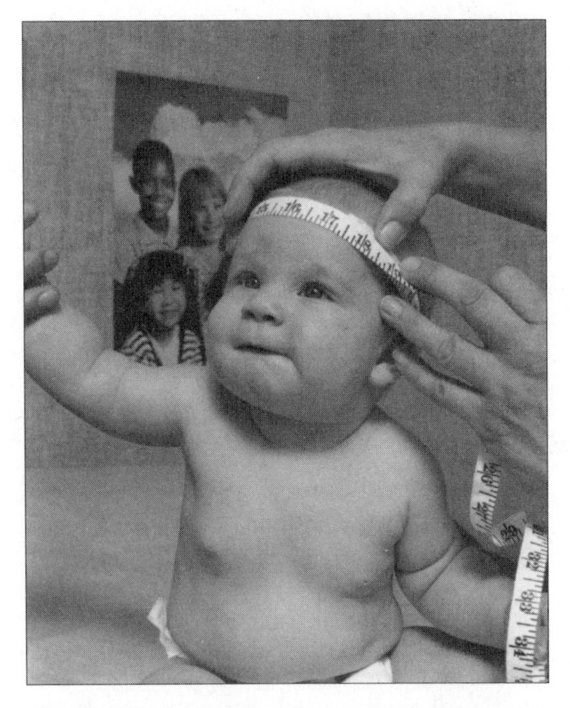

Figure 28–4 Measuring head circumference (From Keir, Wise, and Krebs, Medical Assisting: Administrative and Clinical Competencies, *3rd ed. Delmar Publishers Inc., 1993)*

CHEST CIRCUMFERENCE

Chest circumference is usually measured in children up to 12 months of age. Measure the chest using a paper or flexible tape. Measurement is taken from the midsternal area just under the child's nipples around the back, under the axillae, and around the chest. During childhood, chest circumference exceeds head size by about 5–7 cm (2–3 in.), Figure 28–5.

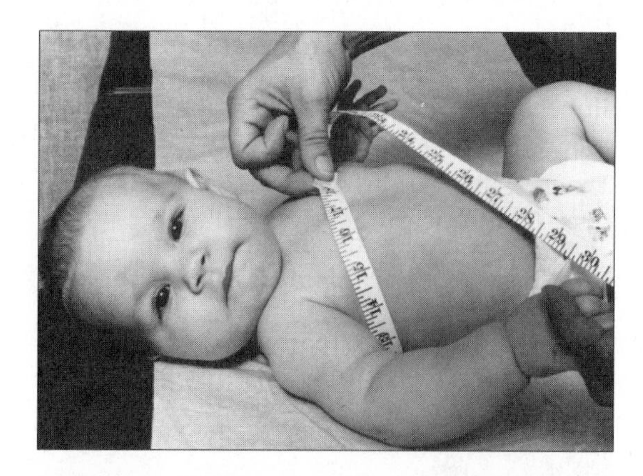

Figure 28–5 Measuring chest circumference (From Keir, Wise, and Krebs, Medical Assisting: Administrative and Clinical Competencies, *3rd ed. Delmar Publishers Inc., 1993)*

TEMPERATURE

Temperature may be measured through oral, rectal, axillary, or tympanic routes. Body temperature can be measured in two scales: Fahrenheit (F) or Celsius (C).

Many types of thermometers are available today. Mercury (glass) thermometers have been replaced in many institutions by digital thermometers, electronic thermometers, tympanic membrane sensors, and plastic strip thermometers, which provide accurate temperature readings in less time.

Electronic thermometers contain an electronic sensing probe covered by a disposable sterile sheath. Temperature (in either Fahrenheit or Celsius) is displayed on a liquid crystal display screen within 15 to 60 seconds, depending on the model used. Recommendations for the length of time a mercury thermometer stays in place vary. The nurse should check the accepted procedure where he or she works.

ORAL TEMPERATURE

The oral route is used for children over 3 years of age. Caution the child against biting down on the thermometer. If a mercury thermometer is used, wait approximately three minutes before removing the thermometer. Do not take an oral temperature if the child has a history of seizures.

RECTAL TEMPERATURE

Rectal temperatures are often taken in infants and toddlers. Place the infant or child either prone or on the side, with the knees flexed, Figure 28–6a. An infant can be placed prone on a parent's lap, Figure 28–6b. Do not force the thermometer. When using a mercury thermometer, allow approximately three to five minutes to obtain an accurate reading, Figure 28–6.

AXILLARY TEMPERATURE

Axillary temperatures are often taken when other methods are not advised. Place the mercury thermometer or probe in the axillary space and have the child hold the arm close to the trunk. If a mercury thermometer is used, keep in place for five minutes before reading the mercury column, Figure 28–7.

PULSE

The **apical pulse**, which is heard at the apex of the heart, is generally preferred over other

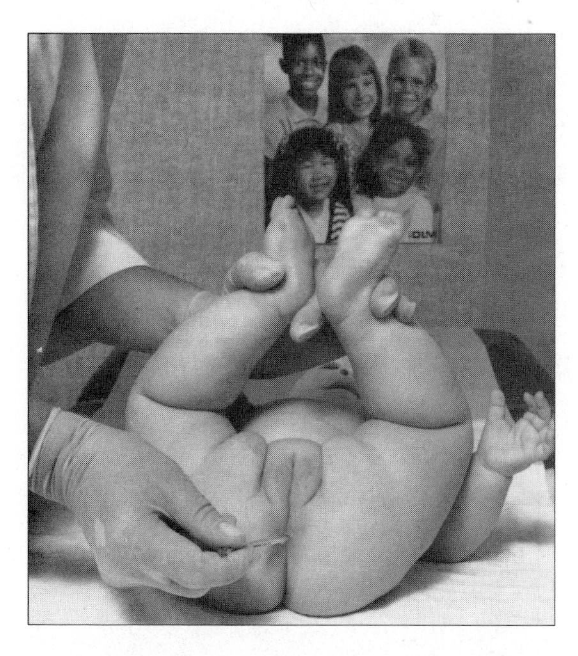

a.

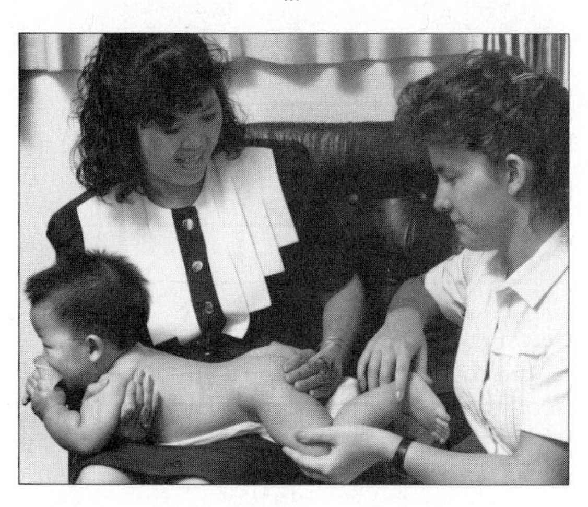

b.

Figure 28–6 *Measuring rectal temperature (From Keir, Wise, and Krebs,* Medical Assisting: Administrative and Clinical Competencies, *3rd ed. Delmar Publishers*

pulse locations for infants and small children (under 5 years of age). A satisfactory pulse can be taken radially (at the thumb side of the wrist,

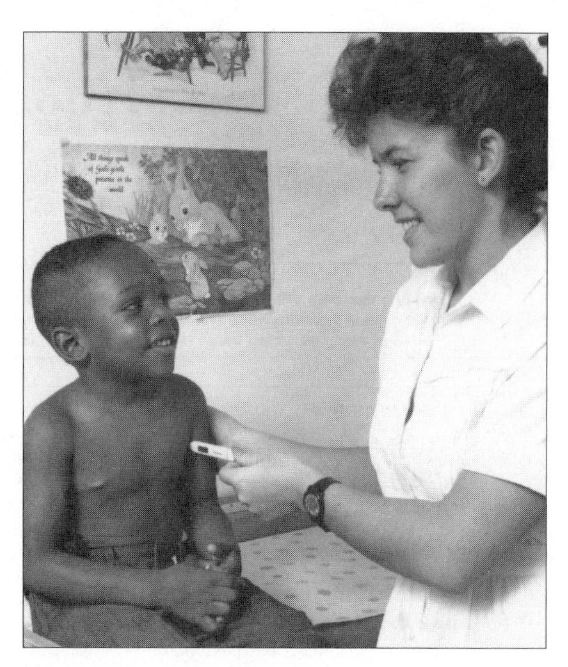

Figure 28–7 *Measuring axillary temperature (From Keir, Wise, and Krebs,* Medical Assisting: Administrative and Clinical Competencies, *3rd ed. Delmar Publishers Inc., 1993)*

above the radial artery) in children over 2. Each "lub-dub" sound is counted as one beat. The pulse is counted for one full minute.

The normal pulse rate varies with age, decreasing as the child grows older, Figure 28–8. The heart rate may also vary considerably among children of the same age and size. The heart rate increases in response to exercise, excitement, anxiety, and fever and decreases to a resting rate when the child is still.

Listen to the heart rate, noting whether the heart rhythm is regular or irregular. Children often have a normal cycle of irregular rhythm associated with respiration called **sinus arrhythmia**. In sinus arrhythmia, the child's heart rate is faster on inspiration and slower on expiration. Record whether the pulse is normal, bounding, or thready.

NORMAL HEART RATE RANGES FOR CHILDREN		
Age	**Heart Rate Range**	**Average Heart Rate**
Infants to 2 years	80–130	110
2 to 6 years	70–120	100
6 to 10 years	70–110	90
10 to 16 years	60–100	85

Figure 28–8

RESPIRATIONS

In older children and adolescents, respiratory rate is counted in the same way as in an adult. In infants and young children (under 6 years of age), however, the diaphragm is the primary breathing muscle. Thus, respiratory rate is assessed by observing the rise and fall of the abdomen. Inspiration, when the chest or abdomen rises, and expiration, when the chest or abdomen falls, are counted as one respiration. Because these movements are often irregular, they should be counted for one full minute for accuracy. Normal respiratory rate varies with the child's age, Figure 28–9.

NORMAL RESPIRATORY RATE RANGES FOR CHILDREN	
Age	**Respiratory Rate per Minute**
1 year	20–40
3 years	20–30
6 years	16–22
10 years	16–20
17 years	12–20

Figure 28–9

BLOOD PRESSURE

Blood pressure measurement is part of routine vital sign assessment. In children 3 years of age and older, blood pressure should be measured annually.

Blood pressure may be measured using mercury gravity, electronic, or aneroid equipment. The size of the blood pressure cuff is determined by the size of the child's arm or leg. A general rule of thumb is that the width of the inflatable bladder should be forty percent of the circumference of the extremity used. If the cuff is too small, pressure will be falsely high; if too large, falsely low. Sometimes it is difficult to hear the blood pressure in an infant or small child. Use a pediatric stethoscope over pulse sites if possible.

If the pulse still cannot be auscultated, the blood pressure can be measured by touch. Palpate for the pulse. Keeping your fingers on the pulse, pump up the cuff until the pulse is no longer felt. Slowly open the air valve, watching the column of mercury, and note the number where the pulse is again palpated. This is called the palpated systolic blood pressure.

NURSING CONSIDERATIONS IN PEDIATRIC ASSESSMENT

- Assess parameters of normal growth: height, weight, chest circumference, and head circumference.
- Observe the child's overall appearance and posture.
- Evaluate the physical findings for degree of wellness.
- Observe the child's mobility during assessment procedures.
- Assess vital signs for degree of wellness.
- Observe how the family and child (patient) perceive and manage health.
- Use the opportunity presented by the pediatric assessment to observe the parent-child relationship.

REVIEW QUESTIONS

A. Multiple choice. Select the best answer.

1. Head circumference is
   a. not routinely measured in children over 3 years of age unless the head size is questionable
   b. usually measured with paper or metal tape
   c. usually measured with cloth tape
   d. normally exceeded by chest circumference in children under 2 years of age

2. The oral route is usually used to measure temperature in
   a. children over 3 years of age
   b. children with a history of seizures
   c. infants over 10 months of age
   d. children under 3 years of age

3. Axillary measurement of temperature is
   a. preferred over rectal and oral methods in infants and children
   b. more accurate than rectal or oral methods
   c. faster than oral or rectal methods
   d. sometimes indicated for the immunocompromised child or the child with a physical disability

4. The normal pulse rate for an infant is
   a. 70–120 b.p.m.
   b. 80–130 b.p.m.
   c. 90–140 b.p.m.
   d. 100–150 b.p.m.

5. When assessing respirations in infants and young children do all of the following except
   a. observe the rise and fall of the abdomen
   b. note whether breath sounds are clear on both sides of the chest
   c. check for flaring and/or retractions
   d. count rise and fall of chest or abdomen as separate respirations

B. True or false. Write *T* for a true statement and *F* for a false statement.

1. ___ The method chosen for taking a child's temperature will be influenced by the height and weight of the child.
2. ___ Chest circumference is usually measured in all children up to 3 years of age.
3. ___ The apical pulse is usually preferred over other pulse locations in infants.
4. ___ Sinus arrhythmia is an abnormal finding that should be reported immediately to the child's physician.
5. ___ Blood pressure should be measured annually in children 3 years of age and older.

SUGGESTED ACTIVITIES

- List and discuss the other types of observations that the nurse will want to make while taking measurements and assessing vital signs of a child.
- Review recommendations for taking temperatures of infants, toddlers, and children using different methods. Discuss the advantages, disadvantages, and precautions for each method.
- Interview three parents to find out what kinds of observations they make about the growth and development of their infants and children. Find out what their expectations are and how they arrived at those expectations. List any opportunities you identify for educating parents.

BIBLIOGRAPHY

Keir, L., B. A. Wise, and C. Krebs. *Medical Assisting: Administrative and Clinical Competencies*, 3rd ed. Albany, NY: Delmar Publishers, 1993.

Margolius, F. R., N. V. Sneed, and A. D. Hollerbach. Accuracy of apical pulse rate measurements in young children. *Nursing Research* 40, no. 6 (1991): 379–380.

Roche, A., et al. Head circumference reference data: Birth to 18 years. *Pediatrics* 7, no. 5 (1987): 706–712.

Seidel, H. M., J. W. Ball, J. E. Dains, and G. W. Benedict. *Mosby's Guide to Physical Examination*, 2nd ed. St. Louis, MO: Mosby-Year Book, 1991.

Wong, D. L. *Whaley & Wong's Essentials of Pediatric Nursing*, 4th ed. St. Louis, MO: Mosby-Year Book, 1993.

CHAPTER

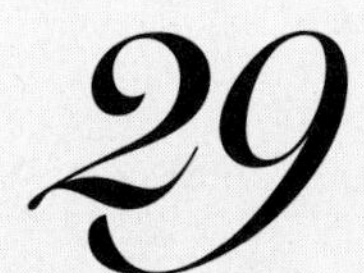

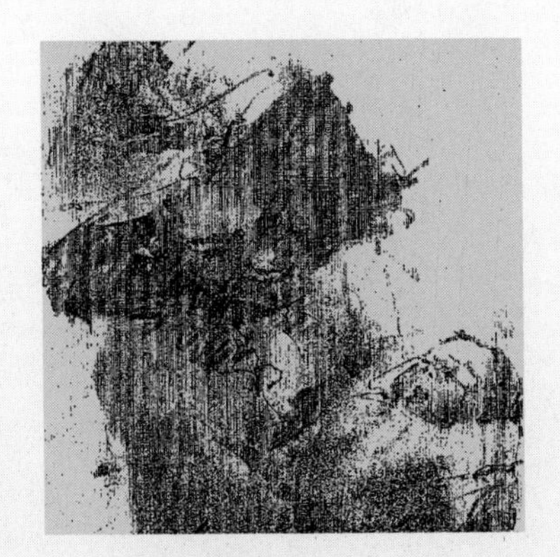

The Hospitalized Child

OBJECTIVES

AFTER STUDYING THIS CHAPTER, THE STUDENT SHOULD BE ABLE TO:

- IDENTIFY THE STRESSORS OF HOSPITALIZATION FOR CHILDREN AT EACH DEVELOPMENTAL STAGE.
- DESCRIBE COMMON BEHAVIORAL REACTIONS TO THESE STRESSORS AT EACH DEVELOPMENTAL STAGE.
- DESCRIBE NURSING INTERVENTIONS TO MINIMIZE THE STRESS OF HOSPITALIZATION FOR CHILDREN.
- DISCUSS THE ROLE OF PLAY IN MINIMIZING THE STRESS OF HOSPITALIZATION.
- IDENTIFY NURSING INTERVENTIONS APPROPRIATE TO SUPPORT PARENTS, GRANDPARENTS, AND SIBLINGS DURING A CHILD'S HOSPITALIZATION.
- DISCUSS SCHOOLING NEEDS DURING HOSPITALIZATION.
- DISCUSS METHODS FOR PREPARING CHILDREN OF DIFFERENT DEVELOPMENTAL STAGES FOR PROCEDURES.
- IDENTIFY STRATEGIES TO HELP CHILDREN COPE WITH THE STRESSORS OF PROLONGED HOSPITALIZATION.

Key Terms

STRESSORS
SEPARATION ANXIETY
PROTEST
DESPAIR
DETACHMENT

Hospitalization is a stressful experience for the child, parents, and siblings and has a profound effect on the family as a unit. In order to provide developmentally appropriate care, nurses must be familiar with age-specific responses to hospitalization and techniques to minimize hospital stressors.

Stressors of Hospitalization

How a child reacts to the stressors of hospitalization is strongly influenced by his or her developmental stage. Erikson's stages of psychosocial development provide a framework for understanding these reactions (refer to Chapter 23). The major **stressors** of hospitalization for children of all ages include separation, loss of control, fear of bodily injury, and pain (Foster et al. 1989, Wong 1993).

Separation from Parents and Familiar People

Infant. Separation from familiar people and routines because of hospitalization is the most disruptive stressor for infants. Young infants under 6 months of age display a response to a change in caretakers, but have not yet developed selective attachment to the primary caretaker. Infants under the age of 6 months who are separated from their mothers are likely to become quiet and subdued.

Providing for the care of the infant's basic needs is the priority of nursing care. Encourage parents to room-in with the infant and to participate in his or her care. These measures provide for continuity of the primary caregiver and help to maintain home routines as much as possible. Talking or singing to the infant, holding, rocking, and cuddling can also help to lessen the stressors of hospitalization.

After 8 months of age, infants have formed an intense attachment to the primary caretaker (usually the mother) and experience **separation anxiety** when separated from the caretaker. Older infants and toddlers who are separated from their mothers experience a pattern of responses that includes protest, despair, and detachment, Figure 29–1. These responses occur when the infant encounters strange people, strange events, and an absence of mothering (Bowlby 1969).

RESPONSE PATTERNS OF HOSPITALIZED CHILDREN

1. **Protest**, a yearning and searching for the mother, characterized by sobbing, crying, and clinging as the mother tries to leave.
2. **Despair**, characterized by sadness, withdrawal, increasing protest at the mother's absence, and growing anger with her for staying away.
3. **Detachment**, an apparent loss of interest in the mother.

When reunited with the mother after a period of separation, the child exhibits intense anxiety, tends to be overpossessive, and is unwilling to be left alone, insisting on staying close to the mother any time he or she suspects the mother will be lost again.

Figure 29–1

During the initial phase of **protest**, the infant cannot be consoled and refuses any attention except from the parent. Crying may cease only with physical exhaustion.

When the act of protest fails to bring the parent back, the second phase, **despair**, becomes evident. The infant withdraws from events and people, rarely resisting anything that is done. This compliant behavior can be misunderstood to be an adaptation to the hospital experience. The infant is likely to cry intensely or have a temper tantrum when parents visit. This response is normal and does not indicate that the parents have no control over the infant or that the child is "better" when the parents are not around.

The third phase, **detachment**, usually occurs after prolonged separation and can result when an infant is cared for by a variety of nurses over an extended period in the hospital. The infant shows interest in the hospital surroundings and no longer appears upset when parents come and go. Although the infant appears to have adapted to the separation, in actuality he or she is repressing feelings for the parent.

It is important to explain to parents that separation anxiety is a normal response. Encourage the parents to room-in and participate in the infant's care. If parents must leave, they should be honest about the need to do so. Bringing belongings from home such as familiar toys and blankets provides the infant with comfort objects.

Toddler and Preschool Child. The behaviors of protest, despair, and detachment continue to occur in response to separation during the toddler and preschool years. In the protest phase, the toddler cries out verbally, clings to parents, and tries to force the parents to stay. The toddler may attack strangers by kicking, biting, pinching, or hitting them. In the despair phase, the toddler is uncommunicative, passive, and uninterested in the environment. Regression to earlier behaviors, such as drinking from a bottle or needing to be diapered, is common. In the detachment phase, the toddler seems to have adjusted to hospitalization, appears happy and friendly, and is less demanding.

The preschool child may refuse to eat and have difficulty sleeping in response to separation. The child frequently asks when the parents will visit and cries quietly for parents when they are gone. Like the toddler, the preschool child may withdraw and regress to earlier behaviors. Breaking toys, hitting other children, and refusing to cooperate are common behaviors of the preschool child who is experiencing separation anxiety. Progression to the stage of detachment is uncommon.

Encourage parents of toddlers and preschool children to room-in and participate in the child's care, maintaining normal routines whenever possible. If parents must leave, encourage them to leave familiar objects with the child. Encourage the child to talk about the parents and home and to express feelings of protest. Avoid blaming or shaming the child for regressing to earlier behaviors. Give parents appropriate information so they can understand that the child's behavior is a normal response to separation. Provide comfort for the child by being physically present and spending time with the child.

School-Age Child. The school-age child is beginning to demonstrate an increased independence from parents. At this age, peers take on increased importance in how children see themselves. School-age children who are hospitalized and separated from their friends may react with feelings of loneliness, isolation, or depression. During hospitalization, school-age children need to have outlets for their energy and creativity. Playroom activities that enable them to be active and noisy may help in the adjustment to hospitalization. Parents remain important supports for the hospitalized school-age child. Although coping mechanisms are developing, under stress the child may revert to more dependent behaviors. Doing so may be distressing to the child, who is attempting to become more independent. Children and families need to understand that these responses to the stress of hospitalization are not unusual.

Adolescent. Adolescents have an increasing sense of self and are influenced by peer groups. Development of relationships and increased independence from parents are important at this stage. Hospitalization is particularly difficult because the adolescent is separated from peer group support. Adolescents usually cope well with short-term separation from home and family. However, during hospitalization, visits and contacts from family and friends are important. Telephone calls can help maintain contact if visits are not possible. Adolescents may develop their own support group with other hospitalized adolescents. Nurses can help this process by encouraging adolescents to meet to discuss their health concerns.

LOSS OF CONTROL

A child who is hospitalized experiences loss of control over certain body functions and over the ability to perform activities of daily living. Behavioral and emotional responses to loss of control include whining, crying, hostility, frustration, and anger. The child may experience depression and apathy if he or she is not allowed to have some control over activities.

Infant. The infant who can sit, crawl, or walk experiences frustration with any physical limitation such as restraints, traction, or confinement to a crib. For this reason it is important to allow the infant as much mobility as possible. Loss of control also results from a change in usual routines, sights, sounds, and smells. Encourage usual family routines and rituals. Play activities and infant stimulation are necessary for continued development of social and motor skills.

Toddler. For the toddler, loss of control results from physical restriction, altered routines and rituals, and dependency (Wong 1993). Again, allow the toddler as much mobility as possible. Because toddlers rely on rituals to provide stability in their lives, maintaining home routines for eating, sleeping, bathing, toileting, and play is important, Figure 29–2. Disruption of these routines may result in regression to earlier behaviors. The toddler

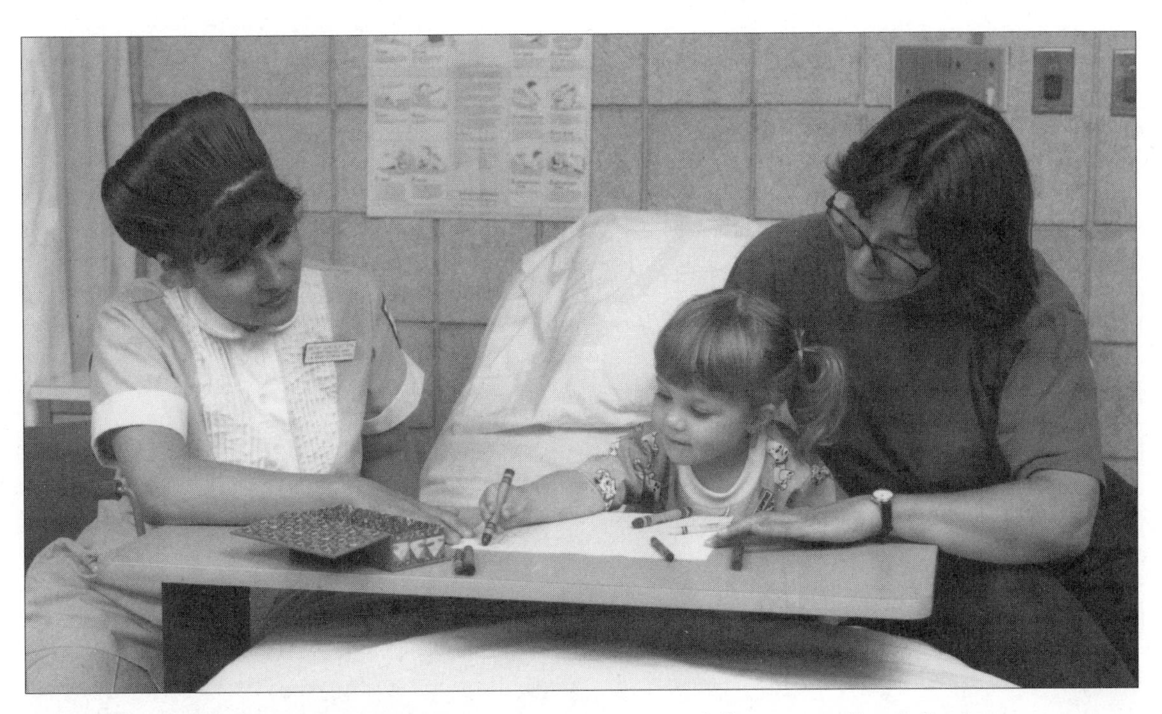

Figure 29–2 *Quiet play, such as coloring, can help the toddler cope with the stressors of hospitalization.*

may throw temper tantrums and be resistant to efforts of the caregiver. The parent's participation in the child's care should be strongly encouraged. Inform parents that some regression may occur and should be accepted without blaming the child.

Preschool Child. The preschool child experiences loss of control in response to physical restriction, altered routines, dependency, and a loss of his or her sense of self-power (Wong 1993). Provide the preschooler opportunities to play, preferably activities that require the use of large muscle groups. If these activities are prohibited because of the child's physical condition, provide appropriate toys and games that allow the child to relieve some of the frustrations of limited mobility.

Preschool children have a tremendous sense of omnipotence and may think of illness and hospitalization as punishment for bad thoughts or deeds. This "magical thinking" results in an exaggerated and frightening view of what is happening to them. Preschoolers may experience feelings of shame, guilt, and fear. Talk to the child about the cause of the illness. Allow the child to be a part of the decision-making process whenever possible in order to provide some sense of control. Choices and decisions may be as simple as what color pajamas to wear or whether the child would prefer to take a medication from a spoon or a medicine cup.

School-Age Child. Hospitalization threatens the school-age child's growing sense of independence. Having to wear pajamas all day or needing assistance with bathing or using a bed pan may be embarrassing and cause the child to feel that he or she has lost control. School-age children need to find ways in which to have some control in the hospital setting. They can be allowed to take part in making deci-

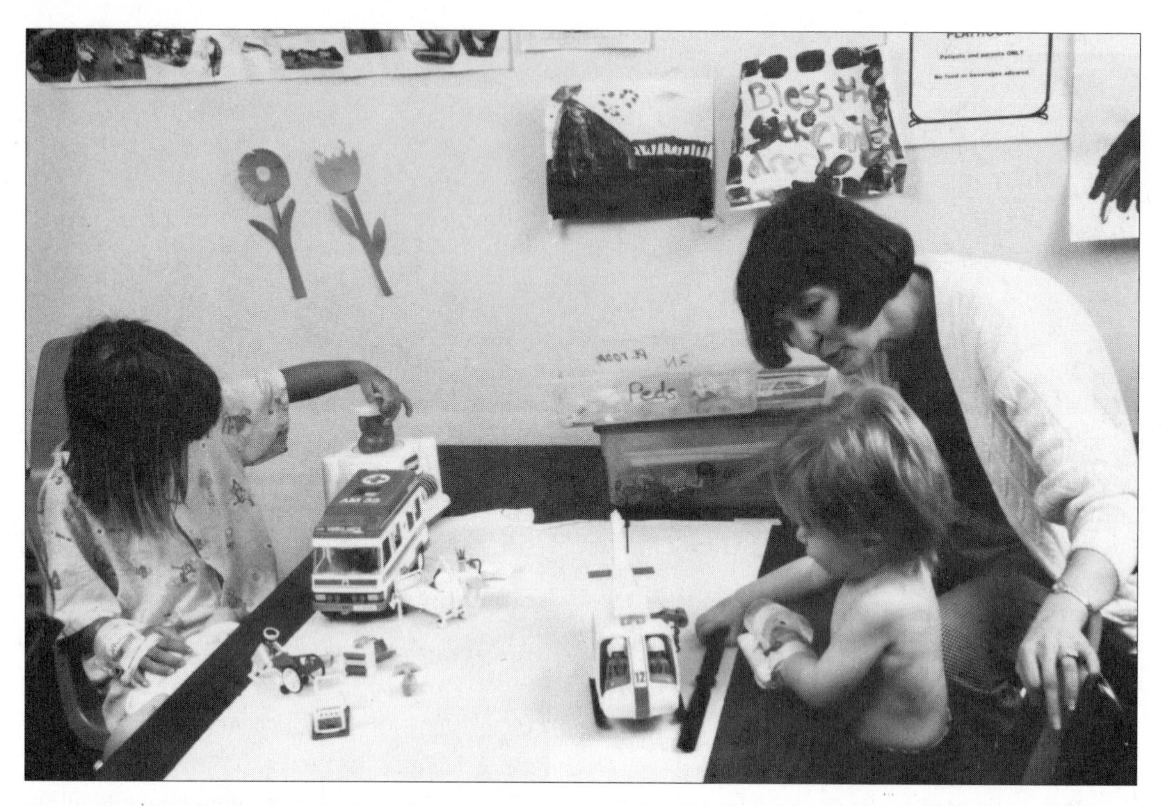

Figure 29–3 *This school-age child is able to express fears about her illness and hospitalization through play involving a toy hospital. A child life teacher looks on, assisting another child.*

sions about activities of daily living or to choose a new hobby to investigate while they are in the hospital.

Children at this age may be reluctant to express concerns or ask questions out of fear of appearing to lack confidence. Help children talk about their concerns by leading them into conversations and letting them know that other children have the same concerns. Children can also be encouraged to express their concerns through games, puppet shows, or art, Figure 29–3. Explanations should be given in terms that are appropriate for the age of the child.

Adolescent. The adolescent is often acutely aware of the loss of control that can occur in the hospital. Adolescents want the nurse and others to relate to them as mature individuals and not to treat them as children. They can be helped to retain their identity by being allowed to wear their own clothes and to decorate their rooms with favorite objects and items. Setting aside an area in the hospital as a teen room with age-appropriate games, books, and other activities helps foster a sense of personal identity and independence, Figure 29–4. Allowing some flexibility in institutional rules can help the adolescent retain a sense of being in control. Letting an adolescent sleep in rather than being awakened for early morning assessments is an example of flexibility. Respecting the adolescent's privacy helps to support a sense of

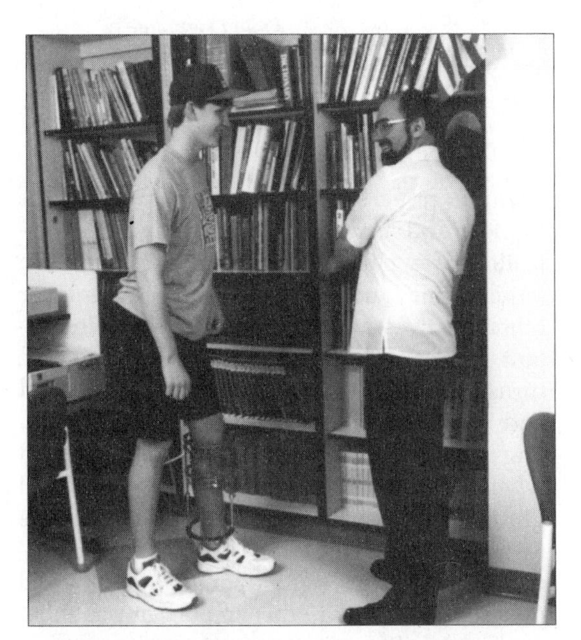

Figure 29–4 *A teen room provides age-appropriate activities for the hospitalized adolescent.*

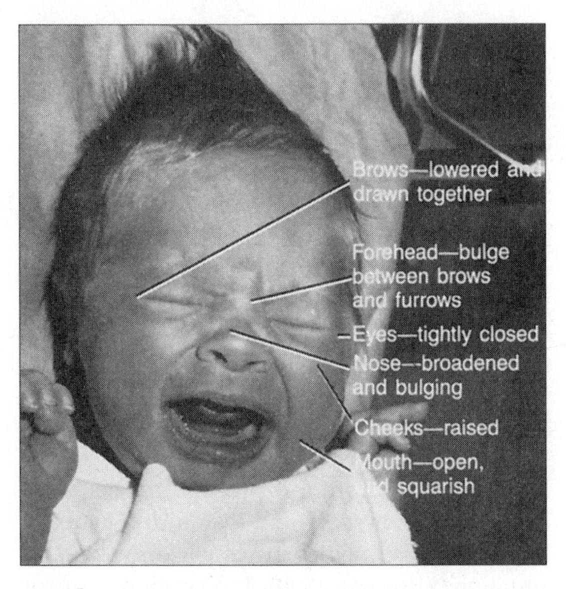

Figure 29–5 *Facial expression of pain in an infant. (From D. L. Wong.* Whaley & Wong's Essentials of Pediatric Nursing, *4th ed. St. Louis, MO: Mosby-Year Book, 1993.)*

independence and control. Programs to maintain normal school and recreational activities also help to give the adolescent control.

BODILY INJURY AND PAIN

All children experience pain; the expression of pain, however, is directly related to a child's age and stage of development. Young children may not know what pain is and will need help describing it. They may refuse to admit pain because of fear of an injection or painful procedure. Parents are usually sensitive to their child's behaviors and should be encouraged to tell the nurse when the child is in pain. Appropriate pharmacological and nonpharmacological pain control methods should be used for children in all age groups and developmental stages (see Chapter 31).

Infant. The facial expression of distress is the most consistent indicator of pain in infants, Figure 29–5. An older infant's responses to pain include loud crying, deliberate withdrawal of the body area, and the facial expression of discomfort. As the infant begins to have prior recall of painful experiences, apprehension and fear of painful events tend to increase. Encourage parents to stay with the infant and to hold and cuddle the infant to provide comfort.

Toddler. Toddlers frequently become overactive and restless with pain. They physically resist a painful stimulus, cry loudly, cling to the parent, and are immensely emotionally upset. Behavioral responses include grimacing, clenching the teeth, biting the lips, rubbing and opening the eyes wide, or acts of physical aggression such a biting, kicking, and hitting (Wong 1993). Encourage the toddler to express pain and provide comfort measures as appropriate. Pain control measures such as distraction and diversion are often useful.

Preschool Child. Preschool children are vulnerable to threats of bodily injury. Fear of bodily harm and mutilation is common and parents should be told that this response is normal at this developmental stage. Intrusive behaviors are very threatening. Preschool children may fear that all their blood will drain out after an injection. Painful procedures and pain may be viewed as punishment for wrongdoing. Allow the preschool child to act out fears with the use of dolls, dramatic play, and, for the older preschooler, with drawings and paintings. Encourage parents to stay with the child during procedures to provide comfort and security.

School-Age Child. School-age children may express concerns about bodily injury and pain by passive requests for help, talking about pain, or trying to delay events that may cause harm or pain to them. They may be afraid of not ever getting well again and of the effects the illness will have on their bodies. Allow the child to ask questions and discuss fears, and explain the child's illness and the reason for procedures in developmentally appropriate language.

Adolescent. The greatest stress of hospitalization for adolescents is the fear of bodily alterations. The nurse needs to be aware of concerns about bodily changes and be able to respond appropriately. Adolescents may fear losing control when they are in pain. Thus, they often react to pain by maintaining their self-control and giving little verbal response. They may be reluctant to discuss their pain, because discussing it would indicate an inability to maintain self-control. Adolescents may also think that nurses should know when they are in pain and that they should not have to ask for pain medication (Favaloro and Touzel 1990). Observe for signs of pain, such as changes in mobility, irritability, or being quiet and withdrawn.

NURSING CARE RELATED TO HOSPITALIZATION

SUPPORT SYSTEMS

An appropriate support system helps to reduce the fear and anxiety that accompany hospitalization of a child or sibling. Today's mobile families may not live near grandparents or other relatives and thus may lack this important support system. Parents may need to take turns spending time with the hospitalized child and juggle work and child care for other siblings. The single parent is especially stressed when a child is hospitalized. In some cultural groups it is common for other family members to assist the family who is experiencing hospitalization. Thus, grandparents, aunts and uncles, cousins, and other important people in the family's life may be present at home or in the hospital to provide support to the family.

SCHOOLING NEEDS

School is an important part of the life of the school-age child and adolescent. Children who are hospitalized, especially for frequent or extended admissions, should be helped to set aside time in which to study and complete schoolwork assignments. The nurse should also work with children and parents to determine whether the child's schooling needs are being met. Some children may need the services of a tutor to assist them with their assignments.

PREPARING FOR PROCEDURES

Preparing children for procedures helps to decrease their anxiety and fear and to increase their coping strategies in response to stressful situations (Broome 1990). Preparation for procedures is geared to the child's developmental level, which determines what information is given and when it is given (Bates and Broome 1986). Painful procedures should be performed in a separate treatment room, so that the child's room will be perceived as a safe place.

Infant and Toddler. Infants and toddlers do not understand lengthy explanations or anticipate actions that will happen to them. Immediately before a procedure is to be performed, give them short explanations and then continue with the procedure. Toddlers may benefit from handling equipment or small replicas of equipment before it is used on them. Dolls can be used to demonstrate what will happen during the procedure.

Preschool Child. Preschool children also benefit from handling equipment used in procedures. Puppets, cartoons, or stories can also be used to demonstrate procedures. Explain in simple terms close to the time at which the procedure will be performed how the procedure will affect the child.

School-Age Child. Plan to prepare the school-age child in advance of the scheduled time so the child has time to comprehend the information. Use correct terminology and diagrams, models, equipment, or videotapes to explain and prepare the child.

Adolescent. Adolescents require explanations and reasons for the procedure. If possible they should be involved in decision making and planning and given the opportunity to learn techniques to help them stay in control during the procedure.

CHILDREN WITH CHRONIC DISEASES OR PROLONGED HOSPITALIZATIONS

Children with chronic diseases or prolonged hospitalizations are at risk for delays or regression in their development. Nurses along with other health team members can develop and implement plans of care that promote the child's development (Lipsi et al. 1991). Encourage children to decorate their hospital rooms — with posters, pictures, cards, or displays of collections such as baseball cards — to make them feel more comfortable with their surroundings. Encourage children to develop new interests to help them occupy their time. Children can be helped to stay in control by developing and maintaining a routine schedule of activities throughout the day.

REHABILITATION

Rehabilitation care involves planning for the long-term needs of hospitalized children. Nurses should be involved in planning and implementing care for children who require rehabilitation in both acute-care hospitals and long-term care facilities.

FAMILY SUPPORT

Families may require support to cope with a child's hospitalization and return home. Nurses should encourage the parents to participate in the child's care. Supporting family members, providing information, and preparing for discharge and home care are important. Recommend community support groups for parents of children with chronic conditions. Support groups provide a place for families to discuss similar concerns and strategies for coping. Resources are also available to help prepare families for hospitalization of a child. The Association for the Care of Children's Health, 7910 Woodmont Avenue, Suite 300, Bethesda, Maryland 20814 is a national resource that provides such information.

REVIEW QUESTIONS

A. Multiple choice. Select the best answer.

1. Katie is 3 years old. She is hospitalized with idiopathic thrombocytopenic purpura. Katie's meals are served on a colorful plate with small utensils that fit easily in her hands. The dietary department has sent small portions of food on her tray. Katie's mother is rooming in and is present when you carry the tray into her room. You should
   a. hand the tray to her mother and ask her to feed Katie
   b. ask Katie who she would like to have help her with her tray
   c. feed Katie, using the small utensils
   d. allow Katie to feed herself

2. Micah is 30 months of age and has been potty trained for 6 months. He is hospitalized for surgical treatment of chronic otitis media. Micah has wet the bed three times since the surgical procedure 12 hours ago. His mother is angry because she had successfully potty trained him before he "came in here." You should
   a. explain to his mother that regression to earlier behaviors is common with hospitalization
   b. cut back on the fluids you are giving him, especially the sodas
   c. get a box of disposable diapers and put one on him
   d. tell the mother it's not your fault he is wetting the bed

3. Connor, 4 years old, is being admitted for same-day surgery for a tonsillectomy. His father helps him put the hospital gown on. Connor begins to cry when he is told to take his underwear off. The most appropriate nursing action is to
   a. tell Connor if he is a "big boy" he can have a lollipop after the procedure
   b. explain to his father that boys this age have a "fear of castration," so this is a normal response
   c. allow Connor to wear his underwear
   d. inform Connor and his father that this is one of the "rules" when someone has surgery

4. When planning care for adolescents in the hospital, the nurse should include all of the following except
   a. privacy
   b. area for them to gather for group activities
   c. allowing them to wear their own clothes
   d. maintaining strict rules restricting visitors

5. Which of the following is the most significant stressor of hospitalization for adolescents?
   a. fear of pain
   b. separation from family
   c. fear of altered body image
   d. fear of bodily injury

B. True or false. Write *T* for a true statement and *F* for a false statement.

1. ___ It is best for everyone if the parents stay outside the treatment room rather than with the toddler during a procedure.
2. ___ A nursing intervention to get a preschooler to take his medication is to tell him to "be a good boy" like his roommate, Jonathan.
3. ___ Infants do not need pharmacological agents for pain control because they experience only minimal pain.
4. ___ Procedures should be explained to children in terms appropriate for their developmental level.
5. ___ Preparing children for painful procedures decreases their fear.

SUGGESTED ACTIVITIES

- Care for hospitalized children of different developmental stages. Compare and contrast children's reactions to illness and hospitalization.
- Invite the parents of a chronically ill child to speak to the class about the needs of families and siblings during hospitalization and after returning home.
- Invite the parents and siblings of a child who was admitted to the hospital because of an emergency situation to talk about their fears and needs during this time of crisis.
- Invite a pediatric staff nurse to discuss common reactions of children to hospitalization and nursing care to minimize the stressors of hospitalization.

BIBLIOGRAPHY

Bates, T., and M. Broome. Preparation of children for hospitalization and surgery: A review of the literature. *Journal of Pediatric Nursing* 1, no. 4 (1986): 230–239.

Bowlby, J. *Attachment and Loss*, vol. 1. New York: Basic Books, 1969.

Bowlby, J. *Attachment and Loss*, vol. 2. New York: Basic Books, 1973.

Broome, M. Preparation of children for painful procedures. *Pediatric Nursing* 16, no. 6 (1990): 537–541.

Carson, D., J. Fravely, and J. Council. Children's prehospitalization conceptions of illness, cognitive development, and personal adjustment. *Child Health Care* 21, no. 2 (1992): 103–110.

Favaloro, R., and B. Touzel. A comparison of adolescents' and nurses' postoperative pain rating and perceptions. *Pediatric Nursing* 16, no. 4 (1990): 414–417, 424.

Foster, R. L., M. M. Hunsberger, and J. J. Anderson. *Family-Centered Nursing Care of Children*. Philadelphia: W. B. Saunders, 1989.

Lipsi, K., K. Clement-Shafer, and C. Rushton. Developmental rounds: An intervention strategy for hospitalized infants. *Pediatric Nursing* 17, no. 5 (1991): 433–437, 468.

Mott, S., S. James, and A. Sperhac. *Nursing Care of Children and Families*. Redwood City: Addison-Wesley, 1990.

Murray, R. B., and J. Zentner. *Nursing Assessment and Health Promotion: Strategies through the Life Span.* Norwalk, CT: Appleton and Lange, 1993.

Vessey, J., and M. Mahon. Therapeutic play and the hospitalized child. *Journal of Pediatric Nursing* 5, no. 5 (1990): 328–333.

Whaley, L., and D. Wong, eds. *Nursing Care of Infants and Children*, 4th ed. St. Louis, MO: Mosby-Year Book, 1991.

Wong, D. L. *Whaley & Wong's Essentials of Pediatric Nursing*, 4th ed. St. Louis, MO: Mosby-Year Book, 1993.

CHAPTER

30

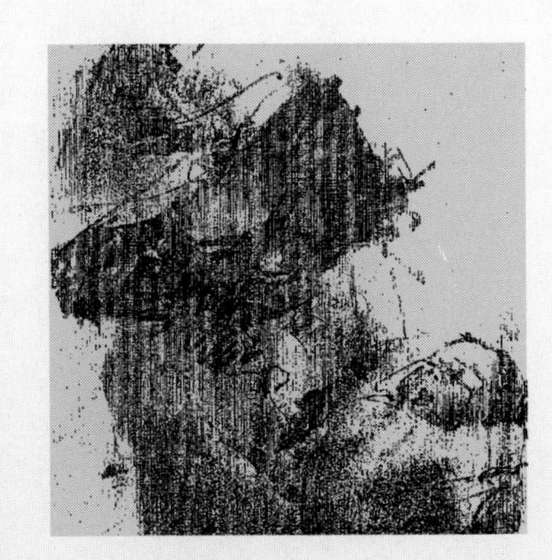

Routine Pediatric Procedures

Objectives

AFTER STUDYING THIS CHAPTER, THE STUDENT SHOULD BE ABLE TO:

- PREPARE CHILDREN AT DIFFERENT DEVELOPMENTAL STAGES FOR PROCEDURES.
- IDENTIFY THE REQUIREMENTS FOR OBTAINING INFORMED CONSENT IN CHILDREN.
- SAFELY RESTRAIN, HOLD, TRANSPORT, AND POSITION A CHILD FOR PROCEDURES.
- ADMINISTER MEDICATIONS TO CHILDREN CORRECTLY AND SAFELY BY DIFFERENT ROUTES.
- APPLY A URINE COLLECTION BAG AND OBTAIN A URINE SPECIMEN.
- ADMINISTER OXYGEN TO A CHILD, USING VARIOUS DELIVERY SYSTEMS.
- SUCTION A TRACHEOSTOMY TUBE IN A CHILD.
- SUCTION AN INFANT'S NOSE USING A BULB SYRINGE.
- ASSIST WITH THE INSERTION OF A NASOGASTRIC OR GASTROSTOMY TUBE.
- ADMINISTER A GAVAGE FEEDING TO A CHILD.

Key Terms

CRADLE HOLD

FOOTBALL HOLD

UPRIGHT HOLD

Nurses who care for hospitalized children need to be familiar with a variety of pediatric procedures performed routinely in the hospital setting. This chapter highlights variations and precautions for the following procedures: informed consent, restraints and positioning, medication administration, specimen collection, oxygen administration, suctioning, nasogastric and gastrostomy tubes, and gavage feeding.

Informed Consent for Children

If a child is a minor, a parent or legal guardian must give written consent for any procedure or treatment. If the parent is unavailable, the person who is assuming the responsibility for the child can give consent for emergency treatment providing he or she has written permission from a parent or legal guardian to authorize care. Verbal consent can be given by a parent or guardian over the telephone provided that two witnesses are listening to the consent. There must be written and signed documentation of the phone call. An emancipated minor may give consent as a mature minor.

Preparing Children for Procedures

Children should be prepared for procedures on the basis of their age, developmental stage, and ability to understand what is being explained to them. The nurse should be honest about the activities and discomfort associated with the specific procedure in order to develop a trusting relationship with the child. Involving parents when appropriate can provide support and comfort to the child (see Chapter 29).

Infant

The infant feels pain and shows signs of anxiety during procedures. Give a pacifier or bottle and hold the infant close to provide comfort.

Toddler

Explain the procedure to the toddler just before it is to be performed. Use simple words and objects, if appropriate. Provide distraction during the procedure and reward the toddler after the procedure is over. Encourage the toddler to express feelings. Provide comfort and support.

PRESCHOOL CHILD

Provide the preschool child with simple verbal explanations about procedures. Let the child handle equipment if possible. Answer all questions as honestly as possible. Preschool children fear bodily harm and mutilation and find invasive procedures threatening. The child may think that a painful procedure is punishment for something he or she did wrong. Encourage the child to talk about fears and anxieties.

SCHOOL-AGE CHILD

The school-age child understands treatments and procedures. Use terminology the child can easily comprehend. The school-age child also fears bodily injury and needs to be encouraged to talk about fears and anxieties.

ADOLESCENT

The adolescent understands explanations about procedures. Answer any questions he or she may have. The adolescent will react to pain by trying to act stoic while maintaining self-control. Encourage the adolescent to discuss fears and anxieties if he or she is willing. Coping methods such as imagery, breathing, or relaxation techniques can be helpful. Involving the adolescent in the decision-making process, when possible, can help the teenager retain a sense of being in control.

RESTRAINTS AND POSITIONING

HIGH-TOP CRIB

Infants and toddlers are usually placed in high-top cribs to protect them from injury in the hospital environment, Figure 30–1.

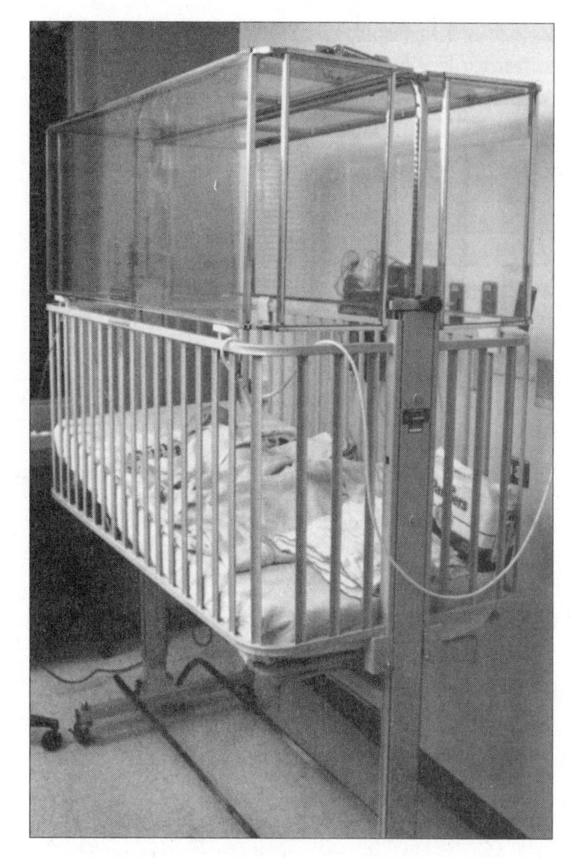

Figure 30–1 *High-top crib*

ELBOW RESTRAINTS

Elbow restraints are used to keep a child from bending an elbow or touching the face, neck, or head. A commercially manufactured restraint or a modified armboard can be used. To apply an elbow restraint:

1. Place the armboard on the ventral side of the arm, extending from midhumerus to midforearm.
2. Wrap Kling around the armboard.
3. Tape in place, Figure 30–2.

PAPOOSE BOARD

The papoose board is a commercially manufactured body restraint consisting of a metal board with cloth wrappings lined with Velcro

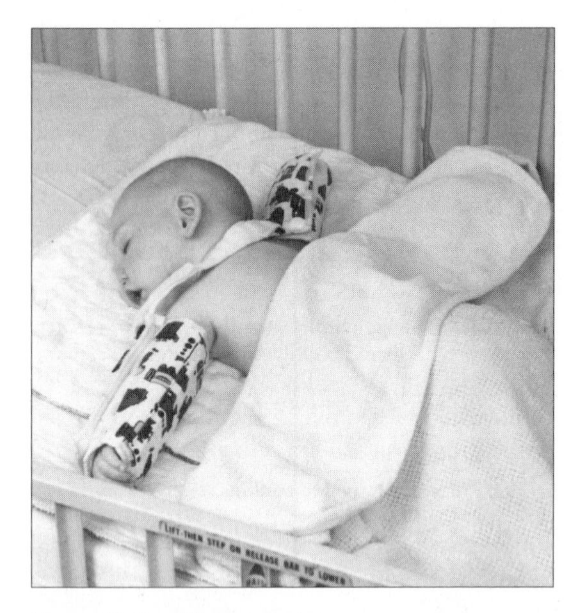

Figure 30–2 *Elbow restraints*

fasteners. The board immobilizes the child's arms and legs. To use a papoose board:

1. Place a towel, small sheet, or small bath blanket over the board.
2. Place the child supine with head at the top of the board.
3. Place the cloth wrappings around the child, securing the Velcro.

MUMMY RESTRAINT

The mummy restraint is used to immobilize an infant's arms and legs. To apply a mummy restraint:

1. Fold down the top corner of a small blanket. Place the infant diagonally on the blanket with neck at the fold, Figure 30–3a.
2. Bring one side of the blanket over the infant's arm, shoulder, and chest, and secure beneath the body, Figure 30–3b. Bring the bottom corner up over infant.
3. Bring the other side over the infant and wrap securely, Figure 30–3c.

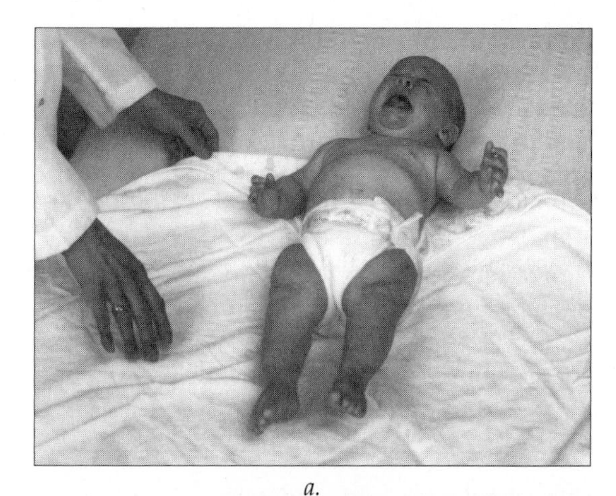

a.

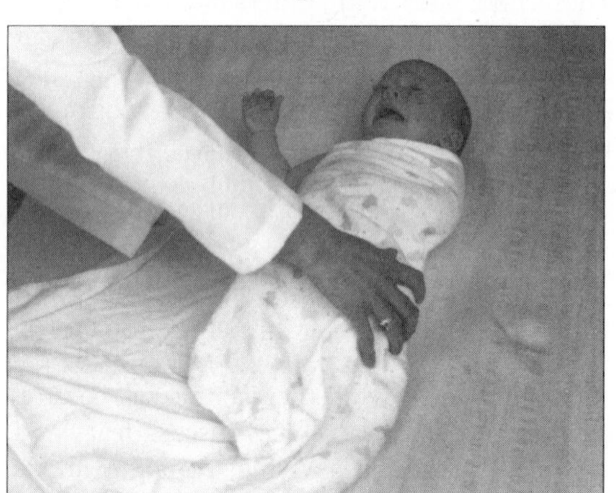

b.

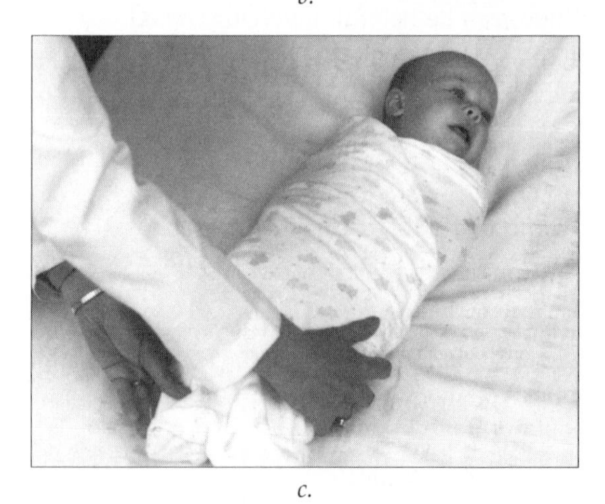

c.

Figure 30–3 *Mummy restraint*

HOLDING AND TRANSPORTING INFANTS

Hospitalized infants need to be held as well as transported to other areas within the hospital. Three positions for safely holding and transporting infants are the **cradle**, **football**, and **upright holds**.

Cradle Hold. The infant is held with head resting in the bend of the nurse's elbow with back supported. The infant's thigh is held by the carrying arm, Figure 30–4a.

Football Hold. The infant's body is supported on the nurse's forearm. The infant's head and neck rest in the nurse's palm. The rest of the infant's body is securely held between the nurse's body and elbow, Figure 30–4b.

Upright Hold. The infant is held upright against the nurse's chest and shoulder. The infant's buttocks are supported by one of the nurse's hands. The other hand and arm support the infant's head and shoulders, Figure 30–4c.

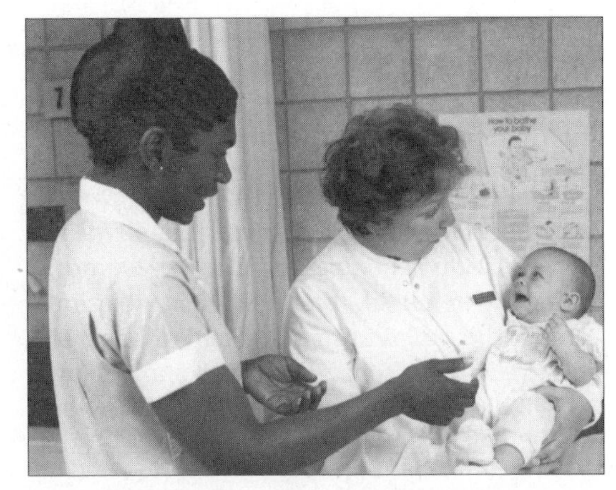

a.

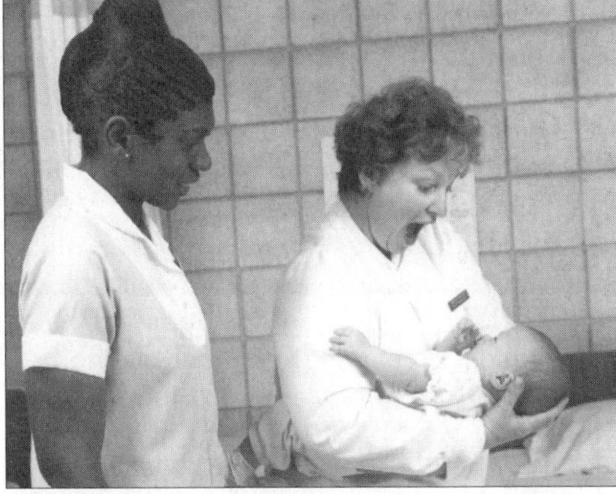

b.

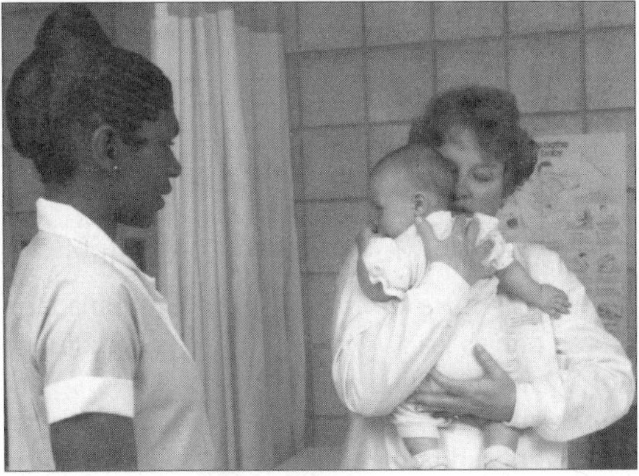

c.

Figure 30–4 *(a) Cradle hold. (b) Football hold. (c) Upright hold.*

POSITIONING FOR A LUMBAR PUNCTURE

A lumbar puncture is used to measure cerebrospinal fluid (CSF) pressure, obtain a sample of CSF, or administer medications, anesthetics, air, or radiopaque contrast material. To position a child for lumbar puncture:

1. Place the child on the side (lateral recumbent) with knees pulled to abdomen and neck flexed to the chin. The back should be arched. An infant can be held in this position by leaning over and holding the neck, buttocks, and thighs in your hands, Figure 30–5. An infant can also be placed in a sitting position with head flexed on the chest. An older child can sit up with neck flexed to the chin and spine arched forward. Lean

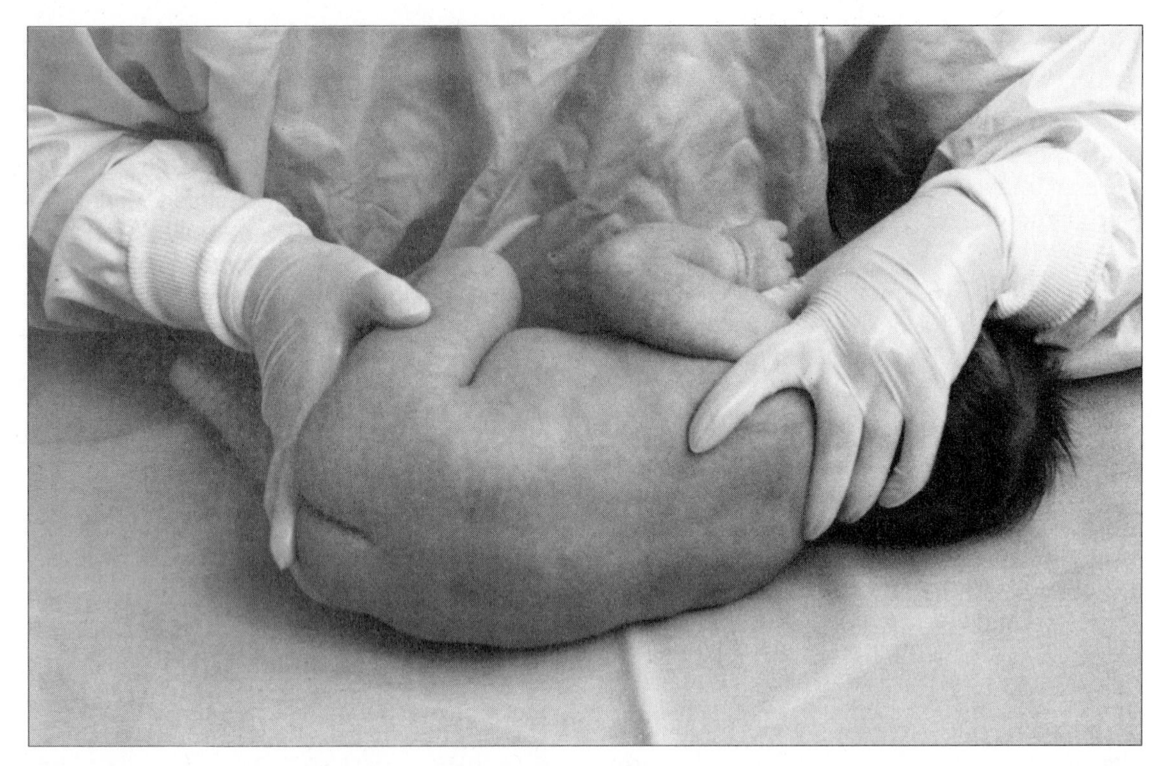

Figure 30–5 *Positioning infant for a lumbar puncture*

over the child with your entire body, using your forearms against the child's legs and buttocks and around the shoulders and head, being careful not to interfere with respiratory effort.

MEDICATION ADMINISTRATION

The nurse should follow the "Five Rights" of proper drug administration before any medication is given:

1. Right drug
2. Right patient
3. Right time
4. Right route
5. Right dose

ROUTES OF ADMINISTRATION

Oral Route. The method of administration depends on the child's age. Liquid medications can be administered by placing small amounts of liquid along the side of an infant's mouth using a plastic syringe, calibrated dropper, medicine cup, or spoon. Wait for the infant to swallow before administering more liquid. Give medications slowly. Alternatively, medication can be put in a nipple from which the infant then sucks. Tablets can be crushed and mixed in juice, syrup, or strained fruit. Toddlers and preschool-age children may need to be held firmly on the nurse or parent's lap.

PRECAUTION: Never put medications into the infant's formula. The infant may not consume the entire feeding, or may ingest so slowly that the medication loses potency. Never give oral medications to a crying child. Aspiration may result.

Intramuscular Route

1. The recommended injection site for infants and children under 3 years of age is the vastus lateralis. The gluteal sites can be used after the child is walking, if hospital policy permits.
2. Have another nurse, assistant, or parent restrain the child during the injection.
3. Put on clean gloves and locate the injection site.
4. Clean the site with alcohol or Betadine using a firm outward circular motion.
5. Firmly grasp the muscle between the thumb and fingers to stabilize and isolate the muscle.
6. Using a dartlike motion, insert the needle quickly at a 90-degree angle. Pull back on the plunger. If no blood is present, inject the medication, withdraw the needle, and massage the area with a dry gauze pad.

   PRECAUTION: Do not cap needle. Discard in a puncture-resistant container using universal precaution recommendations.

Intravenous Route

Preparation

1. Check the intravenous insertion site for patency, redness, blanching, and edema.
2. Check specific dilution recommendations.
3. Check medication compatibility with intravenous fluids that the child is receiving.
4. Check administration rate.
5. Check length of time drug can be administered.

Administration

1. Intravenous medications for infants and children should be put in a volutrol, burette, or soluset and administered through a continuous infusion pump to ensure accurate administration.
2. Set time of infusion.
3. Flush line after medication has infused.

Eye Drops

1. Place the child in a supine or sitting position with head extended.
2. Put on clean gloves.
3. Pull the child's lower lid down with one hand while your other hand rests on the child's head.
4. Place drops or ointment into the lower conjunctival sac starting from the inner canthus.
5. Close the eyelids to prevent leakage of medication after administration.
6. Dry the inner canthus of the eye and position the child's head in the midline to prevent excessive medication from getting into the other eye.

Ear Drops

1. Place the child in a supine position with head turned exposing the ear upward.
2. For a child under 3 years of age, pull the pinna gently down and back to straighten the ear canal.
3. For the child older than 3 years, pull the pinna up and back.
4. Instill drops into the ear canal.
5. Have the child remain in the same position for a few minutes to help the medication drain into the ear canal.
6. A cotton plug may be put loosely in the ear to prevent the medication from draining out.

SPECIMEN COLLECTION

BLOOD

Blood samples of children are obtained by venipuncture or capillary stick. The child is restrained in a supine position on a bed or stretcher.

Venipuncture. The sites most frequently used are the antecubital fossa and forearm. The dorsum of the hand or foot may also be used. The external jugular and femoral vein are used when it is difficult to obtain blood from traditional sites.

Capillary Stick. The sites include the plantar surface of the heel for newborns and children under the age of 1 year, the great toe, the ear lobe or the palmar surface of the tip of the third or fourth finger for children over 1 year.

> **PRECAUTION:** Universal precautions should be used whenever blood is drawn from any patient.

URINE

Infant. Urine collection bags are used to obtain a urine specimen from infants and toddlers who are not yet toilet trained. The bags are clear plastic with adhesive tabs. To apply a collection bag correctly:

1. Put on clean gloves.
2. Wash and dry the perineum, genitalia, and surrounding skin.
3. Remove paper covering adhesive, Figure 30–6a.
4. Attach the bag, using the adhesive tabs — for girls stretch the perineum and apply the bag around the labia, Figure 30–6b; for boys place the penis and scrotum inside the bag, Figure 30–6c.
5. Seal tightly to protect against leaks. Put the child's diaper back on carefully.
6. Check the bag frequently and as soon as the child urinates, gently pull the bag away from the skin.

OXYGEN ADMINISTRATION

FACE MASK

A face mask delivers high concentrations of oxygen effectively. Several types of masks are available. The mask should extend from the bridge of the child's nose to the cleft of the chin. The mask should fit snugly on the face, but no pressure should be put on the eyes.

NASAL CANNULA

The nasal cannula delivers a low flow and low concentration of oxygen. The prongs of the cannula are placed in the child's nares, allowing the child to be mobile.

BLOW-BY

Blow-by oxygen is used when the child needs low concentrations of oxygen with humidification. The oxygen cannula is held under the child's nose.

TRACHEOSTOMY COLLAR

A tracheostomy collar is a plastic collar that goes over a tracheostomy tube. It provides humidified air or oxygen and keeps the airway warm and moist.

> **PRECAUTION:** Watch for fluid collection in the tubing and take precautions so that fluid does not drain into the tracheostomy.

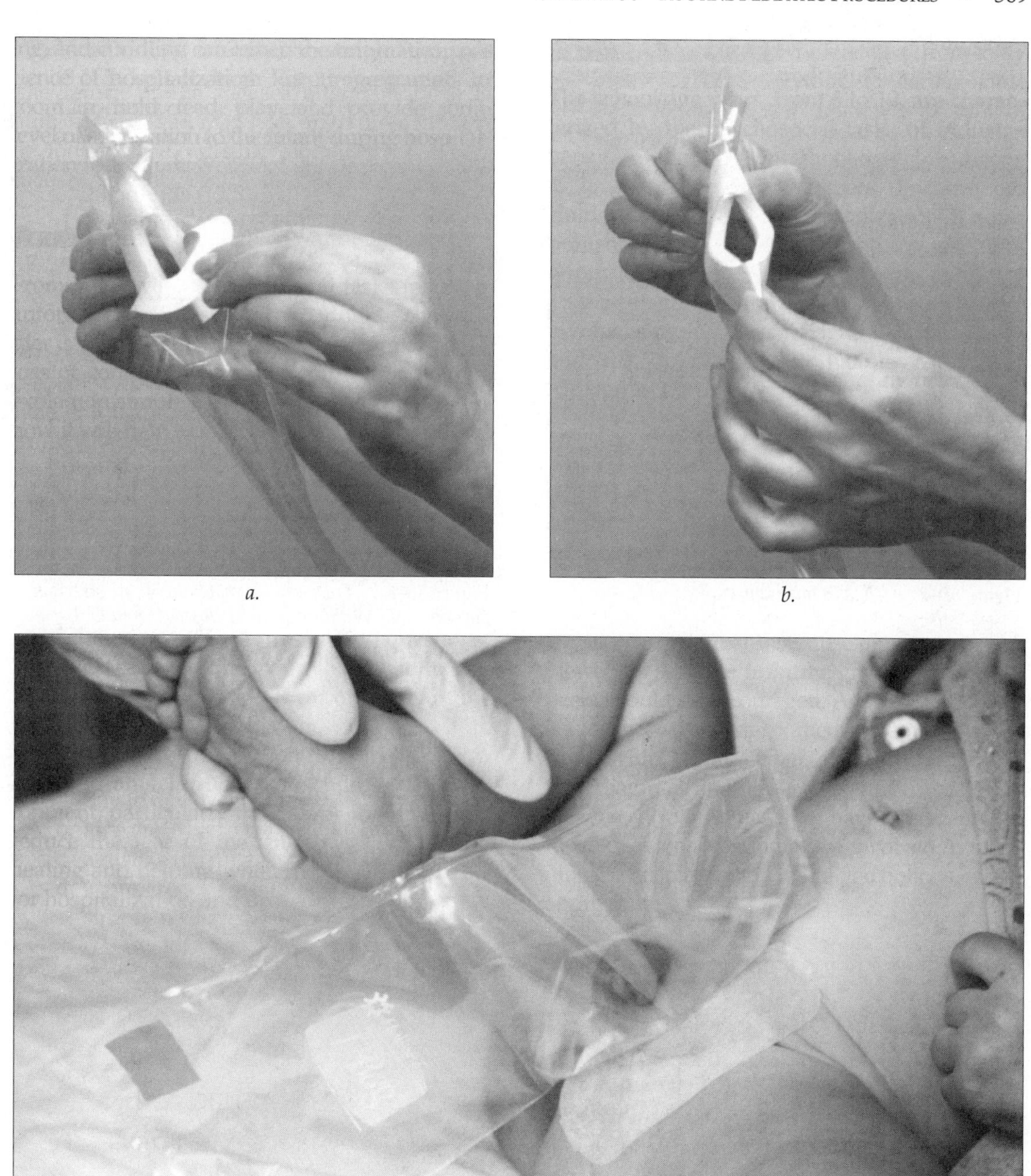

a.

b.

c.

Figure 30–6 *Applying a urine collection bag. (a) Removing paper covering adhesive. (b) Bending and opening the collection bag. (NOTE: Although gloves are recommended when placing a urine collection bag on an infant, it is difficult to remove the paper covering using gloves. Gloves must be worn, however, when touching the infant's perineal area.) (c) Collection bag applied. (a and b from B. Hegner and E. Caldwell.* Nursing Assistant: A Nursing Process Approach, *6th ed. Albany, NY: Delmar Publishers, 1992.)*

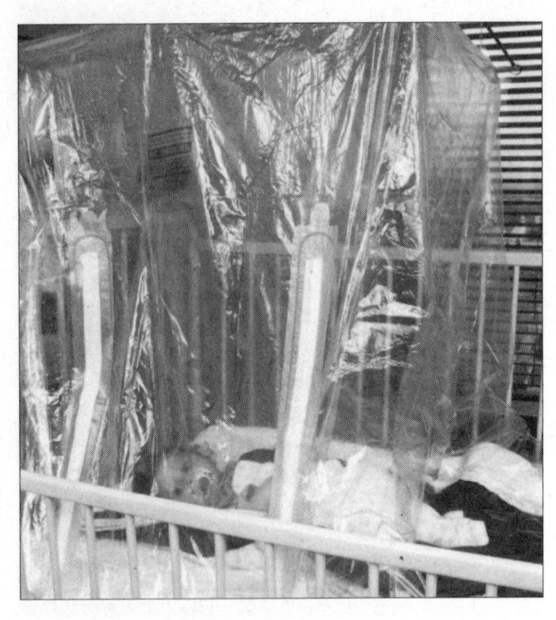

Figure 30–7 *Child in mist tent*

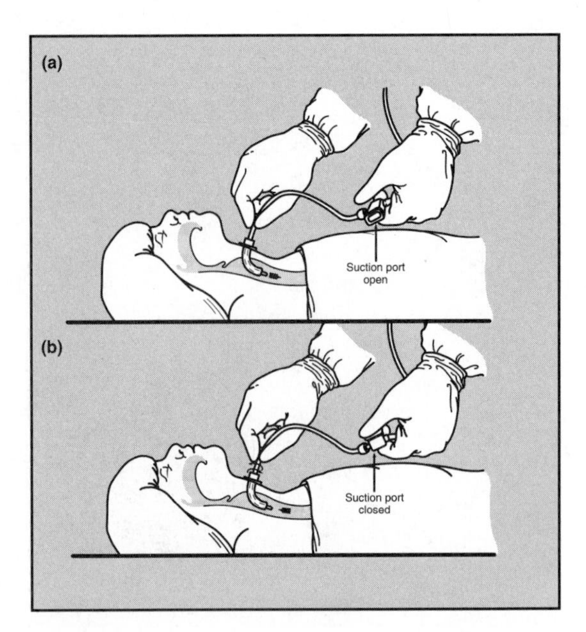

Figure 30–8 *Tracheostomy suctioning. (a) Insertion, port open. (b) Withdrawal, port closed. (From D. L. Wong.* Whaley & Wong's Essentials of Pediatric Nursing, *4th ed. St. Louis, MO: Mosby-Year Book, 1993.)*

MIST TENT (OXYGEN TENT)

The mist tent delivers oxygen concentrations of 35% to 40% and is an effective way to deliver humidified oxygen, Figure 30–7. Tuck the tent under the mattress to reduce oxygen loss. Check the child's clothes and blankets frequently and change when damp.

SUCTIONING

Suctioning may be necessary to maintain a patent airway in a pediatric patient. Children with tracheostomies will require tracheostomy tube suctioning. Infants, who are obligatory nose breathers, may require suctioning to remove excessive nasal secretions.

USING A BULB SYRINGE

A bulb syringe is used to suction excess secretions from an infant's nose. To use a bulb syringe:

1. Squeeze the bulb before placing the tip into the infant's nose, Figure 30–9a.
2. Place the tip of the bulb syringe into the infant's nares or mouth.
3. Be sure there is a seal and release the bulb, Figure 30–9b.
4. Remove the syringe and expel the contents.

NASOGASTRIC AND GASTROSTOMY TUBES

Nasogastric tubes are inserted to provide liquid feedings for the child who cannot swallow, to decompress the stomach, or to wash out (or lavage) the stomach. Gastrostomy tubes are inserted to provide liquid feedings to the child requiring long-term tube feeding.

PROCEDURE

Suctioning a Tracheostomy Tube

Purpose: Tracheostomy tube suctioning is required in order to keep the child's airway open and free from mucous plugs and increased secretions.

Equipment:

- Catheter kit containing sterile suction catheter, sterile cup, and sterile gloves. The size of the catheter used for suctioning depends on the size of the tracheostomy tube in place. The diameter of the catheter should be one-half the diameter of the tracheostomy tube.
- Sterile normal saline
- Clean gloves
- The equipment at the bedside should include replacement tracheostomy tubes, Ambu bag, oxygen, and suction equipment.

Preparation:

1. Turn on the wall suction and set as ordered.
2. Turn on oxygen source and attach to the Ambu bag.

Procedure:

1. Put the sterile glove on your dominant hand. Put a clean glove on the other hand.
2. Using sterile technique, remove the catheter from the paper sheath.
3. To test the suction equipment, place the end of the catheter in a cup of sterile saline.
4. Hyperventilate the child before and after suctioning with 100% oxygen if ordered by the physician.
5. Insert the catheter with the suction port open no more than 0.5 cm below the edge of the tracheostomy tube, Figure 30–8a.
6. Withdraw the catheter slowly, rotating the catheter while covering the suction port, Figure 30–8b.
7. Remove catheter and irrigate with sterile water.
8. If secretions are thick, a few drops of sterile saline (0.5 to 2 mL) injected into the tube can help to loosen them.

PRECAUTION: Do not suction for longer than 5 to 10 seconds. Allow the child to rest between aspirations to prevent hypoxia.

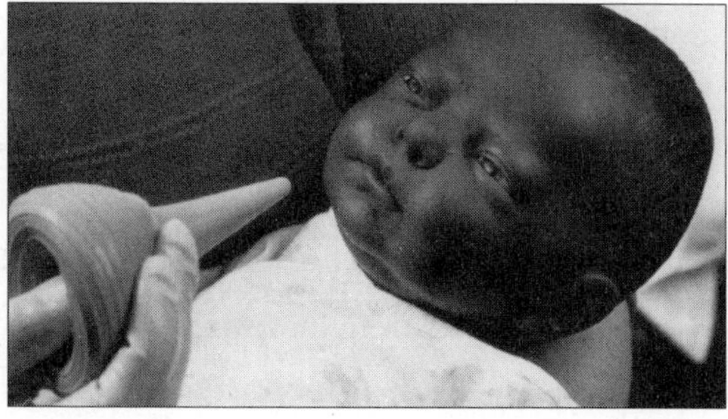

a.

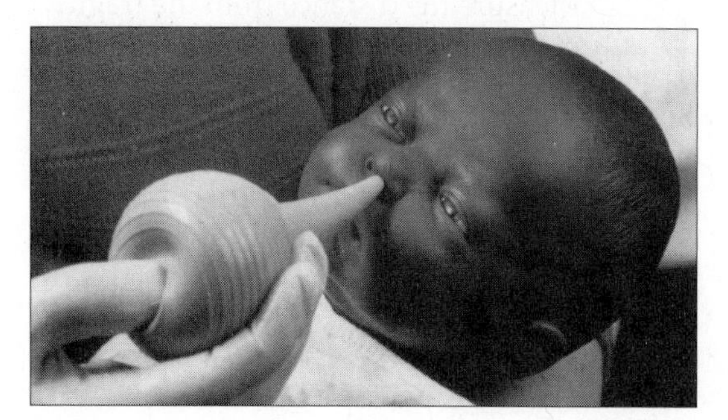

b.

Figure 30–9 *(a) Squeezing the bulb syringe. (b) Releasing the bulb syringe.*

GASTROSTOMY TUBES

Gastrostomy tubes are surgically placed in the stomach in children needing long-term feedings. To provide proper care for a gastrostomy tube:

1. Monitor the insertion site for any irritation or infection.
2. Clean area daily and apply an antibiotic ointment.
3. Apply a dressing when needed.
4. Tape the tube carefully to prevent the tube from dislodging and causing erosion or enlargement of the insertion site.
5. Clamp the tube when not in use.

GASTROSTOMY FEEDING BUTTON

The gastrostomy button is a small flexible device made out of silicone rubber that may be used as an alternative to a gastrostomy tube in the patient requiring long-term tube feedings.

PROCEDURE

Nasogastric Tubes

Purpose: Nasogastric tubes are inserted through the nose into the stomach and are used for alimentation or decompression and emptying of the stomach.

Equipment:

- Appropriate-size tube
- Suction
- Tape
- Stethoscope
- 20-mL syringe, gauze, and clean gloves

Preparation:

1. Place the child in a supine position. Elevate the head of the bed, if possible.
2. Measure the distance from the tragus of the ear to the mouth and then to the xiphoid process to determine the distance to the stomach. Mark the tube.

Procedure:

1. Put on clean gloves.
2. Lubricate the tube with water-soluble lubricant or sterile water.
3. Insert the tube into the child's nares or mouth.
4. If using the nose, advance the tube along the floor of the nasal passages.
5. If using the mouth, direct the tube toward the back of the throat.
6. Have the child swallow while the tube is being inserted to make placement easier.
7. Advance the tube until you have reached the mark.
8. Check the tube for placement by aspirating stomach contents and checking pH or by injecting a small amount of air through the syringe while at the same time auscultating over the stomach. You will hear growling sounds if the tube is properly placed.
9. Tape securely in place and attach to the child's nose or cheek with tape.
10. To remove the tube, place the child in Fowler's position. Unfasten the tape, and gently pull from the oropharynx.

A well-established gastrostomy site is required. A mushroom-like tip holds the button in place, and two flat wings help to keep it against the abdominal wall. A one-way valve inside the button at the gastric opening prevents reflux of stomach contents.

GAVAGE FEEDING

A gavage feeding is given through a tube that has been placed into the stomach through either the nose or mouth. The size of the tube used for the feeding depends on the thickness of the feeding and the size of the child.

PROCEDURE

Gavage Feeding

Purpose: Infants and children are fed by gavage because of congenital anomalies, to supplement oral feedings, and after surgery. Feedings can be intermittent or continuous, and administration can be performed by gravity or pump. (Refer to Chapter 19 and Figure 19–9.)

Equipment:

- Sterile water for irrigation of the tube
- A stethoscope to check tube placement
- An asepto syringe or 10-, 20-, or 30-mL syringes
- The formula or solution
- If the feeding is to be administered by gravity, an IV pole may be used.

Procedure:

1. Place the infant or child in an upright position if possible. If not, place the child on the back or right side with head and chest elevated.
2. Check the placement of the tube before each feeding by aspirating stomach contents or by injecting a small amount of air through the syringe while at the same time auscultating over the stomach. You will hear growling sounds if the tube is properly placed.
3. Formula should be administered at room temperature.
4. Start the flow slowly to ensure patency. The feeding should take approximately 30 minutes to complete.
5. Flush the tube with sterile water (1–5 mL, depending on the size of the tube).
6. When the feeding is complete, clamp the tube. If the tube is to be removed, clamp or pinch and withdraw quickly.
7. Position the child on the right side after feeding for about 1 hour to prevent aspiration or vomiting.

REVIEW QUESTIONS

A. Multiple choice. Select the best answer.

1. Which of the following is not a recommended method for holding or transporting an infant?
   a. cradle hold
   b. football hold
   c. mummy hold
   d. upright hold
2. Todd, 5 years old, is scheduled to receive an intramuscular injection. The preferred administration site for a child of Todd's age is the
   a. vastus lateralis
   b. gluteus maximus
   c. vastus medialis
   d. biceps brachii
3. The diameter of the catheter used for suctioning a tracheostomy tube should be
   a. one-quarter the diameter of the tube
   b. one-third the diameter of the tube
   c. one-half the diameter of the tube
   d. two-thirds the diameter of the tube
4. Which of the following delivery modes would provide the highest concentration of oxygen?
   a. face mask
   b. nasal cannula
   c. mist tent
   d. blow-by
5. Which of the following is not a commonly used site for venipuncture?
   a. antecubital fossa
   b. dorsum of the hand
   c. dorsum of the foot
   d. femoral vein

B. True or false. Write *T* for a true statement and *F* for a false statement.

1. ___ Toddlers benefit from simple explanations of procedures.
2. ___ When administering ear drops to a 4-year-old child, pull the pinna down and back.
3. ___ Oral medications should never be put in an infant's formula.
4. ___ When suctioning a tracheostomy tube, the nurse may safely apply suction for up to 15 seconds at a time.
5. ___ The formula used for gavage feeding should be administered at room temperature.

SUGGESTED ACTIVITIES

- Select a procedure. Practice explaining the procedure to children of different developmental stages. What differences are necessary?
- Spend time in an out-patient department or emergency room observing how children are restrained for procedures.
- Practice carrying and transporting a life-size infant doll or mannequin.
- Make a list of the different routes for administering medications to children and identify safety precautions that should be taken.
- List the differences in technique when applying a urine collection bag to a boy or girl.
- Practice using a bulb syringe on an infant mannequin.

BIBLIOGRAPHY

Bindler, R. M., and L. B. Howry. *Pediatric Drugs and Nursing Procedures*. Norwalk, CT: Appleton and Lange, 1991.

Broadwell Jackson, D., and R. B. Saunders. *Child Health Nursing*. Philadelphia: J. B. Lippincott, 1993.

Heiney, S. P. Helping children through painful procedures. *American Journal of Nursing*, November (1991): 20–24

Rice, J., and E. G. Skelley. *Medications and Mathematics for the Nurse*, 7th ed. Albany, NY: Delmar Publishers, 1993.

Skale, N. *Manual of Pediatric Nursing Procedures*. Philadelphia: J. B. Lippincott, 1992.

Speer, K. M., and C. L. Swann. *The Addison-Wesley Manual of Pediatric Nursing Procedures*. Redwood City, CA: Addison-Wesley, 1993.

Wong, D. L. *Whaley & Wong's Essentials of Pediatric Nursing*, 4th ed. St. Louis, MO: Mosby-Year Book, 1993.

CHAPTER

31

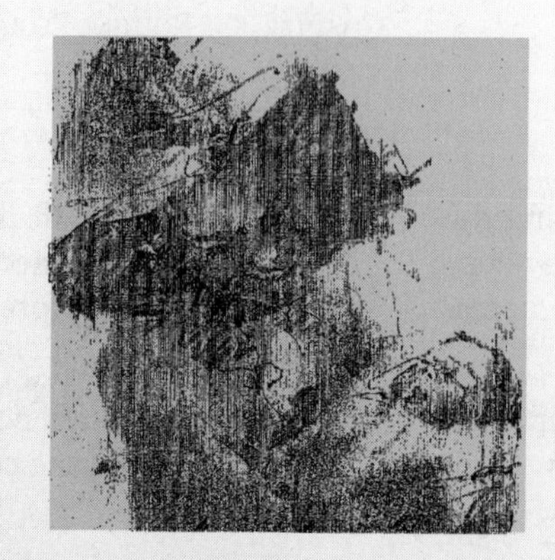

The Pediatric Surgical Patient

OBJECTIVES

AFTER STUDYING THIS CHAPTER, THE STUDENT SHOULD BE ABLE TO:

- DEFINE THE ROLE OF THE NURSE IN THE PREOPERATIVE AND POSTOPERATIVE CARE OF THE PEDIATRIC SURGICAL PATIENT.
- IDENTIFY SIGNIFICANT STRESSORS ASSOCIATED WITH SURGERY THAT PRODUCE ANXIETY FOR CHILDREN.
- DESCRIBE NURSING CARE THAT MAY REDUCE THE PSYCHOLOGICAL AND PHYSICAL STRESS OF SURGERY FOR THE CHILD AND FAMILY.
- DESCRIBE PREOPERATIVE NURSING PROCEDURES.
- DISCUSS THE IMPLICATIONS OF PREOPERATIVE TEACHING FOR THE POSTOPERATIVE RECOVERY PERIOD.
- DESCRIBE POSTOPERATIVE NURSING CARE OF THE CHILD.
- DISCUSS PEDIATRIC POSTOPERATIVE PAIN MANAGEMENT.
- IDENTIFY NURSING CONSIDERATIONS IN DISCHARGE PLANNING FOR THE POSTSURGICAL PEDIATRIC PATIENT.

Key Terms

PREOPERATIVE CARE
PREOPERATIVE TEACHING
PREOPERATIVE CHECKLIST
POSTOPERATIVE CARE
PAIN MANAGEMENT
POSTOPERATIVE EXERCISES

Conditions requiring surgery are as stressful for children and families as hospitalization (refer to Chapters 27 and 29). With today's focus on cost containment and advances in surgical technology, nurses do not have a great deal of time to prepare children and their families for the surgical experience. Pediatric surgery can take place in a traditional hospital setting, in an out-patient surgical suite associated with the hospital, or in a free-standing surgical center. Many children now go home soon after recovery from anesthesia. The nurse needs to assist the child through the surgical experience and help the child return to optimal functioning.

Preoperative Care

Preoperative care is the care given to the child and family in preparation for the forthcoming surgery. Children require emotional and physical preparation as part of preoperative care. The specific care will depend on the reason for the surgery and the individual needs of the child. Figure 31–1 summarizes preoperative nursing care of the child.

Psychological Aspects

Providing emotional support is as important as the preparation given for hospital procedures. When planning care, the nurse should be aware of the six stressors that produce anxiety for the child before and after surgery: (1) admission, (2) blood testing, (3) the day before surgery, (4) preoperative injections, (5) transport to the operating room, and (6) return from the postanesthesia area (Visintainer and Wolfer 1975).

Preoperative teaching is designed to reduce preoperative anxiety and promote a positive postoperative outcome. Rehearsing surgical events with the inclusion of known stressors has been shown to decrease the trauma of the surgical experience. Preoperative teaching helps children use their coping skills and feel in control of a difficult situation (Kennedy and Riddle 1989). In addition, children who receive emotional support and understand procedures generally experience fewer complications of surgery than children who do not receive support or information (Yale 1993). Materials used and timing of delivery must take into account the child's developmental stage:

NURSING CARE PLAN: Preoperative Care

PATIENT PROBLEM	GOAL(S)
Anxiety or fear (child) related to surgery (separation anxiety, fear of the unknown, or lack of knowledge)	Before surgery, the child will demonstrate minimal insecurity and anxiety. The child will be relaxed before entering the operating room.
Anxiety or fear (parents) caused by potentially life-threatening condition of child	The parents will be able to explain the child's forthcoming surgery and the hoped-for response.
Potential injury resulting from surgery	Before the child goes to surgery, legal authorization will be signed and included on the chart. Before surgery, all necessary physical preparation will be completed.

Figure 31–1 *Nursing care plan for preoperative care of the child undergoing surgery*

Nursing Intervention	Rationale
Before the surgery, explain what will be happening and what the child's role will be. Use age-appropriate teaching materials. Orient the child to unfamiliar surroundings. Explain where the parents will be.	Knowledge decreases anxiety, which in turn decreases the amount of medication needed for anesthesia and promotes postoperative recovery.
Administer preoperative medication (preferably oral) if ordered. Place the child in a quiet room. Allow parents to stay with the child. Allow parents and a favorite toy or object to accompany the child.	Intramuscular injections are stressful. Allowing parents and significant objects to accompany the child utilizes the child's own coping strategies and decreases separation anxiety.
Include important family members in preoperative teaching.	Increased knowledge decreases anxiety. When the parents feel secure and trusting the child is more likely to feel secure as well.
Discuss informed consent with parent or legal guardian. Check document for correct surgical procedure and correct date. Witness signature of parent or legal guardian. Place on chart.	Parent or legal guardian must give verbal or written consent for surgery for children under 18 years of age (with exceptions).
Administer any preparations designed to cleanse the bowel, antibiotics, and preoperative medications, as ordered.	Enemas or irrigating solutions cleanse the bowel of normal bacteria.
Dress the child in hospital gown (if possible allow to wear underwear or pajama bottoms).	Clothing must be unrestrictive to allow full visualization during surgery. Underclothing or pajama bottoms are very important to children and can be removed after anesthesia.

PATIENT PROBLEM	GOAL(S)
	During surgery, the child will experience no complications due to aspiration, allergies, anemia, bleeding, or infection.
	The child will arrive safely in the operating room.

Figure 31–1 *continued*

- *Infants* and toddlers can be told about the procedure as it begins.
- *Preschoolers* benefit from rehearsals and trips to the areas involved before surgery.
- *School-age children* benefit from films in which peers model behavior. They can be taught about the surgical procedure and routine up to a week before the surgery.
- *Adolescents* can be taught about the surgical procedure as soon as it is scheduled. Provide clear explanations and teach stress-reduction techniques. Discuss particular fears related to surgery (anesthesia, venipuncture).

If pain is an expected result of the surgical procedure, children need to be honestly told of

NURSING INTERVENTION	RATIONALE
Remove any makeup, prostheses, or orthodontic devices.	All items that could harm the child during surgery must be removed.
Bathe child, groom hair, and brush teeth. Check for loose teeth. Record any skin lesions or breaks in the skin.	Bathing decreases the number of microorganisms on the skin. Bathing is also comforting.
Prepare operative site according to physician's orders.	Antimicrobial soaps and removal of hair further decrease the chance of infection.
Give the child nothing to eat or drink after the time designated by the physician's orders. Have the child void before taking preoperative medication.	Undigested food if vomited could be inhaled into the lungs causing aspiration pneumonia.
Take and record vital signs.	Changes in vital signs may indicate pain or fever. They also provide a baseline for comparison in recovery period.
Check laboratory reports for hemoglobin, white blood count, reduced platelets, or prolonged bleeding time.	Surgery would be postponed if there was a potential for hemorrhage related to inability of the blood to clot.
Check identification band. Put side-rails up or use safety straps when conveying. Do not leave child unattended.	Children are susceptible to injury during transport, especially when premedicated for surgery.

the possibilities beforehand. They need to know that the pain will not last long. Older children are capable of using imaging or relaxation techniques to cope with painful situations (Berde 1989).

Parents will be anxious and need support and guidance before and after the surgical procedure. Including parents in the child's preoperative teaching helps them understand and cope with their child's responses to the experience. Although not always permitted, the presence of parents before surgery has a calming effect on the child. Many hospitals allow parents to stay with the child until the induction of the anesthesia and then to be present when the child awakens from anesthesia, Figure 31–2. Parents should be offered the option of staying with their child when policy permits.

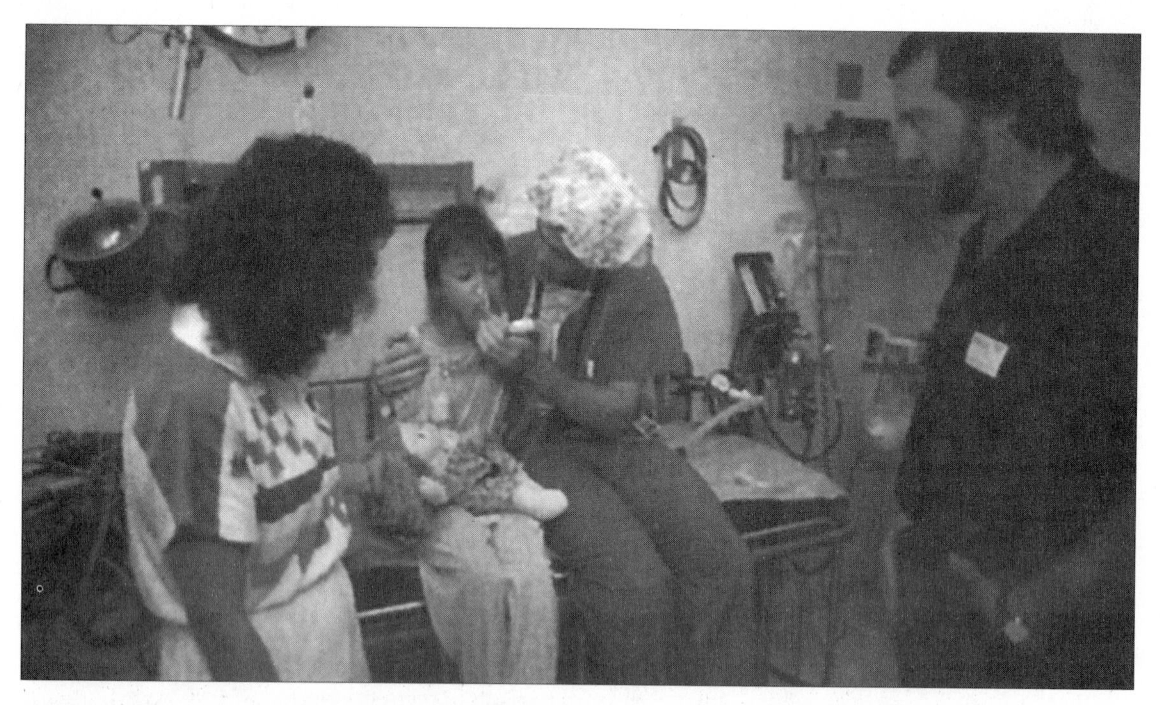

Figure 31–2 *Parents with child undergoing anesthesia (From D. L. Wong.* Whaley & Wong's Essentials of Pediatric Nursing, *4th ed. St. Louis, MO: Mosby-Year Book, 1993.)*

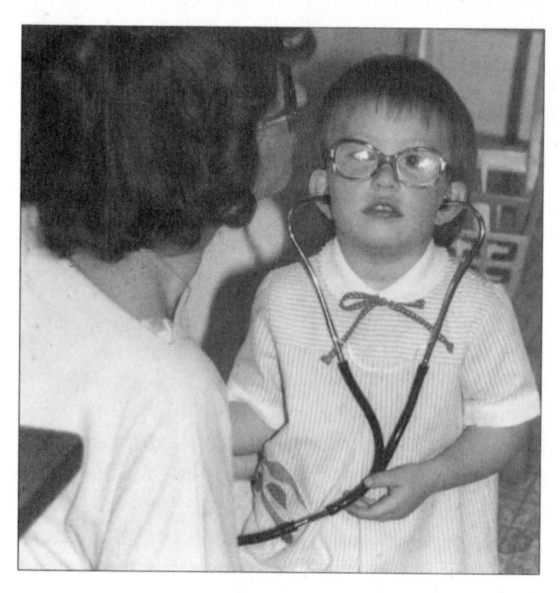

Figure 31–3 *Allowing the child to play with hospital equipment helps to lessen anxiety.*

Most children when asked state that they want their parents present (Murphy 1992).

Allowing children the opportunity to see and play with equipment, such as stethoscopes, blood pressure cuffs, and oxygen masks, helps to lessen their anxiety, Figure 31–3. Sometimes it is helpful to rehearse the child's surgery using a favorite doll. Drawings are an enjoyable activity for children of all ages and can offer invaluable information about a child's perceptions and fears, Figure 31–4. This information can help nurses to correct misconceptions and lessen the child's anxieties before surgery (O'Malley and McNamera 1993).

PHYSICAL ASPECTS

In addition to psychological care, children usua.

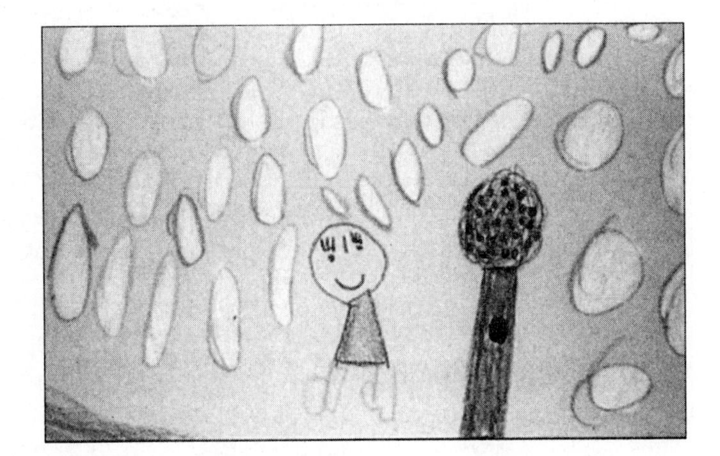

Hooray Hooray it's my operation day
Soon I will be better than I can go
out and play.

b.

Figure 31–4 *These two drawings illustrate children's conceptions of the surgical experience. (a) Trees drawn with knotholes represent a child's fear of invasive procedures. (b) This child's mother has added her feelings about surgery to his drawing. (From M. E. O'Malley and S. T. McNamera. Children's drawings.* AORN Journal *57, 1993.)*

ally require various types of physical care before surgery. The steps of the preoperative process are usually arranged in what is known as a **preoperative checklist**, Figure 31–5. When preparing the child for surgery, the nurse notes when each step of the checklist has been accomplished.

The physician determines the fluid and nutritional needs of the child before surgery. Generally, no milk or solid foods are given after midnight of the night before surgery. But clear liquids (if ordered) can be given up to about two hours before surgery. Infants in particular should not go for longer than four hours

SAMPLE PREOPERATIVE CHECKLIST

- Consent forms witnessed, signed, and in chart
- Identification band in place
- Laboratory tests completed and results in chart
- Allergies clearly noted in chart
- Vital signs obtained and recorded
- NPO before surgery
- Voided before surgery
- Prescribed medications given
- Eyeglasses and any prostheses, including orthodontic devices, removed
- Mouth checked for loose teeth
- Operative site bathed and cleansed, if ordered

Figure 31–5

without fluids. In order for the child to be well hydrated, an intravenous line is started. Careful attention must be given to IV drip rates to avoid overhydration.

POSTOPERATIVE CARE

Postoperative care includes the physical as well as emotional care given in the postanesthesia room (PAR; also referred to as the postanesthesia care unit or the recovery room) and on the nursing unit during recovery from the surgical procedure. After the surgical procedure, the child is closely monitored in the postanesthesia area. Once sufficiently recovered from anesthesia, the child is either transferred back to the room or discharged home. The child should be awake, alert, and have stable vital signs, and any nausea, vomiting, or pain should be under control before release from the postanesthesia area. Figure 31–6 summarizes postoperative nursing care of the child.

TRANSFERRING THE CHILD

When a child is transferred from the postanesthesia area back to the room, the transferring nurse is responsible for giving a report on the child's status, including: (1) what was done during the surgery, (2) what anesthesia was administered, (3) whether any medications have been given, and (4) what orders the physician has written. The child's level of consciousness, vital signs, dressings and wounds, tubes, IV lines, and comfort level are assessed.

ARRIVAL ON NURSING UNIT

Close supervision is important. Changes in vital signs or behavior may signal life-threatening complications such as shock, hemorrhage, or malignant hyperthermia. Priority assessments during this period are airway, breathing, and circulation. Careful documentation and communication are essential (Whaley and Wong 1991).

PAIN MANAGEMENT

A common misconception is that children have a higher pain threshold than adults. They do not. Children are, however, often undermedicated for postoperative pain because of their inability to provide a description of pain.

The child's level of comfort should be assessed, and analgesics given accordingly. Change in behavior is the best indicator that a child may need pain medication. Assessment tools such as the Faces rating scale (Figure 31–7) can help the nurse and the child determine the quality of the child's postsurgical pain (Wong and Baker 1988). The nurse asks the child to pick the face that most closely describes the pain he or she is feeling. Keep in mind that fear of injections may prevent a child from acknowledging pain. Reassure the child that pain medication does not have to involve a "shot."

Effective **pain management** occurs when medications are given at regular intervals rather than on an as-needed basis. Children as young as 7 years of age benefit from patient-controlled analgesia (a drug-delivery system that allows patients to administer pain medication as they need it).

Nonpharmacological pain control methods may be used with analgesics, to increase their effectiveness, or alone when the child has minimal pain. These methods include distraction, cutaneous stimulation (rubbing, massage), transcutaneous electrical nerve stimulation (TENS), relaxation, hypnosis, imagery, and application of heat and cold. The presence of parents is also an important source of comfort for children in pain.

Pain needs to be controlled in order for the child to be able to perform effectively **postoperative exercises**, such as coughing and deep breathing, early ambulation, or leg exercises. These exercises stimulate circulation and respiration, thereby preventing atelectasis and blood stasis. Children who receive adequate pain management have less anxiety and recover more quickly than those who do not (Bender et al. 1990).

Mastery over painful and stressful events is important to children. During the recovery period, they need time to work through the experience. Play, drawing, and storytelling provide excellent means for expression and allow the child to discuss fears and perceptions.

WOUND CARE

Children usually return from surgery with surgical dressings in place. Compression is accomplished with elasticized bandages. If bleeding is controlled, the wound may be covered with a clear dressing. This dressing protects the wound, allows healing, and is easily viewed and cleaned (Failla and Vega-Cruz 1991).

The initial surgical dressing is usually not changed by the nurse, but it can be reinforced if bleeding occurs. Careful measurements and documentation regarding the dressing and drainage are essential. Any drains connected to the wound should be assessed for patency and amount of drainage. Careful aseptic technique must be exercised when handling or changing dressings.

DISCHARGE PLANNING

Discharge planning should include parents, other caregivers, and the extended family, as appropriate. The child's developmental stage, parents' educational level, and the extent of the surgery must be considered when giving discharge instructions. Reinforce verbal instructions about wound care, diet, activity, and pain management with written instructions. Additional considerations include proximity of the home to health care services, available support services, and the financial needs of the family (Hamilton and Vessey 1992).

NURSING CARE PLAN: Postoperative Care

PATIENT PROBLEM	GOAL(S)
Potential injury resulting from surgery or anesthesia	The child will return safely from surgery with least amount of stress possible. The child's wound will heal and be free of infection. The child will not develop complications of surgery.
Pain	The child will rest quietly and exhibit minimum evidence of pain.

Figure 31–6 Nursing care plan for postoperative care of the child undergoing surgery.

NURSING INTERVENTION	RATIONALE
Place the child in bed in position of safety and comfort. Follow physician's orders.	Measures to provide safety and comfort minimize trauma of transfer to hospital room.
Perform careful handwashing. Keep wound clean and dry.	Handwashing is the first line of defense against microorganisms.
Follow hospital procedure regarding changing dressings. Apply antibacterial medications as ordered. Record any unusual appearance or drainage.	Clean dry dressings inhibit growth of microorganisms. Antimicrobial medications and soaps fight infection. Redness, drainage, or swelling may be signs of infection.
Change diapers carefully to prevent contamination.	Careful disposal of diapers decreases the child's chance of developing an infection.
Check carefully for excessive bleeding. Monitor carefully for stable vital signs. Assist with early ambulation. Help the child to void.	Early detection of complications allows for prompt intervention. Common complications of surgery may be shock, respiratory depression, hemorrhage, and infection. Changes in vital signs may be the first clue. Early ambulation increases circulation and stimulates respiration.
Keep the child NPO until awake.	Until bowel sounds return nothing should be given by mouth to decrease the chance of aspiration and gastric distention.
Assess pain frequently using assessment tools as well as physiological responses (e.g., heart rate and blood pressure).	Children may have difficulty communicating that they have pain. Unrelieved pain has negative physical and psychological effects.
Administer analgesics as prescribed and evaluate their effectiveness. Administer antiemetics as ordered. Include nonpharmacological pain relief (e.g., ice, imaging, and breathing techniques).	Prevention of pain is best. Severe pain is difficult to manage. Continuous administration of opioid analgesics gives optimum pain relief.

PATIENT PROBLEM	GOAL(S)
Potential for inadequate hydration	The child will take in and retain sufficient fluids to maintain adequate hydration.
Potential for inadequate nutrition	The child will receive adequate nourishment.

Figure 31–6 *continued*

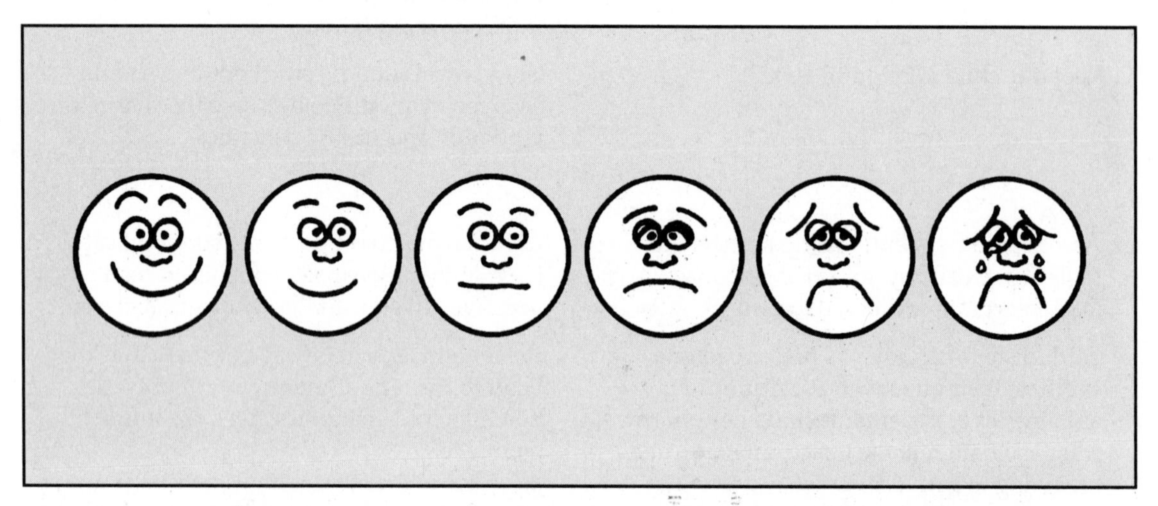

Figure 31–7 *Faces rating scale (From D. L. Wong.* Whaley & Wong's Essentials of Pediatric Nursing, *4th ed. St. Louis, MO: Mosby-Year Book, 1993.)*

NURSING INTERVENTION	RATIONALE
Check for signs of dehydration (e.g., shiny, tight dry skin, less output than expected for age).	Skin should be warm, dry and supple.
Obtain weight measurement daily. Record intake and output. Weigh all diapers.	Helps ensure an accurate record of fluid status. An infant should have 6 to 8 wet diapers a day.
Offer fluids as soon as ordered or as child can tolerate them.	
Encourage the child with favorite drinks, ice chips, frozen pops (no red drinks or frozen pops if bleeding needs to be evaluated).	Providing favorite drinks improves fluid intake.
Ensure a nutritious, age-appropriate diet during recovery period.	A well-balanced diet promotes healing.

NURSING CARE RELATED TO THE PRE- AND POSTOPERATIVE PERIOD

- Provide knowledgeable nursing care during the pre- and postoperative period.
- Anticipate stressful pre- and postoperative events and give appropriate nursing care to lessen the trauma of known stressors.
- Provide honest, developmentally appropriate explanations of pre- and postoperative procedures and routines.
- Prepare the child for pre- and postoperative procedures and allow him or her to rehearse, handle equipment, and visit the surgical area.
- Assess the child's understanding of preoperative teaching. (For example, have the child point to the part of the body that will be operated on.)
- Monitor the child postoperatively for changes in vital signs and assist in postoperative exercises.
- Observe the child for pain and use both pharmacological and nonpharmacological interventions for pain control.

REVIEW QUESTIONS

A. Multiple choice. Select the best answer.

1. The nurse is responsible for all of the following preoperative events except
   a. taking a nursing history and physical examination
   b. rehearsing expected procedures and events
   c. obtaining baseline vital signs
   d. informing the child and family about the advantages and risks of the surgery

2. Of the following preoperative information, which would be most important for psychological support of an infant?
   a. favorite foods
   b. normal comforting pattern
   c. birth date
   d. number of siblings

3. The pediatric surgical patient can be expected to perceive which of the following as the most stressful?
   a. preoperative teaching, visiting the operating room, examining a stethoscope
   b. meals, parental visitation, trips to the playroom
   c. roommates, primary care nurse, transport to the laboratory in a wagon
   d. admission, blood testing, transport to surgery on a cart

4. The nurse demonstrates nursing interventions to lessen the psychological trauma of the child and family when he or she
   a. asks the mother to leave during preoperative procedures
   b. includes the mother during preparation of the child for the preoperative procedure
   c. keeps hospital equipment out of sight until the procedure has begun
   d. gives significant toys to family member for safe keeping

5. All of the following interventions help children master difficult situations except
   a. avoiding telling the child about the unpleasant effects of surgery
   b. allowing the child to rehearse surgical events
   c. giving age-appropriate information about the surgical procedures
   d. telling the child there will be medicine for the "hurt"

6. Of the following, which would be important for the anesthesiologist to know?
   a. the child's normal bedtime
   b. the child's last bowel movement
   c. the child's loose third molar
   d. the child's favorite sport

7. Timmy, 4 years old, clings to his teddy bear and refuses to get onto the surgical cart. What is the best solution?
   a. Firmly tell Timmy he must get on the cart — it is hospital policy.
   b. Postpone the surgery until Timmy is ready to go.
   c. Ask the physician to come talk to Timmy.
   d. Allow Timmy's parents to pull him to surgery in the unit wagon.

8. All of the following are normal preoperative procedures except
   a. antibacterial bath
   b. preoperative medication
   c. completion of preoperative checklist
   d. blood transfusion

9. The nurse prepares to receive a pediatric patient from the postanesthesia area. The priority assessment will be
   a. pain level
   b. respiratory status
   c. intravenous infusion site
   d. patency of drainage tubes

10. When will the nurse give the child something to drink?
    a. as soon as the child is awake
    b two hours after admission to room
    c. as soon as the child is awake enough to swallow and the physician's orders permit
    d. eight hours after surgery

11. Early ambulation after surgery accomplishes which of the following?
    a. diverts the child from the surgical pain
    b. stimulates respiratory and circulatory function
    c. assures early hospital dismissal
    d. increases the chance of postsurgical complications

SUGGESTED ACTIVITIES

- Visualize how the surgical experience looks and feels to a child (choose a specific age: toddler, preschool child, etc.). Identify stressors and actions that might help to alleviate the child's fear and anxiety.
- Collect and compare several pre- and postoperative checklists. What items do all checklists have in common? How do they differ? Make suggestions for additions or deletions.
- Write for the following free materials:
  - Faces scale (send a stamped self-addressed business envelope to Ms. C. Baker, 4412 St. Thomas Drive, Oklahoma City, OK 73120)
  - Pain management materials (AHCPR Publications Clearinghouse, P.O. Box 8547, Silver Spring, MD 20907; or call 1-800-358-9295)

BIBLIOGRAPHY

Acute Pain Management Guideline Panel. *Acute Pain Management in Infants, Children, and Adolescents: Operative and Medical Procedures. Quick Reference Guide for Clinicians.* AHCPR Pub. No. 92-0020. Rockville, MD: Agency for Health Care Policy and Research, Public Health Service, U.S. Department of Health and Human Services, 1992.

Bender, L. H., K. Weaver, and K. Edwards. Postoperative patient-controlled analgesia in children. *Pediatric Nursing* 16 (1990): 549–557.

Berde, C. B. Pediatric postoperative pain management. *Pediatric Clinics of North America* 36 (1989): 921–937.

Failla, S., and P. Vega-Cruz. Ask the O.R. *American Journal of Nursing* 91 (1991): 26–27.

Hamilton, B., and J. Vessey. Pediatric discharge planning. *Pediatric Nursing* 18 (1992): 475–478.

Jacox, A., B. Ferrell, G. Heidrich, N. Hester, and C. Measkowski. Managing acute pain. *American Journal of Nursing* 92 (1992): 49–55.

Kennedy, D., and I. Riddle. The influence of the timing of preparation on the anxiety of preschool children experiencing surgery. *Maternal-Child Nursing Journal* 18 (1989): 117–131.

Konings, K. Preop use of Golytely in pediatrics. *Pediatric Nursing* 15 (1989): 473–474.

Murphy, E. K. OR nursing law: Issues regarding parents in the operating room during their children's care. *AORN Journal* 56 (1992): 120–124.

O'Malley, M. E., and S. T. McNamera. Children's drawings. *AORN Journal* 57 (1993): 1074–1089.

Visintainer, M. A., and J. A. Wolfer. Psychological preparation for surgical pediatric patients: The effects of children's and parents' stress responses and adjustment. *Pediatrics* 56, no. 2 (1975): 187–202.

Whaley, L. F., and D. L. Wong. *Nursing Care of Infants and Children*, 4th ed., pp. 1184–2101. St. Louis, MO: Mosby-Year Book, 1991.

Wong, D., and C. Baker. Pain in children: Comparison of assessment scales. *Pediatric Nursing* 14, no. 1 (1988): 9–17.

Yale, E. Preoperative teaching strategy. *AORN Journal* 57 (1993): 901-908.

UNIT

viii

The Dying Child

CHAPTER

32

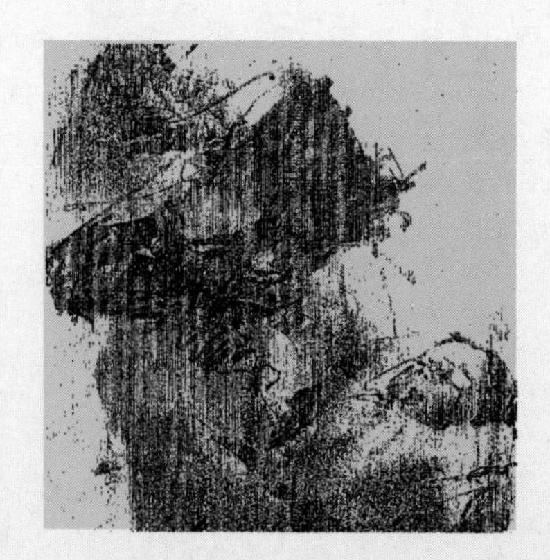

Caring for the Dying Child

OBJECTIVES

AFTER STUDYING THIS CHAPTER, THE STUDENT SHOULD BE ABLE TO:

- IDENTIFY THE CHILD'S CONCEPT OF DEATH AT VARIOUS DEVELOPMENTAL STAGES.
- DEFINE THE STAGES OF GRIEVING, ACCORDING TO KUBLER-ROSS.
- DESCRIBE COMMON RESPONSES OF PARENTS OF A DYING CHILD:
- DESCRIBE COMMON RESPONSES OF SIBLINGS OF A DYING CHILD.
- DISCUSS SOURCES OF SUPPORT FOR THE DYING CHILD AND FAMILY.
- DESCRIBE HOSPICE CARE.
- OUTLINE NURSING CONSIDERATIONS IN THE CARE OF THE DYING CHILD.

KEY TERMS

MAGICAL THINKING

ANTICIPATORY GRIEVING

HOSPICE CARE

The death of a child is difficult for both families and health care providers to face. The life of a child who dies is often viewed as having been unjustly cut short. Helping dying children and their families to cope with and accept the child's death is one of the greatest challenges facing nurses. To provide effective and supportive care, the nurse must understand children's perceptions of death at varying ages, stages of grieving, and parental and sibling responses. The nurse should also be knowledgeable about resources that can provide support to the family of a dying child.

CHILDREN'S PERCEPTION OF DEATH AND DYING

As we grow older, we learn about death from our environment and those around us. Death is a part of life. We begin to develop a concept of death that changes with each developmental stage. Some children are exposed to death when a family member dies. Other children learn about death by observing the life cycles of the insects, birds, and animals around them. It is important to remember that all children experience life uniquely and develop at individual rates. Furthermore, all children express and handle feelings and cope with illness and death in their own way.

INFANCY AND TODDLERHOOD

Concept of Death. Infants and toddlers appear to have no real concept of death. Because young children live in the present, it is impossible for them to comprehend the absence of life. Death is perceived as a separation from loved ones.

Reactions to Death and Dying. Infants respond to the behaviors of those around them. Thus, they may respond with distress to the emotional and physical distress of others, especially their parents' reactions of sadness, anxiety, depression, or anger.

Toddlers, who lack a true concept or understanding of death, will persist in seeking to speak with or visit a person who has died. It is important to emphasize that the dead person will return only in the child's thoughts and memories.

Terminally ill toddlers fear separation from their parents. Because ritualism is extremely important in the life of the toddler, any change in the ill child's routines can produce anxiety.

PRESCHOOL YEARS

Concept of Death. During the preschool period, between 3 and 5 years of age, children gradually develop the concept of nonexistence, of "life" and "not life." However, death is seen as reversible and temporary. Death may be seen as a kind of sleep, a temporary separation. To the preschooler, death is unpleasant because it separates people.

Reactions to Death and Dying. Preschool children have a tremendous sense of omnipotence, which leads them to believe that their thoughts and deeds can cause an event to occur. This belief is termed **magical thinking**. They may think that their thoughts caused the death of another. Similarly, preschoolers who become seriously ill may believe that the illness is punishment for their thoughts and actions.

The terminally ill preschooler's greatest fear concerning death is separation from parents. Preschoolers may fear going to sleep and never waking up. They may also associate "going to sleep" under anesthesia for surgical procedures with death (for example, a pet may have been "put to sleep"). For this reason, the presence of parents during painful or traumatic procedures is often helpful.

SCHOOL-AGE YEARS

Concept of Death. Children between the ages of 5 and 9 tend to personify death. Death is seen as a person such as an angel, ghost, God, skeleton, or a monster, who is either living or dead, with either good or bad intentions, who causes people to die. Children may have nightmares about these figures. They tend to believe that their own death can be avoided by personal ingenuity and efforts (for example, by running faster than death or locking the door to keep death out). From age 9 or 10 through adolescence, children begin to comprehend that death is inevitable, universal, and irreversible, and that they too will die someday, Figure 32–1.

Reactions to Death and Dying. School-age children continue to attribute the cause of death to misdeeds or bad thoughts and feel intense guilt and responsibility for the event. They tend to fear the possibility of death more than its occurrence. Bodily mutilation is especially feared.

It is important for school-age children to assimilate all the facts about death into a concrete logical framework. They want to know what happens to the dead body, who dresses it, and how the body feels. This information helps them to understand what will happen to them if they should die.

To achieve independence, self-worth, and self-esteem, seriously ill school-age children need to understand what is happening to them and to participate in what is done for them. Dying represents a loss of control over every aspect of living. Anticipatory preparation is effective and very necessary. Fear, exhibited as verbal uncooperativeness, may be erroneously interpreted as rude, impolite, or stubborn behavior. In reality, this verbal behavior is a plea for control and power.

ADOLESCENCE

Concept of Death. Adolescents have a mature understanding of death and yet still are influenced by remnants of magical thinking. Possible feelings of guilt and shame can be alleviated by making it clear that thoughts and activities do not cause diseases such as cancer.

Reactions to Death and Dying. Adolescents have more difficulty than other age groups in dealing with death. Some teenagers cope with death by expressing appropriate emotions, talking about the loss, and resolving the grief.

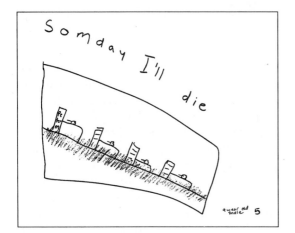

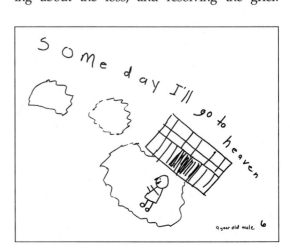

Figure 32–1 *These pictures illustrate the school-age child's concept of death. (Courtesy of Darlene McCown, Ph.D., R.N., P.N.P.)*

Others may appear undisturbed by the event, extremely angry, or unusually silent and withdrawn. Expect and accept these personal expressions of anger, fear, and sadness. Nurses can also be role models for parents in communicating with the adolescent.

The developmental task of adolescence is to establish an identity by finding out who one is, what one's purpose is, and where one belongs. Adolescents strive for group acceptance as well as independence from parental constraints. The crisis of a life-threatening illness may make an adolescent feel isolated from peers and unable to communicate with parents for emotional support. Any suggestion of being different or of ceasing to be is a threat.

Often the adolescent becomes emotionally attached to a nurse or physician. Parents may not understand this attachment and may even resent it. Reassure them that this is a normal occurrence for many adolescents who face a life-threatening illness.

The physical changes that occur with a life-threatening illness are especially troublesome for adolescents, who are oriented to the present. Physical changes are of more concern than the prognosis for future recovery.

It is important to allow the adolescent maximum self-control and independence during hospitalization. Answer the adolescent's questions honestly and respect the need for privacy and solitude.

STAGES OF GRIEVING

The stages of grieving identified by Elisabeth Kubler-Ross (1969) can be applied to older school-aged children and adolescents with a life-threatening illness, as well as their parents and siblings. These stages represent behaviors that surface as the individual attempts to cope with the anticipated loss.

- *Denial* and *isolation* are the initial reactions, during which the individual reacts with shock and disbelief. Denial serves as a protective buffer against overwhelming anxiety.
- *Anger* usually follows denial and is a reaction that occurs with the recognition of the reality of the diagnosis. Anger may be expressed as envy and resentment of the living. It may also be displaced onto others: "The doctor is no good"; "The nurse's didn't care." This stage may occur and recur anytime during the course of an illness.
- *Bargaining* occurs when the individual tries to postpone the inevitable. The individual usually bargains for an extension of life, preferably without pain.
- *Depression* may center on past losses, such as loss of hair from chemotherapy, or on anticipated losses, such as impending death.
- *Acceptance*, the final phase, is a time of inner peace and resolution in which the individual is no longer angry or depressed, recognizing that death is a certainty. This stage occurs only if the individual works through the earlier stages of grieving.

PARENTS' RESPONSES

Death of a loved one is always painful. The death of a child, however, is especially difficult to accept. In our culture, we expect to live to old age and associate dying with having lived a full life. Thus, children's deaths are viewed as unnatural and even unfair.

When a child dies unexpectedly, the parents are at first overwhelmed, experiencing shock and disbelief. The grieving process may last for weeks, months, or even years. Parents need reassurance that their feelings are normal and expected. If the death was preventable, parents will need to deal with feelings of guilt before they can begin to resolve and accept the loss.

When a child is diagnosed with a terminal illness, most parents react with shock at the time the diagnosis is given. This reaction is commonly followed by denial, and then guilt.

"If only we'd come to the doctor sooner" is a common reaction. Anger is typical. Parents may displace anger onto others, particularly health care professionals. Nurses who care for the child may be seen as competitors for the child's attention. It is important that nurses respect the parents' feelings and allow for these expressions of anger.

Anticipatory grieving occurs as parents begin to accept the loss of their child and increases in intensity until the child's death. Typically, the mother is most intensely involved with the ill or dying child. The father may feel left out or escape by concentrating on work. During the anticipatory grieving phase, it is important for the nurse to help parents maintain a bond with and provide comfort for their child.

SIBLINGS' RESPONSES

Siblings of terminally ill children experience changes in family routines as parents spend time with the ill child, often away from the home and possibly in another community. Even very young children who do not fully understand the implications of death are aware that something serious is going on. They experience not only separation from their brother or sister, but also separation from their parents.

The healthy siblings may feel unloved and respond by increasing their demands on parents. They may express feelings of resentment, anger, anxiety, depression, fear of the ill child's death, fear of their own death, jealousy, guilt, psychological and physical isolation from their parents, and a wide variety of behaviors aimed at obtaining attention from the parents (Walker 1990). These behaviors occur at a time when the parents are already under stress from the emotions and responsibilities of caring for the dying child. It is important to reassure siblings that they will continue to be loved and cared for.

Young children are unable to understand cause-and-effect relationships. They may think that they caused the death, viewing death as a punishment or the result of their angry thoughts. Siblings may express angry feelings toward the child who has died. Anger also may be turned inward, resulting in depression. It is important that parents recognize that anger is a normal part of the grief process and anticipate and accept these feelings.

As appropriate, siblings should be encouraged to visit the ill child. If they wish to participate, they should also be included in care of the dying child.

COMMON STRESSORS OF TERMINAL ILLNESS

Children who experience a life-threatening illness usually have some awareness that they are seriously ill, whether or not their parents or health care providers have actually discussed their condition with them. Potential stressors for terminally ill children include inadequate information about their disease and its treatment, not understanding what they hear, and not being informed as the disease progresses (Hymovich and Hagopian 1992). Dying children need to be able to share in honest communication. It is inadvisable to lie to children in an effort to "protect" them from the knowledge that they are dying. How, when, and what children are told are extremely important (Walker 1993).

RESOURCES FOR CARE OF THE ILL OR DYING CHILD

SUPPORT GROUPS

Support groups can provide emotional support to the parents and siblings of ill or dying children. These groups, composed of families who are coping with or have experienced a similar illness or loss, provide a forum for expressing and understanding feelings of grief and loss (Wheeler and Limbo 1990). Family support systems and friends are also very important during the crisis of the illness and after the death of a child.

SPIRITUAL SUPPORT

Spiritual beliefs about life and death become more important as the child and family begin to face the reality of the child's death. These beliefs can provide great comfort and support (Mott et al. 1990). Parents and other family members may request the presence of clergy or hold prayer sessions for the dying child. Nurses must take care to support the beliefs of the family and not impose their own personal beliefs on others.

HOSPICE AND HOME CARE

Hospice care provides holistic care and support for the patient with a terminal illness. This care may take place in the family's home, in a hospice center, or in a facility that applies the hospice concept. The goal of hospice care is to enable the individual to live life as fully as possible; free of pain; with respect, choices, and dignity; supported and cared for by his or her family. In this caring atmosphere, the patient and family can be assisted in the grieving process and in the preparation for death.

Hospice care of children is provided by an interdisciplinary team that provides a continuum of care and facilitates the role of the parents as the primary caregivers. Whether the care takes place in the home or in a hospice center, the hospice team is available to the family around the clock. Hospice care includes pain control measures and emotional support for the child and family members.

NURSING CONSIDERATIONS

EMOTIONAL NEEDS OF THE DYING CHILD

The dying child has the same emotional and developmental needs as other children of the same age and requires an environment that meets those needs. A key component of nursing care is promoting the child's and family's feelings of trust and security in the hospital staff. This component of nursing care is especially important when caring for the dying child. Perhaps the most important nursing intervention is that of explaining what death is, if the child asks. Nurses should answer only those questions asked by the child and should ensure that their answers are appropriate to the child's developmental stage (Petix 1987). Figure 32–2 is a nursing care plan for the child who is terminally ill or dying.

AWARENESS OF PERSONAL FEELINGS

The nurse develops a close relationship with the child and family who are facing death. The death of a child can be especially difficult for nurses who, like others in our society, do not expect children to die. There is a sense of helplessness and failure when a child dies. It is important that the nurse understand his or her perceptions of death and dying and realize that these perceptions have been defined by circumstances and specific situations in his or her life.

Nurses often react in much the same way as the family when a child is diagnosed with a fatal illness. Denial serves to protect the nurse from being overwhelmed by the reality of impending death. Anger may be expressed when the nurse finds that he or she has been assigned to care for the terminally ill child. Nurses may also feel anger toward family members who are demanding and seemingly unappreciative of their care. Recognition of these feelings may lead to a sense of guilt.

NURSING CARE PLAN: Terminally Ill or Dying Child

PATIENT PROBLEM	GOAL(S)	NURSING INTERVENTION	RATIONALE
Anticipatory grieving (family)	The family will receive comfort and supportive care from the nursing staff.	Identify the family's stage of grieving. Convey an attitude of caring to the family.	The stage of grieving affects how the nurse relates to the family's actions and concerns.
		Give parents and siblings an opportunity to express and clarify feelings.	Provides the family with a safe outlet for feelings and clarifies concerns that may be unnecessary.
		Provide information about the child's status.	Being informed about the child's status increases the family's sense of security and control.
		Help the family deal with their feelings.	Providing an opportunity to express and clarify feelings may help to minimize stress.
		Involve family members in planning the child's care and in decision making when possible.	Participation enables family members to come to terms with the reality of the child's illness.
		Provide privacy for the family and provide for the physical comfort of the child and family.	Communicates genuine concern for the child and family.

Figure 32–2 *Nursing care plan for the child who is terminally ill or dying*

PATIENT PROBLEM	GOAL(S)	NURSING INTERVENTION	RATIONALE
		Encourage family members to talk to the child.	Having parents explain and talk with the child about the illness and hospitalization experience opens family communication.
Fear and anxiety	The child will experience a reduction in fear and anxiety through the empathetic care of the nursing staff.	Be open and honest in communication with the child: • Answer only the questions asked. • Explain death to the child, if asked. • Tell the truth in simple terms. • Use the language of the child.	The child who is informed about the illness and treatment feels less isolated and is better able to cope.
		Be a good listener and observer.	Provides a safe, acceptable outlet for feelings.
		Give the child the opportunity to discuss fears and prognosis. Reassure the child that he or she will not be left alone to die.	Acknowledgment of the child's fears and concerns decreases fear and anxiety and prevents the child from experiencing feelings of isolation and alienation.

Figure 32–2 *continued*

PATIENT PROBLEM	GOAL(S)	NURSING INTERVENTION	RATIONALE
Ineffective family coping	The family will identify stressors of the child's illness and possible coping strategies.	Encourage the family's involvement in the child's care, as desired, and assist them to care for their child.	Involvement gives family members a sense of control and comfort in knowing they did something to help the child.
		Provide opportunities for expression and clarification of feelings.	Allowing the family to communicate feelings helps them to accept and deal with their emotions.
		Include siblings in discussions of the child's prognosis and course of the disease. Include what is known about the disease; emphasize that none of the siblings' thoughts or actions could have caused it and that other family members won't "catch" the disease.	Siblings have increased feelings of self-worth when they assume responsibilities for the ill child. Including siblings makes them feel less isolated and reassures them that someone cares about them and about what is happening to them.
		Explore with the family the stressors they have experienced and discuss how they have coped.	Helps the family to identify coping skills that have worked for them and gives them courage to face what is ahead.

Figure 32–2 *continued*

Nurses may experience alternating feelings of hope and despair. Another common reaction is ambivalence. Nurses need to accept that they cannot be all things to all people and they need support too. The nurse's role is unique, and the privilege of providing care, comfort, and compassionate support to a child and family can be very fulfilling.

REVIEW QUESTIONS

A. Multiple choice. Select the best answer.

1. Samantha, 11 years of age, is terminally ill with leukemia. One quiet night Samantha asks the nurse, "What will it be like when I die?" The best response by the nurse would be,
   a. You need to have your parents explain that to you.
   b. Samantha, everything is going to be okay. You don't need to worry.
   c. I'm too busy to talk about such hard times right now. I'll be back later.
   d. Samantha, tell me what you think it will be like.

2. A preschool child who becomes very ill is likely to perceive this illness as
   a. punishment for bad thoughts or deeds
   b. a bogeyman who has come to get him
   c. insignificant
   d. frightening because it may lead to body mutilation

3. Nine-year-old Mario is dying of osteosarcoma. He tells the nurse that he doesn't want his friends to think he looks "different" from anyone else. The nurse working with Mario realizes that his fear associated with dying is fear of
   a. being separated from his parents
   b. rejection
   c. mutilation
   d. losing his hair

4. Krista's grandmother has died. When her parents go to check on Krista at bedtime, her door is locked. She tells her parents that she is afraid of the "ghost that took Grandma away." In what age group is this concept of death common?
   a. toddlerhood
   b. preschool age
   c. early school age
   d. adolescence

5. Jamie is crying and states that it is her fault that her baby brother died. During what developmental period are children likely to feel guilt that their bad thoughts or deeds are sufficient to have caused an illness or death?
   a. toddlerhood
   b. preschool years
   c. early school age
   d. adolescence

B. True or false. Write *T* for a true statement and *F* for a false statement.

1. ____ Of all age groups, the school-age child by far has the most difficult time dealing with death, including his or her own death.

2. ____ The adolescent is less concerned with present physical changes than with the prognosis for future recovery.

3. ____ Siblings may respond with a wide range of emotions during the dying child's illness.

4. ____ Young children are unable to understand cause-and-effect relationships.

5. ____ Young children know they are seriously ill even if no one has discussed this fact with them.

SUGGESTED ACTIVITIES

- Schedule clinical hours with a nurse who specializes in pediatric oncology. Observe strategies that he or she uses with children of different developmental stages.
- Review case situations of nurses working with dying children and discuss what the nurse may be feeling, as well as appropriate interventions in these situations.
- Interview a nurse or social worker who works with children who have life-threatening illnesses about the emotional aspects of working with these children and their families.
- Speak with a grief counselor about family responses to the death of a child.

BIBLIOGRAPHY

Armstrong-Dailey, A. Children's hospice care. *Pediatric Nursing* 16, no. 4 (1990): 337–339, 409.

Bowden, V. Children's literature: The death experience. *Pediatric Nursing* 19, no. 1 (1993): 17–21.

Bowlby, J. *Attachment and Loss*, vol. 1. New York: Basic Books, 1969.

Bowlby, J. *Attachment and Loss*, vol. 2. New York: Basic Books, 1973.

Castiglia, P. Death of a sibling. *Journal of Pediatric Health Care* 2, no. 4 (1988): 211–213.

Foster, R. L., M. M. Hunsberger, and J. J. Tackett Anderson. *Family-Centered Nursing Care of Children*. Philadelphia: W. B. Saunders, 1989.

Gibbons, M. B. A child dies, a child survives: The impact of sibling loss. *Journal of Pediatric Care* 6, no. 2 (1992): 65–72.

Hymovich, D., and G. Hagopian. *Chronic Illness in Children and Adults: A Psychosocial Approach.* Philadelphia: W. B. Saunders, 1992.

Kubler-Ross, E. *On Death and Dying*. New York: Macmillan, 1969.

Lawson, L. V. Culturally sensitive support for grieving parents. *Maternal Child Nursing* 15 (March/April, 1990): 76–79.

McCown, D. When children face death in a family. *Journal of Pediatric Health Care* 2, no. 1 (1988): 14–19.

Mott, S., S. James, and A. Sperhac. *Nursing Care of Children and Families*. Redwood City, CA: Addison-Wesley, 1990.

National Institute of Mental Health. *Caring about Kids: Talking to Children about Death*. Publication no. (ADM) 79-838. Washington, D.C.: U.S. Department of Health, Education and Welfare, 1979.

Petix, M. Explaining death to school-age children. *Pediatric Nursing* 13, no. 6 (1987): 394–396.

Phillips, M. Support groups for parents of chronically ill children. *Pediatric Nursing* 16, no. 4 (1990): 404–406.

Walker, C. Siblings of children with cancer. *Oncology Nursing Forum* 17, no. 3 (1990): 355–360.

Walker, C. L. The child who is dying. In D. Broadwell Jackson and R. B. Saunders, eds. *Child Health Nursing*. Philadelphia: J. B. Lippincott, 1993.

Whaley, L., and D. Wong. *Nursing Care of Infants and Children*, 4th ed. St. Louis, MO: Mosby-Year Book, 1991.

Wheeler, S. R., and R. Limbo. Blueprint for a perinatal bereavement support group. *Pediatric Nursing* 16, no. 4 (1990): 341–347.

Wong, D. L. *Whaley & Wong's Essentials of Pediatric Nursing*, 4th ed. St. Louis, MO: Mosby-Year Book, 1993.

CHAPTER

33

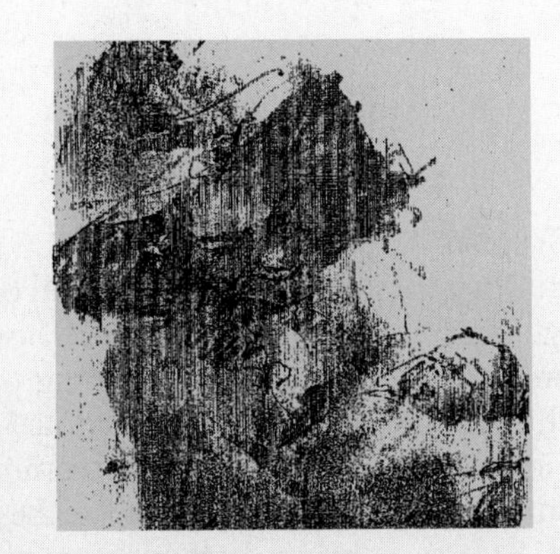

Sudden Infant Death Syndrome

Objectives

AFTER STUDYING THIS CHAPTER, THE STUDENT SHOULD BE ABLE TO:

- STATE THE INCIDENCE OF SIDS IN THE UNITED STATES.
- IDENTIFY MATERNAL AND INFANT FACTORS THAT APPEAR TO PLACE INFANTS AT RISK FOR SIDS.
- DESCRIBE COMMON RESPONSES OF FAMILIES OF INFANTS WHO DIE FROM SIDS.
- IDENTIFY SPECIFIC INTERVENTIONS FOR THESE FAMILIES.
- IDENTIFY SUPPORT GROUPS AVAILABLE FOR FAMILIES OF AN INFANT WHO DIES OF SIDS.
- IDENTIFY NURSING CARE RELATED TO THE FAMILY OF AN INFANT WITH SIDS.

Key Terms

SUDDEN INFANT DEATH SYNDROME

CRIB DEATH

COT DEATH

SLEEP APNEA

Sudden infant death syndrome (SIDS), also called **crib death** or **cot death**, is the sudden death of an infant under 1 year of age that remains unexplained following a complete autopsy investigation and review of the history. SIDS is the leading cause of death in children between the ages of 1 and 12 months in the United States. Between 7,000 and 8,000 infants die of SIDS each year.

CAUSE

The cause of SIDS is unknown, although the following pattern of risk factors appears to predispose an infant to SIDS: low socioeconomic status, mother younger than 20 years, multiple pregnancies with short intervals between births, twin or triplet birth, male infant, and low birth weight. Other factors that have been linked with SIDS are:

- *Season and time of day*: SIDS occurs most often in winter and between midnight and 9 A.M.
- *Sleep*: Most deaths are unobserved and are thought to occur during sleep.
- *Illness*: SIDS is often preceded by a mild upper respiratory illness.
- *Race*: It is most common among Native American infants, followed by black, hispanic, and white infants; the lowest incidence is among Asian infants.
- *Family recurrence*: It is four to five times more common among siblings of an infant who died of SIDS, although no genetic link has been found (Rudolph 1991).

Research has focused on the possibility that SIDS infants have as-yet-unidentified neurological or respiratory alterations that result in abnormal breathing. For the past 20 years, researchers have also investigated whether there is a connection between SIDS and **sleep apnea**. Sleep apnea is the cessation of breathing for brief periods during sleep. The link between the prone (abdominal) sleeping position and an increased risk of SIDS prompted the American Academy of Pediatrics to recommend that healthy infants sleep supine or on the side. The exceptions are infants with respiratory problems or infants with gastric reflux who require special positioning. Infants with a history of sleep apnea who have required resuscitation, and siblings of SIDS victims often are monitored at home in an effort to prevent SIDS. The majority of SIDS victims, however, have no symptoms before death.

FAMILY RESPONSES

Typically the infant is found in the morning, dead in the crib. Parents may find the infant huddled in a corner, underneath the sheet or blanket, with blood-tinged, frothy fluid coming from the nose and mouth. The infant's position and wet, stool-filled diaper indicate a sudden, convulsive death. Parents commonly report having heard no cries or other sounds of distress during the night.

The first response of parents is to call for help. Efforts may be made to resuscitate the infant. When these fail, the focus of emergency personnel is shifted to the family. Parents commonly feel guilt, confusion, grief, and anger, and question whether they could have done something to prevent the infant's death. For this reason, police and emergency personnel should be able to provide appropriate information about SIDS; in particular, that the cause of SIDS is unknown, it occurs unexpectedly, and it cannot be predicted or prevented.

Figure 33–1 provides a summary of nursing interventions that can be used in assisting the family of an infant who has died of SIDS.

PROVIDING SUPPORT FOR THE FAMILY OF A SIDS INFANT

- Provide private area for parents and support persons to say "goodbye." Obtain a rocking chair and enough chairs for family and friends present. Place a "Do Not Disturb" sign on the door.
- Wrap the infant in a clean blanket, comb the hair, wash the face, swab the mouth, and apply petroleum jelly to the lips before bringing the infant to parents.
- Make sure parents are seated and an ammonia ampule is available (in case they faint) before placing infant on the lap. Gently remind them that the infant's skin will feel cool and bluish "blood" bruises may be visible.
- Provide a lock of hair, handprints, and footprints of the infant to the parents for a memory book. Obtain these while preparing the infant for viewing; offer them before the family leaves the hospital.
- Collect all personal items belonging to the infant and any written information (names of resource persons, SIDS support groups) for the parents to take with them before they leave the hospital.

Figure 33–1

SUPPORT GROUPS

SIDS affects all family members, including the siblings and grandparents of the infant. Many hospitals have follow-up programs in which nurses call or visit the family to provide support and answer questions about the infant's death. Other individuals who were close to the infant, such as babysitters, may also benefit from psychological support and counseling.

Group therapy is recommended for all families of SIDS victims. Most communities have a local support group that includes other parents of SIDS victims. Nurses can also refer parents to the National Foundation for Sudden Infant Death Syndrome, 8240 Professional Place, Landover, MD 20785; telephone (301) 459-3388, 24-hour hotline (800) 221-7437.

Nurses are often deeply affected by the death of a seemingly healthy infant and should be encouraged to express their feelings about the infant's death and the resuscitation effort.

NURSING CARE RELATED TO FAMILY OF INFANT WITH SIDS

- Remember that an autopsy is required by law in most states when a child's death is unexplained.
- Reassure parents of a confirmed SIDS infant that they are not responsible for the infant's death and would not have been able to prevent it.
- Help the family begin the grief process.
- Provide emotional support for parents, siblings, and other family members.
- Refer parents to appropriate local support groups.
- Recommend resources for obtaining information about SIDS.
- Consider child abuse as a cause of death when an infant dies unexpectedly (even if the thought makes you uncomfortable).

REVIEW QUESTIONS

A. Multiple choice. Select the best answer.

1. Sudden infant death syndrome is characterized by which of the following?
   a. involves the death of an infant under 1 year
   b. occurs most often between 9 P.M. and midnight
   c. is explained only after a complete autopsy
   d. is preceded by high-pitched cry of infant

2. Which of the following is a risk factor that appears to predispose an infant to sudden infant death syndrome?
   a. low socioeconomic status of parent(s)
   b. high birth weight
   c. older mother
   d. female infant

3. Which of the following does not refer to sudden infant death syndrome?
   a. SIDS
   b. sleep apnea
   c. cot death
   d. crib death

4. In the United States, sudden infant death syndrome is the leading cause of death in children between 1 and 12 months of age. How many deaths does it cause each year?
   a. 7,000–8,000
   b. 3,000–6,000
   c. 70,000–80,000
   d. 30,000–60,000

5. Research on sudden infant death syndrome finds which of the following factors to be linked to its occurrence?
   a. It occurs most often in summer.
   b. It is most common among Asian infants.
   c. It is often preceded by diarrhea and vomiting.
   d. It is more common among siblings of an infant who died of SIDS.

6. Which of the following is typical of sudden infant death syndrome?
   a. Infant appears to have been neglected by parents.
   b. Blood-tinged, frothy fluid is found coming from nose and mouth.
   c. Infant's death is preceded by a severe viral illness.
   d. Infant is found stretched out, face up, with back arched upward.

7. What information should a nurse tell parents concerned about sudden infant death syndrome?
   a. Continuous monitoring can prevent these deaths.
   b. Research will soon identify the cause.
   c. It cannot be predicted.
   d. It can be prevented through altered nutritional and lifestyle practices.

8. The nurse can play a key role in helping the grief-stricken parents by doing which of the following?
   a. counseling the family to avoid viewing the infant
   b. avoiding mention of the need for an autopsy
   c. allowing the family to hold or touch the infant, if desired
   d. suggesting that family members put the death behind them and move on with their lives

9. The nurse might recommend any of the following support resources for parents and others close to the deceased infant except
   a. National Foundation for Sudden Infant Death Syndrome
   b. group therapy
   c. hospital follow-up programs
   d. Alcoholics Anonymous

10. Research into the cause of sudden infant death syndrome has centered on the following
    a. a connection with sleep apnea
    b. gastrointestinal alterations
    c. infant alcoholism
    d. congenital anomalies

SUGGESTED ACTIVITIES

- Discuss your feelings about death with your classmates. Identify ways in which those feelings will help or hinder you in dealing with people who have different beliefs. List methods you can use to help make your reactions more effective and supportive.
- Discuss with your classmates your feelings about the sudden and unexplained death of an infant. Identify ways in which this type of death differs from others. List ways in which you can demonstrate your sensitivity.
- Interview someone who has been involved in a professional capacity with the death of an infant from SIDS. Find out what problems health care workers have in dealing with the sudden, unexplained death of an infant. Discuss ways in which you can prepare yourself or support other health care workers for this situation.
- The nurse must consider child abuse as a possible cause of death when an infant dies unexpectedly. Discuss how you would handle this possibility in an actual situation with the family of a child who had just died.

BIBLIOGRAPHY

Broadwell Jackson, D., and R. B. Saunders, eds. *Child Health Nursing*. Philadelphia: J. B. Lippincott, 1993.

Rudolph, A. M. *Rudolph's Pediatrics*, 19th ed. Norwalk, CT: Appleton & Lange, 1991.

Wong, D. L. *Whaley & Wong's Essentials of Pediatric Nursing*, 4th ed. St. Louis, MO: Mosby-Year Book, 1993.

Zylke, J. W. Sudden infant death syndrome: Resurgent research offers hope. *Journal of the American Medical Association* 262 (1989): 1565.

UNIT

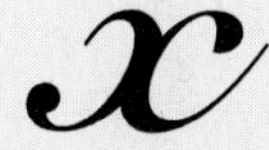

Common Pediatric Conditions

CHAPTER

34

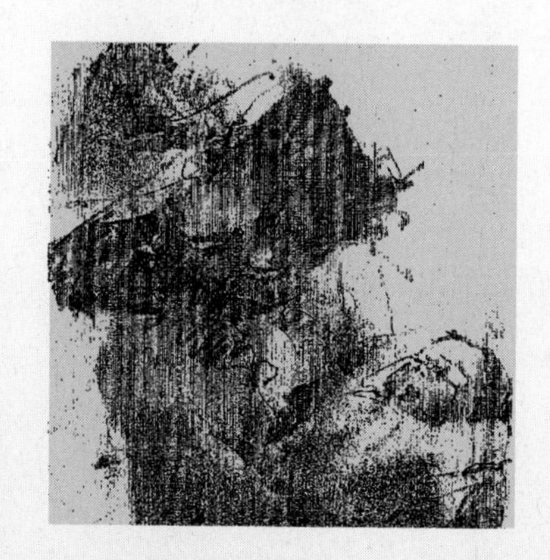

Communicable and Infectious Diseases

OBJECTIVES

AFTER STUDYING THIS CHAPTER, THE STUDENT SHOULD BE ABLE TO:

- DIFFERENTIATE BETWEEN COMMUNICABLE AND INFECTIOUS DISEASES.
- DESCRIBE THE LINKS IN THE CHAIN OF INFECTION.
- LIST THE FOUR STAGES OF INFECTION.
- IDENTIFY MEASURES THAT HEALTH CARE PROVIDERS CAN TAKE TO PREVENT THE SPREAD OF INFECTION.
- DESCRIBE SEVERAL TYPES OF ISOLATION AND EXPLAIN THEIR USE.
- IDENTIFY SEVERAL COMMUNICABLE AND INFECTIOUS DISEASES OF CHILDHOOD, INCLUDING THEIR CAUSATIVE AGENTS, TRANSMISSION, INCUBATION PERIOD, CONTAGIOUS PERIOD, PREVENTION, SIGNS AND SYMPTOMS, TREATMENT, AND NURSING CARE.
- DISCUSS THE CAUSE, INCIDENCE, AND SYMPTOMS OF ACQUIRED IMMUNODEFICIENCY SYNDROME, AND DESCRIBE THE TREATMENT AND NURSING CARE OF CHILDREN WITH THIS DISORDER.

KEY TERMS

COMMUNICABLE DISEASES
INFECTIOUS DISEASES
HOST
CHAIN OF INFECTION
CAUSATIVE AGENT
PATHOGEN
RESERVOIR
PORTAL OF EXIT
TRANSMISSION
DIRECT CONTACT
INDIRECT CONTACT
PORTAL OF ENTRY
SUSCEPTIBLE HOST
PRODROMAL PHASE
BARRIER
ISOLATION

Communicable diseases are diseases that are spread from one person to another either directly or indirectly. **Infectious diseases** are diseases that are caused by microorganisms that invade the body and then reproduce and multiply. Disease is caused by damage to the cells, secretion of a toxin, or an antigen-antibody reaction in the **host** (a person who harbors the infectious organism). Infectious diseases are the fifth most common cause of death in the United States and account for half of all health care visits (Foster et al. 1989, Grimes 1991). By law, many communicable diseases must be reported to the local health department.

THE INFECTIOUS PROCESS

THE CHAIN OF INFECTION

The process of the development of infectious disease in humans is called the **chain of infection**. This chain must be intact for an organism to produce an infectious disease. Conversely, to prevent infection, one of the links of the chain must be broken. The links in the chain of infection are the causative agent, reservoir, portal of exit, transmission, portal of entry, and susceptible host, Figure 34–1.

The **causative agent** (also called a **pathogen**) is the organism that causes the disease. The most common causes of disease in children are viruses, bacteria, parasites, and fungi. The **reservoir** is where the organism grows and reproduces. The reservoir can be someone with the disease, someone carrying the disease, an animal, or the environment.

The **portal of exit** refers to the method by which the infectious organism leaves the reservoir. It can leave through bodily secretions from the respiratory, genitourinary, or intestinal tract; feces; blood; saliva; tears; draining wounds; and vaginal secretions.

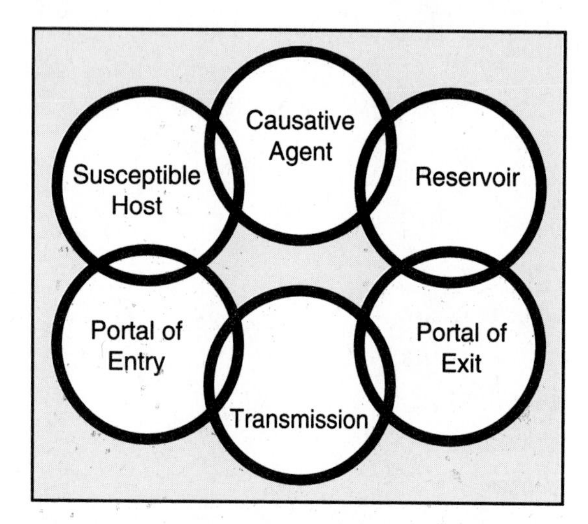

Figure 34–1 The chain of infection (Adapted from Hegner and Caldwell, Nursing Assistant: A Nursing Process Approach, *6th ed. Delmar Publishers Inc., 1992)*

Transmission refers to the spread of pathogens, by either direct contact or indirect contact, by airborne spread, by inanimate objects (such as soil, food, bedding, towels, and combs), or by vectors (such as insects). **Direct contact** refers to actual physical contact (person-to-person, body-to-body), as in the spread of sexually transmitted diseases. **Indirect contact** occurs as a result of organisms that live on animate or inanimate objects. The object becomes a common vehicle and has the potential to infect many people.

The **portal of entry** is the means by which the organism enters the host. It may enter through breaks in the skin or mucous membranes, ingestion, inhalation, or across the placenta in utero. A **susceptible host** is a person at risk for contracting an infectious disease. Several risk factors contribute to the individual's susceptibility to infection and to the severity of the resulting disease. These include:

- age
- sex
- underlying diseases
- immunizations and vaccinations
- heredity
- nutritional status
- living conditions

STAGES OF INFECTION

Infection occurs in four identifiable stages: the latent period, incubation period, communicability period, and disease period. The length of each stage varies, depending on the pathogen and the susceptibility of the host. The latent period begins when the body is invaded by the pathogen and ends when the person begins to shed the pathogen (communicability period). The incubation period begins when the pathogen invades the body and ends when the disease process starts. During this period, the pathogen multiplies within the individual. The communicability period begins when the latent period ends and continues for as long as the pathogen is present. The disease period follows the incubation period. During this stage, the individual may or may not have symptoms (Grimes 1991). The earliest phase of the developing disease or condition is referred to as the **prodromal phase**.

INFECTION CONTROL AND PRECAUTIONS

UNIVERSAL PRECAUTIONS

An essential component of disease prevention is infection control. The Centers for Disease Control and Prevention (CDC) recommends that blood and body fluid precautions be used for all patients. Nurses need to protect themselves from exposure to infectious agents in the blood or other body fluids of patients. This protection involves the use of a **barrier**, such as gloves, gown, mask, and protective eyewear. The goal of universal precautions is to minimize the risk of exposure to the blood and body fluids of all patients regardless of their isolation precaution status or diagnosis. Universal precautions to take in all clinical settings are presented in Figure 34–2.

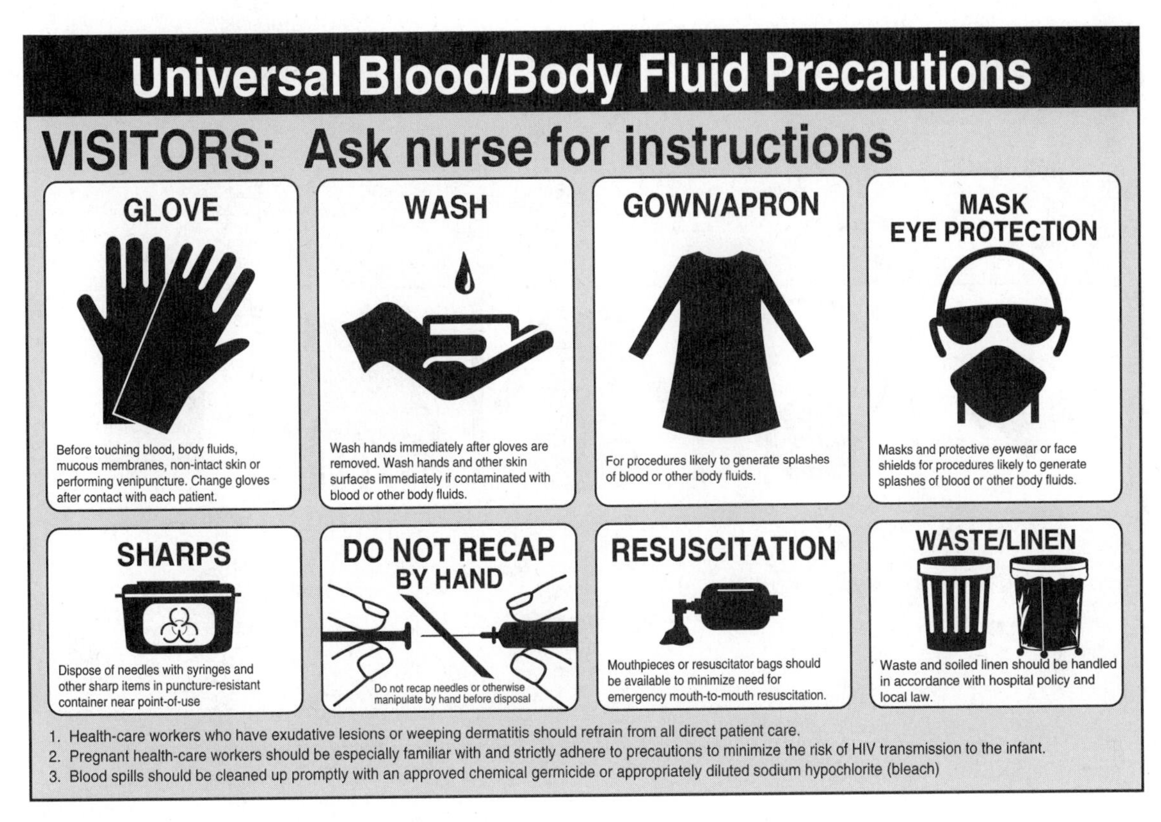

Universal Blood/Body Fluid Precautions
VISITORS: Ask nurse for instructions
GLOVE
Before touching blood, body fluids, mucous membranes, non-intact skin or performing venipuncture. Change gloves after contact with each patient.
WASH
Wash hands immediately after gloves are removed. Wash hands and other skin surfaces immediately if contaminated with blood or other body fluids.
GOWN/APRON
For procedures likely to generate splashes of blood or other body fluids.
MASK
EYE PROTECTION
Masks and protective eyewear or face shields for procedures likely to generate splashes of blood or other body fluids.
SHARPS
Dispose of needles with syringes and other sharp items in puncture-resistant container near point-of-use
DO NOT RECAP BY HAND
Do not recap needles or otherwise manipulate by hand before disposal
RESUSCITATION
Mouthpieces or resuscitator bags should be available to minimize need for emergency mouth-to-mouth resuscitation.
WASTE/LINEN
Waste and soiled linen should be handled in accordance with hospital policy and local law.
1. Health-care workers who have exudative lesions or weeping dermatitis should refrain from all direct patient care.
2. Pregnant health-care workers should be especially familiar with and strictly adhere to precautions to minimize the risk of HIV transmission to the infant.
3. Blood spills should be cleaned up promptly with an approved chemical germicide or appropriately diluted sodium hypochlorite (bleach)

Figure 34–2 *(Courtesy of BREVIS Corporation)*

ISOLATION

Children are placed in short-term **isolation** for infectious diseases, for chemotherapy, and because of immunodeficiency diseases. The CDC has established isolation guidelines designed to protect patients and staff from acquiring communicable diseases. The purpose of placing a child in isolation is to interrupt the chain of infection by preventing the transmission of microbes. The type of isolation or precaution used depends on the disease and its mode of transmission. The following categories are used for diseases that require isolation precautions:

respiratory isolation
strict isolation, Figure 34–3
contact isolation
enteric precautions
drainage/secretion precautions
acid-fast bacillus (AFB) isolation (tuberculosis)
blood and body fluid precautions

The nurse must follow hospital policy where he or she works for isolation guidelines, procedures, and precautions. All hospital health care providers and personnel need to be responsible for and practice proper isolation techniques to protect patients, the environment, and themselves. The most important of these techniques are:

- *Handwashing*: the most important means of preventing the spread of infection for all isolation precautions

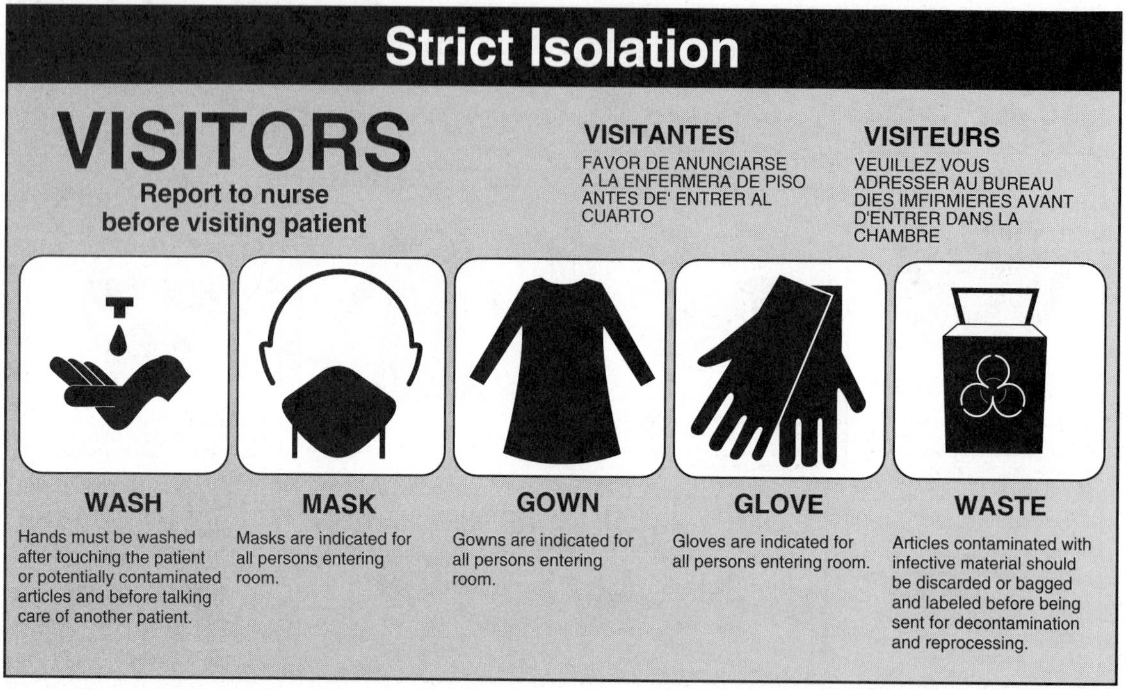

Strict Isolation

VISITORS
Report to nurse
before visiting patient

VISITANTES
FAVOR DE ANUNCIARSE
A LA ENFERMERA DE PISO
ANTES DE' ENTRER AL
CUARTO

VISITEURS
VEUILLEZ VOUS
ADRESSER AU BUREAU
DIES IMFIRMIERES AVANT
D'ENTRER DANS LA
CHAMBRE

WASH
Hands must be washed after touching the patient or potentially contaminated articles and before talking care of another patient.

MASK
Masks are indicated for all persons entering room.

GOWN
Gowns are indicated for all persons entering room.

GLOVE
Gloves are indicated for all persons entering room.

WASTE
Articles contaminated with infective material should be discarded or bagged and labeled before being sent for decontamination and reprocessing.

Figure 34–3 *Strict isolation is used for children with diseases such as smallpox, diphtheria, and chickenpox. (Courtesy of BREVIS Corporation)*

- *Gowns*: worn to prevent self-contamination
- *Gloves*: worn whenever there is exposure to body fluids
- *Face mask*: worn whenever there is exposure to droplet secretions
- *Equipment*: disposable equipment should be used whenever possible
- *Needle safety*: needles should be placed in an appropriate rigid, puncture-resistant container or receptacle
- *Containment of articles:* contaminated articles (linens, equipment, trash) should be bagged, labeled, and disposed of according to hospital guidelines for specific isolation precautions

Children in isolation are at risk for loneliness and depression resulting from lack of social interaction. The following nursing interventions can help to prevent or reduce this social isolation.

- Encourage parents and siblings to visit and to bring in the child's favorite toys from home.
- Encourage patients, especially teenagers, to call friends.
- Reassure small children that they can talk to the nurse using the intercom in their room.
- Spend extra time with the child, reading a story or playing a game.

Be sure the child and parents understand that they must abide by the isolation precautions for the safety of the patient and others.

COMMUNICABLE AND INFECTIOUS DISEASES OF CHILDHOOD

Figure 34–4 describes communicable and infectious diseases of childhood, along with their treatment and nursing care. The incidence of some of these diseases has been reduced because of the development of vaccines that are routinely administered to infants and children (see Chapter 25). Improved preventive measures have reduced the incidence of other diseases. Nurses who work in pediatrics should become familiar with the signs and symptoms of these diseases.

ACQUIRED IMMUNODEFICIENCY SYNDROME

Description. Acquired immunodeficiency syndrome (AIDS) is a multisystem disorder that occurs in adults and children infected with human immunodeficiency virus (HIV-1), one of a family of viruses called retroviruses. The virus causes gradual destruction of the body's immune system. As a result, the patient becomes immunocompromised and is at risk for serious infection and invasion by any pathogen.

HIV is transmitted through sexual contact, sharing contaminated needles, and through injection or transfusion. HIV has been found in blood, semen, vaginal secretions, and in breast milk (in low concentrations). Approximately 80% of HIV-infected children are under the age of 13 years (Rudolph 1991).

In the pediatric age group, infection with HIV occurs:

- in infants of infected mothers (through blood, amniotic fluid, or breast milk)
- in children who received blood and blood products from HIV-infected donors before mandatory screening was instituted in March 1985
- in adolescents who abuse intravenous (IV) drugs and participate in homosexual or heterosexual activities without precautions

Symptoms. The time between infection and illness can be as long as 10 years. Diagnosis is based on the clinical presentation of symptoms and is confirmed by serological tests or viral cultures or both. AIDS in children is primarily a disease of infants and presents with the following symptoms:

- hepatosplenomegaly
- lymphadenopathy
- oral candidiasis
- failure to thrive
- weight loss
- diarrhea
- chronic eczema
- fever of unknown origin

Treatment. Children with AIDS suffer from a chronic disease that affects many body systems, resulting in acute exacerbations. There is no cure. Treatment is supportive and focuses on preventing infection, maintaining good nutrition, and treating specific symptoms. Zidovudine (AZT) syrup has been authorized for use in children from 3 months to 12 years who have either HIV-associated symptoms or a T-lymphocyte cell count of less than 400 (Spratto and Woods 1993).

Nursing Care. Nurses should always follow universal precautions to minimize exposure to HIV (see earlier discussion). Nurses who care for infants, children, and teenagers with AIDS should reassure parents that "extensive follow-up of household contacts of both adults and children with AIDS has failed to demonstrate any evidence of HIV transmission via shared living space, kitchens, or bathrooms or through casual contact" (Last 1992). Nurses play an important role in educating the public to reduce fear, panic, prejudice, and discrimination related to the disease and its causes.

Because of the life-threatening nature of the disorder, psychosocial support to families of children with AIDS is an essential part of care. Depending on their symptoms and the progression of the disease, children may be relatively symptom-free or require supportive home care. Encourage parents to keep infected children in school as long as possible. Nurses can play an important role in providing information to school officials, teachers, schoolmates, and their parents to help them understand that HIV transmission does not occur through normal daily contact.

COMMUNICABLE AND INFECTIOUS DISEASES OF CHILDHOOD

Disease	Signs and Symptoms	Treatment and Nursing Care
Chickenpox *Agent*: Varicella, herpes zoster virus *Transmission*: Airborne; direct contact with an infected person *Incubation period*: 10–21 days (average of 14–15 days) *Communicability period*: From 1 to 2 days before the onset of the rash to 5–6 days after *Prevention*: Isolation of infected patients; a live attenuated varicella vaccine is being tested in the United States	1–2 days before the rash, patient develops a low-grade fever and malaise. Rash starts as macules on an erythematous base, progresses to papules, and then to clear fluid-filled vesicles approximately 2–4 mm in diameter. Unruptured vesicles become purulent and dry and crust over. Crust may remain for 1–3 weeks. Lesions are not confined to the skin and can develop on any mucosal surface. Fever is present during rash peak and disappears by the time vesicles have dried or crusted over.	Maintain strict isolation in hospital. Provide relief of itching (oatmeal baths, Caladryl lotion, Benadryl, cool environment). Fever management. Encourage fluids (fruit-flavored popsicles, soft drinks, ice cubes). Keep children busy so they don't have time to itch (coloring, painting, finger-painting, playing games). Keep patient's fingernails short and clean.
Diphtheria *Agent: Corynebacterium diphtheriae* *Transmission*: Droplet (from active cases or carriers) *Incubation period*: 1–7 days *Communicability period*: Variable (usually 2 weeks), until bacilli are no longer present in discharge and lesions *Prevention*: Active immunization with diphtheria toxoid (see Chapter 25)	Respiratory tract and skin infections. Disease can be either mild or severe. Sore throat, difficulty swallowing, low-grade fever. THROAT: Erythema, localized exudate or a membrane, which may occur as a patch, cover entire tonsil, or spread to cover the soft and hard palates and the posterior portion of the pharynx. Membrane may be whitish and wipe off easily or be thick, blue-white to gray-black, and adhere. Attempts to remove the membrane result in bleeding. Enlarged cervical lymph nodes.	Maintain strict isolation in hospital. Corticosteroids. Antibiotics. Fever management. Airway maintenance. Monitor breathing pattern. Provide oxygen as prescribed.

Figure 34–4

COMMUNICABLE AND INFECTIOUS DISEASES OF CHILDHOOD

Disease	Signs and Symptoms	Treatment and Nursing Care
Erythema infectiosum (fifth disease) *Agent*: Parvovirus B19 *Transmission*: Droplet *Incubation period*: 6–14 days *Communicability period*: Unknown *Prevention*: None	First symptom is a rash, which appears in three stages. FIRST STAGE: Red, maculopapular, coalesces on the cheeks, looking like a "slapped face" with circumoral pallor; disappears in 1–4 days. SECOND STAGE: A day after face rash appears, a red maculopapular rash appears on arms, legs, and trunk; rash proceeds from proximal to distal surface; can last 1 week or more. THIRD STAGE: Rash fades but can reappear if skin is irritated or exposed to heat or cold.	No specific treatment. Provide comfort measures. Temperature control (acetaminophen). Relieve itching with antipruritics. Explain the three phases of the rash to parents.
Hepatitis B (HBV) *Agent*: Hepadnaviridae *Transmission*: Direct or indirect contact with blood, semen, sexual contact; by direct access to the circulation through breaks in the skin or passages through mucous membranes, blood products, infected needles, infected mothers to newborns, person-to-person spread, interpersonal contact over long periods of time, between siblings and adults *Incubation period*: 45–180 days (average of 60–90 days) *Communicability period*: During incubation period and throughout clinical course of disease *Prevention*: Hepatitis B vaccine (see Chapter 25)	Onset is insidious, including malaise, weakness, anorexia. Diagnosis can be made only by serological testing.	Maintain strict isolation in hospital. Maintain bed rest. Maintain fluid balance. Provide high-caloric liquids, encourage small frequent feedings. Watch for bruising and bleeding. Educate parents about the disease and its transmission and make clear that untreated infection can result in chronic active hepatitis and cirrhosis.

Figure 34–4 *continued*

COMMUNICABLE AND INFECTIOUS DISEASES OF CHILDHOOD

Disease	Signs and Symptoms	Treatment and Nursing Care
Lyme disease (tickborne bacterial infection) *Agent: Borrelia burgdorferi* spirochete *Transmission*: Tick bite; ticks live in wooded areas and grasslands; infected ticks are carried by wild animals (birds, mice, raccoons, deer) and by domestic animals (cats, dogs, horses, cows); tick bite is not painful; tick transmits infected spirochetes when it draws blood for nourishment. *Incubation period*: 3–32 days *Communicability period*: Not communicable *Prevention*: Avoid tick-infested areas; wear appropriate dress outdoors (long pants; socks that overlap pant cuffs, closed-toe shoes); use bug repellents; frequently inspect clothing, skin, and hiking equipment after return from tick-infested areas	INITIAL SIGNS: Slowly expanding red rash called erythema migrans. Starts as a flat or raised red area. May progress to partial central clearing, or develop blisters or scabs in the center, or have a bluish discoloration. OTHER EARLY SIGNS WITH OR WITHOUT RASH: Fatigue, headache, stiff neck, jaw discomfort, pain or stiffness in muscles or joints, slight fever, swollen glands or conjunctivitis. If untreated, can result in arthritis, joint pain and swelling, and heart and nervous system complications.	Antibiotics (tetracycline or doxycycline for children over 8; penicillin or erythromycin for younger children). Remove tick carefully: Do not try to pull tick off skin. Place a few drops of alcohol on tick or take a cotton-tipped applicator covered with petroleum jelly and smear the jelly all over the tick. This smothers the tick, which then begins to withdraw from the skin. Once the tick begins to withdraw, it can be removed. Reassure parents that not all ticks carry the spirochete that causes Lyme disease.

Figure 34–4 *continued*

COMMUNICABLE AND INFECTIOUS DISEASES OF CHILDHOOD

Disease	Signs and Symptoms	Treatment and Nursing Care
Measles (rubeola) *Agent*: Paramyxovirus group (a single-stranded RNA virus) *Transmission*: Airborne; large respiratory droplets; close contact between patients and susceptible persons *Incubation period*: Average 10–12 days (range of 8–16 days) *Communicability period*: One of the most contagious diseases; infectious during prodromal phase and for the first few days of the rash (from 4 days before to 4 days after the onset of the rash) *Prevention*: Live attenuated virus vaccine (see Chapter 25)	Fever, malaise, followed by cough, coryza, and conjunctivitis. Maculopapular rash usually appears approximately 14 days after infection and typically 2–4 days after onset of prodromal symptoms. Rash starts on the face and hairline and then spreads to the trunk and extremities. Temperature elevation occurs 1–3 days after rash onset. Rash lasts 5–7 days. BUCCAL MUCOSA: small bluish-white spots on a red background (Koplik's spots) seen on buccal mucosa 2 days before and after the onset of the rash.	Maintain strict isolation in hospital until day 5 of rash. Maintain bed rest. Relieve itching with antipruritics. Fever management. Encourage fluids. Advise parents that child's eyes can be sensitive to light.
Mononucleosis (acute viral infection) *Agent*: Epstein-Barr virus (EBV) of the herpesvirus family *Transmission*: Direct contact with infected oropharyngeal secretions (saliva, kissing) *Incubation period*: 4–6 weeks (30–50 days) *Communicability period*: Saliva remains infective for up to 18 months *Prevention*: None	Febrile illness, sore throat, malaise, fatigue, myalgia, generalized lymphadenopathy, splenomegaly. Symptoms resolve within 2–3 weeks.	Corticosteroids (prednisone). Maintain bed rest. Treat sore throat and fever. Advise parents that it may take up to 3–4 weeks for child to feel normal.

Figure 34–4 *continued*

COMMUNICABLE AND INFECTIOUS DISEASES OF CHILDHOOD

Disease	Signs and Symptoms	Treatment and Nursing Care
Mumps (infectious parotitis) *Agent*: Myxovirus group (RNA virus) *Transmission*: Droplet; direct contact *Incubation period*: 14–21 days (average of 18 days) *Communicability period*: Virus may be excreted 7 days before to 9 days after clinical onset of disease *Prevention*: Live attenuated virus vaccine (see Chapter 25)	PRODROMAL PHASE: Anorexia, headache, vomiting, myalgia lasting 12–48 hours. Mild to moderate fever, painful unilateral or bilateral parotid gland swelling, orchitis. Inflammation of other salivary organs.	Corticosteroids, if indicated. Antipyretics (acetaminophen) for pain and fever. Encourage fluids. Maintain bed rest.
Pertussis (whooping cough) *Agent*: *Bordella pertussis* *Transmission*: Droplet; one of the most contagious diseases *Incubation period*: 7–10 days (range of 4–21 days) *Communicability period*: Begins approximately 1 week after exposure; child is most infectious during the early stages *Prevention*: Active immunization with killed-cell vaccine (see Chapter 25)	Spasmodic, paroxysmal coughing (the sudden onset of repeated violent coughs without intervening respirations). FIRST 1–2 WEEKS: runny nose followed by shallow, irregular nonproductive coughing; changes into deep spasms of paroxysmal coughing; vomiting and inspiratory whooping.	Antibiotics. Corticosteroids. Fever management. Encourage fluids.

Figure 34–4 *continued*

COMMUNICABLE AND INFECTIOUS DISEASES OF CHILDHOOD

Disease	Signs and Symptoms	Treatment and Nursing Care
Poliomyelitis *Agent*: Three serotypes of poliovirus *Transmission*: Pharyngeal secretions and feces, primarily via oral-fecal route (where sanitation and personal hygiene are poor) *Incubation period*: 7–24 days (range of 3–36 days) *Communicability period*: Infectious for up to several weeks before symptoms develop; virus is excreted in pharyngeal secretions for a few days and in the stool for several weeks *Prevention*: Trivalent vaccine (oral polio virus [OPV] or inactivated polio vaccine [IPV]) (see Chapter 25)	Virus is introduced into mouth, where it replicates in the oropharyngeal mucosa and in the Peyer's patches in the ileum. Virus enters bloodstream and central nervous system (CNS), where it attacks the motor neurons of the spinal cord and occasionally the brain stem. Infection of these cells results in death of the lower motor neurons and flaccid paralysis of the muscles they innervate. In cases of limited CNS involvement, symptoms include fever, meningeal irritation (stiff neck and back), or fever, malaise, headache with nausea, vomiting, sore throat.	Maintain strict isolation in hospital. Fever management. Encourage fluids. Physical therapy, positioning, and range-of-motion exercises are important. Maintain bed rest. Sedatives, if indicated. Hot, moist packs to muscles in spasm. Follow-up home care arrangements on discharge.

Figure 34–4 *continued*

COMMUNICABLE AND INFECTIOUS DISEASES OF CHILDHOOD

Disease	Signs and Symptoms	Treatment and Nursing Care
Rabies (acute viral infection of the CNS) *Agent*: Rhabdoviridae; two types (urban, in dogs; wild, in wildlife) *Transmission*: After inoculation, the virus enters the wound and travels along the nerves from the point of entry to the CNS *Incubation period*: Highly variable (average of 6 weeks); determined by the location of the bite and the distance the virus must travel to the brain *Communicability period*: Not communicable *Prevention*: Rabies immune globulin (RIG) of human origin or antirabies serum (ARS) of equine origin should be given to all persons bitten by animals in whom rabies cannot be excluded and for nonbite exposures to animals suspected or proved to be rabid	Runs its course in 1 week. HYDROPHOBIA: Swallowing is difficult, produces painful contracture of the muscles of deglutition, leading to a reflex contraction at the sight of liquids. Periods of excitability (mania) and quiet. Usually results in death.	Follow guidelines for rabies prophylaxis: DOMESTIC DOG AND CAT: (1) If healthy and available for 10 days of observation at time of attack: thoroughly clean bite with soap and water; no further treatment is needed, unless animal develops rabies. (2) Rabid or suspected rabid: administer RIG. WILD ANIMAL: Regard as rabid unless proved negative by laboratory test; administer RIG. LIVESTOCK, RODENTS, RABBITS: Consider individually; consult local and state public health officials. Bites of rodents or rabbits and hares almost never call for rabies prophylaxis.

Figure 34–4 *continued*

COMMUNICABLE AND INFECTIOUS DISEASES OF CHILDHOOD

Disease	Signs and Symptoms	Treatment and Nursing Care
Roseola infantum (exanthem subitum) *Agent*: Herpes virus type 6 *Transmission*: Unknown; disease of infants and toddlers (6 months–3 years) *Incubation period*: Unknown *Communicability period*: Unknown *Prevention*: None	Very high fever for 3–4 days followed by rash. Irritability. Macules and papules appear first on the trunk and spread to face, neck, and extremities. Rash can last from 24 to 48 hours.	Fever management. Reassure parents that rash will disappear in a few days.
Rubella (German or 3-day measles) *Agent*: RNA virus of the togavirus group *Transmission*: Direct contact; droplet *Incubation period*: 14–21 days *Communicability period*: Begins about 7 days before onset of rash and lasts for 4 days after *Prevention*: Primary rubella infection induces lifelong immunity; live attenuated virus vaccine (see Chapter 25)	Nonspecific maculopapular rash lasting 3 days or less. Appears on face; progresses to neck, trunk, and legs. GENERALIZED LYMPHADENOPATHY: Postauricular, suboccipital, and posterior cervical lymph nodes. Itching, occasionally low-grade fever, headache, malaise, coryza, sore throat, anorexia.	Fever management (antipyretics, tepid sponge bath). Pain management (acetaminophen). Isolate child from pregnant women. Encourage fluids (popsicles, soft drinks).

Figure 34–4 *continued*

COMMUNICABLE AND INFECTIOUS DISEASES OF CHILDHOOD

Disease	Signs and Symptoms	Treatment and Nursing Care
Scarlet fever (scarlatina) *Agent*: Group A beta-streptococcal disease resulting from infection with strains of beta-hemolytic streptococci *Transmission*: Respiratory secretions; caused primarily by intimate or direct contact *Incubation period*: 24–48 hours *Communicability period*: Not communicable *Prevention*: None	Occurs primarily in children 2–18 years old, most often in winter and spring. Characterized by erythematous skin rash; blanches on pressure; most visible on the neck, chest, skinfolds; peeling of skin (tips of toes and fingers). Strep throat, fever, pain, swelling, beefy redness of pharynx with exudate and tender cervical nodes, strawberry tongue. If untreated, can cause acute rheumatic fever and glomerulonephritis.	Encourage fluids. Antibiotics (penicillin is the drug of choice; erythromycin). Fever management. Advise parents of the importance of taking antibiotics for the full number of days prescribed. Advise parents of the importance of follow-up throat cultures, if indicated.

Figure 34–4 *continued*

COMMUNICABLE AND INFECTIOUS DISEASES OF CHILDHOOD

Disease	Signs and Symptoms	Treatment and Nursing Care
Tetanus (lockjaw) *Agent*: *Clostridium tetani* (anaerobic, gram-positive rod that exists in both vegetative and spore forms) *Occurrence*: Not a communicable disease; occurs as a complication of puncture wounds, compound fractures, abrasions, burns, injections, surgery, animal bites, gastrointestinal infections, abortions, abscesses, and chronic skin ulceration *Etiology*: Spores can survive for years; found in soil, dust, animal feces, and less commonly in human feces and on human skin; organisms thrive on necrotic tissue and lack of oxygen; exotoxin travels along motor neurons and is disseminated through bloodstream; fixes to gangliosides in skeletal muscle, spinal cord, brain, autonomic nervous system *Incubation period*: From trauma to onset of symptoms, 2 days–3 weeks (usually 6–8 days) *Communicability period*: Not communicable *Prevention*: Active immunization with tetanus toxoid (see Chapter 25)	Clinical disease is a result of the effects of the neurotoxin on various receptors. EARLY SIGNS: Stiffness or cramps in muscles around wound; deep tendon hyperreflexia; stiffness of neck, jaw; facial pain. PROGRESSIVE DISEASE: Change of facial expression, sudden contractures of muscle groups (opisthotonos). Laryngeal, diaphragmatic, and intercostal muscle spasms may produce acute respiratory failure.	Antitoxin serum therapy. Medications (sedatives, psychotherapeutics, antianxiety agents, muscle relaxants). Monitor for breathing difficulties. Maintain airway. High fatality rate; teach parents the importance of child's receiving tetanus immunization and the importance of wound cleaning.

Figure 34–4 *continued*

COMMUNICABLE AND INFECTIOUS DISEASES OF CHILDHOOD

Disease	Signs and Symptoms	Treatment and Nursing Care
Typhoid fever (acute bacterial disease) *Agent*: *Salmonella typhi* (natural pathogen of humans only) *Transmission*: Most often traced to ingestion of food or water contaminated with human waste *Incubation period:* 7–21 days (average of 14 days) *Communicability period*: CARRIERS: Following treated or untreated infection; *S. typhi* is carried in the stool for 1–2 months *Prevention*: Killed-cell vaccine; enteric coated capsule now available (mutant strain); UNPLEASANT SIDE EFFECTS: fever, headache, myalgia, malaise, localized pain and swelling	Fever, malaise, chills, headache, generalized aches in muscles and joints. Enlarged spleen. Leukopenia and small discrete rose-colored spots (caused by bacterial emboli in the skin capillaries) may appear on the trunk. Abdominal distention and tenderness.	Antimicrobial therapy (chloramphenicol, trimethoprim-sulfamethoxazole, ampicillin, amoxicillin, cephalosporins). Maintain strict isolation; enteric precautions should be taken. Instruct parents and visitors to avoid use of child's toilet.

Figure 34–4 *continued*

REVIEW QUESTIONS

A. Multiple choice. Select the best answer.

1. If you were trying to explain the difference between an infectious disease and a communicable disease to a patient, which of the following would be the best statement?
   a. Communicable diseases are more serious than infectious diseases.
   b. Communicable diseases spread, either directly or indirectly, between people; infectious diseases are caused by organisms invading a body directly, then multiplying to produce the disease.
   c. Many infectious diseases have to be reported to local health departments; communicable diseases do not.
   d. Disease is caused by damage to the cells, secretion of a toxin, or an antigen-antibody reaction in the host.
2. Which of the following stages of infection may occur simultaneously?
   a. latent period and incubation period
   b. latent period and communicability period
   c. incubation period and disease period
   d. latent period and disease period
3. Universal precautions are designed primarily to
   a. minimize the risk of exposure to patients with AIDS
   b. be used in high-risk clinical situations
   c. protect health care providers from terminally ill patients
   d. minimize the risk of exposure to blood and body fluids of all patients
4. Children are placed in isolation to interrupt the chain of infection by preventing the spread of microbes. Which of the following would *not* be a reason for placing a child in short-term isolation?
   a. infectious disease
   b. immunodeficiency disease
   c. an allergic reaction
   d. chemotherapy
5. Most children with acquired immunodeficiency syndrome (AIDS) are
   a. adolescents
   b. school-age children
   c. preschool children
   d. infants
6. Which of the following childhood diseases has the longest incubation period?
   a. diphtheria
   b. chickenpox
   c. hepatitis B
   d. measles
7. Parvovirus is the agent responsible for which disease?
   a. fifth disease
   b. measles
   c. mononucleosis
   d. mumps
8. Angela, 6 years old, has complained of a headache and queasiness for the past two days and now has developed a moderate fever and parotid gland swelling. These signs and symptoms are characteristic of
   a. fifth disease
   b. mumps
   c. Lyme disease
   d. rabies
9. Marco's mother brings him to the walk-in clinic. He has a low-grade fever and rash, with clear, fluid-filled vesicles. The nurse suspects that Marco has
   a. rubella
   b. chickenpox
   c. measles
   d. roseola
10. Which of the following diseases is usually transmitted by droplet?
    a. hepatitis
    b. poliomyelitis
    c. tetanus
    d. diphtheria

SUGGESTED ACTIVITIES

- Children in isolation can become lonely and depressed. Suggest three techniques that might be used to relieve loneliness for infants, children, or adolescents.
- If you work with children, you are apt to be asked many questions about communicable diseases. Develop a memory-assisting system for remembering five facts about a particular disease. Share your system with other students.
- Develop a poster display to teach other students about AIDS.

BIBLIOGRAPHY

Foster, R. L., M. M. Hunsberger, and J. J. Tackett Anderson. *Family-Centered Nursing Care of Children*. Philadelphia: W. B. Saunders, 1989.

Gershon, A. A. Herpesvirus. *Emergency Medicine* (November, 1991): 105–115.

Grimes, D. *Infectious Diseases*. St. Louis, MO: Mosby-Year Book, 1991.

Holcroft, C. Acyclovir approved for childhood chickenpox. *Nurse Practitioner* 17, no. 5 (1992).

Last, J. M., and R. B. Wallace. *Public Health and Preventive Medicine*, 13th ed. Norwalk, CT: Appleton & Lange, 1992.

Pilliteri, A. *Maternal and Child Health Nursing*. Philadelphia: J. B. Lippincott, 1992.

Rudolph, A. M. *Rudolph's Pediatrics*, 19th ed. Norwalk, CT: Appleton & Lange, 1991.

Sharts-Engel, N. C. An overview of maternal-child infectious diseases (1976–1990). *American Journal of Maternal-Child Nursing* 16 (1991): 58.

Spratto, G. R, and A. L. Woods. *RN's NDR '93*. Albany, NY: Delmar Publishers, 1993.

Weingarten, C. T., and S. M. Gomberg. Measles: Again an epidemic. *Pediatric Nursing* 18, no. 4 (1992): 369–371.

Wong, D. L. *Whaley & Wong's Essentials of Pediatric Nursing*, 4th ed. St. Louis, MO: Mosby-Year Book, 1993.

CHAPTER

35

Integumentary Conditions

Objectives

AFTER STUDYING THIS CHAPTER, THE STUDENT SHOULD BE ABLE TO:

- NAME FIVE SKIN CONDITIONS THAT AFFECT INFANTS AND TODDLERS AND DESCRIBE THEIR CAUSES, SYMPTOMS, TREATMENT, AND NURSING CARE.
- NAME FOUR SKIN CONDITIONS THAT AFFECT PRESCHOOL AND SCHOOL-AGE CHILDREN AND DESCRIBE THEIR CAUSES, SYMPTOMS, TREATMENT, AND NURSING CARE.
- NAME TWO SKIN CONDITIONS THAT AFFECT ADOLESCENTS AND DESCRIBE THEIR CAUSES, SYMPTOMS, TREATMENT, AND NURSING CARE.
- NAME FOUR TYPES OF BURNS, AND IDENTIFY THE MOST COMMON.
- DESCRIBE ONE METHOD USED TO ASSESS THE EXTENT OF A BURN INJURY.
- IDENTIFY THE AMERICAN BURN ASSOCIATION CRITERIA FOR BURN SEVERITY.
- DISCUSS THE CARE OF CHILDREN WITH MINOR BURNS.
- IDENTIFY TWO GOALS OF BURN WOUND CARE AND DESCRIBE TREATMENT MEASURES FOR BURN WOUNDS.
- IDENTIFY NURSING CONSIDERATIONS IN CARE OF THE BURNED CHILD.

Key Terms

PRIMARY IRRITANT

ALLERGEN

ANAPHYLAXIS

KERION

COMEDONES

ESCHAR

Integumentary conditions occur frequently in children of all ages. The nurse needs to be able to accurately identify these conditions and understand their causes and treatment. Effective treatment of skin conditions often requires that children receive long-term care and follow-up or adhere to a specific treatment plan. For this reason, teaching the parents and child about the condition, its cause, and its treatment is an important aspect of nursing care for many skin conditions.

Burns are a common cause of injury in children, especially young children (see Chapter 26). Most burn injuries are minor and do not require hospital admission. Major burns, however, are serious injuries that require skilled medical and nursing care.

Overview of the System

The skin and its accessory structures — hair, nails, and glands — make up the integumentary system. The skin performs several important functions: protection, body temperature regulation, excretion, sensation, and vitamin D production.

The two principal layers of the skin are the epidermis and dermis. The epidermis, which helps to protect the body against bacterial invasion, is the outermost nonvascular layer of the skin. The dermis — containing nerves, nerve endings, sebaceous and sweat glands, and hair follicles — is the thicker, inner layer of the skin that lies below the epidermis. Below the dermis is the subcutaneous fatty tissue (sometimes called the hypodermis), consisting of loose connective tissue (muscle and fat), Figure 35–1.

Lesions are common presenting signs of many integumentary conditions. Primary skin lesions are illustrated in Figure 35–2 (page 574).

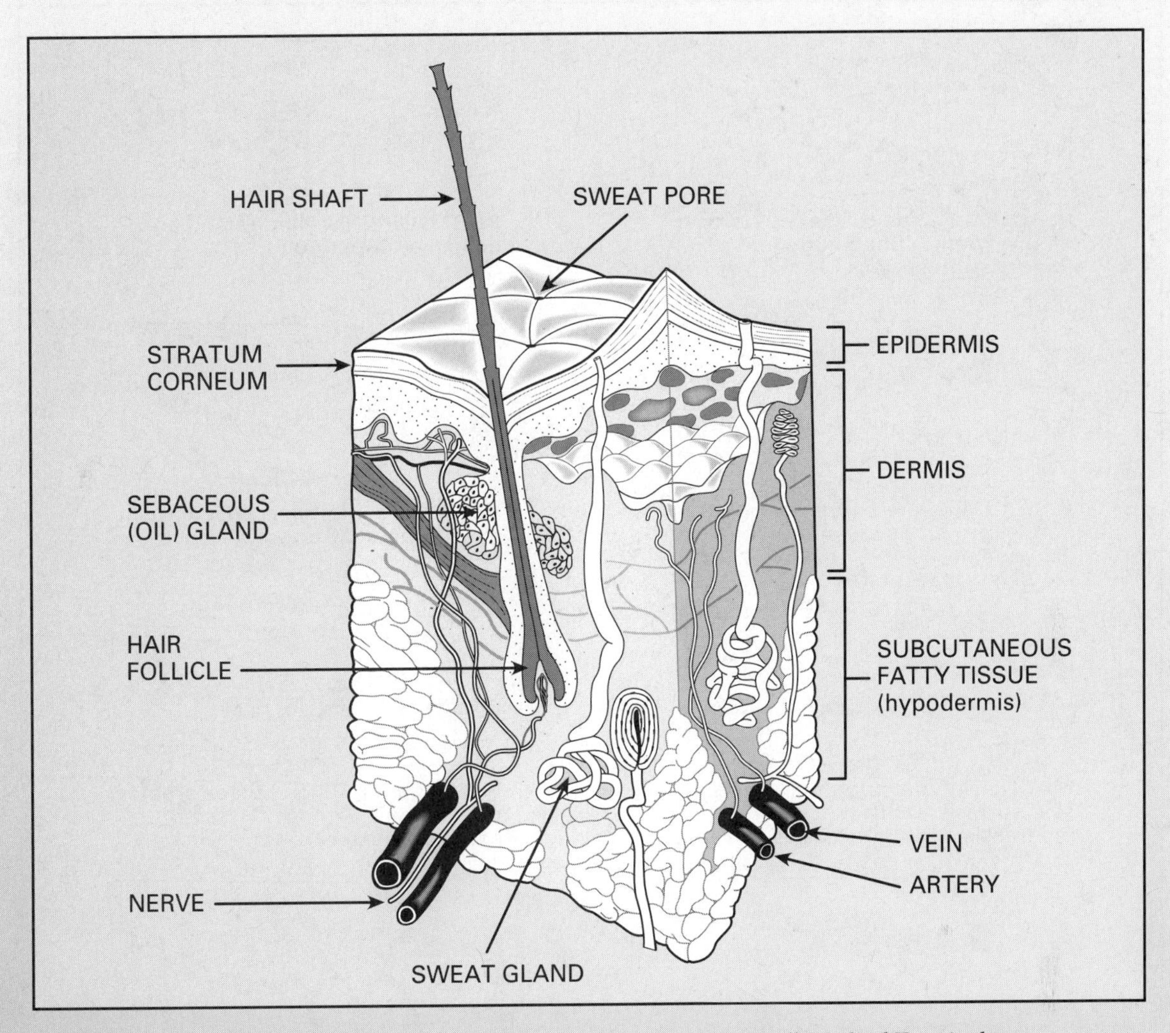

Figure 35–1 *Cross section of the skin (Adapted from Smith, Davis, and Dennerll,* Medical Terminology: A Programmed Approach, *6th ed. Delmar Publishers Inc., 1991)*

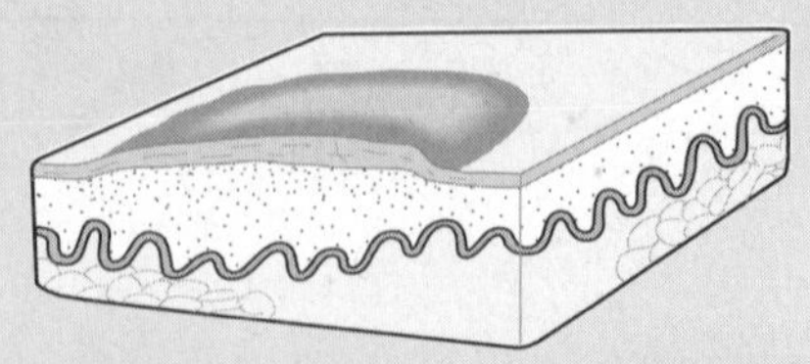

PLAQUE - Raised thickened portion of skin, well-defined edge and a flat or rough surface.
ex. psoriasis, eczema

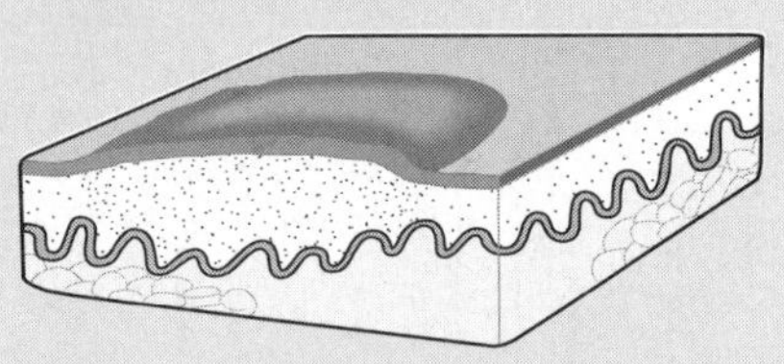

WHEAL - Elevated area, irregular shape formed as a result of localized skin edema
ex. hives, insect bites

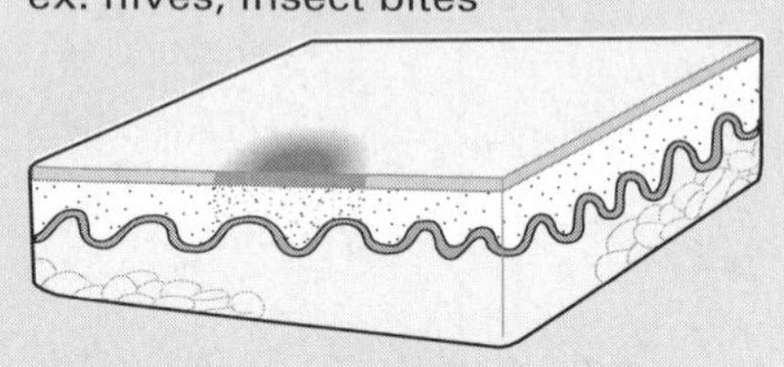

MACULE - A flat spot, flush with the skin surface, a different color.
ex. freckle, rash of measles, roseola

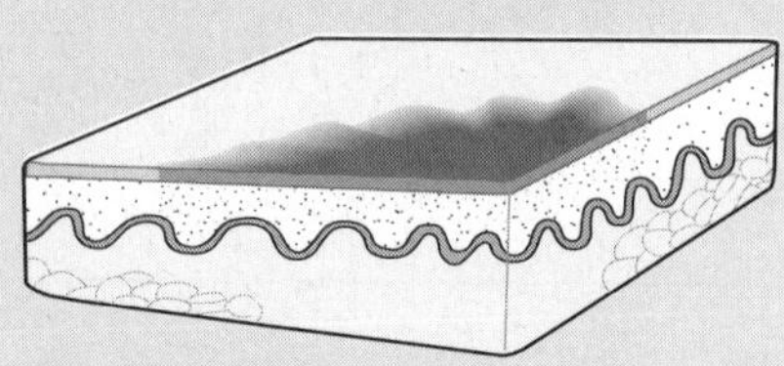

PATCH - Flat surface tissue that differs from surrounding area in color, texture
ex. port wine mark.

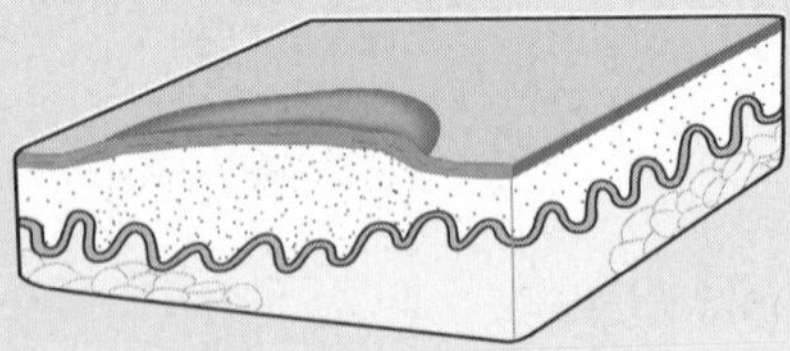

PAPULE - A raised spot on the surface of the skin
ex. flat wart, nevus

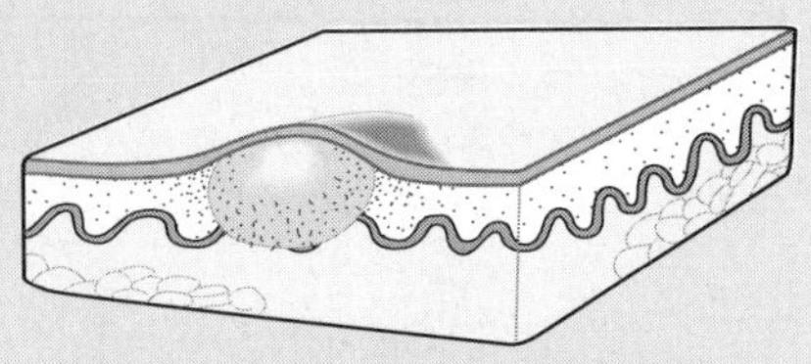

PUSTULE - Pus-filled raised area
ex. acne, impetigo

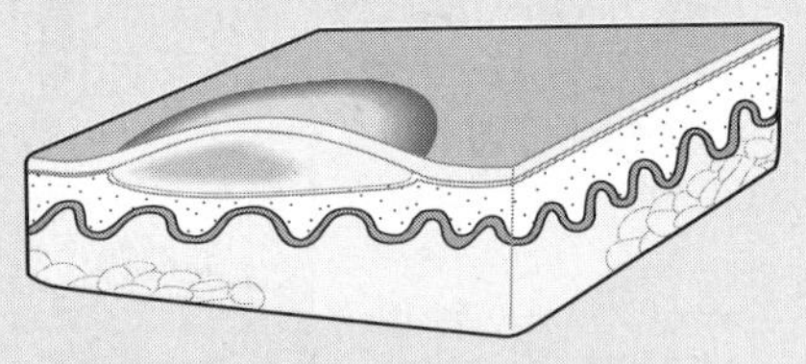

VESICLE - Fluid-filled raised area.
ex. blister, chickenpox, herpes simplex

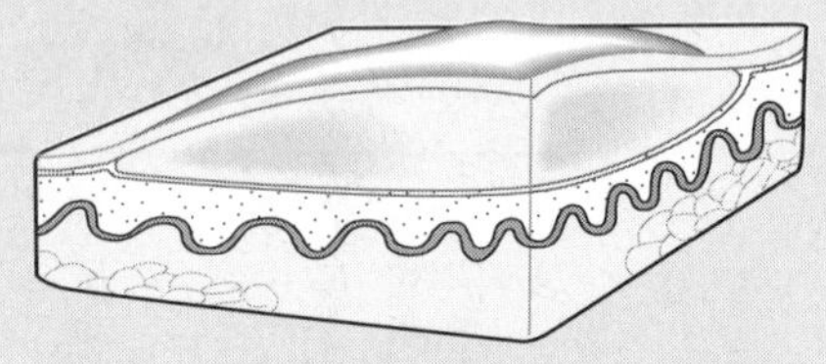

BULLA - Fluid-filled blister greater than 1 cm
ex. large blister

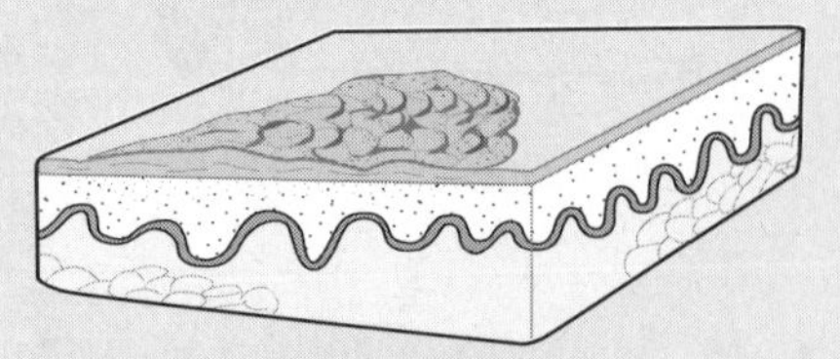

SCALE - Excess dead epidermal cells.
ex. Seborrheic dermatitis

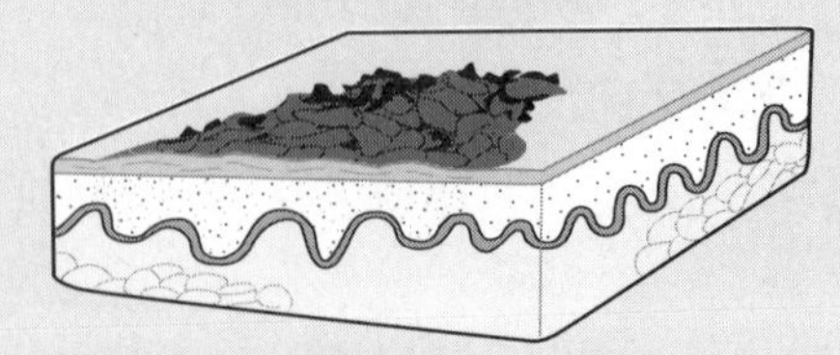

CRUST - A collection of dried serum and cellular debris
ex. eczema, impetigo

Figure 35–2 *Primary skin lesions*

INFANT AND TODDLER

MILIARIA RUBRA

Miliaria rubra, also called prickly heat or heat rash, is caused by plugging of the sweat ducts. Sweat leaks into the surrounding skin when exposed to heat and high humidity, causing fine red papules or vesicles, inflammation, and a stinging or prickling sensation. The rash is most often found in areas prone to sweating, such as the neck, groin, and axillae, and underneath clothing. Lesions usually heal by themselves; however, an anti-inflammatory lotion may be prescribed. A cool environment and lightweight clothing should be encouraged.

CONTACT DERMATITIS

Contact dermatitis is an inflammation of the skin caused by a **primary irritant** or **allergen** contact. Primary irritants are chemical substances such as bleaches, dyes, soaps, detergents, and gasoline. Common allergens are poison ivy, oak, and sumac; wool; fur; shoe leather; nickel; and rubber (latex). Recently, cases of reactions to latex have been reported, ranging from contact dermatitis to **anaphylaxis**, a hypersensitivity response to a previously encountered antigen (Fritsch and Fredrick Pilat 1993). Latex is found in gloves, catheters, airway equipment, monitors, intravenous equipment, plastic syringes, and adhesive tape.

A primary irritant contact dermatitis develops within a few hours after contact, peaks in 24 hours, and disappears. An allergic contact dermatitis can take as long as 18 hours to appear, peaks between 48 and 72 hours, and can last for two to three weeks. The basic features of the skin lesions are erythema, edema, and a papulovesicular rash in patches or streaks. Pain, pruritus, and burning may be present. Treatment includes avoiding further contact with the allergen, topical steroids, and antihistamines to reduce itching.

DIAPER DERMATITIS

Diaper dermatitis, or diaper rash, is the most common irritant contact dermatitis in infancy. It is usually caused by prolonged contact of the skin with urine and stool. It may also occur as a result of inadequate cleansing of the diaper area; contact with detergents, ointments, or soaps; or friction.

Symptoms can include erythema, edema, vesicles, and weeping involving the perineum, genitals, and buttocks, with extension to the inner thighs. *Candida albicans* (monilia) is the causative organism in 80% of diaper rashes that last longer than four days (Rosenstein and Fosarelli 1989). Figure 35–3 shows the typical lesions of a monilial diaper rash.

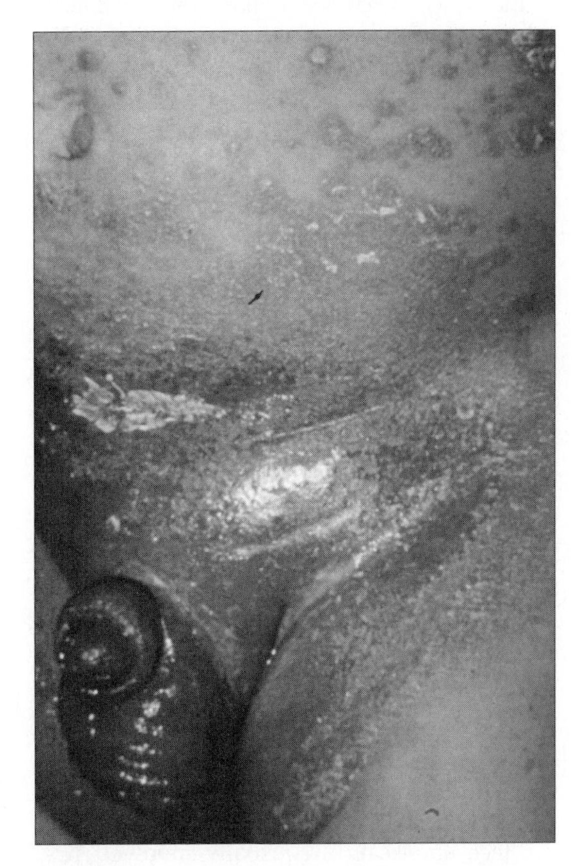

Figure 35–3 *Monilial diaper rash (Courtesy of the Centers for Disease Control and Prevention, Atlanta, GA)*

Treatment includes frequent diaper changes, avoidance of plastic pants, exposing the diaper area to the air, cleansing the diaper area at each diaper change, and applying protective ointment (Balmex, A&D, Desitin). Caution parents to avoid using commercially available baby wipes, because the alcohol in these products will further dry and irritate the inflamed area.

SEBORRHEIC DERMATITIS

Seborrheic dermatitis is a chronic, inflammatory skin disease. It consists of erythematous, scaling, crusting lesions that can be greasy or dry and yellow in appearance. Lesions occur in areas that are rich in sebaceous glands, such as the scalp, face, back, behind the ear and in creases. The eyebrows and eyelashes also can be involved.

This condition is commonly seen in newborns and infants (as cradle cap) and at puberty (as dandruff or flaking). Treatment consists of topical steroids (except for cradle cap), shampoos (such as Head & Shoulders or Sebulex), and antibiotics, when indicated.

ATOPIC DERMATITIS (ECZEMA)

Description. Atopic dermatitis (eczema) is a general term used to describe chronic superficial inflammation of the skin in different types of patients. Atopic dermatitis has been associated with allergy and is thought to have a hereditary tendency. It is one of the most common skin disorders in children (Zitelli and Davis 1991).

Symptoms. Atopic dermatitis can be divided into three clinical phases (infantile, childhood, and adolescent) based on the age of the child and the distribution of the lesions.

1. *Infantile*: Lesions, typically red, itchy papules and plaques, are followed by crusting. The face and scalp are usually involved first (Figure 35–4); later the rash may spread to the extensor aspects of the extremities, buttocks, thighs, anogenital region, and trunk.
2. *Childhood*: Lesions are typically dry, papular, more thickened, and pruritic. Areas involved are the wrists, ankles, antecubital and popliteal fossae, and the back and sides of the neck. Sometimes the soles of the feet are involved (atopic feet) and there is erythema, cracking, and pain.
3. *Adolescent*: Lesions are pruritic and have a thickened, hardened appearance with varying degrees of erythema and scaling. Areas involved are the hands (most often), eyelids, neck, feet, and flexor areas.

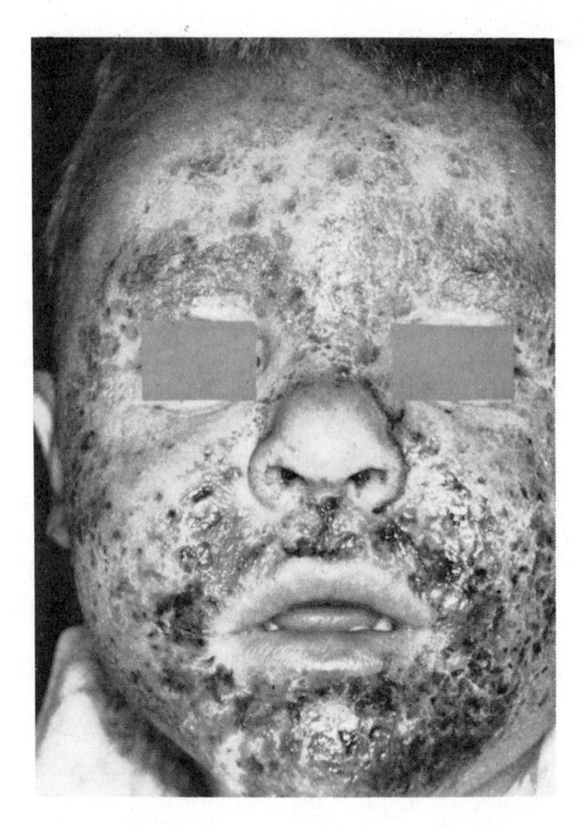

Figure 35–4 *Infantile eczema (From Stewart, Danto, and Maddin,* Dermatology, *4th ed. C. V. Mosby, St. Louis, 1978)*

Treatment. Treatment focuses on reducing inflammation and preventing secondary infection by hydrating the skin, which helps to relieve itching.

Acute Condition

- If weeping is present, wet compresses (cotton cloth soaked in aluminum acetate solution) are applied to the area.
- Systemic antibiotics are prescribed if superimposed infection is suspected.
- Topical steroids (triamcinolone) may be prescribed for maintenance therapy of mild dermatitis of the face and intertriginous areas.
- Apply emollients to dry, scaling, or fissured eruptions.
- Use oatmeal baths (Aveeno) to soothe inflammation.
- Antipruritics (Vistaril, Atarax) may be prescribed to relieve itching.

Chronic Condition

Parents should be taught the following measures:

- Dress the child in cotton clothes and avoid wool clothing and perfumed soaps.
- Wash the child with mild soap (Dove, Tone).
- Apply steroid cream or lotion in small amounts frequently.
- Use prescribed medications when needed to relieve pain.

Nursing Care. The nurse should teach the parents and child about the causes of atopic dermatitis and how to prevent frequent occurrences. Counsel parents about diet, clothing, and the use of soaps and lotions. Encourage compliance with the treatment plan. Treatment failures can be frustrating for both parents and child. Emphasize the importance of not scratching the lesions to avoid secondary infection. Keeping the nails clean and cutting fingernails and toenails short reduces the chance of infection. Advise parents of young children to have the child wear cotton gloves or socks on the hands to prevent scratching, especially at bedtime.

PRESCHOOL AND SCHOOL-AGE CHILD

IMPETIGO

Impetigo is a highly contagious, superficial infection of the skin caused by *Streptococcus* and *Staphylococcus* organisms. The most common sites are the face, extremities, hands, and neck.

In a group A streptococcal infection, the lesion begins as a papule that changes to form a small, thin-walled vesicle with an erythematous halo. At first, the vesicle is filled with clear fluid, which later becomes cloudy; the vesicle then ruptures, forming a superficial honey-colored crust. In staphylococcal infection, the initial macule may form small, thin-walled pustules or the larger flaccid bullae known as bullous impetigo. Lesions may coalesce over time, and satellite lesions may form.

Impetigo commonly causes pruritus, burning, and secondary enlargement and tenderness of the regional lymph nodes. Treatment involves the use of systemic antibiotics (penicillin, erythromycin), when indicated. Scrubbing lesions with hexachlorophene (pHisoHex) and applying topical antibiotics aid in control of lesions but do not cure the infection. Teach parents to keep the child's fingernails short and clean. Applying a topical bactericidal ointment (Bactoban) aids in reducing secondary infection.

RINGWORM

Ringworm refers to a group of fungal infections of the skin, hair, and nails. These highly contagious infections occur in all age groups and are usually spread from person to person or from animal to person. There are three common causative organisms: trichophyton, microsporum, and epidermophyton.

The most common types of infection (identified by the Latin word *tinea* and a word indicating the area affected) are:

- *Tinea capitis*: a fungal infection of the scalp and hair, characterized by scaling and patchy hair loss. Sometimes the short broken-off hairs result in inflammation with a boggy patch and pustules (called a **kerion**).
- *Tinea corporis*: a superficial fungal infection of the smooth hairless skin of the body, called "ringworm" because of the characteristic round lesions with central clearing and a scaly, annular border. More than one lesion may be present, Figure 35–5.
- *Tinea cruris* ("jock itch"): a fungal infection that occurs on the inner aspects of the thighs and scrotum.
- *Tinea pedis* ("athlete's foot"): a fungal infection of the foot and toes, characterized by fissuring and pinhead-sized lesions.

Diagnosis is made by observation; by using an ultraviolet light (Wood's lamp) to look at the lesions, which fluoresce if ringworm is present; by examining scrapings from the lesion in a potassium hydroxide (KOH) preparation under the microscope; and by fungal cultures.

Treatment is similar regardless of the causative organism, but differs with the site and extent of the infection. Topical therapy is used for localized skin infection; systemic therapy for widespread skin infection and infection of the scalp, hair, or nails (Rosenstein and Fosarelli 1989). If the hair or nails are involved, griseofulvin is the treatment of choice (Hathaway et al. 1993).

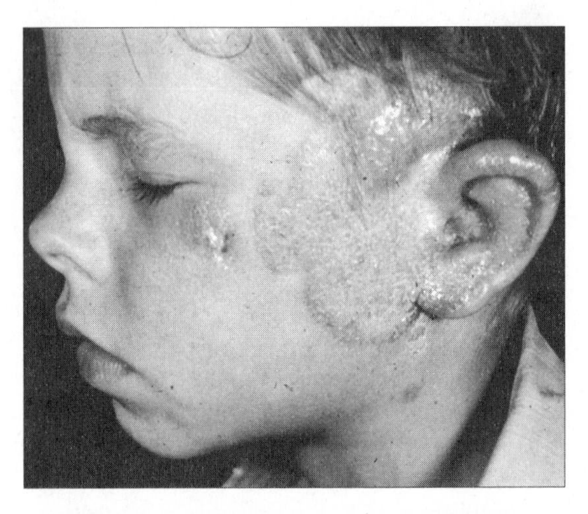

Figure 35–5 *Ringworm (tinea corporis) of the face and scalp (Courtesy of the Centers for Disease Control and Prevention, Atlanta, GA)*

PEDICULOSIS CAPITIS (LICE)

Description. Pediculosis capitis is an infestation of the scalp by lice. The female louse, Figure 35–6, lays eggs at the base of the hair shaft close to the skin, where the warmth of the scalp provides the heat necessary for incubation. The eggs (nits) can be seen as oval, white, 0.5-mm dots attached firmly to the hair shaft. They are usually located about 0.5–1 cm from the scalp but sometimes run the entire length of the hair shaft.

Symptoms. Itching is the primary symptom. Head lice can be found anywhere on the scalp,

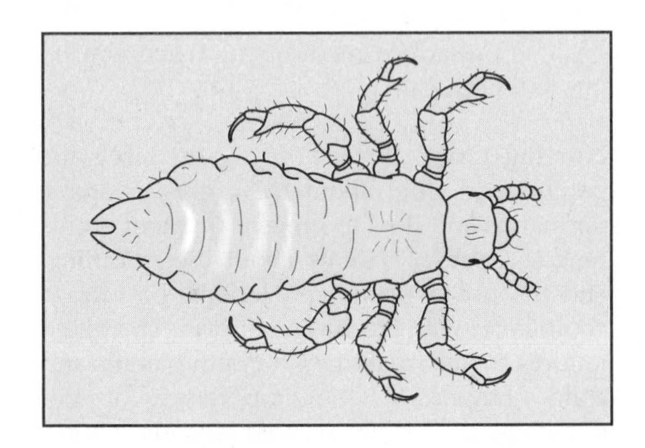

Figure 35–6 *The female head louse (enlarged)*

but are most often seen on the back of the head and neck and behind the ears. Scratching causes inflammation and secondary bacterial infection, with pustules, crusting, and cervical adenopathy. The eyelashes may be involved, causing redness and swelling. Although nits resemble dandruff, they are cemented to the hair rather than easily moved along the hair shaft, as is dandruff (Habif 1990).

Treatment. Treatment consists of washing the hair with a pediculicide, such as lindane (Kwell) shampoo. Parents should be told to use approximately 30 mL of the shampoo; work into a lather; rub for five minutes; then rinse and dry with a towel. The dead nits will remain attached to the hair until removed. To remove the nits, the hair should be combed with an extra-fine-toothed comb. Vinegar compresses applied to the hair for 15 minutes will help to remove the nit shells.

Nursing Care. Reassure the parents and child that anyone can become infested with lice. Notify the child's school, day-care center, babysitter, and parents of playmates, because lice are easily transmitted from child to child. Teach parents how to prevent the spread of lice and reinfestation, Figure 35–7.

SCABIES

Scabies is a contagious infestation caused by the mite *Sarcoptes scabiei*. Infestation begins when a fertilized female mite burrows into the stratum corneum (dead horny layer of the epidermis; see Figure 35–1) to bury her eggs. The burrow enlarges from several millimeters to a few centimeters in length during her 30-day life cycle (Habif 1990).

Symptoms include pruritic papules, vesicles, pustules, and linear burrows. An eczematous eruption caused by hypersensitivity to the mite is sometimes seen. Secondary infection can also occur.

The linear burrow is the diagnostic sign of scabies. It consists of a small, scaly, linear lesion with pinpoint vesicles at the end, in which the female mite lives (Zitelli and Davis 1991). Areas of involvement include the webs of the fingers, axillae, flexures of the arms and wrists, belt line, nipples, genitals, and lower buttocks. In infants, the palms, soles of the feet, head, and neck can be affected. Diagnosis is made by examining microscopically scrapings

PREVENTING PEDICULOSIS (LICE)

- Soak combs, brushes, and hair accessories in pediculicide such as lindane (Kwell) for 1 hour or in boiling water for 10 minutes.
- Machine wash all washable clothing, towels, and bed linens in hot water and dry in a hot dryer for at least 20 minutes. Dry clean nonwashable items.
- Thoroughly vacuum carpets, car seats, pillows, stuffed animals, rugs, mattresses, and upholstered furniture.
- Seal nonwashable items in plastic bags for 14 days if unable to vacuum or dry clean.
- Instruct children not to share combs, hats, or scarves.

***Figure* 35–7** *(Adapted from Clore, Dispelling the common myths about pediculosis,* Journal of Pediatric Health Care, *1989)* from a burrow or an unscratched papule and observing a mite, egg, or mite feces.

Treatment consists of applying a scabicide such as lindane (Kwell, Scabene), available as a cream, lotion, or shampoo. The scabicide is applied from the neck down and washed off after six to eight hours.

Because lindane becomes concentrated in the central nervous system, it is not recommended for use on infants. Eurax lotion is used, instead. Like lindane, Eurax is applied from the neck down, but it is applied nightly for two nights and washed off 24 hours after the second application. Infants sometimes need to be retreated in 7 to 10 days. To prevent the infant from touching the body and then putting the fingers in the mouth, keep the hands covered during treatment.

All family members should be treated at the same time as the affected child. In addition, advise parents to wash all clothing and bed linens to prevent reinfestation.

BITES AND STINGS

Bites. Children frequently are bitten by animals as well as other children. Animal bites include bites from dogs, cats, snakes, and arthropods. It is not unusual for a child to be bitten by the family pet while playing. Examples of common arthropod bites are those of spiders, ticks, scorpions, mites, and centipedes. Bites of the black widow and brown recluse spiders are the most dangerous. Tick bites can transmit Lyme disease (see Chapter 34) and Rocky Mountain spotted fever.

Human bites usually occur while children are fighting with one another. These bites easily become infected by organisms that are part of the normal flora of the mouth.

Stings. Children are most frequently stung by bees, wasps, and ants. Common symptoms include pain, redness, itching, and swelling. Some children, however, may have severe allergic reactions, resulting in anaphylactic shock.

Treatment. Treatment usually consists of cool compresses, local cleansing of the affected area, and application of a disinfectant. Oral antihistamines can be given to control swelling and reduce itching.

ADOLESCENT

ACNE

Description. Acne, a disorder of the hair follicle and its oil gland, is a common problem for adolescent boys and girls. Acne occurs primarily in the sebaceous follicles of the face, neck, shoulders, upper chest, and back. The sebaceous glands secrete excessive oil or sebum, which is deposited at the openings of the glands. Obstruction of the sebaceous follicle openings produces the lesions of acne.

Symptoms. The three major types of acne are:

- *Comedomal acne*: characterized by open (white head) and closed (black head) **comedones**, which are caused by an accumulation of keratin and sebum within the opening of a hair follicle.
- *Papulopustular acne*: characterized by rupture of the follicular walls, producing papules and pustules.
- *Cystic acne*: characterized by nodules and cysts that are scattered over the face, chest, and back. This type of acne requires vigorous treatment and can lead to severe scar formation.

Treatment. It is important for the nurse to understand the psychosocial impact that acne can have on the developing adolescent. Parents should be encouraged to seek medical care for the teenager with acne and not dismiss the condition as simply a part of the growing process. Acne appears at a time when the adolescent is attempting to build a new identity and form close relationships with members of the opposite sex. Acne may affect adversely the teenager's body image and self-esteem. Encouraging the teenager to talk, listening to his or her concerns, and offering emotional support and reassurance that this condition will not last forever are important aspects of care (Habif 1990).

Treatment involves the use of topical and oral agents, alone or in combination. Topical agents such as vitamin A (retinoid) cream and benzoyl peroxide are frequently prescribed, along with oral antibiotics. Topical agents are applied to the entire affected area in order to treat existing lesions and prevent new lesions from developing.

Nursing Care. Patient education is an important component of nursing care. The nurse should explain the cause of acne and the treatment plan to the adolescent.

Dispel myths about diet and dirt as causative factors, for example, that eating chocolate or fried foods causes pimples. Adolescent girls who use cosmetics should be advised to use nongreasy lotions and water-based products. The psychosocial impact of acne must not be overlooked. Explain that no drug will prevent the adolescent from developing additional lesions and that the results of treatment will not be visible for four to eight weeks. Reinforce the importance of follow-up visits and of complying with the treatment plan. Caution adolescents who are using retinoid agents to avoid or minimize exposure to sunlight, as the skin is more susceptible to burning.

HERPES SIMPLEX INFECTIONS

Herpes simplex is a viral infection caused by two different herpes viruses. Type 1 herpes causes most oral, skin, and cerebral infections. Type 2 herpes causes most genital and congenital infections (Hathaway et al. 1993). Herpes simplex type 1 infection is more commonly seen in children.

Individuals with primary infections shed the virus in saliva, urine, stool, or from skin lesions. Intimate contact, shared eating utensils, and respiratory droplets are major modes of spread. Parents frequently pass the virus on to their children (Zitelli and Davis 1991).

Most children with symptomatic type 1 herpes are under 5 years of age and have an illness characterized by fever, malaise, localized vesicular lesions, and regional adenopathy. Symptoms in infected infants include high fever, irritability, and drooling. Children may also develop primary gingivostomatitis, characterized by multiple oral ulcers on the gingiva, tongue, buccal mucosa, and lips. Pharyngeal ulcers may occur in older children.

Vesicular lesions, also called "cold sores" or "fever blisters," often begin with a tingling or burning sensation of the upper or lower lip, followed by the appearance of grouped vesicles on an erythematous base. Within 24 hours, the vesicles usually begin to scab and form a crust, and the lesions resolve completely within about a week.

Treatment is symptomatic and involves keeping the lesions clean and dry, and providing pain relief if indicated.

BURNS

Burns are the second leading cause of unintentional injury and death in children and annually claim the lives of 1,200 children in the United States. In all, 60,000 children are hospitalized each year for treatment of burns. Child abuse is suspected in approximately 16% of these cases (Eichelberger et al. 1993).

CAUSES

Burn injuries are caused by exposure to thermal, chemical, electrical, or radioactive agents.

- Thermal burns are the most common type of burn and result from direct contact with flame, flash (blow torch), hot liquids (coffee, tea, grease), and grills, Figure 35–8.
- Chemical burns result from contact with or ingestion of agents that burn or irritate the skin surface, mucous membranes, or intestinal organs.
- Electrical burns result from contact with electrical cords, wall sockets, and appliances such as blow dryers and curling irons, Figure 35–9.
- Radiation burns result from contact with radioactive substances that give off alpha, beta, and gamma rays, causing tissue damage. X-rays are gamma rays, and the damage they cause can be severe.

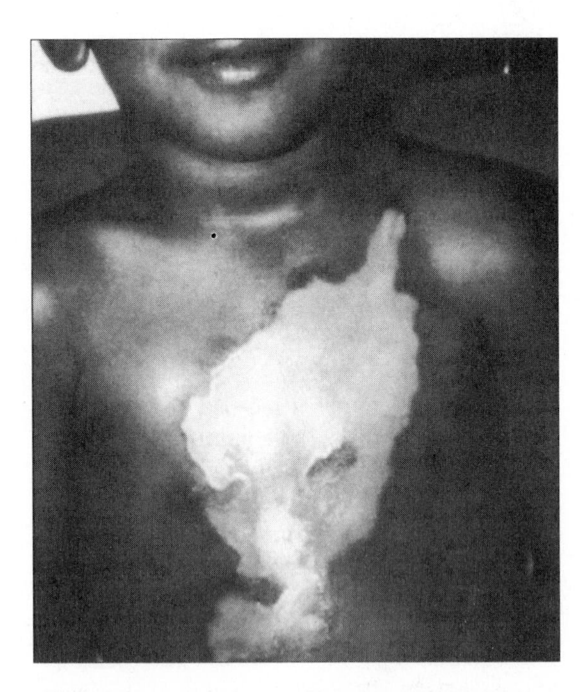

Figure 35–8 *A scald burn caused by hot liquid decreases in width where the liquid drained down the chest to form an arrow point. (From Eichelberger, Ball, Pratsch, and Runion,* Pediatric Emergencies: A Manual for Prehospital Care Providers, *1992. Reprinted by permission of Prentice-Hall, Englewood Cliffs, NJ)*

CLASSIFICATION

The classification and severity of the burn are assessed by evaluating the following:

- type of burn
- duration of contact
- depth of burn injury; that is, superficial (first-degree), partial thickness (second-degree), or full thickness (third-degree), Figure 35–10
- areas affected, expressed as a percentage of body surface area (BSA); the Lund and Browder formula, Figure 35–11, is widely used to estimate the extent of burn injuries in children
- age and health of the child
- preexisting illness or condition

Burns are further identified as minor, moderate, or severe according to the American Burn Association criteria for burn severity.

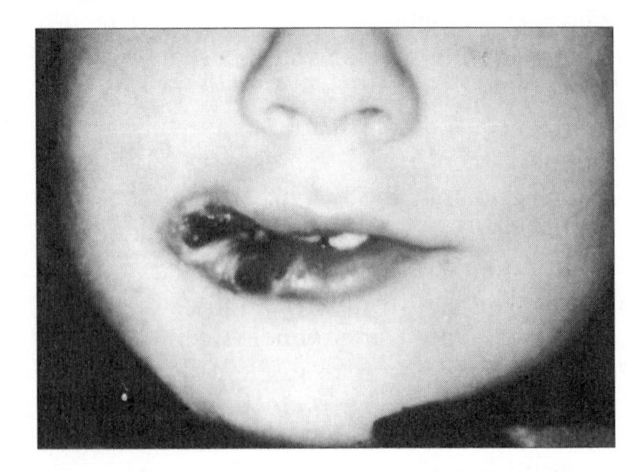

Figure 35–9 *Burn from biting an electrical cord (From Eichelberger, Ball, Pratsch, and Runion,* Pediatric Emergencies: A Manual for Prehospital Care Providers, *1992. Reprinted by permission of Prentice-Hall, Englewood Cliffs, NJ)*

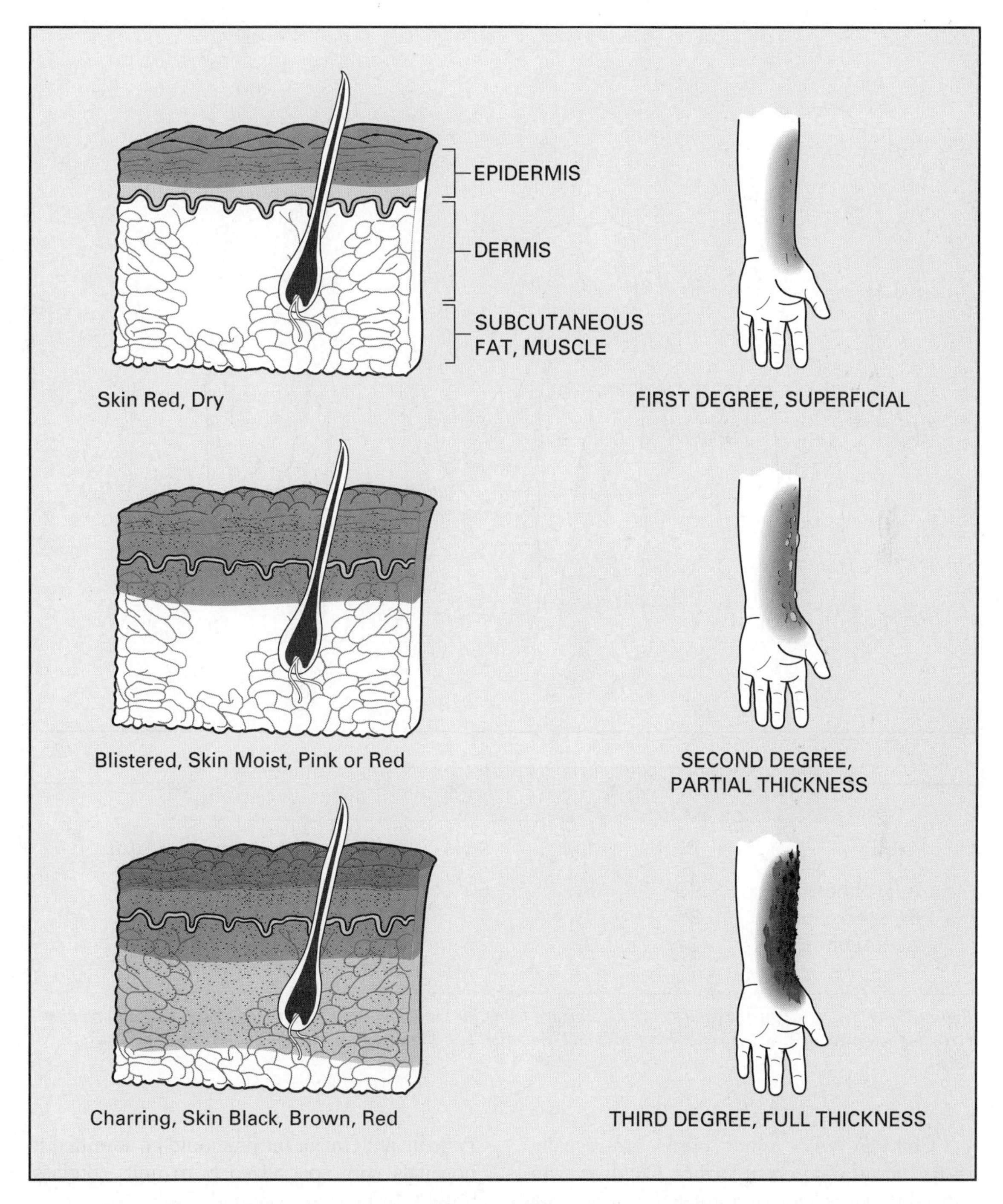

Figure 35–10 *Burn depth classification (Adapted from Eichelberger, Ball, Pratsch, and Runion,* Pediatric Emergencies: A Manual for Prehospital Care Providers, *1992. Reprinted by permission of Prentice-Hall, Englewood Cliffs, NJ)*

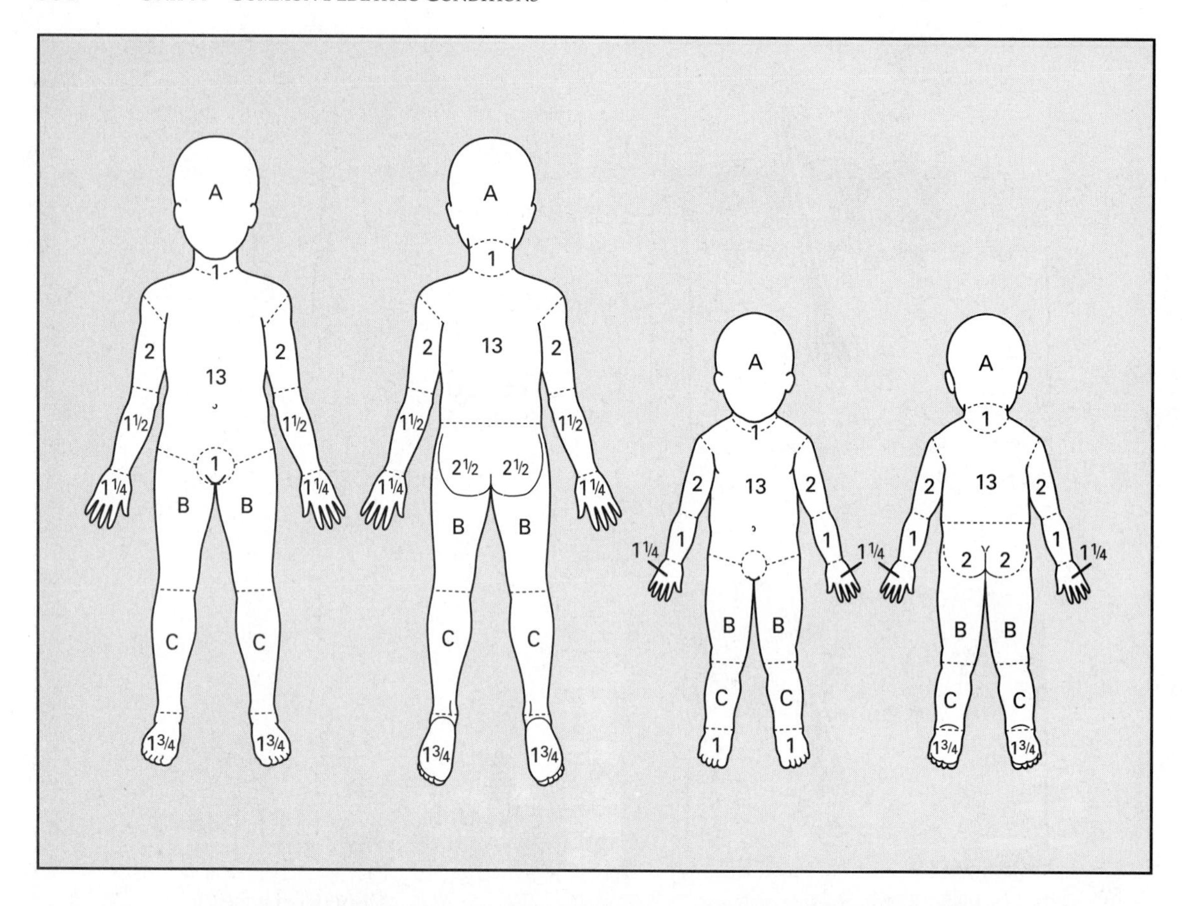

RELATIVE PERCENTAGES OF AREAS A, B, AND C, BY AGE

Area	Birth	1 yr	5 yrs	10 yrs	15 yrs	Adult
A (½ of head)	9½	8½	6½	5½	4½	3½
B (½ of one thigh)	2¾	3¼	4	4½	4½	4¾
C (½ of one leg)	2½	2½	2¾	3	3¼	3½

Figure 35–11 *The extent of a child's burn is estimated using the Lund and Browder formula, which indicates relative percentages of areas affected. (Adapted from Artz and Moncrief,* The Treatment of Burns, *2nd ed. W. B. Saunders, 1969)*

Children with minor burns are usually treated in an out-patient facility. Children with moderate burns should be treated in a hospital that has a staff trained to deliver burn care. Patients with major burns should be admitted to hospitals with specialized burn units (Budassi Sheehy 1990).

CARE OF MINOR BURNS

Nurses who work in clinics or other outpatient facilities are frequently called on to provide care to children with minor burns. Interventions include the following actions.

- Remove restrictive clothing and jewelry.
- Assess the extent of the burn.
- Soak the affected area in a mild antiseptic soap solution.
- Debride only open blisters; leave closed blisters intact.
- Cover the wound with an antimicrobial agent and a bulky dressing.
- Determine whether the child's tetanus immunization is up to date.
- Instruct parents in the use of antibiotics, if prescribed, and analgesia for pain relief.
- Instruct parents to keep the dressing clean and dry, to elevate the burned area or extremity for 24 hours, and to return to the facility in two days (Budassi Sheehy 1990).

CARE OF MAJOR BURNS

The child with a major burn injury who is admitted to a hospital requires immediate assessment and skilled medical and nursing care. Major burns cause significant disruption to essential body systems. Immediate care requires the following actions.

- Provide for the child's immediate survival from the burn incident.
- Monitor respiratory status and maintain a patent airway.
- Be aware of the signs of shock and monitor vital signs closely.
- Take every precaution to keep an intravenous line open.
- Assess for bleeding.

During hospitalization, the child needs skilled and sensitive nursing care to provide pain relief, provide nutritional support, control infection, ensure adequate hydration, prevent electrolyte imbalances, and promote wound and tissue healing. Throughout the recovery period, the nurse acts to encourage physical mobility, promote normal growth and development, and provide emotional support for the child and family.

BURN WOUND CARE

Once the child has been stabilized, a treatment plan is established to care for the burn wound. Two primary goals of wound care are to protect the child from infection and promote healing of the wound. Burn wound care involves several procedures: cleansing the wound, hydrotherapy (whirlpool), application of burn dressings, surgical excision of **eschar** (the tough, leathery scab that forms over severely burned areas), debridement, and skin grafting. All of these procedures are frightening and painful, and emotional support of the child and family are important aspects of care.

Topical Treatment. Burns may be treated by open therapy or closed therapy. Open therapy involves exposing the burn to air and applying a topical medication directly to the wound. In closed therapy, the burn is covered first with a topical medication and then with a fine mesh gauze. Topical antibacterial agents reduce the number of bacteria present on the burn. The most common topical burn medications are Silvadeen, Sulfamylon, aqueous silver nitrate, Povidone-iodine, and bacitracin or triple antibiotic ointment.

Debridement. In second- and third-degree burns, debridement is begun as soon as possible to reduce the chance of infection. Hydrotherapy, tub baths, soaks, or showers are used before debridement to soften and loosen eschar. Because debridement is very painful, pain medication is given before the procedure.

Children need emotional support, understanding, and sensitive nursing care to cope with these difficult and painful treatment periods.

Skin Grafting. Third-degree burns involve complete destruction of the epidermis and dermis. Because no epithelial cells remain, skin grafting is necessary. Grafts may be temporary or permanent.

There are three types of skin grafts:

- *Allograft*: fresh cadaver skin, which provides the best temporary skin graft. Allograft covering renders the burn pain-free and reduces the bacterial count on the burn surface.
- *Xenograft (heterograft)*: a temporary skin covering (usually pigskin) that is commercially available.
- *Autograft*: a layer of skin from the epidermis and part of the dermis (called a split-thickness graft) that is removed from an unburned portion of the child's body and then placed on the burn wound. Autograft provides a permanent skin covering.

Contractures and Scars. Third-degree burns commonly heal with contractures and scars. Areas commonly affected by contractures are the hands, joints of the arms and legs, neck, face, calves, and legs. Preventive measures and treatment vary. Aggressive physical therapy should start as soon as the child can tolerate it.

NURSING CONSIDERATIONS IN CARE AND REHABILITATION OF THE BURNED CHILD

Care of the burned child is challenging. The child who has been burned is frightened, anxious, and in pain. Thus, the relationship that is established with the child is an integral part of the care that nurses provide.

The rehabilitative process begins at the time of hospital admission. Burns have a significant impact on the child, family, and nursing staff. It is important that each individual deal with his or her feelings about the injury and that open communication be encouraged throughout hospitalization and the rehabilitation phase.

Parents need to be encouraged to discuss the circumstances surrounding the burn injury. Feelings of guilt should be addressed so that the parents can become active participants in the child's care. Parents are encouraged to visit as often as possible, to provide emotional support to the child, and to assist with various aspects of physical care, such as dressing changes and baths. Most important, parents should not be afraid to touch and hold the child and to show love and affection no matter how badly disfigured the child initially appears. If indicated, social services, support groups, and pastoral care representatives can be recommended to families needing support.

Burned children experience intense pain during dressing changes, hydrotherapy, debridement, and positioning. The nurse helps the child through painful procedures by providing emotional support and understanding. Because major burns often require extended hospitalization with slow physical recovery, the nurse becomes a key member of the child's support group, along with parents and family.

How a child responds to the events that caused the burn, and to pain, treatments, and the possibility of disfigurement will depend on his or her age and developmental stage. Throughout the healing process, the nurse needs to keep in mind the child's developmental stage.

REVIEW QUESTIONS

A. Multiple choice. Select the best answer.

1. Which of the following disorders is apt to be seen in all age groups?
   a. diaper dermatitis
   b. ringworm
   c. acne
   d. seborrheic dermatitis
2. A common presenting sign of impetigo is
   a. formation of a thin-walled lesion that ruptures, forming a honey-colored crust
   b. greasy or dry scaling lesions
   c. a widespread, erythematous rash
   d. papular lesions with a thickened, hardened appearance
3. Jamie, 9 years old, has recently developed tinea corporis. This infection is characterized by
   a. fungal infection of the head and scalp
   b. round lesions with central clearing and a scaly border
   c. vesicular lesions with weeping
   d. fissuring and pinhead-sized lesions
4. Which major type of acne is most likely to lead to severe scar formation?
   a. cystic acne
   b. papulopustular acne
   c. comedomal acne
   d. sebaceous acne
5. Symptomatic type 1 herpes is most commonly seen in
   a. children over 5 years of age
   b. adolescents who contract the infection through intimate contact
   c. children under 5 years of age
   d. school-age children who contract the infection from friends
6. The Lund and Browder formula is used to determine
   a. duration of contact
   b. depth of burn injury
   c. type of burn
   d. extent of burn
7. Which of the following might be used as a topical burn medication?
   a. betadine solution
   b. cortisone
   c. retinoid cream
   d. lindane
8. The most common types of burns are
   a. chemical
   b. electrical
   c. thermal
   d. radiation

B. Match the term in column I to the correct definition in column II.

Column I

1. atopic dermatitis
2. pediculosis capitis
3. xenograft
4. allograft
5. impetigo

Column II

a. a highly contagious bacterial infection of the skin, most commonly seen on face, limbs, hands, and neck
b. the best temporary skin graft; made of fresh cadaver skin
c. a chronic, inflammatory skin disease characterized by crusting lesions in areas rich in sebaceous glands
d. a commercially available temporary skin covering, usually pigskin
e. an infection caused by the laying of eggs or nits

SUGGESTED ACTIVITIES

- Make up teaching tools that can be used with parents of children in a particular age group (infants and toddlers, preschool and school-age, or adolescent) to help parents learn how to prevent, identify, and treat skin diseases common to the age group.
- Interview parents or children who have experienced one of the skin disorders discussed in the chapter. Find out about the feelings of the parent(s) or child, the reaction of others to the child, and the approaches to coping that were chosen by parent(s) or children.
- Interview a nurse who has worked on a burn unit. Find out about techniques that the nurse has used to make the experience less traumatic for burned children and their parents. Find out how the nurse deals with his or her own feelings and stress.

BIBLIOGRAPHY

Adamski, D. B. Assessment and treatment of allergic response to stinging insects. *Journal of Emergency Nursing* 16 (1990): 70–80.

Betz, C. L., and E. C. Poster. *Mosby's Pediatric Nursing Reference*, 2nd ed. St. Louis, MO: Mosby-Year Book, 1992.

Broadwell Jackson, D., and R. B. Saunders. *Child Health Nursing*. Philadelphia: J. B. Lippincott, 1993.

Budassi Sheehy, S. *Mosby's Manual of Emergency Care*, 3rd ed. St. Louis, MO: Mosby-Year Book, 1990.

Budassi Sheehy, S., J. A. Marvin, and C. D. Jimmerson. *Manual of Clinical Trauma Care: The First Hour*, St. Louis, MO: Mosby-Year Book, 1989.

Castiglia, P. T. Acne. *Journal of Pediatric Health Care* 3 (1989): 259–261.

Clore, E. R. Dispelling the common myths about pediculosis. *Journal of Pediatric Health Care* 3 (1989): 28–33.

Eichelberger, M. R., J. W. Ball, G. S. Pratsch, and E. Runion. *Pediatric Emergencies: A Manual for Prehospital Care Providers*. Englewood Cliffs, NJ: Brady/Prentice-Hall, 1992.

Fritsch, D. F., and D. M. Fredrick Pilat. Exposing latex allergies. *Nursing '93* 23, no. 8 (1993): 46–48.

Habif, T. *Clinical Dermatology: A Color Guide to Diagnosis and Therapy*, 2nd ed. St. Louis, MO: Mosby-Year Book, 1990.

Hathaway, W. E., W. W. Hay, Jr., J. R. Groothuis, and J. W. Paisley. *Current Pediatric Diagnosis and Treatment*, 11th ed. Norwalk, CT: Appleton & Lange, 1993.

Park, B. R., and D. Smith. Treatment of head lice and scabies in children. *Pediatric Nursing* 15 (1989): 522–524.

Rosenstein, B. J., and P. D. Fosarelli. *Pediatric Pearls: The Handbook of Practical Pediatrics*. St. Louis, MO: Mosby-Year Book, 1989.

Rudolph, A. M. *Rudolph's Pediatrics*, 19th ed. Norwalk, CT: Appleton & Lange, 1991.

Wong, D. L. *Whaley & Wong's Essentials of Pediatric Nursing*, 4th ed. St. Louis, MO: Mosby-Year Book, 1993.

Zitelli, B. J., and H. W. Davis. *Atlas of Pediatric Physical Diagnosis*, 2nd ed. St. Louis, MO: Mosby/Gower, 1991.

Conditions of the Eyes and Ears

Objectives

After studying this chapter, the student should be able to:

- Briefly describe strabismus and discuss its symptoms, treatment, and nursing care.
- Describe the cause, symptoms, and implications of several common childhood eye conditions.
- Describe several types of trauma to the eye.
- Discuss the implications of visual impairment and identify methods of vision assessment in childhood.
- Briefly describe otitis media and discuss its symptoms, treatment, and nursing care.
- Describe several types of trauma to the ear.
- Discuss the implications of hearing impairment and identify methods of hearing assessment in childhood.

Key Terms

diplopia
photophobia
visual acuity
occlusion therapy
visual field
tympanometry
myringotomy

Conditions of the eyes and ears are among the most common disorders affecting infants and young children. Because normal vision and hearing are essential for learning, assessment and treatment of eye and ear problems are important aspects of pediatric care. Vision and hearing screening are performed routinely throughout childhood. Problems such as strabismus, amblyopia, glaucoma, and cataracts should be diagnosed and treated promptly to prevent decrease or possible loss of vision. Children are also treated for infectious conditions, such as conjunctivitis or otitis media, and injuries to the eye and ear.

Overview of the Eye

The eye consists of external structures (eyelid, conjunctiva, lacrimal glands) that serve to protect and lubricate the globe of the eye, Figure 36–1a and internal structures that make vision possible. Internal structures of the eye include the sclera, cornea, pupil, iris, lens, aqueous and vitreous humor, and retina, Figure 36–1b.

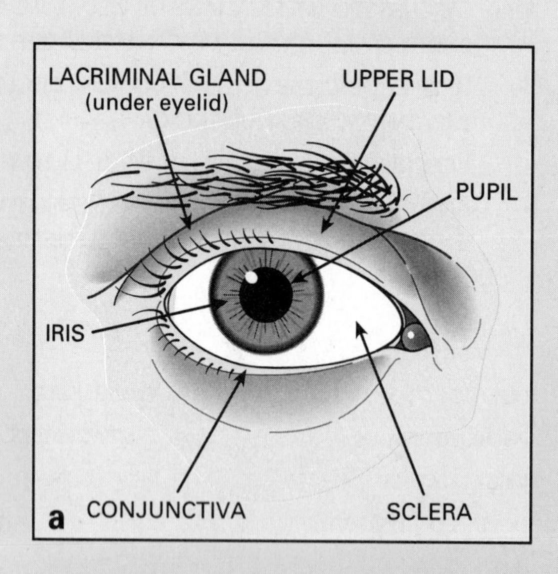

Figure 36–1 *(a) External view of the eye. (b) Cross section of the eye. (b adapted from Smith, Davis, and Dennerll,* Medical Terminology: A Programmed Approach, *6th ed. Delmar Publishers Inc., 1991)*

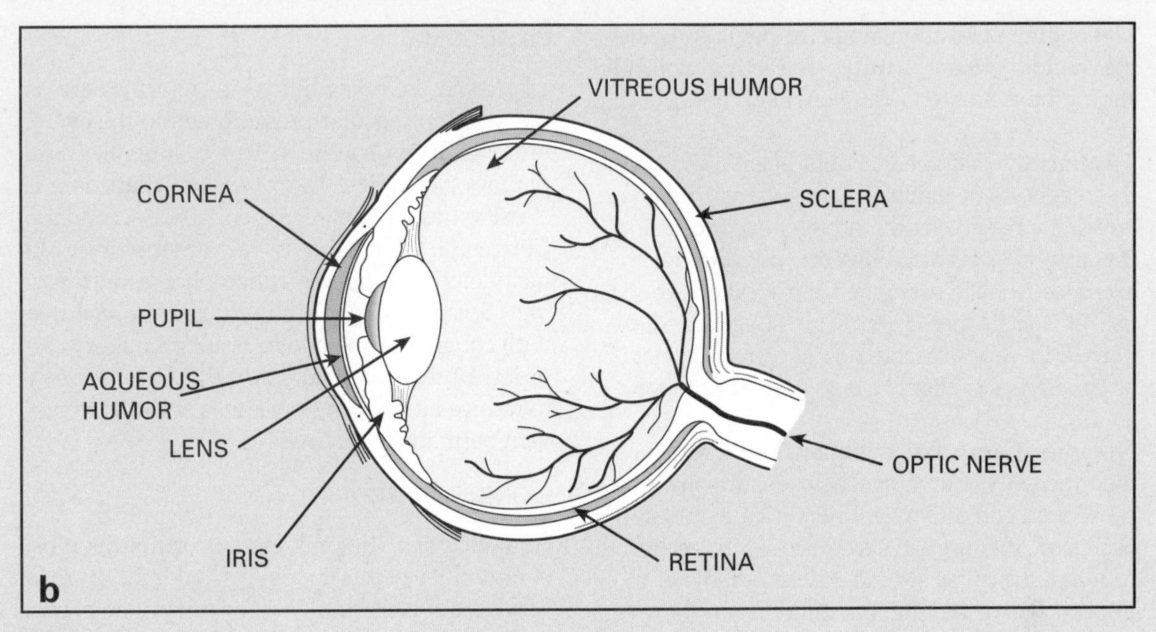

Figure 36–1 *continued*

Conditions of the Eye

Strabismus

Description. Strabismus refers to misalignment (crossing) of the eyes. Although commonly termed "cross-eye," the condition may affect one or both eyes, and it may involve eyes turning inward (esotropia), outward (exotropia), upward (hypertropia), or downward (hypotropia), Figure 36–2. Strabismus may occur as a result of muscle imbalance, poor vision, or a congenital defect (Hathaway et al. 1993).

Symptoms. The child with strabismus may develop a squint or frown in an attempt to focus the eyes. Difficulty occurs when the child attempts to shift the focus from one distance to another. The child has trouble picking up objects and cannot see print or moving objects clearly. Common symptoms are double vision (**diplopia**), extreme sensitivity to light (**photophobia**), dizziness, and headache. Diagnosis is often made by inspection of the child's eyes.

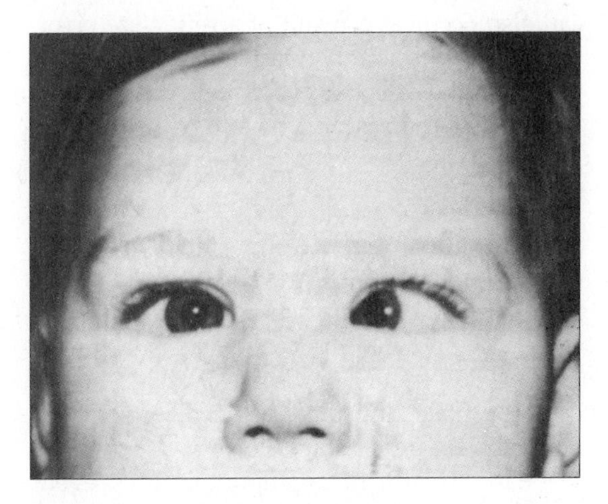

Figure 36–2 *Strabismus (esotropia) (From Newell,* Ophthalmology: Principles and Concepts, *7th ed. Mosby-Year Book, St. Louis, 1992)*

The degree of fixation, angle of deviation, and the child's **visual acuity** (refractive ability) should be evaluated (Vaughan et al. 1992).

Treatment. Treatment should begin as soon as the diagnosis is made. Treatment may involve wearing a patch over the stronger eye (**occlusion therapy**) to prevent amblyopia, performing eye exercises to help strengthen the weaker eye, or use of special prescription glasses or medications. If these approaches do not correct the deviation, surgery to align the eyes may be necessary.

Nursing Care. Once strabismus has been identified, the nurse can help ensure that the prescribed corrective treatment is carried out. If occlusion therapy or eye exercises have been ordered, the nurse should advise parents of the importance of having the child wear the eye patch or perform the exercises as prescribed.

AMBLYOPIA

Amblyopia, also known as "lazy eye," is a condition of reduced vision in one or both eyes. The most common cause is untreated strabismus, which causes the brain to suppress the visual image in the deviating eye. Amblyopia can also occur as a result of a refractive error. The child with amblyopia has reduced visual acuity in the affected eye. Treatment consists of patching, glasses, and visual exercises.

CATARACTS

A cataract is an opacity (or clouding) of the crystalline lens, which prevents the passage of light to the retina. Cataracts may occur in one or both eyes and may be congenital or acquired (the result of trauma or diseases). Children with cataracts have difficulty seeing objects clearly and may lose peripheral vision.

Early treatment is important to prevent long-term visual impairment. Treatment consists of surgery to remove the cloudy lens and fitting the child with removable contact lenses or glasses a few days after surgery.

GLAUCOMA

Glaucoma is a condition in which there is increased intraocular pressure within the eye. If untreated, this condition can eventually cause partial or complete loss of vision. Glaucoma is classified as primary (congenital) or secondary. Congenital glaucoma is rare. Symptoms can include corneal opacity, photophobia, and tearing. Secondary glaucoma occurs in children with congenital, metabolic, or inflammatory disorders of the eye (Rudolph 1991). Early surgery to reduce intraocular pressure is essential to prevent permanent blindness.

CONJUNCTIVITIS

Conjunctivitis, or "pink eye," is one of the most common eye conditions in children. It may result from bacterial, viral, or fungal infections; from allergic reactions; or from physical or chemical irritants (Hathaway et al. 1993). Symptoms include diffuse redness of the conjunctiva with a watery or purulent discharge from the eye. Vision is usually normal.

The treatment of conjunctivitis depends on the cause. Treatment of bacterial conjunctivitis involves identifying the causative organism, by smear or culture, and administering either a broad-spectrum antibiotic or ophthalmic drops or ointment. Conjunctivitis is extremely contagious. The nurse should instruct parents to wash hands after touching the child or giving eye drops or ointment and to keep the child's wash cloth and towels separate from those of other family members.

RETINOBLASTOMA

Retinoblastoma is a congenital, malignant tumor that occurs in the first two years of life. It is the most common retinal tumor occurring in childhood. The initial sign is the presence of a white reflex, or cat's eye reflex, in place of the normal red reflex. Early diagnosis and treatment are essential to prevent spread through the optic nerve and orbital tissues. Enucleation is the treatment of choice.

TRAUMA

Trauma to the eye may take many forms. The most common are foreign bodies, injury to the eyelid and cornea, burns, and child abuse.

Foreign Bodies. Foreign bodies are often found in the conjunctiva, cornea, and intraocular areas. A foreign body can usually be removed without difficulty from the conjunctiva using a moist cotton applicator or gauze pad. Before attempting to remove an object from the cornea, an anesthetic should be applied. More deeply imbedded foreign bodies are serious injuries that require ophthalmologic examination and prompt treatment (Hathaway et al. 1993). The nurse should instruct parents never to try to remove an object that has penetrated the eye.

Injuries to the Eyelids. Bruises to the eyelid should always be carefully assessed to determine whether there is any injury to the globe. Bruises can be treated initially using cold compresses to reduce bleeding and swelling. If the child sustains any type of laceration to the eyelid, referral should be made to an ophthalmologist.

Corneal Injuries. The cornea may be injured through abrasion or laceration. The child with a corneal abrasion is usually extremely uncomfortable. Treatment involves instillation of a mild paralyzing agent (cycloplegic) to the cornea, use of an antibiotic ointment, and patching of the eye for two to four days. The child with a corneal laceration should be referred to an ophthalmologist. Treatment involves suturing, observation for infection, and systemic antibiotics and tetanus toxoid, if laceration occurred with a contaminated object.

Burns. Burns that affect the external or internal structures of the eye are serious injuries. Burns to the eyelids should be treated like burns to any other part of the skin (see Chapter 35).

Chemical burns of the cornea and conjunctiva should be treated as an emergency, with tap water irrigations and topical anesthetics. The upper lid should be everted carefully and flushed thoroughly. Any child who suffers a severe chemical burn of the eye should be hospitalized and seen by an ophthalmologist.

Ultraviolet burns of the cornea can be caused by welders flash, exposure to snow on the ski slopes, or a treatment lamp or sunlamp. These burns cause severe pain and tearing and are treated using topical anesthetic, analgesics, antibiotic ointment, and eye patches.

Infrared burns, which can result from unfiltered observation of an eclipse or exposure to and penetration of x-rays, also require referral to an ophthalmologist. Infrared burns are serious injuries that can result in a permanent loss of vision.

Child Abuse. Injury to the eye may also be caused by child abuse. Common signs of such eye trauma include bruises of the eyelids, conjunctival bleeding, bleeding within the aqueous humor, and retinal hemorrhage. The nurse should refer a child with any of these symptoms to an ophthalmologist for a thorough examination. (Child abuse is discussed in more detail in Chapter 26.)

VISUAL IMPAIRMENT

The function of the external and internal eye structures and related cranial nerves makes vision possible. Early diagnosis of a visual impairment is important, because vision is an essential sense for learning. Vision assessment should be a routine component of the child's physical examination. Evaluation should include screening children at risk because of heredity, maternal rubella infection, or prematurity; observing for behaviors that indicate a vision problem; and testing of visual acuity and **visual field** (area of vision).

It is recommended that routine eye examinations be performed shortly after birth, at 6 months, at 4 years, at 5 years, and then every two years until age 16. Color vision testing should be performed between the ages of 8 and 12 years (Vaughan et al. 1992). The Snellen alphabet chart and the "E" chart are commonly used to test distance vision, Figure 36–3a,b. The child with a visual acuity score of 20/200 or less in the good eye after correction or a visual field of no greater than 20 degrees in the better eye is termed legally blind.

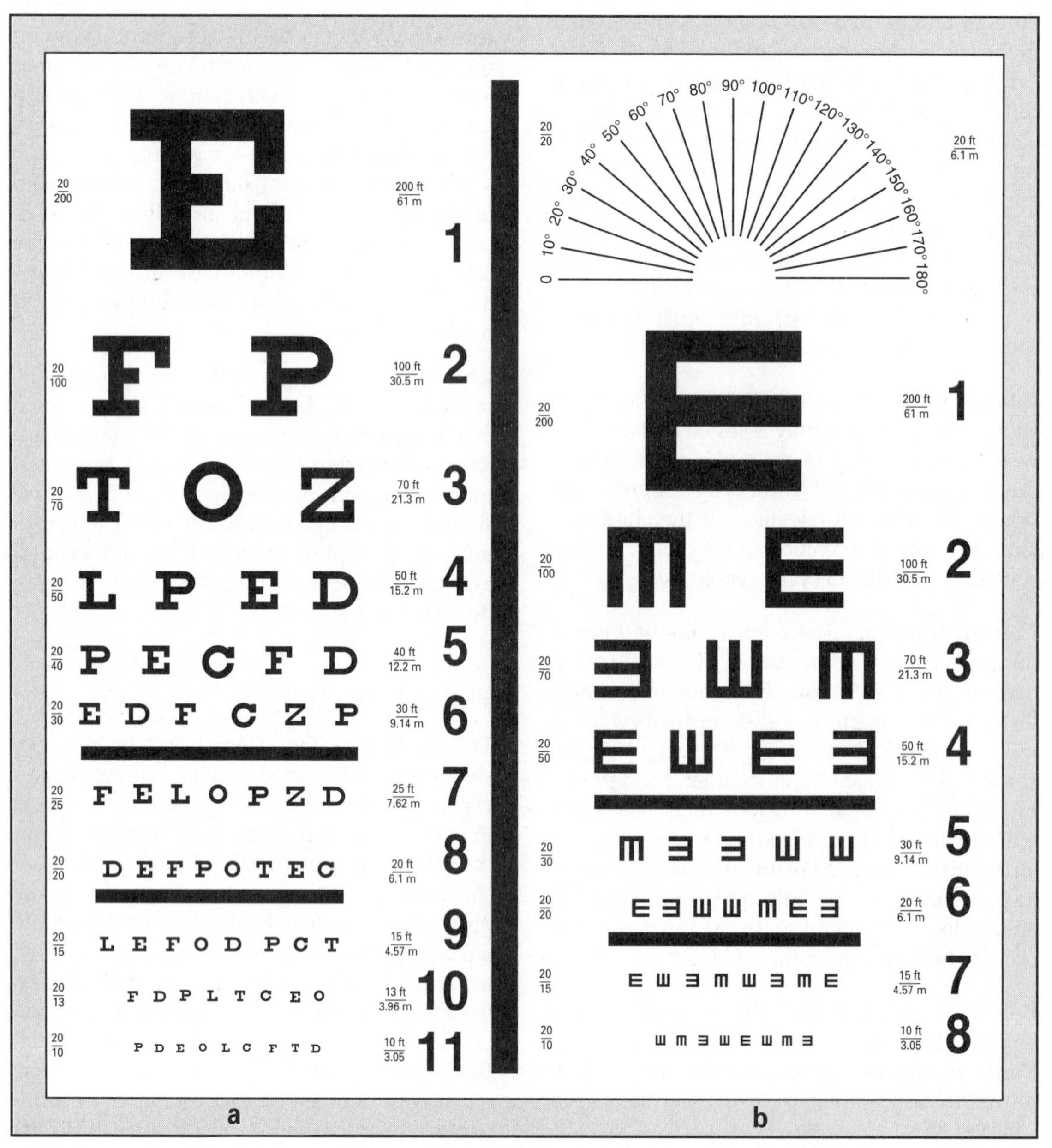

Figure 36–3 *(a) Snellen alphabet chart for testing distance vision. (b)* E *test for testing distance vision in illiterate patients, particularly preschool children. (Courtesy of the National Society to Prevent Blindness)*

Overview of the Ear

The ear is composed of three parts: the outer (or external) ear, the middle ear, and the inner ear, Figure 36–4a,b. The external auditory canal leads to the tympanic membrane, which separates the outer ear from the middle ear. The middle ear, made up of the ossicles (malleus, incus, and stapes), transmits sound from the tympanic membrane to the inner ear, composed of the cochlea and semicircular canals. The eustachian tube connects the middle ear to the pharynx and serves to equalize pressure inside the ear with that of the outside environment.

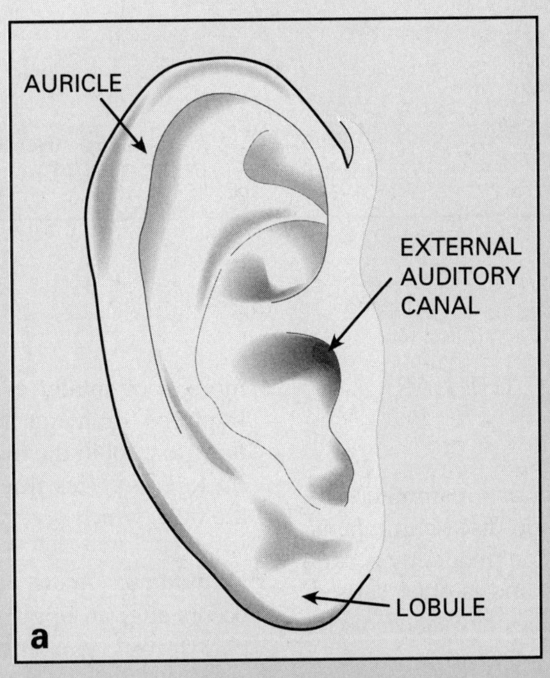

Figure 36–4 *(a) External view of the ear. (b) Cross section of the ear. (b adapted from Smith, Davis, and Dennerll,* Medical Terminology: A Programmed Approach, *6th ed. Delmar Publishers Inc., 1991)*

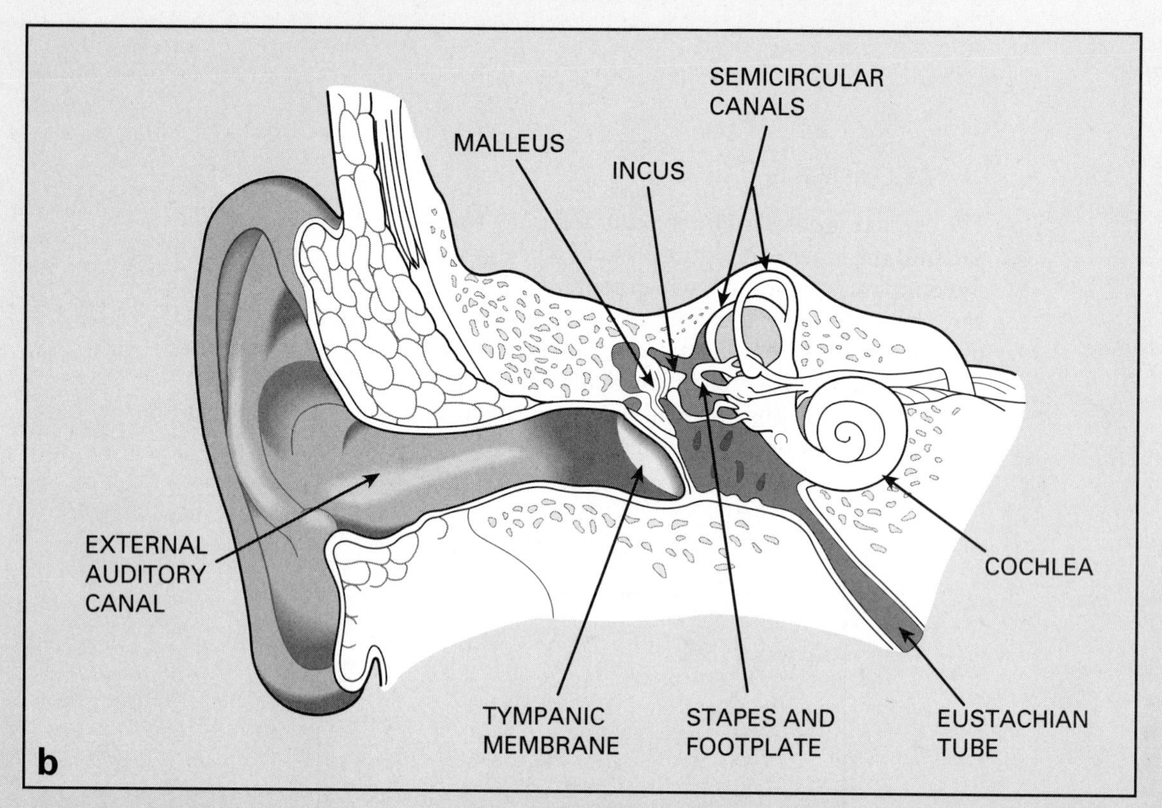

Figure 36–4 *continued*

Conditions of the Ear

Otitis Media

Description. Otitis media, an inflammation of the middle ear, is a common disease in infants and young children. Infection frequently occurs during the winter months and is often caused by *Streptococcus*, *Haemophilus*, or *Staphylococcus* organisms.

Otitis media occurs as an acute or chronic disorder. The acute form develops rapidly and resolves within about three weeks. Chronic otitis media is defined as an infection that lasts more than three months.

Infants and children are prone to otitis media because the eustachian tube is angled more horizontally in children than in adults. Impaired drainage in the tube causes secretions to pool in the middle ear, allowing bacteria to grow. This fluid causes pressure within the tube, which is very painful.

Symptoms. Acute otitis media frequently occurs after an upper respiratory infection. Ear pain, fever, crying, fussiness, irritability, pulling at the affected ear, and loss of appetite are common symptoms. There may be visible drainage from the ear.

Otoscopic examination reveals an immobile, red tympanic membrane. Landmarks are either poorly visible, absent, or distorted, depending on whether fluid is present in the middle ear space. **Tympanometry** (measurement of the internal ear pressure) is often performed to confirm the diagnosis. Because recurrence or persistence of otitis media places infants and children at risk for permanent ear damage or hearing loss, early identification is essential.

Treatment. Treatment consists of systemic antibiotics, antibiotic ear drops, analgesics, or antipyretic drugs to help reduce symptoms of fever and pain. Most children improve within two to four days. The child should be examined after the completion of antibiotic therapy for complications or residual hearing impairment. Some children may require **myringotomy** (surgical incision of the eardrum) and insertion of tympanostomy (PE) tubes to relieve symptoms of severe pain and to promote drainage.

Nursing Care. Nurses should be aware of the possibility of otitis media when caring for children with upper respiratory infections. In addition to the treatment measures outlined above, parents may be instructed to have the child lie on the affected side, to encourage drainage from the ear.

Parents should be advised of the possibility of temporary hearing loss (sometimes lasting several months), which may accompany acute otitis media. To help prevent future occurrences, the nurse should teach parents to place infants in an upright position for feedings, avoid propping bottles, and never allow the infant or young child to go to bed with a bottle. Parents should also teach small children how to blow their noses, as this clears out the eustachian tube, preventing pooling of secretions.

TRAUMA

Children frequently sustain trauma to the ear. Common forms of trauma are abrasions, lacerations, rupture of the tympanic membrane, and insertion of a foreign body.

Abrasions and Lacerations. Children may cause abrasions or lacerations of the ear canal by inserting sharp objects into the ear. Injuries can also be caused by parents' attempts to remove ear wax. In all cases, the tympanic membrane should be examined to ensure that it is free of injury. Abrasions and lacerations of the canal tend to heal readily; therefore, as long as the tympanic membrane is uninjured, no treatment is necessary. Lacerations to the outer ear require sutures.

Rupture of the Tympanic Membrane. A perforation of the tympanic membrane can occur as a result of a head injury, a blow to the side of the head and ear, or the insertion of a sharp, pointed object such as a stick, paper clip, bobby pin, or ballpoint pen into the ear canal. The child should be referred to an otolaryngologist, because these injuries do not heal spontaneously.

Foreign Bodies. Children may intentionally or unintentionally put almost any object into the ear. Objects that are frequently found include paper, wadded tissue, beads, earring parts, and insects. An initial attempt may be made to remove the foreign body by pulling on the earlobe to straighten the ear canal and then gently shaking the child's head. If this method fails, various other measures may be used to try to remove the object, including use of a cotton-tipped applicator coated with warmed wax, forceps, or irrigation. If the object is large or wedged in the ear canal, the child should be referred to an otolaryngologist for treatment (Hathaway et al. 1993).

HEARING IMPAIRMENT

Hearing is essential for normal speech development and learning. For this reason, hearing evaluation should be performed frequently in children from infancy through adolescence.

Each year, approximately 1,000 children are born deaf in the United States (Riley 1987).

Hearing loss may also occur during early childhood as the result of birth trauma, maternal rubella infection, chronic otitis media, meningitis, or antibiotics that damage cranial nerve VIII.

Screening is essential for early detection and diagnosis of hearing impairment. Attainment of hearing and speech milestones is used as an initial hearing screen. Sometimes hearing is assessed by watching the child's reaction to various auditory stimuli. Preschool children can be tested using earphones and pure tone audiometry.

REVIEW QUESTIONS

A. Multiple choice. Select the best answer.

1. Andrea, 8 years old, has diplopia and photophobia and complains to her mother of frequent headaches. These are symptoms of
   a. strabismus
   b. amblyopia
   c. glaucoma
   d. cataract
2. The white reflex is an initial sign of what disorder?
   a. glaucoma
   b. amblyopia
   c. retinoblastoma
   d. corneal laceration
3. Treatment for amblyopia might include all of the following except
   a. wearing a patch over the weak eye
   b. performing eye exercises to help strengthen the weaker eye
   c. surgery to align the eyes
   d. use of prescription glasses
4. A foreign body can usually be removed without difficulty from the
   a. conjunctiva
   b. cornea
   c. aqueous humor
   d. sclera
5. Color vision assessment is usually performed
   a. at birth, 6 months, and 4 years of age, and every 2 years thereafter
   b. at birth, 6 years, and 12 years of age
   c. between the ages of 8 and 12 years
   d. when a child enters school (5 to 6 years of age)
6. Michael, 5 years old, has acute otitis media. This condition
   a. requires surgical treatment using myringotomy
   b. is a congenital defect of the eustachian tube
   c. occurs frequently in summer months
   d. may be caused by *Haemophilus* organisms
7. The middle ear consists of the
   a. auricle, tympanic membrane, and ossicles
   b. ossicles, cochlea, and semicircular canals
   c. tympanic membrane and eustachian tube
   d. malleus, incus, and stapes

B. Match the term in column I to the correct description in column II.

Column I	Column II
1. amblyopia	a. increased pressure within the eye
2. glaucoma	b. a congenital, malignant tumor that occurs in the first two years of life
3. cataract	c. "lazy eye"; reduced vision in one or both eyes
4. retinoblastoma	d. clouding of the crystalline lens
5. conjunctivitis	e. redness and discharge caused by infection, allergic reaction, or physical irritant

SUGGESTED ACTIVITIES

- Make a poster or give a presentation on ways of preventing trauma to the eyes or ears.
- Discuss the importance of the eyes and ears in childhood development. Interview a special education teacher or a parent to find out how children with vision or hearing impairments compensate.
- There are a number of inspirational biographies of vision-, speech-, or hearing-impaired people. Read one of those biographies and demonstrate how the inspirational story can be used in a health care setting.
- Interview a health care worker who is involved with vision- or hearing-impaired clients. Ask what kind of differences exist between children who have been impaired since birth and those who develop an impairment later in life. Discuss the implications for you as a nurse dealing with those children or their families.

BIBLIOGRAPHY

Bluestone, C. D. Modern management of otitis media. *Pediatric Clinics of North America* 36 (1989): 1371–1387.

Broadwell Jackson, D., and R. B. Saunders. *Child Health Nursing*. Philadelphia: J. B. Lippincott, 1993.

Budassi Sheehy, S. *Mosby's Manual of Emergency Care*, 3rd ed. St. Louis, MO: Mosby-Year Book, 1990.

Fisher, M. C. Conjunctivitis in children. *Pediatric Clinics of North America* 34 (1987): 1447–1456.

Hathaway, W. E., W. W. Hay, Jr., J. R. Groothuis, and J. W. Paisley. *Current Pediatric Diagnosis and Treatment*, 11th ed. Norwalk, CT: Appleton & Lange, 1993.

Newell, F. W. *Ophthalmology: Principles and Concepts*, 7th ed. St. Louis, MO: Mosby-Year Book, 1992.

Riley, M. A. *Nursing Care of the Child with Ear, Nose, and Throat Disorders*. New York: Springer, 1987.

Rosenstein, B. J., and P. D. Fosarelli. *Pediatric Pearls: The Handbook of Practical Pediatrics*. St. Louis, MO: Mosby-Year Book, 1989.

Rudolph, A. M. *Rudolph's Pediatrics*, 19th ed. Norwalk, CT: Appleton & Lange, 1991.

Vaughan, D. G., T. Asbury, and P. Riordan-Eva. *General Ophthalmology*, 13th ed. Norwalk, CT: Appleton & Lange, 1992.

Wong, D. L. *Whaley & Wong's Essentials of Pediatric Nursing*, 4th ed. St. Louis, MO: Mosby-Year Book, 1993.

CHAPTER

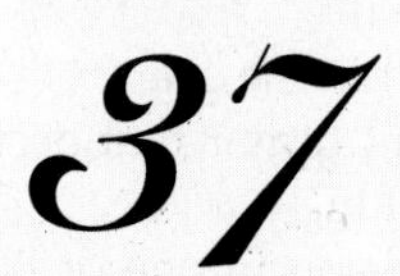

Cardiovascular Conditions

Objectives

AFTER STUDYING THIS CHAPTER, THE STUDENT SHOULD BE ABLE TO:

- DIFFERENTIATE BETWEEN CONGENITAL AND ACQUIRED HEART DISEASES AND GIVE AN EXAMPLE OF EACH.
- DESCRIBE THE CHANGES THAT TAKE PLACE IN THE CARDIOVASCULAR SYSTEM AT BIRTH.
- DIFFERENTIATE BETWEEN CYANOTIC AND ACYANOTIC HEART DEFECTS AND GIVE EXAMPLES OF EACH.
- DISCUSS COMMON DIAGNOSTIC PROCEDURES PERFORMED ON CHILDREN WITH CONGENITAL HEART DISEASE.
- DISCUSS THE CAUSES, SYMPTOMS, TREATMENT, AND NURSING CARE OF CONGESTIVE HEART FAILURE.
- DISCUSS THE CAUSES, SYMPTOMS, TREATMENT, AND NURSING CARE OF SYSTEMIC HYPERTENSION.
- DISCUSS THE CAUSES, SYMPTOMS, TREATMENT, AND NURSING CARE OF RHEUMATIC FEVER.

Key Terms

CONGENITAL HEART DISEASE
ACQUIRED HEART DISEASE
ACYANOTIC HEART DISEASE
CYANOTIC HEART DISEASE
BACTERIAL ENDOCARDITIS
CONGESTIVE HEART FAILURE
CHOREA

Cardiovascular conditions are some of the most serious illnesses that affect children. These conditions most often affect the child's heart and great vessels. A **congenital heart disease** develops during fetal development and is present at birth. The majority of these defects are diagnosed within the first month of life. An **acquired heart disease** occurs after birth as a result of complication of another disease.

Families of children diagnosed with congenital heart disease often experience anxiety, fear, and guilt because of their lack of understanding about their child's disease and its treatment (Kashani and Higgins 1986). The nurse can play an instrumental role by providing emotional support to parents. This support can include active listening, family referral to a counselor or therapist, teaching the family about their child's disease and its treatment, or referral to support groups in the community.

Overview of the System

The cardiovascular system is composed of the heart (Figure 37–1), arteries, veins, and capillaries. The main function of the heart is to pump blood throughout the body and to the lungs, oxygenating and carrying nutrients to the cells and removing the waste products of metabolism.

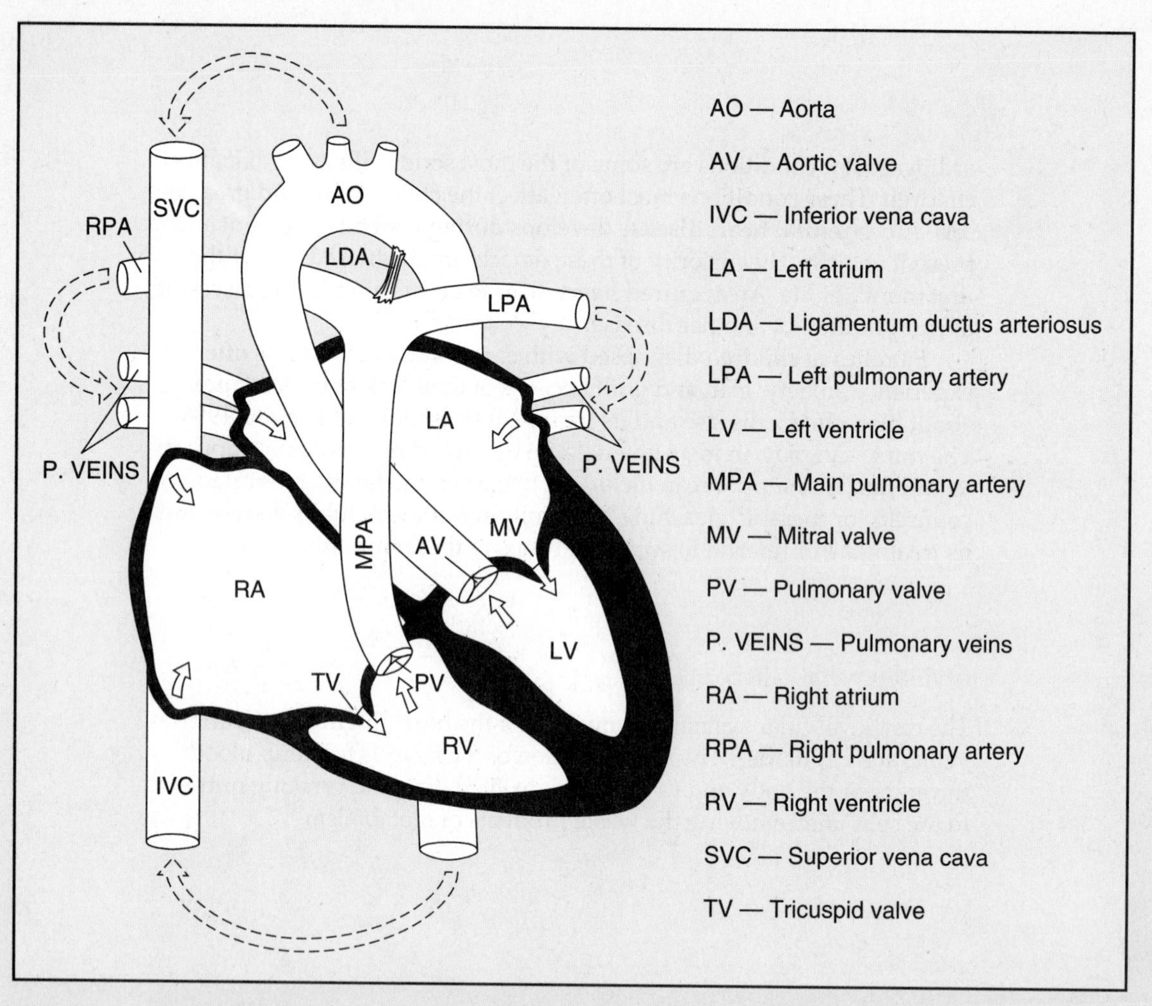

Figure 37–1 *Anatomy of the heart (Courtesy Ross Laboratories)*

Postnatal Circulation

At birth, the circulation of blood through the cardiovascular system changes. When an infant takes his or her first breath, the lungs fill with air. The lungs are now responsible for oxygenating the blood. The three fetal shunts — the ductus venosus, foramen ovale, and ductus arteriosus — that enabled the majority of blood to bypass the liver and the lungs are no longer needed and will, within days or weeks, cease to function.

The ductus venosus constricts at birth and closes within 48 hours. As the infant breathes air into the lungs, the pulmonary vascular resistance (flow of blood into the lungs) decreases. This decreased resistance results in closure of the foramen ovale within several weeks of birth. The ductus arteriosus constricts at birth and, in most infants, closes anatomically within the first several days of life. It can take months, however, for total closure to occur, and the ductus arteriosus can reopen under stressful conditions such as hypoxemia or acidosis.

INFANT

CONGENITAL HEART DISEASE

Description. Congenital heart disease occurs in 8 to 10 of 1,000 live births (Hazinski 1992). Ninety percent of congenital heart diseases in children are a result of multifactorial inheritance (genetic or environmental factors). The most common causes are maternal alcoholism, rubella during the first trimester of pregnancy, insulin-dependent diabetes, and maternal trimethadione ingestion (Daberkow and Washington 1989). The majority of congenital heart diseases develop during the fourth through seventh weeks of fetal life, because it is during this time that the heart is forming. Refer to Chapter 4 for a discussion of fetal circulation.

Classification. Congenital heart diseases are classified as either acyanotic or cyanotic. **Acyanotic heart disease** is usually associated with defects that increase the flow of blood to the lungs. Blood flows from the left to the right side of the heart, where it is oxygenated and mixes with unoxygenated blood. No change in the infant's skin coloring is noted. The most common acyanotic heart defect is a ventricular septal defect.

Cyanotic heart disease is usually associated with defects that result in the mixing of unoxygenated blood with oxygenated blood. The child's skin is bluish because of the unoxygenated blood circulating through the systemic circulatory system. Cyanotic heart defects may also be caused by an obstruction in the aorta or the left side of the heart. The most common cyanotic heart defect is tetralogy of Fallot.

Symptoms and Treatment. Several of the most common acyanotic and cyanotic heart defects of children are illustrated in Figure 37–2. Figure 37–3 (page 605) summarizes signs and symptoms and treatment for these defects. The defects can occur alone or in combination with each other.

Diagnosis is made by both invasive and noninvasive methods. Noninvasive methods include history, physical examination, chest x-ray, electrocardiogram (ECG), and echocardiogram. Invasive methods include cardiac catheterization and angiography.

Cardiac catheterization involves the insertion of a radiopaque catheter under fluoroscopy. The catheter is usually inserted through the femoral artery or vein into the heart, allowing visualization of the valves, chambers, and great vessels, as well as measurement of pressures and oxygen saturations within the heart. If angiography is performed at the same time, a contrast dye is injected through the catheter to observe blood flow through the heart. Nursing care for a child undergoing cardiac catheterization is summarized in Figure 37–4 (page 610).

Children with congenital heart defects are at risk for developing congestive heart failure and bacterial endocarditis. Congestive heart failure occurs when the heart fails to compensate for changes in blood flow and fails to pump blood efficiently through the heart (see Congestive Heart Failure, below). Bacterial endocarditis is a bacterial infection of the valves or the inner lining of the heart. It occurs most often in children with valvular abnormalities, prosthetic valves, and heart defects that produce turbulent blood flow and after cardiac surgery in which a catheter was placed within the heart.

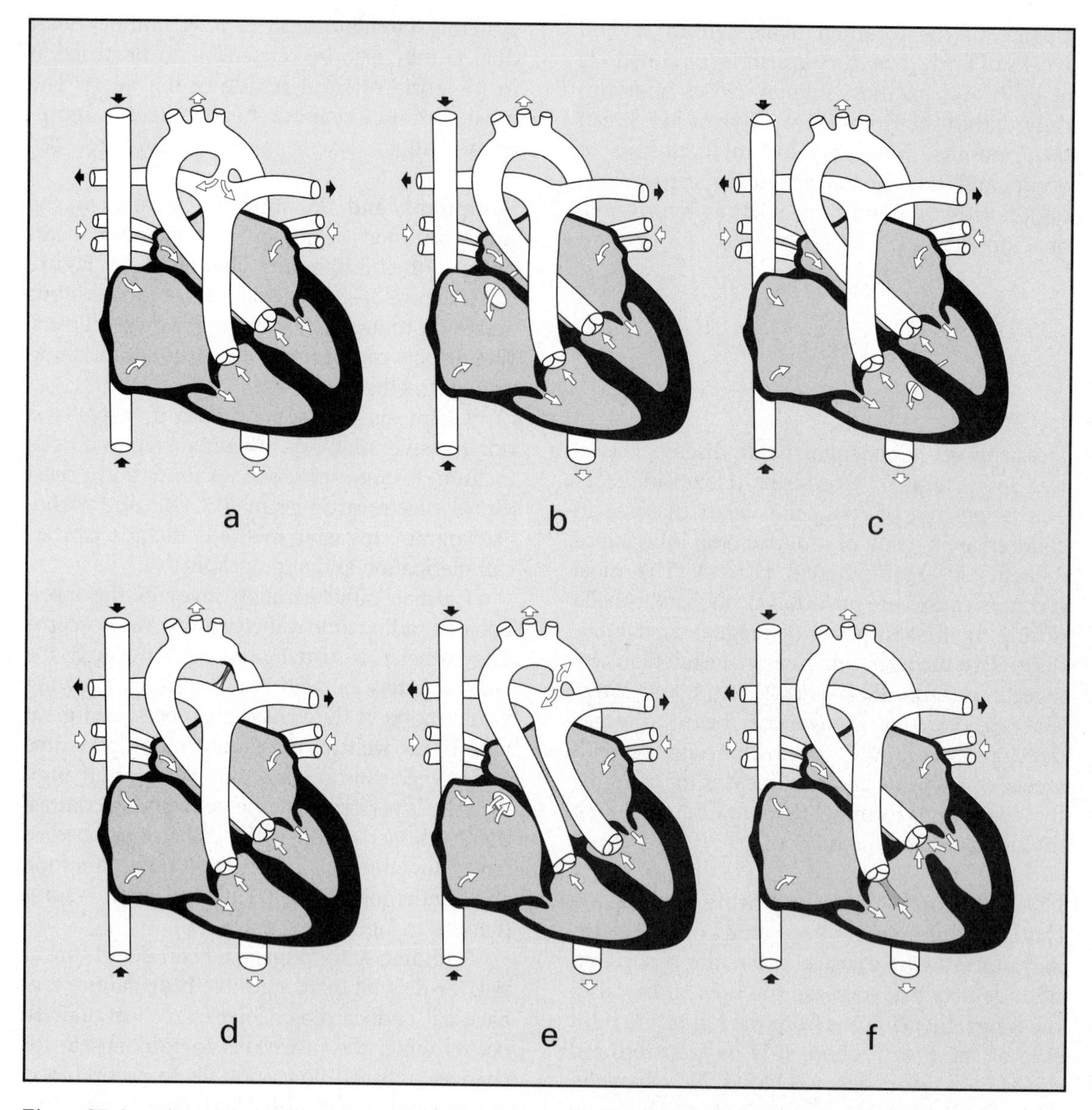

Figure 37–2 *Acyanotic (a–d) and cyanotic (e–f) heart defects (a) Patent ductus arteriosus (b) Atrial septal defects (c) Ventricular septal defect (d) Coarctation of the aorta (e) Complete transposition of the great vessels (f) Tetralogy of Fallot (Courtesy Ross Laboratories)*

CONGENITAL HEART DEFECTS

ACYANOTIC DEFECTS

Patent Ductus Arteriosus

Description		Signs and Symptoms
The ductus arteriosus is a remnant of fetal circulation. It closes shortly after birth and becomes a ligament. Failure of the ductus to close results in a continued flow of blood from the aorta to the pulmonary artery (a left-to-right shunting of blood). Blood flow to the lungs is increased. Premature infants are most at risk Figure 37–2a.		*Newborn:* Respiratory distress, congestive heart failure *Older Child:* Murmur, increased oxygen consumption, bounding pulses, widening pulse pressure, dyspnea
Atrial Septal Defect		
An abnormal opening in the wall or septum between the atria. With the change in blood flow after birth, pressures are higher on the left side of the heart than on the right. Blood flows from the left atrium to the right atrium then to the right ventricle, pulmonary artery, and into the lungs. Blood flow is increased to the lungs, Figure 37–2b.		Most children with an atrial septal defect are asymptomatic. Symptoms include systolic murmur, increased number of respiratory infections, decrease in normal exercise tolerance, delayed physical growth, congestive heart failure (uncommon), and cardiac enlargement.

Figure 37–3

continues

CONGENITAL HEART DEFECTS

Ventricular Septal Defect

Description	Signs and Symptoms	Treatment
An abnormal opening in the septum between the ventricles, causing blood to flow from the left ventricle to the right ventricle then to pulmonary artery and into the lungs, Figure 37–2c.	Symptoms vary with the size of the defect. Small or moderate-sized defects usually produce no symptoms and most close spontaneously, usually within the first year of life. Large defects usually are more serious. The child with a large ventricular septal defect has an increased amount of blood flow to the lungs. It may take 1 to 2 months before a child begins to have symptoms of congestive heart failure. Symptoms may include murmur, tachypnea, feeding difficulties, excessive perspiration, tachycardia, mild cyanosis, slow physical growth, splenomegaly, and irritability.	ASYMPTOMATIC INFANT/CHILD SURGICAL MANAGEMENT: Defect is closed with synthetic patch. SYMPTOMATIC INFANT/CHILD MEDICAL MANAGEMENT: Treatment of symptoms of congestive heart failure *Surgical management:* Palliative surgery includes banding of pulmonary artery (a piece of prosthetic material is tied around the main pulmonary artery to constrict blood flow to the lungs). Complete repair involves closing the defect with a prosthetic patch.

Figure 37–3 *continued*

Congenital Heart Defects

Description	Signs and Symptoms	Treatment
Coarctation of the Aorta		
A narrowing in the lumen of the aorta that obstructs blood flow to the lower extremities and body, while blood flow to the head and upper extremities is increased, Figure 37–2d.	Symptoms depend on the severity of the defect, the anatomical location, and the presence of other heart defects. *Infant:* Congestive heart failure, failure to thrive *Older Child:* Systolic murmur, hypertension, episodes of sudden or unexplained nosebleeds, frequent headaches, leg fatigue, full bounding pulses in upper extremities (increased blood pressure), weak or absent pulses in lower extremities (decreased blood pressure), and visible pulsation	*Surgical management:* Removal of the narrowed segment. End-to-end anastomosis of the aortic segments or insertion of a graft between the two ends of the aorta
Pulmonary Stenosis		
A narrowing at the entrance to the pulmonary artery that obstructs blood flow to the lungs, causing enlargement of the right ventricle (right ventricular hypertrophy) and decreased blood flow to the lungs.	Murmur, cardiomegaly, cyanosis (with severe stenosis), and right ventricular failure (with severe stenosis)	*Surgical management:* Valvotomy (surgical valve replacement) *Nonsurgical management:* Balloon angioplasty during cardiac catheterization to dilate valve

Figure 37–3

continues

CONGENITAL HEART DEFECTS

CYANOTIC DEFECTS

Complete Transposition of the Great Vessels

Description	Signs and Symptoms	Treatment
Reversal of the anatomical positions of the pulmonary artery and aorta, establishing two separate circulatory systems. The aorta originating from the right ventricle is pumping unoxygenated blood throughout the body, and the pulmonary artery originating from the left ventricle is pumping oxygenated blood to the lungs, Figure 37–2e.	Cyanosis, tachypnea, full bounding arterial pulses, poor physical growth, clubbing of fingers and toes	*Nonsurgical management:* Prostaglandins are continuously given intravenously to keep ductus arteriosus open. During cardiac catheterization a balloon atrial septostomy (Rashkind procedure) is performed, which creates an opening between the atria. These two openings allow unoxygenated blood to mix with oxygenated blood, which then circulates throughout body. *Surgical management:* Arteries may be switched to their original position (Jalene procedure) using cardiopulmonary bypass, or a large, single atrium may be created (Mustard procedure), allowing diversion of systemic blood flow to left side of heart and to pulmonary artery. Also allows pulmonary blood flow to be diverted to right side of heart and to aorta.

Figure 37–3 *continued*

Congenital Heart Defects

Tetralogy of Fallot

Description	Signs and Symptoms	Treatment
Consists of four heart defects: (1) ventricular septal defect, (2) right ventricular hypertrophy, (3) right ventricular outflow obstruction, and (4) overriding aorta, Figure 37–2f.	Cyanosis, poor physical growth, systolic murmur, hypoxic spells, polycythemia, activity intolerance, and squatting	*Surgical management:* Palliative procedures are usually performed initially to increase blood flow to the lungs by an anastomosis between the subclavian artery and the pulmonary artery. Either a Blalock-Tussing shunt or a Modified Blalock-Tussing shunt is performed. Complete correction to close the ventricular septal defect and relieve right ventricular outflow obstruction will take place usually between the ages of 8 months and 3 years if infant or child is stable. Corrective surgery may take place sooner if the infant or child has severe hypoxemia, severe polycythemia, a decrease in exercise intolerance, or an increase in hypercyanotic spells (Hazinski 1992).

Figure 37–3

NURSING CARE: CARDIAC CATHETERIZATION

Precatheterization

Nursing care before catheterization centers on support and teaching:

1. Teach the child and family about the procedure. Preparation of the child must be based on the child's cognitive and developmental level.
2. A visit to the catheterization laboratory is one of the most helpful ways to educate both the child and family.
3. If a visit is not possible, showing the child a picture book with photographs of the room and equipment can be helpful. Allow the child and family to ask questions to help relieve anxiety.

Postcatheterization

1. Assess the child's vital signs.
2. Assess circulation to the extremity in which the catheter was introduced. For example, if the femoral vein is used (most common), the leg and foot are examined.
3. Compare both extremities for capillary filling time, color, temperature, edema, and sensation.
4. Keep the child on bed rest until at least 6 hours after the catheterization.
5. Assist the child to keep the extremity in which the catheter was inserted straight until ambulation is possible.
6. Assess the pressure dressing for signs of bleeding. If blood is noted on the dressing, notify the physician immediately.

Figure 37–4 *Nursing care for the child undergoing cardiac catheterization*

Nursing Care. Depending on the defect, nursing care may involve administration of medication, pre- and postsurgical care, and patient and family teaching about the defect and its treatment. Nursing care is directed toward improving cardiac output, reducing energy expenditure, promoting physical growth, and reducing the family's fears. Early identification of the signs and symptoms of congenital heart disease and identification of changes in the child's condition are important aspects of nursing care. Encourage the family to avoid overprotecting the child. Emphasize that the child should participate in normal age-appropriate activities and rest when he or she is tired. Figure 37–5 summarizes nursing care for the child with a congenital heart defect.

CONGESTIVE HEART FAILURE

Description. **Congestive heart failure** is not a disease, but rather a condition in which the blood supply to the body is insufficient to meet the body's metabolic demands. Congenital heart defects are the most common cause of congestive heart failure in children. Other causes include severe anemia, arrhythmias, and weak or damaged heart muscle.

Congestive heart failure can occur on either the left or the right side of the heart. Right-sided heart failure occurs when the right ventricle has difficulty pumping blood into the pulmonary artery. Blood then backs up on the right side of the heart and into the inferior and superior venae cavae. Left-sided heart failure occurs when the left ventricle is unable to pump adequate amounts of blood into the aorta, causing blood to back up into the lungs. Because children's hearts are small, they frequently have both left- and right-sided heart failure.

Symptoms. Signs and symptoms of congestive heart failure include feeding difficulties, tachypnea, tachycardia, rales, hepatomegaly, splenomegaly, cardiomegaly, dyspnea, activity intolerance, decreased urine output, diaphoresis, slow growth pattern (failure to thrive), periorbital edema, poor peripheral circulation with cool extremities, and respiratory distress, Figure 37–6 (page 614).

Treatment. Congestive heart failure is treated with medications. Digoxin is the drug of choice in children older than 1 month of age. Digoxin slows the child's heart rate, which increases the heart's force of contraction and the output of blood from the ventricles, Figure 37–7 (page 615). Diuretics such as furosemide (Lasix), spironolactone (Aldactone), and thiazides are given to reduce edema. Potassium supplements and potassium-rich diets may be used with diuretic therapy to reduce the chance of hypokalemia.

Nursing Care. The goal of nursing care is to limit the child's expenditure of energy. The nurse should cluster care so that the child has periods of uninterrupted rest. Try to meet the needs of the crying or fussy child as soon as possible. Encourage the child to take time to rest or take naps throughout the day. The child's room should be "neutral thermic," that is, neither too hot nor too cold. This temperature allows the child to use as little energy as possible for thermoregulation. Positioning the child in a semi-Fowler's position prevents pressure on the diaphragm, allowing gas exchange from increased lung expansion.

The child's intake and output should be strictly monitored often during each shift. Any significant difference between fluid that has been ingested and urine that has been excreted must be reported. Weigh the child at the same time every day to assess fluid status.

When feeding an infant with congestive heart failure, limit oral feedings to 20 to 30 minutes and burp infant after every 15 to 30 mL of formula. Many infants with congestive heart failure are given concentrated high-carbohydrate formulas containing 24 to 30 calories per ounce. Gavage feeding is sometimes necessary. Children should be encouraged to eat high-calorie, low-sodium, and high-nutrient foods. A nutritionist can be helpful in educating the family about the nutritional needs of the child.

Parent education is an important part of nursing care. Parents need to know about administration of medication as well as how to conserve the child's energy during feedings and activities.

SCHOOL-AGE CHILD AND ADOLESCENT

SYSTEMIC HYPERTENSION

Hypertension refers to a consistent state of elevated blood pressure. Specifically, the systolic or the diastolic blood pressure is above the 95th percentile for the age and the sex of the child on more than three separate occasions (Broadwell Jackson and Saunders 1993).

Hypertension is categorized as either primary (essential) or secondary. Primary hypertension refers to a chronic increase in blood pressure that is not a result of any underlying disease or illness. Secondary hypertension results from another disease or illness.

NURSING CARE PLAN: Congenital Heart Disease

PATIENT PROBLEM	GOAL(S)
Failure to gain weight, respiratory difficulties with eating (tachypnea, retractions, nasal flaring)	The child will have an adequate intake of nutrients and calories.
Activity and exercise intolerance, fatigue on exertion, respiratory distress, tachycardia	The child will have reduced oxygen needs and reduced strain on the heart.

Figure 37–5 Nursing care plan for congenital heart disease

NURSING INTERVENTION	RATIONALE
Monitor caloric intake, daily weights, strict intake and output.	Daily weights enable monitoring of weight gain or loss.
Hold infant in a semi-upright position to feed.	Semi-upright position allows for better lung expansion and easier breathing.
Allow infant to rest after 15–30 mL of formula.	The more energy the child uses, the more oxygen is needed.
Feed at the first sign of hunger. Give small, frequent feedings every 2–3 hours. Alternate oral and gavage feedings. Provide a quiet environment with little stimulation during feeding.	Calories (energy) used for crying cannot be used to gain weight.
Educate family and child about diet therapy (high-calorie, high-carbohydrate, low-sodium, high-iron).	Helps ensure an adequate intake of nutrients.
Cluster nursing care to allow for periods of uninterrupted rest.	Rest gives the child energy to eat and play.
Attend to the child's crying or call light immediately. Place toys or personal items within easy reach. Position the child in semi-Fowler's position with loose unrestrictive clothing.	An increase in activity increases the body's need for oxygen.
Keep the temperature in the child's room neutral (not too hot or too cold).	An increase in the child's temperature increases metabolic rate, which in turn increases oxygen needs.

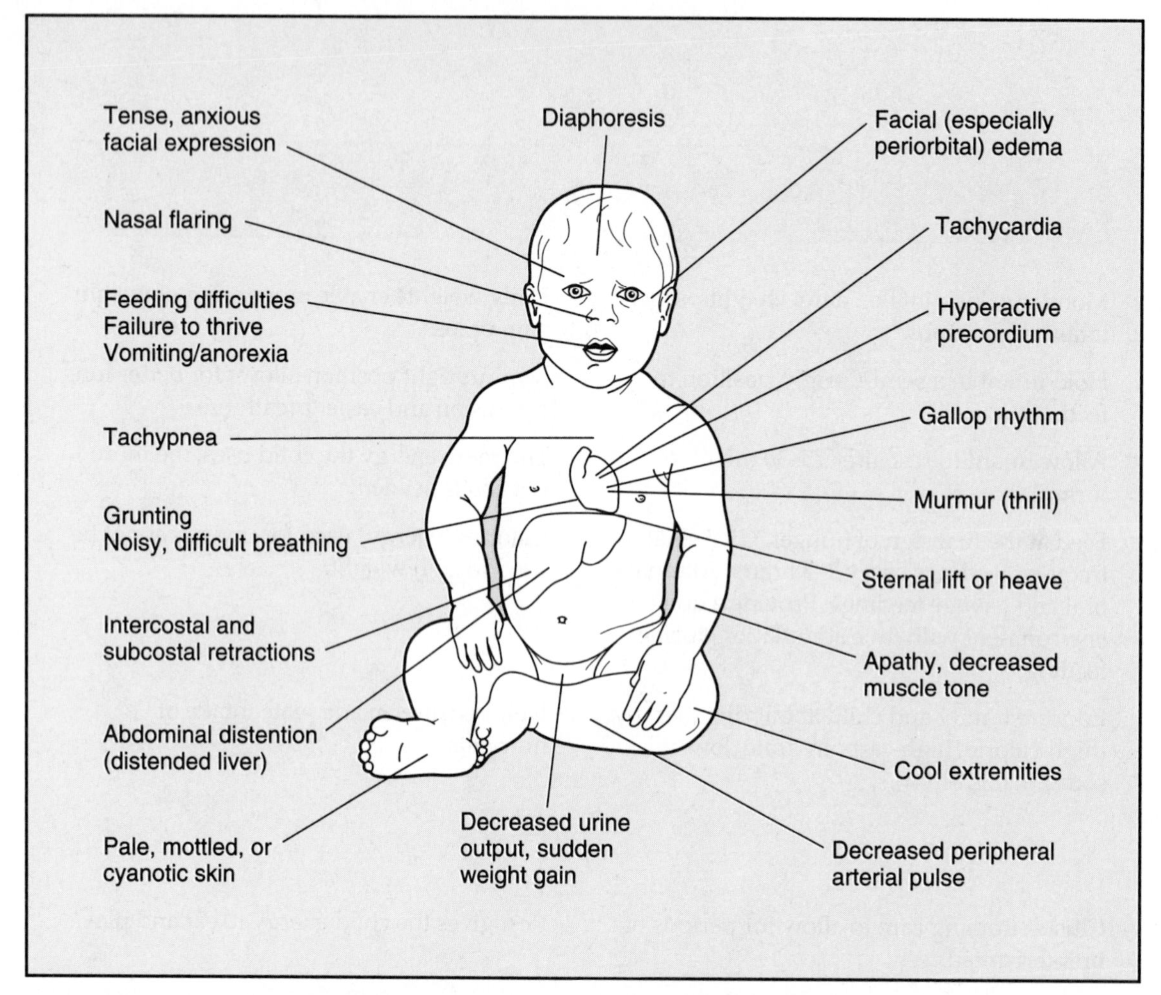

Figure 37–6 *Infant with congestive heart failure, physical assessment findings. (Adapted from* Critical Care Nurse 2, *no. 5, 1982, with permission from American Association of Critical-Care Nurses, Aliso Viejo, CA)*

In the United States, it is estimated that 1% to 2.5% of children between 3 and 18 years of age have hypertension. Genetics, race, sex, and environmental factors such as obesity, emotional stress, and excessive salt ingestion are thought to contribute to the development of hypertension. Treatment includes stress reduction, physical exercise, a salt-reduction diet, and medications (Broadwell Jackson and Saunders 1993).

RHEUMATIC FEVER

Description. Rheumatic fever is the most common acquired heart disease of young children and adolescents. It is a systemic inflammatory disease that affects primarily the heart, joints, brain, and skin. The damage to the heart usually involves the mitral valve and, as the disease progresses, the myocardium.

The disease usually develops about two to three weeks after an untreated group A beta-

DIGOXIN ADMINISTRATION TIPS

1. Check apical pulse for 1 full minute before administration.
2. Hold administration of digoxin if the pulse is less than 90 to 110 beats per minute (b.p.m.) for infants and less than 70 to 80 b.p.m. for older children or physician instructed limits.
3. Give digoxin on an empty stomach (1 hour before or 2 hours after eating) to increase absorption of medication.
4. If child vomits within 15 minutes after receiving digoxin, repeat the dose once. If the child vomits again, notify the physician.
5. Check serum potassium levels before administering digoxin. Low potassium levels can enhance the toxic side effects of digoxin.
6. Observe child for signs and symptoms of digoxin toxicity such as nausea and vomiting, diarrhea, anorexia, tachycardia, bradycardia, arrhythmias, and hypotension.
7. Give medication at regular times 12 hours apart.
8. If two or more doses are missed, notify the physician.
9. Keep medication in locked cabinet.
10. Never double or increase dosage of medication.

Figure 37–7

streptococcal infection (strep throat pharyngitis). Antibodies formed to combat the toxin released by the streptococci react with tissue antigens, resulting in damage to various body organs. Young school-age children are often exposed to streptococcal infections, especially during the winter and early spring. However, only 3% or fewer children with strep throat infections develop rheumatic fever. This low incidence implies that hereditary or environmental factors play a role in increasing susceptibility to the disease.

Symptoms. Initial symptoms may include fatigue and joint tenderness. Symptoms can progress to include carditis, polyarthritis, erythema marginatum, subcutaneous nodules, and chorea. Carditis, the most serious clinical symptom, occurs in over 50% of children with rheumatic fever. Approximately 10% of children develop **chorea**, also known as St. Vitus dance, which is characterized by involuntary, rapid movements of the muscles of the face and limbs (Broadwell Jackson and Saunders 1993).

Treatment. The Jones criteria are used to differentiate rheumatic fever from other illnesses with similar symptoms, Figure 37–8. A throat culture is taken to identify the presence of group A beta-streptococci. A rising or elevated antistreptolysin-O (ASO) titer identifies the presence of antibodies to streptococci.

The goals of treatment are to eradicate the streptococcal infection, prevent permanent car-

JONES CRITERIA (UPDATED 1992)*

Major Manifestations	Minor Manifestations	Supporting Evidence of Antecedent Group A Streptococcal Infection
Carditis	*Clinical Findings*	Positive throat culture or rapid streptococcal antigen test
Polyarthritis	Arthralgia	Elevated or rising streptococcal antibody titer
Chorea	Fever	
Erythema marginatum	*Laboratory Findings*	
Subcutaneous nodules	Elevated acute phase reactants	
	Erythrocyte sedimentation rate	
	C-reactive protein	
	Prolonged PR interval	

*If supported by evidence of preceding group A streptococcal infection, the presence of two major manifestations, or of one major and two minor manifestations indicates a high probability of acute rheumatic fever.

Figure 37–8 *Guidelines for the diagnosis of initial attack of rheumatic fever. (Data from Committee on Rheumatic Fever, Endocarditis, and Kawasaki Disease of the Council on Cardiovascular Disease in the Young, American Heart*

diac damage, reduce inflammation, and manage associated symptoms. Treatment includes administration of oral penicillin for 10 days. If the child is allergic to penicillin, erythromycin is prescribed. Aspirin or corticosteroids may be given to decrease the inflammatory process.

Nursing Care. Nursing care includes teaching the child and parents about the illness and its treatment and providing emotional support. Emphasize to the parents the importance of the child's receiving the complete 10-day course of antibiotics. Diversional activities should be provided for the child who may be on bed rest. These include books, tapes, puzzles, and art projects. Children with carditis are cautioned to avoid strenuous physical exercise for two to three months after the signs of cardiac inflammation have disappeared.

REVIEW QUESTIONS

A. Multiple choice. Select the best answer.

1. Bobby, age 4 months, is admitted for a cardiac catheterization that is to be performed tomorrow morning. Which of the following statements would best indicate that Bobby's mother understands about the procedure?
   a. "A cardiac catheterization takes only 10 minutes to perform, and Bobby will go home tomorrow afternoon."
   b. "Bobby's catheterization will be performed in his room by his pediatrician."
   c. "Bobby's catheterization will help his doctors to diagnose his heart problem."
   d. "The catheterization that the doctors are doing tomorrow will take a picture of Bobby's heart."

2. Sally, 18 days old, is diagnosed with a heart defect. Her parents ask you what caused her heart problem. Your best response would be which of the following?
   a. "Sally's heart problem was caused by something you did wrong during your pregnancy."
   b. "Sally's heart problem developed during your last trimester from some type of virus you came in contact with."
   c. "I don't know. Maybe you should ask her doctor."
   d. "Sally's heart problem was probably caused by a combination of physical and environmental factors during your pregnancy."

3. Which of the following is not an acyanotic heart defect?
   a. patent ductus arteriosus
   b. coarctation of the aorta
   c. tetralogy of Fallot
   d. atrial septal defect

4. Glenn, age 2 years, is diagnosed with coarctation of the aorta. Which of the following clinical symptoms would you expect to find?
   a. high blood pressure in the lower extremities and low blood pressure in the upper extremities
   b. low blood pressure in the lower extremities and high blood pressure in the upper extremities
   c. low blood pressure in the lower extremities and low blood pressure in the upper extremities
   d. high blood pressure in the lower extremities and high blood pressure in the upper extremities

5. Which of the following is *not* a duct in fetal circulation?
   a. foramen ovale
   b. ductus venosus
   c. ductus ovale
   d. ductus arteriosus

6. A child with congenital heart disease should be on what type of diet?
   a. High-calorie, high-carbohydrate, low-sodium
   b. High-calorie, high-carbohydrate, high-sodium
   c. Low-calorie, moderate-carbohydrate, low-sodium
   d. High-calorie, moderate-carbohydrate, low-sodium

7. The best position in which to place Molly, a 6-month-old infant with congestive heart failure, after feeding is
   a. prone, semi-Fowler's
   b. flat, prone
   c. Trendelenburg, prone
   d. supine, semi-Fowler's

8. Stephanie, 5 years old, will undergo a cardiac catheterization tomorrow morning. Which of the following approaches would best prepare Stephanie for the procedure?
   a. Tell Stephanie that the doctors will cut a small hole in her leg and thread a small catheter into her so the doctors can see her heart.
   b. Allow Stephanie and her family to visit the catheterization lab the evening before and provide masks, needles, syringes, gowns, and stethoscopes for a supervised play session after the tour.
   c. Show Stephanie pictures of her heart in a book and describe the procedure to her.
   d. Don't tell Stephanie anything until she is ready to go to her catheterization because preparing her the day before will upset her too much.
9. Common signs and symptoms of congestive heart failure include all of the following except
   a. feeding difficulties
   b. clubbing of the fingers
   c. tachycardia
   d. tachypnea
10. Sarah is a 4-month-old infant with congestive heart failure. Before giving Sarah her 8 A.M. dose of digoxin, you auscultate her heart rate. Her apical pulse is 84. What should you do?
    a. Give the medication first and then tell her physician.
    b. Hold the medication, because her heart rate is less than 90 b.p.m.
    c. Wait an hour and then give the medication.
    d. Hold her medication and notify her physician.

SUGGESTED ACTIVITIES

- Spend a day in a cardiac catheterization laboratory observing the procedure.
- Spend a day in a cardiology clinic. Interview children with congenital heart defects and their parents about what it is like to live with a heart disease.
- Attend a support group meeting for parents of children with congenital heart defects.
- Spend a day in the echocardiogram laboratory to observe diagnostic testing for heart disease.
- Visit the local offices of the American Heart Association and the March of Dimes to learn their purpose in relation to congenital heart disease. Assess parent teaching materials available from each organization.

BIBLIOGRAPHY

Adams, F., G. Emmanouilides, and T. Riemenschneider. *Moss' Heart Disease in Infants, Children, and Adolescents*, 4th ed. Baltimore: Williams and Wilkins, 1989.

Agamalian, B. Pediatric cardiac catheterization. *Journal of Pediatric Nursing* 1 (1986): 73–79.

Bowlen, J. Helping children and their families cope with congenital heart disease. *Critical Care Quarterly* 8 (1985): 65–74.

Broadwell Jackson, D., and R. B. Saunders. *Child Health Nursing*. Philadelphia: J. B. Lippincott, 1993.

Callow, L. A new beginning: Nursing care of the infant undergoing the arterial switch operation for transposition of the great arteries. *Heart & Lung* 18 (1989): 248–257.

Daberkow, E., and R. Washington. Cardiovascular diseases and surgical intervention. Pp. 427–465 in G. Merenstein and S. Gardner, eds. *Handbook of Neonatal Intensive Care*, 2nd ed. St Louis, MO: C. V. Mosby, 1989.

Foster, R. L. R., M. M. Hunsberger, and J. J. T. Anderson. *Family-Centered Nursing Care of Children*. Philadelphia: W. B. Saunders, 1989.

Garson, A., J. Bricker, and D. McNamara. *The Science and Practice of Pediatric Cardiology*, vol. 2, pp. 671–690. Philadelphia: Lea and Febiger, 1990.

Guyton, A. *Human Physiology and Mechanisms of Disease*, 5th ed. Philadelphia: W. B. Saunders, 1992.

Hagedorn, M., and S. Gardner. Physiologic sequelae of prematurity: The nurse practitioner's role. Part III. Congestive heart failure. *Journal of Pediatric Health Care* 4 (1990): 229–236.

Hazinski, M. *Nursing Care of the Critically Ill Child*, 2nd ed. St. Louis, MO: Mosby-Year Book, 1992.

Kashani, I., and S. Higgins. Counseling strategies for families of children with heart disease. *Pediatric Nursing* 12 (1986): 38–40.

Liebman, J., and M. Freed. Cardiovascular system. Pp. 445–491 in R. Behrman and R. Kliegman, eds. *Nelson's Essentials of Pediatrics*. Philadelphia: W. B. Saunders, 1990.

Moore, K. *The Developing Human: Clinically Oriented Embryology*, 4th ed. Philadelphia: W. B. Saunders, 1988.

Page, G. Tetralogy of Fallot. *Heart & Lung* 15 (1986): 390–399.

Wong, D. *Whaley & Wong's Essentials of Pediatric Nursing*, 4th ed. St. Louis, MO: Mosby-Year Book, 1993.

CHAPTER

38

Respiratory Conditions

OBJECTIVES

AFTER STUDYING THIS CHAPTER, THE STUDENT SHOULD BE ABLE TO:

- NAME THREE RESPIRATORY CONDITIONS THAT AFFECT INFANTS AND DISCUSS THEIR CAUSES, SYMPTOMS, TREATMENT, AND NURSING CARE.
- NAME THREE RESPIRATORY CONDITIONS THAT AFFECT TODDLERS AND DESCRIBE THEIR CAUSES, SYMPTOMS, TREATMENT, AND NURSING CARE.
- IDENTIFY THE AGE GROUP MOST AT RISK FOR FOREIGN BODY ASPIRATION AND DESCRIBE APPROPRIATE NURSING ACTION FOR THIS EMERGENCY.
- DISCUSS THE CAUSES, SYMPTOMS, TREATMENT, AND NURSING CARE OF ASTHMA
- NAME SEVERAL OTHER RESPIRATORY CONDITIONS THAT AFFECT PRESCHOOL AND SCHOOL-AGE CHILDREN AND DISCUSS THEIR CAUSES, SYMPTOMS, TREATMENT, AND NURSING CARE.

Key Terms

- RETRACTIONS
- STEATORRHEA
- INTUSSUSCEPTION
- SWEAT TEST
- STRIDOR
- LARYNGOSPASM
- ALLERGIC SHINER
- NASAL SALUTE
- TRIGGER

Respiratory illnesses are common throughout early childhood. In most children, these illnesses produce mild symptoms that can be managed at home. In chronic conditions, such as asthma, teaching the parents and child about the disease and its management is an important part of nursing care. Serious respiratory illnesses are potentially life-threatening and require skilled medical treatment and nursing care.

Overview of the System

The process of oxygenation and gas exchange is accomplished by the coordinated efforts of the neurological, cardiovascular, and respiratory systems. The respiratory system includes upper airway and lower airway structures, Figure 38–1.

The upper airway consists of the mouth, nose, pharynx, epiglottis, larynx, and trachea. Inspired air is normally warmed, moistened, and filtered before it enters the trachea and descends into the lower airway. Nasal cilia and mucus are the first line of defense against large, inhaled particles such as dust, pollen, and water. The palatine tonsils and adenoids fight harmful organisms by trapping and destroying them.

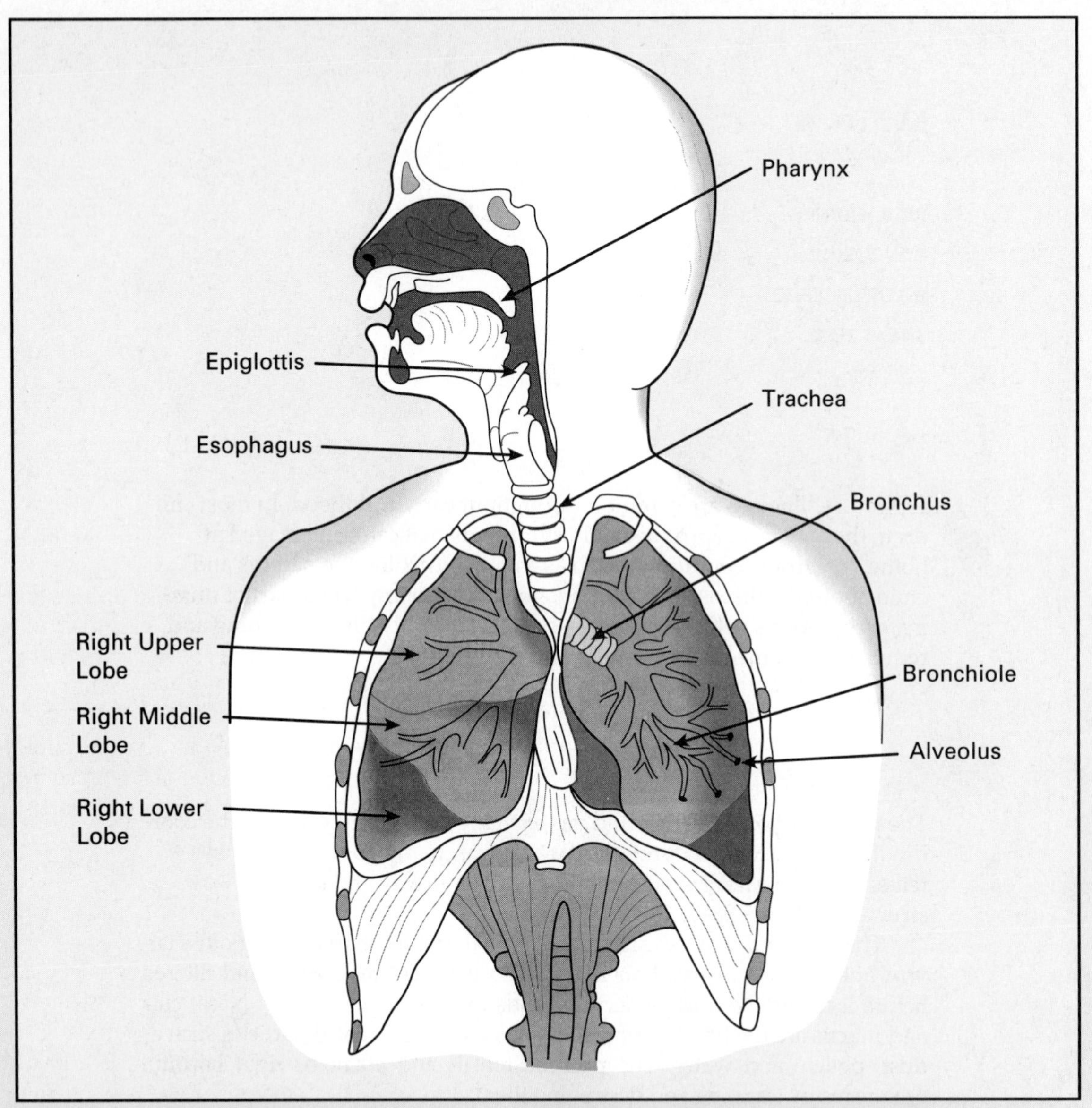

Figure 38–1 *The respiratory system (Adapted from G. L. Smith, P. E. Davis, and J. T. Dennerll.* Medical Terminology: A Programmed Text, *6th ed. Albany, NY: Delmar Publishers, 1991.)*

The lower airway consists of the two mainstem bronchi, one each on the right and left side, that further branch into bronchioles and alveoli throughout both lungs (DeJong and McCandless 1983).

INFANT

BRONCHIOLITIS

Description. Bronchiolitis occurs when an infecting agent causes inflammation and obstruction of the bronchioles. It is a frequent cause of hospitalization of infants and children under 2 years of age. The respiratory syncytial virus (RSV) is the most common cause. RSV is transmitted through direct or close contact with respiratory secretions of infected individuals.

Symptoms. The child has a history of rhinitis, a cough, and a low-grade fever for a few days before developing more frequent coughing, rales, wheezing, and labored breathing. Respirations are rapid, shallow, and accompanied by nasal flaring and **retractions** (a visible drawing in of the soft tissues of the chest), signs of severe distress.

Treatment. Treatment includes oxygen, fluid therapy, airway support, and rest. Medications may be given by aerosol to open up the airways. Most children are managed at home.

Nursing Care. If the child is hospitalized, nursing care consists of observation, administration of oxygen, hydration, and supportive airway measures. Observe the child frequently and watch for any worsening of respiratory symptoms. Grouping nursing tasks decreases stress and promotes rest.

Explain procedures to parents to help reduce their anxiety. Watching a child who is in respiratory difficulty is frightening for parents, and they need emotional support and reassurance that their child will get better.

Oxygen is administered using a mist tent, nasal cannula, or face mask (see Chapter 30). Holding the infant upright or elevating the head of the bed helps the child to breathe more easily and helps to drain mucus from the upper airways. Pulmonary hygiene and nebulized medications are usually administered by a respiratory therapist. The infant's nasal passages can be kept clear and open by using a bulb syringe (see Chapter 30). Acetaminophen may be given to control temperature. Adequate fluid intake is important to maintain fluid balance.

PNEUMONIA

Pneumonia is an inflammation of the lungs that occurs most often in infants and young children. It can involve a lobe of the lung or be spread throughout the lung and may be bacterial or viral in origin. Differentiating between viral and bacterial forms of pneumonia is important in order to establish an appropriate treatment plan.

Symptoms can include elevated temperature, cough, dyspnea, tachypnea, decreased breath sounds, pain on inspiration, and malaise.

Treatment is supportive and includes antibiotics, administration of oxygen if indicated, pulmonary care, hydration, and medication for pain (acetaminophen). The *Hemophilus influenzae* b (Hib) conjugate vaccine is recommended beginning at age 2 months as a preventive measure against *H. influenzae* pneumonia (Chapter 35). Nursing care is supportive and similar to that for the child with bronchiolitis.

CYSTIC FIBROSIS

Description. Cystic fibrosis is inherited as an autosomal recessive disorder. It is primarily a disorder of the exocrine glands that affects many body systems. In 1989, chromosome 7 was identified as the cystic fibrosis gene (Collins 1992), making genetic counseling and prenatal diagnosis possible. The disorder occurs most often in Caucasian children.

Symptoms. Symptoms include a chronic cough and frequent respiratory infections. Coughing occurs in an attempt to clear the lungs of thick, sticky mucus, which provides an environment conducive to bacterial growth, accounting for the frequency of respiratory infections.

Infants often present with meconium ileus. **Steatorrhea** (fatty stools) is a characteristic finding because blocked pancreatic ducts do not secrete the enzymes necessary to digest fats and proteins. Because essential nutrients are excreted in the stool, children with cystic fibrosis have difficulty maintaining and gaining weight. They may develop **intussusception** (telescoping of the bowel) or a prolapsed rectum because the large, bulky stools are difficult to pass.

Delayed bone growth, short stature, and a delayed onset of puberty are common. Metabolic function is altered as a result of imbalances created by excessive electrolytes lost in perspiration, saliva, and mucus.

Sterility in males is common because of blockage in or absence of the vas deferens. In females, increased mucus secretions block the passage of sperm, making conception difficult (George 1990, Landon and Rosenfeld 1984).

Treatment. Diagnosis is made on the basis of two positive sweat tests. The **sweat test** analyzes the sodium and chloride content of the child's sweat. Elevated values are diagnostic of cystic fibrosis. The goals of treatment are to maintain adequate respiratory function, prevent infection, and encourage exercise and good nutrition. With improved treatment, children with cystic fibrosis now survive into adulthood. Overwhelming infection and multisystem changes, however, ultimately result in respiratory failure and death.

Nursing Care. Chest physiotherapy, consisting of postural drainage and chest percussion, is usually performed one to four times per day before eating and before bed to help drain mucus from the lungs, Figure 38–2. Medications administered by aerosol treatments are frequently used before postural drainage to help loosen secretions.

Digestive problems resulting from malabsorption can be treated with pancreatic enzyme supplements and dietary modification. Pancreatic enzymes are taken orally with all meals and snacks, and they can be mixed in applesauce or strained fruits for young children. Enzyme replacement is important to reduce bulky stools and to promote adequate weight gain. Water-soluble multivitamins are recommended to prevent vitamin deficiency.

Because children with cystic fibrosis lose a lot of salt in their sweat, parents should be told to add extra salt to food and to encourage salty snacks. Salt tablets should be taken only if prescribed by a physician.

The nurse can play an important role in helping parents to understand and deal with issues related to body image, digestive problems, and the need for frequent hospitalizations. Genetic counseling should be encouraged.

The nurse should refer the family if appropriate to social and other support services to assist them in dealing with the financial burdens from frequent hospitalizations, the purchase of medications and supplies, and the cost of medical follow-up. The Cystic Fibrosis Foundation, 6931 Arlington Rd., Suite 200, Bethesda, MD 20814, 800-FIGHTCF, is a source for information about cystic fibrosis.

Figure 38–3 summarizes nursing care for the child with cystic fibrosis.

TODDLER

BRONCHITIS

Bronchitis is an inflammation of the bronchi that usually occurs during a respiratory illness. Bronchitis is caused most often by a virus, but it also can result from invasion of bacteria or in response to an allergen or irritant.

Symptoms include a coarse, hacking cough, which increases in severity at night, rhonchi, and wheezing. The child may complain of chest and rib pain because of the deep and frequent coughing.

Treatment consists of rest, humidification, and hydration to provide relief from coughing. Expectorants and cough suppressants are occasionally prescribed. Nursing care is primarily supportive.

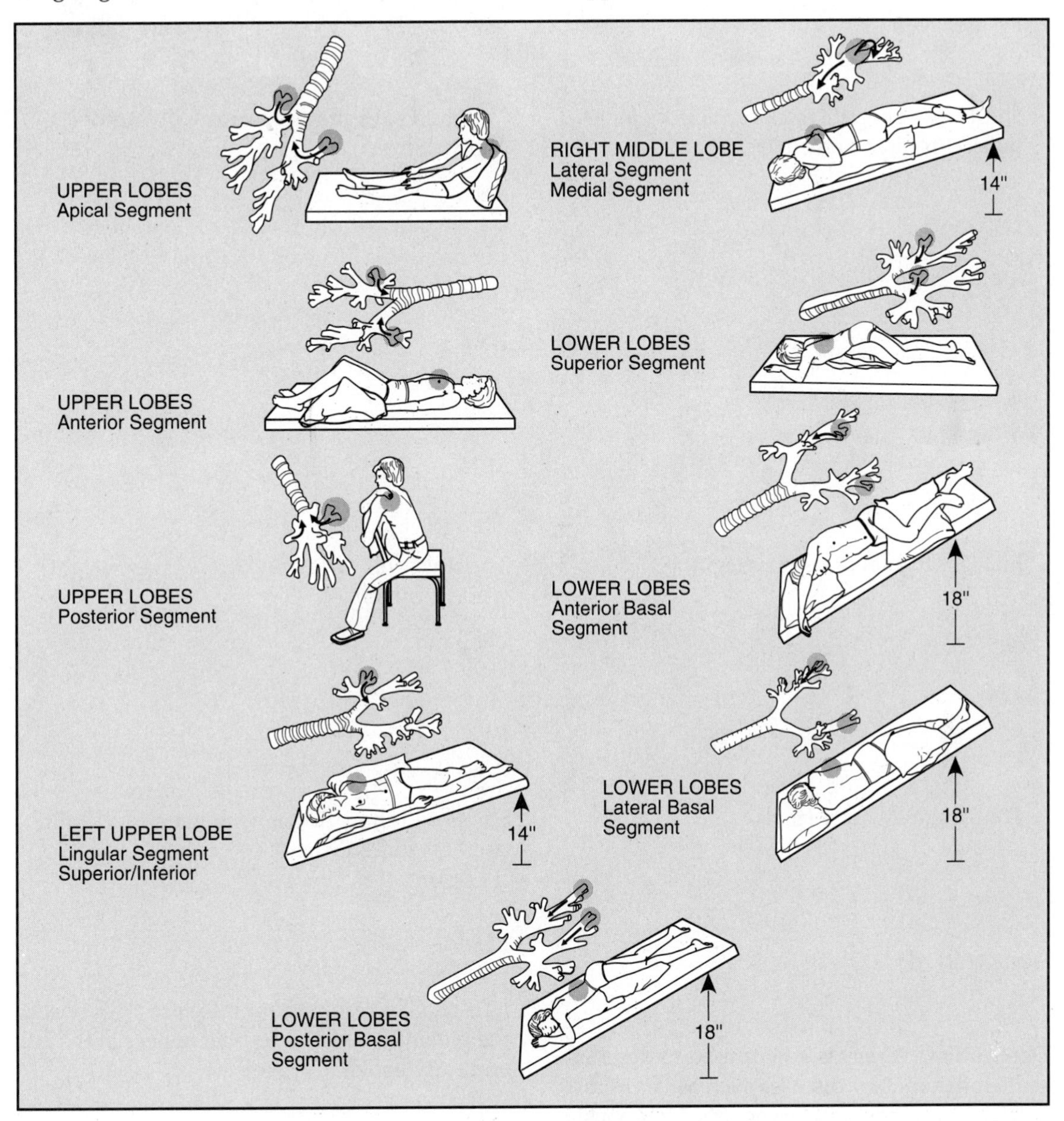

Figure 38–2 *Postural drainage (From Datalizer Slide Charts, Addison, IL)*

NURSING CARE PLAN: Cystic Fibrosis

PATIENT PROBLEM	GOAL(S)
Shortness of breath, thick respiratory secretions, chronic, productive cough	The child's respiratory status will improve and stabilize.
Inability to gain or retain weight	The child will maintain current body weight while hospitalized.
Foul, frequent, fatty stools	Stools will show firmer consistency and will decrease in frequency.

Figure 38–3

CROUP

Description. *Croup* is a term used to describe acute inflammatory diseases such as laryngitis, bacterial tracheitis, and laryngotracheobronchitis (LTB) that result from swelling of the epiglottis, larynx, trachea, and bronchi. Acute viral LTB usually results from infection with one of the parainfluenza viruses that appear in the fall and early winter.

Symptoms. Croup usually has an acute onset after an upper respiratory infection. The child

NURSING INTERVENTION	RATIONALE
Assess respiratory status and vital signs as ordered.	Determines respiratory baseline.
Provide oxygen, nebulizer treatments, and pulmonary hygiene (postural drainage and chest percussion).	Pulmonary therapies thin and mobilize respiratory secretions.
Observe and support child during severe coughing episodes. Encourage rest.	During coughing spells, emotional support and respiratory assessment are essential.
Provide mouth care.	Mouth care removes foul taste.
Encourage appropriate handwashing and disposal of tissues.	Personal hygiene habits often need reinforcement.
Monitor daily weight using same scale at same time of day.	Establishes a baseline, enabling weight trends to be followed.
Administer pulmonary care before meals and evening snack.	Pulmonary care before meals improves respiratory effort and appetite.
Administer prescribed enzymes with all meals and snacks. Keep a record of quality and quantity of stools.	Appropriate enzyme therapy promotes firmer stools and reduced frequency.

continues

has inspiratory **stridor** (a high-pitched sound created by narrowing of the airway), a "barking" cough, a low-grade fever, and hoarseness. **Laryngospasms** (involuntary vibrating contractions of the muscles of the larynx) contribute to both increased hoarseness and stridor. If symptoms are not treated obstruction worsens and the child may develop air hunger, retractions, and respiratory distress.

Treatment. Children are treated at home unless they have expiratory stridor, respiratory

PATIENT PROBLEM	GOAL(S)
Low self-esteem and feelings of powerlessness, resulting from body changes and prolonged hospital stay	The child will have increased self-esteem and demonstrate independence through participation in own care before discharge.

Figure 38–3 *continued*

difficulty, or dehydration. Treatment is supportive. Cool mist helps to moisturize irritated airways and decreases mucosal swelling. Nebulized racemic epinephrine is given to relieve airway obstruction by reducing edema (Hathaway et al. 1993).

Nursing Care. Nursing care consists of good observation skills, keeping the child's airway open, encouraging fluids, rest, reducing stress, and providing emotional support. Intubation equipment should be kept at the bedside. Report any change in the child's respiratory status immediately. Encourage parents to help keep the child calm and quiet by holding the child on their lap or even sitting in the mist tent with the child. The parents and child are usually fearful, anxious, and apprehensive because of the child's respiratory difficulty. Reassure parents that the child will get better.

EPIGLOTTITIS

Description. Epiglottitis, an inflammation of the epiglottis, is most often caused by bacterial invasion of the soft tissue of the larynx by *Hemophilus influenzae* b. Diagnosis is usually made by lateral neck x-ray, which shows a narrowed airway and enlarged, rounded epiglottis. Epiglottitis requires immediate intervention to prevent possible respiratory arrest.

Symptoms. Symptoms include fever, sore throat, hoarseness or a muffled voice, difficulty swallowing, and inspiratory stridor. Throat pain, swelling, and difficulty swallowing cause the child to drool. Epiglottitis can rapidly progress to a life-threatening condition because edema can occur within minutes, obstructing the airway by blocking the trachea. A child who previously was noisily breathing

NURSING INTERVENTION	RATIONALE
Encourage child to be involved in (and responsible for, if appropriate) own treatment plan. Offer choices for nutritious meals and allow preadolescent and adolescent to take enzymes on his or her own.	Preadolescents and adolescents need to have some control and independence related to activities of daily living. Choices improve feelings of self-worth.
Encourage child to dress in own clothes and continue school work. Encourage interaction with other children of same age and provide a means for child to contact peers. Obtain pass permission for out-of-hospital breaks (long hospital stay).	Age-related social needs should be recognized and promoted during hospitalization.
Encourage child to verbalize concerns about future.	Providing emotional support and active listening show concern.

will suddenly become wide-eyed, still, and silent. A quiet child is the sign of a potentially dangerous situation.

Treatment. The goal of treatment is to maintain a patent airway. The airway is most often kept open by inserting an endotracheal tube, preferably in the operating room.

Nursing Care. Children are usually admitted to the intensive care unit when an endotracheal tube is in place. Intravenous antibiotics are given, and the child is placed in a mist tent. Suctioning may be necessary. Nursing care consists of keeping the child's airway open, maintaining adequate hydration, keeping the child in a quiet environment, and eliminating stress. The nurse needs to provide emotional support to the child and parents. Keeping parents informed of the child's condition helps to reduce their stress and fear. Reassure parents that prompt intervention usually results in rapid resolution of symptoms (Hathaway et al. 1993).

FOREIGN BODY ASPIRATION

It is not unusual for infants and young children to explore objects by putting them in their mouths. For this reason, children between the ages of 6 months and 4 years are most at risk for aspiration of a foreign body. The child may have symptoms such as coughing, choking, gagging, and wheezing.

How severe the obstruction is depends on the size and consistency of the object and where it lodges in the respiratory tract. Common causes of airway obstruction include foods such as nuts, popcorn, hot dogs, and raw vegetables; small toy parts or objects such as beads, safety pins, coins, and buttons; and latex balloon pieces.

Foreign bodies lodged above the trachea usually can be coughed out easily. If the child is unable to cough out the object, chest and back thrusts or the Heimlich maneuver can be used (see Chapter 26). Objects that lodge in the trachea can be life-threatening.

Radiopaque objects can be seen on x-ray. Fluoroscopy and fiberoptic bronchoscopy are sometimes used to help with the location, identification, and removal of the foreign body.

The nurse needs to report any change in the child's respiratory status immediately. Parents need emotional support and understanding until the child is out of danger. Teach the parents and family how to child-proof their home. Recommend that parents learn cardiopulmonary resuscitation (CPR) and how to assist a choking child using the Heimlich maneuver (see Chapter 26).

PRESCHOOL AND SCHOOL-AGE CHILD

EPISTAXIS (NOSEBLEED)

Epistaxis, or nosebleed, is common in childhood and occurs frequently in school-age children. The most common source of bleeding is from Kiesselbach's plexus, an area of plentiful veins located in the anterior nares. The most common causes of nosebleed are nosepicking, foreign bodies, trauma, and dryness.

Children are frequently brought to the emergency room or clinic by a parent who has been unable to stop the nose from bleeding. The child and parent may be apprehensive and scared. The nurse should have the child sit upright with the head tilted forward to prevent blood from dripping down the back of the throat.

A cotton ball or swab soaked with Neo-Synephrine, epinephrine, thrombin, or lidocaine may be inserted into the affected nostril to promote vasoconstriction if the bleeding does not stop. Sometimes the nostril has to be cauterized with silver nitrate after the bleeding has stopped.

The child is admitted to the hospital if the bleeding cannot be controlled. One or both nostrils are packed with petroleum jelly gauze. The packing usually remains in place between one and seven days. Hematocrit or hemoglobin is assessed if the child has had significant bleeding. The child's blood pressure should be monitored.

Instruct parents that the child should avoid strenuous exercise, bending over and stooping for long periods of time, hot drinks, and hot baths or showers for the next three to four days. Elevate the child's head on pillows. The child who experiences frequent nosebleeds should be evaluated for underlying causes.

ACUTE NASOPHARYNGITIS

Nasopharyngitis, better known as the "common cold," is caused most often by one of the rhinoviruses or coronaviruses but may also be caused by group A beta-streptococcus.

Symptoms include a red nasal mucosa and clear nasal discharge. The child may also have an infected throat with enlarged tonsils. Vesicles may be seen on the soft palate and in the pharynx. Symptoms can last up to 10 days or longer.

Treatment is supportive. Infants can be treated with normal saline nose drops given every three to four hours, followed by suctioning with a bulb syringe (see Chapter 30). Suctioning is especially helpful before feeding. Normal saline nose drops, decongestants, or nasal sprays can be used for older children. Antihistamines may be helpful for children with profuse nasal drainage.

Instruct parents to use a cool mist vaporizer to help thin mucus secretions and decrease airway swelling. Give acetaminophen to reduce fever. Offer the child fluids to maintain hydration. Fluid intake can be encouraged by providing favorite noncitrus drinks, frozen pops, and ice chips.

STREPTOCOCCAL PHARYNGITIS (STREP THROAT)

Description. A "strep throat" is the result of an infection caused by group A beta-streptococcus. It affects the pharynx and tonsils and is seen most commonly in children 4 to 7 years of age.

Symptoms. Symptoms include a red throat, pain on swallowing, pharyngeal exudate, lymphadenopathy, and fever. A child who has difficulty swallowing, drools, or appears to be having respiratory distress should be seen by a physician immediately.

Treatment. Diagnosis is made by a positive throat culture. Children who are symptomatic are usually treated before the culture results are received. They are given oral penicillin for 10 days or an injection of long-acting penicillin G benzathine (Bicillin). Children who are allergic to penicillin are treated with erythromycin. Children should be treated within seven days of a positive throat culture. A follow-up throat culture after the medication therapy is complete is recommended to ensure that the strep bacteria have been eliminated completely. If a strep throat is not treated or the full course of antibiotics is not taken, complications such as rheumatic fever, rheumatic arthritis, or acute glomerulonephritis can occur.

Nursing Care. Children are usually treated on an out-patient basis. Symptoms should begin to subside approximately 24 hours after the start of penicillin therapy. Emphasize to parents that the full course of antibiotic therapy should be completed as instructed. Acetaminophen reduces fever and helps relieve throat pain. Ice chips, frozen pops, and favorite beverages should be given frequently and in small amounts. Preventing dehydration is important. In children with repeated episodes of strep throat, removal of tonsils and adenoids is frequently recommended.

TONSILLITIS AND ADENOIDITIS

Description. Tonsillitis refers to chronic infection and enlargement of the palatine tonsils. Adenoiditis is a viral or bacterial infection causing enlargement of the pharyngeal tonsils.

Symptoms. Frequent throat infections, persistent redness of the anterior pillars, and enlargement of the cervical lymph nodes are common symptoms. The inflamed adenoids are associated with snoring and disrupted sleep patterns. Many children have associated ear infections and related hearing loss.

Treatment. Treatment for tonsillitis is the same as for pharyngitis. Children who have chronic tonsillitis are candidates for tonsillectomy. If the adenoids are enlarged, they may be removed at the same time. Both tonsillectomy and adenoidectomy continue to be controversial procedures and the end results need to be carefully evaluated against the potential for complications (Hathaway et al. 1993).

Nursing Care. The nursing care of children with tonsillitis is similar to that for children with pharyngitis (see above). If surgery is indicated, the nurse should prepare the child and parents through pre- and postoperative teaching (see Chapter 31). The greatest postoperative threat, after removal of the tonsils or adenoids, is bleeding. Good observation skills are essential during the first 24 hours after surgery. Watch for hemorrhage at the back of the throat. Oral fluids keep the pharynx moist and provide necessary hydration. Warn parents that 7 to 10 days after surgery, the suture scabs will loosen. Any bleeding from the child's nose or mouth at this time should be reported to the physician for prompt evaluation.

NURSING CARE PLAN: Asthma

PATIENT PROBLEM	GOAL(S)
Rapid breathing, wheezing, retractions, and a cough	The child's respiratory status will improve and stabilize.
Dehydration	The child will be adequately hydrated before discharge.
Anxiety (parent) caused by lack of knowledge about asthma management at home	Parents will be able to explain and provide asthma care before discharge.

Figure 38–4

NURSING INTERVENTION	RATIONALE
Assess respiratory status and vital signs as ordered.	Determines respiratory baseline.
Provide oxygen and elevate head of bed.	Ordered oxygen and positioning improve oxygenation, easing breathing and energy expenditure.
Encourage parents to stay with child and provide quiet, calm environment for rest and sleep.	Parents' presence usually reassures child and decreases anxiety in the unfamiliar hospital setting.
Assess IV site and maintain IV fluid infusion.	Initially, the intravenous route will replenish fluids and allow the child to rest.
Check urine specific gravity and carefully monitor intake and output.	Hydration is evaluated by quality and quantity of urine output and vital sign stability.
Offer fluids as ordered when child is able to take oral fluids.	Ability to tolerate fluids signals improvement.
Explain cause and common symptoms of asthma.	Increased knowledge decreases anxiety.
Give parents written information about asthma and its treatment. Identify possible side effects of treatment.	Written information can be referred to later.
Refer parents to asthma support group and American Lung Association for further information.	Provides support and comfort.

ALLERGIC RHINITIS

The most common cause of chronic nasal congestion in children is allergic rhinitis. Symptoms include sneezing, nasal congestion, watery discharge, mouth breathing, **allergic "shiners"** (dark circles under the eyes or discoloration more than normal), and a **nasal salute** (wiping the nose with the heel of the hand).

Treatment consists of minimizing or avoiding exposure to allergens; administering antihistamines, oral decongestants, or topical agents (cromolyn, steroids); and immunotherapy to identify and desensitize the child to known allergens.

ASTHMA

Description. Asthma is a reactive airway disease that occurs in infants, children, and adolescents. It is a chronic condition with acute exacerbations. The stimulus (**trigger**) that precedes an asthmatic episode can be a substance or condition. Asthmatic triggers include exercise, infection, allergens, food additives, irritants, weather, and emotions.

During an asthma attack, increased mucus production, airway swelling, and mucus plugging of small airways occur in response to a trigger. Repeated episodes of muscle spasms, mucosal edema, and mucus plugging can cause the airway to become chronically scarred and irritated, resulting in air trapping.

Symptoms. The child experiencing an asthma attack has rapid and labored respirations. Nasal flaring, retractions, audible expiratory wheezing, and a productive cough may be present. Because the airways are narrowed and partially blocked, a state of hypoxia exists. The child may appear tired and anxious because of difficulty with breathing.

Treatment. The diagnosis of asthma is confirmed through pulmonary function studies such as spirometry and peak flow rates. A spirometer is used to measure the volume of air the lungs can move in and out. The use of a peak expiratory flow rate (PEFR) meter can assist in the management of asthma by helping to identify when obstruction occurs. This device measures the child's ability to forcefully push air out of the lungs. Skin testing may be done to identify allergens that act as asthma triggers.

The overall goal of treatment is to help the child achieve near-normal respiratory function while continuing normal growth and development. Pharmacological and supportive therapies are used to reverse the airway obstruction and promote respiratory function.

Nursing Care. If the child is having difficulty breathing, oxygen may be required. Humidified oxygen can be given by nasal cannula or face mask. Having the child sit in a semi-Fowler's or upright position helps the child to breathe more easily.

Medications are often given by aerosol because they are absorbed quickly and response time is relatively short. Intravenous medications are also given. Drug levels should be monitored frequently. Keep the child in a quiet room and group tasks in order to avoid repeatedly disturbing the child.

Adequate hydration is essential to help thin mucus plugs trapped in the narrowed airways. Intake, output, and specific gravity should be monitored to evaluate the child's hydration status. Offer the child fruit-flavored juices, flavored ices, and favorite beverages when possible.

Supporting and educating the parents and child help them cope with and understand the disease, medication therapy, and the need for lifestyle changes. Parents need to be taught prevention and treatment of asthma and how to avoid frequent hospitalization. Refer parents to local support groups and to the American Lung Association.

Figure 38–4 (page 632) summarizes nursing care for the child with asthma.

TUBERCULOSIS

Tuberculosis is an infectious disease caused by *Mycobacterium tuberculosis*. Transmission is through infectious particles called droplets. Symptoms include a chronic cough, anorexia, weight loss or failure to gain weight, and fever.

The child, immediate family, and suspected carriers should be skin tested for tuberculosis. Intradermal testing using purified protein derivative (PPD) (the Mantoux test) is considered the most accurate test. Active cases of pulmonary tuberculosis are required by law to be reported to public health agencies.

Treatment consists of antitubercular and corticosteroid medications, adequate nutrition, and rest. Parents need to be told about the importance of complying with drug therapy, since treatment may last 6 to 12 months.

REVIEW QUESTIONS

A. Multiple choice. Select the best answer.

1. The structures most responsible for trapping and destroying harmful organisms in the respiratory tract are the
   a. bronchi
   b. tonsils and adenoids
   c. alveoli
   d. cilia

2. The infant with bronchiolitis is most likely to have which of the following clinical findings?
   a. retractions
   b. inspiratory stridor
   c. laryngospasm
   d. thick, tenacious mucus

3. Intussusception is a common finding in children who have
   a. pneumonia
   b. asthma
   c. cystic fibrosis
   d. tuberculosis

4. The treatment of choice for the child with croup to decrease mucosal swelling is
   a. immediate surgery
   b. suctioning of the airway
   c. positioning the child flat on the back
   d. cool humidified air via mist tent

5. A strep throat is a serious infection in children and requires prompt medical therapy because
   a. bleeding can occur without warning
   b. children cannot tolerate the severe throat pain
   c. left untreated, the heart and kidneys may be damaged
   d. the causative organism can cause sterility

6. Danielle, 5 years old, is brought to the emergency department by her parents. She is feverish and has a sore throat, difficulty swallowing, and inspiratory stridor. These are symptoms of
   a. croup
   b. epiglottitis
   c. bronchiolitis
   d. strep throat

7. The nasal salute is a symptom associated with
   a. allergic rhinitis
   b. bronchiolitis
   c. cystic fibrosis
   d. pneumonia

8. Which of the following respiratory conditions is frequently associated with ear infections and related hearing loss?
   a. allergic rhinitis
   b. strep throat
   c. tonsillitis and adenoiditis
   d. pneumonia
9. Pulmonary function studies and peak flow rates are used to diagnose which of the following respiratory conditions?
   a. pneumonia
   b. cystic fibrosis
   c. tuberculosis
   d. asthma
10. Which of the following is true concerning the medication therapy for a child with tuberculosis?
   a. There is no medication for the tuberculosis organism.
   b. The child must be hospitalized until the entire course of medication is completed.
   c. The medications have no side effects.
   d. The medication needs to be given for up to 12 months.

SUGGESTED ACTIVITIES

- Before caring for children with a respiratory disorder, review CPR and Heimlich maneuver procedures (Chapter 26). Ask parents if they know how to perform CPR. Encourage parents to learn CPR, and tell them where they can take classes.
- Contact the Cystic Fibrosis Foundation to obtain information on some aspect of care that interests you. Ask for professional and lay resources and compare the contents of all the booklets you obtain.
- Interview a child with asthma and his or her parents. Identify and compare the concerns that each one has about living with asthma. Which concerns are similar? Which ones are different? Can you make recommendations for alleviating any concerns they have?

BIBLIOGRAPHY

Collins, F. S. Cystic fibrosis: Molecular biology and therapeutic implications. *Science* 256 (1992): 774–779.

DeJong, S., and S. McCandless. The respiratory system. Pp. 21–87 in J. B. Smith, ed. *Pediatric Critical Care.* New York: Wiley and Sons, 1983.

George, M. R. CF: Not just a pediatric problem anymore. *RN* 9 (1990): 60–65.

Hathaway, W. E., W. W. Way, Jr., J. R. Groothuis, and J. W. Paisley. *Current Pediatric Diagnosis and Treatment,* 11th ed. Norwalk, CT: Appleton and Lange, 1993.

Landon, C., and R. G. Rosenfeld. Short stature and pubertal delay in male adolescents with cystic fibrosis. *American Journal of Diseases in Children* 138, no. 4 (1984): 388–391.

National Asthma Education Program, Expert Panel Report. *Guidelines for the Diagnosis and Management of Asthma.* Bethesda, MD: U.S. Department of Health and Human Services, 1991.

Rosenstein, B. J, and P. D. Fosarelli. *Pediatric Pearls: The Handbook of Practical Pediatrics.* Chicaco: Year Book Medical Publishers, 1989.

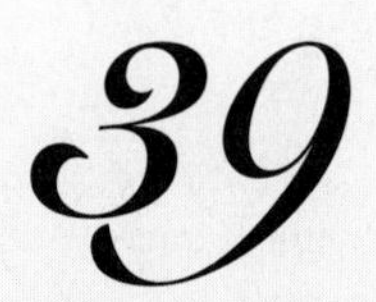

CHAPTER 39

Digestive and Metabolic Conditions

Objectives

After studying this chapter, the student should be able to:

- Name a common oral infection of infancy and discuss its symptoms, treatment, and nursing care.
- Recognize symptoms of colic and discuss treatment and nursing care of this condition.
- Identify common causes of diarrhea in infants and children and discuss treatment and nursing care of this condition.
- Identify three types of dehydration and discuss symptoms, treatment, and nursing care of this condition.
- Compare and contrast the symptoms, treatment, and nursing care of gastroesophageal reflux and pyloric stenosis.
- Differentiate between two conditions causing bowel obstruction in infants and children.
- Identify the two most common types of hernias in infants and discuss their treatment and nursing care.
- Identify two common intestinal parasites in toddlers and preschool children and discuss treatment of these diseases.

- Identify factors that place children at risk for foreign body ingestion and discuss treatment of a child who has ingested a foreign body.
- Discuss the symptoms, treatment, and nursing care of lead poisoning.
- Name two conditions that affect school-age children and adolescents, and discuss their causes, symptoms, treatment, and nursing care.

Key Terms

FECALITH
POLYURIA
POLYDIPSIA
POLYPHAGIA
KETONURIA
KETOACIDOSIS

Digestive and metabolic conditions involve alterations in functioning of the gastrointestinal and endocrine systems. These conditions have the potential to interfere with nutritional intake and fluid balance, resulting in symptoms ranging from electrolyte imbalances to impaired growth and even death. It is important for the nurse to be able to identify and recognize the presenting symptoms of these conditions in order to facilitate early intervention and prevent potentially life-threatening complications.

Overview of the System

The gastrointestinal (GI) system consists of the structures of the oral cavity, pharynx, esophagus, stomach, small intestine, large intestine, liver, and gallbladder, Figure 39–1. The GI system enables the body to ingest, digest, and metabolize nutrients.

The endocrine system consists of glands and organs that secrete hormones that act on cells in other parts of the body. The pancreas functions to

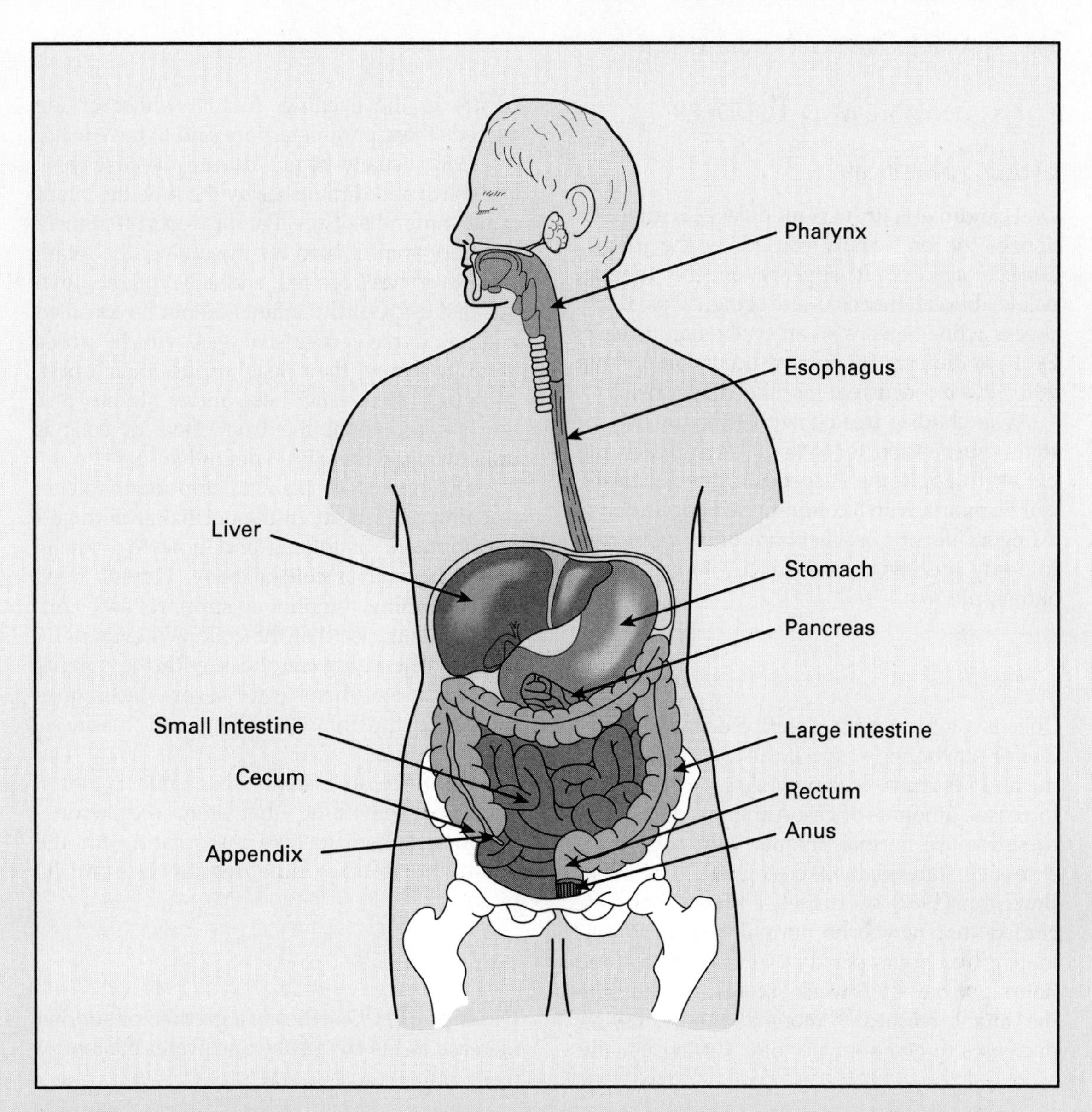

Figure 39–1 *The gastrointestinal system (Adapted from G. L. Smith, P. E. Davis, and J. T. Dennerll.* Medical Terminology: A Programmed Text, *6th ed. Albany, NY: Delmar Publishers, 1991.)*

regulate blood glucose and meet the digestive needs of the body. The pancreatic hormones glucagon and insulin, produced in the beta cells of the islets of Langerhans, play an important role in glucose metabolism. When disease, infection, or trauma interferes with the functioning of the pancreas, both glucose metabolism and digestion can be impaired. This is the case in diabetes mellitus, discussed later in this chapter.

INFANT AND TODDLER

ORAL CANDIDIASIS

Oral candidiasis (thrush, moniliasis) is an infection of the oral cavity caused by the fungus *Candida albicans*. It appears on the tongue, palate, buccal mucosa, and gingiva as thick, cheesy white patches on an erythematous base. Oral candidiasis frequently occurs in infants who have a concurrent monilial diaper rash.

The child is treated with nystatin (Mycostatin) suspension for 7 to 10 days. Teach the parent to apply the suspension directly to the child's mouth with a cotton-tipped applicator or a finger. Nursing mothers are often instructed to apply nystatin cream directly to the areola and nipple area.

COLIC

Colic is a term used to describe certain behaviors of newborns — specifically, excessive crying and fussiness — sometimes associated with increased amounts of gas. Although crying and fussiness are normal, infants with colic have excessive, unexplained crying and fussiness. Brazelton (1962) conducted a study that concluded that newborns normally cry approximately two hours per day, increasing to three hours per day by 6 weeks of age. By the time the infant reaches 3 months of age, crying decreases to one hour per day. Crying usually occurs in the evening. Infants whose crying exceeds these parameters are said to have colic.

Colic usually begins during the first week after birth and diminishes by the time the infant is 3 to 4 months of age. Parents report that there is no apparent reason for the crying; the infant is not wet, has been fed, and is having no obvious distress. Colicky infants cannot be consoled and often have excessive gas, which causes them to draw their legs up to their chest. Although there have been many studies and much speculation, the true cause of colic is unknown and there is no definitive "cure."

The nurse can play an important role in teaching parents about the normal growth and development of infants and how to manage and cope with a colicky baby. Parents need understanding, emotional support, and constant reassurance that the colic will eventually resolve. The nurse can work with the parents and encourage them to try several techniques to reduce the infant's crying and fussiness, Figure 39–2.

Reinforce to parents that colic is not a result of something that they did wrong. Encourage them to take turns caring for the infant and to take "time out" away from the infant.

DIARRHEA

Description. Diarrhea is a gradual or sudden increase in the frequency and water content of

CALMING A COLICKY BABY

- Decrease stimulation
- Swaddle infant and place in a darkened room
- Rock, walk, or place infant in a swing
- Offer infant a pacifier
- Play soft music
- Hold infant close
- Take infant for a ride in a car

Figure 39–2

stools. It is a common occurrence in infants and children. Episodes of diarrhea can be acute, chronic, or recurrent.

Acute diarrhea can have a bacterial, viral, or noninfectious cause. The most common pathogens are *Shigella* (bacillary dysentery), *Salmonella*, and *Escherichia coli* ("traveler's diarrhea"). *Shigella* is frequently found in day-care centers and crowded living conditions. All three bacterial pathogens are transmitted via the fecal-oral route and invade, colonize, and reproduce in the child's intestinal tract (Grimes 1991).

The most common viruses causing diarrhea are rotavirus (also causes fever and vomiting; occurs in the winter and is usually the cause of diarrhea in hospital outbreaks and day-care centers), enterovirus (also causes vomiting and respiratory symptoms), and the Norwalk virus (lasts 24 to 48 hours and can occur in epidemic proportions).

Noninfectious causes of acute diarrhea include acute poisoning (lead and iron) and reactions to antibiotics (ampicillin).

Chronic diarrhea (lasting more than two weeks) can result from infectious and noninfectious conditions. Examples of infectious conditions are amebiasis and giardiasis. Examples of noninfectious conditions are ulcerative colitis, regional enteritis, Hirschsprung's disease, lactase deficiency, and malabsorption. Diarrhea is the most frequent cause of dehydration in infants and children. Its potential to cause a life-threatening medical emergency should not be underestimated (see later discussion).

Symptoms. The infant or child with diarrhea has frequent watery bowel movements with or without mucus or blood. The child may also have symptoms associated with gastroenteritis, such as vomiting, fever, and abdominal pain.

Treatment. Diagnosis is made on the basis of the history, physical examination, and laboratory data. The history helps to identify the duration, frequency, amount, and consistency of the stools as well as characteristics (e.g., presence of blood or mucus, color [black or pale], greasiness, and odor). A diet history is taken to assess for lactose intolerance as well as allergic reactions to medications (such as antibiotics). Ask parents about any recent travel and whether anyone else in the child's household has diarrhea (Rosenstein and Fosarelli 1989). A stool culture may be performed to identify the causative organism. Electrolytes are evaluated to assess the child's potential for dehydration.

The goals of treatment are to replace and correct any fluid and electrolyte imbalances and to maintain adequate nutrition. Children are usually managed as out patients and are not hospitalized unless they have moderate to severe dehydration. Lactose-containing formulas and milk are usually stopped. Breast-fed infants can continue to nurse. If the infant is not dehydrated and is tolerating oral feedings, a soy formula or an electrolyte solution (Pedialyte, Lytren) may be given. Older children are also given oral glucose and electrolyte solutions.

Nursing Care. The nurse can play an important role in the care of the infant or child with diarrhea both in the out-patient and hospital setting. Care of the hospitalized child includes recording intake and output, monitoring IV fluids, encouraging oral fluids, preventing skin breakdown, teaching parents how to care for the child after discharge, and providing emotional support.

The most important aspect of out-patient care is teaching the parents how to care for the child at home. Mothers who are breast feeding should be encouraged to continue and told that the infant may have a slight increase in stooling initially but that eventually the diarrhea will resolve. Teach parents never to dilute electrolyte solutions. Older children should be encouraged to drink fluids such as cola, ginger ale, and fruit-flavored juices or ices. The infant's diet can slowly be advanced from electrolyte solutions to a nonlactose formula (Isomil). Both infants and children can then slowly progress to the so-called BRATS diet (bananas, rice cereal, applesauce, toast, saltines). Encourage parents to call their health care provider if they have any questions about managing the child's condition.

Reinforce to parents the importance of good hygiene, especially thorough handwashing after bowel movements, after changing diapers, and before handling any food.

DEHYDRATION

Description. Dehydration occurs when the body loses excessive amounts of body fluids (especially water). From birth until the onset of puberty, total body weight is more than half fluid. Thus, any sustained reduction in fluid intake or increase in fluid loss can place a child at risk for dehydration.

Normally, fluid loss occurs through the skin (evaporation), lungs, and urine. The body needs a certain amount of water every day to maintain normal fluid and electrolyte balance, Figure 39–3. This need is based on body weight.

Illness alters the child's metabolic status, increasing fluid requirements. Fever, sweating, and diarrhea result in increased fluid losses. In addition, infants and children usually do not take in the same amounts of fluids when they are sick as when they are well.

When dehydration occurs, the child's extracellular volume decreases, causing decreased tissue perfusion and impaired renal function. This can result in metabolic acidosis or alkalosis, respiratory acidosis or alkalosis, and electrolyte alterations such as potassium imbalances.

DAILY FLUID NEEDS

Body Weight	Fluid Need
3–10 kg	100 mL/kg
11–20 kg	50 mL/kg
More than 20 kg	20 mL/kg

Figure 39–3

Fluid loss is expressed as a percentage of total body weight, as follows:

- Mild dehydration: fluid loss is less than 3% to 5% of body weight
- Moderate dehydration: fluid loss is less than 6% to 9% of body weight
- Severe dehydration: fluid loss is more than 10% of body weight

Dehydration is further described as isotonic, hypotonic, or hypertonic, depending on the electrolyte composition of the plasma. In isotonic dehydration, equal amounts of water and sodium are lost, but electrolytes are otherwise normal. In hypotonic dehydration, more electrolytes than water are lost. In hypertonic dehydration, more water than electrolytes is lost.

Symptoms. Symptoms depend on the degree of dehydration. Characteristic findings in mild or moderate dehydration can include lack of tears, dry mucous membranes, decreased skin turgor, pale or mottled color, decreased urinary output. Findings in severe dehydration include tachycardia, low blood pressure, and sunken anterior fontanelle.

Treatment. Diagnosis is based on history, physical examination, and laboratory data. Physical examination should include assessment of the infant's or child's weight, compared with previous weight, if possible, as well as vital signs, blood pressure, and intake and output. Infants should be assessed for a depressed fontanelle and sunken eyes.

The goals of treatment are to replace and restore normal fluid and electrolyte balance, correct any acid-base imbalance, and meet the child's nutritional requirements.

The child is treated with oral rehydration therapy or given intravenous fluids. Many commercially prepared solutions are available to treat a child with mild or moderate dehydration. It is important that the child be given adequate amounts (concentrations) of water, sodium, chloride, potassium, and glucose to replace losses.

Nursing Care. The child should be monitored frequently for a change in color, increased pulse, decreased urine output, and decreased or low blood pressure. These findings are signs of problems with perfusion that could lead to a medical emergency.

Teach parents how to recognize the signs and symptoms of dehydration and what to watch for during the rehydration period. Parents should offer the child 1 to 3 teaspoons (5 to 15 mL) of fluids every 10 to 15 minutes and then increase fluids slowly, as tolerated. Ice chips and frozen juice pops can also be offered to the child. Parents should weigh diapers and count the times that the child urinates or has a bowel movement, if indicated. Advise parents to call the health care provider if they have difficulty getting the child to take fluids.

GASTROESOPHAGEAL REFLUX

Gastroesophageal reflux (GER) is a spontaneous, effortless regurgitation that occurs when the lower esophageal sphincter relaxes, allowing gastric contents to flow backward into the esophagus. Although infants normally have some effortless spitting up of gastric contents, GER should be considered when an infant has recurrent regurgitation or vomiting associated with irritability.

Diagnosis is made in infants under 6 months of age by barium swallow (which shows the backflow of barium from the stomach to the esophagus), esophageal pH probe monitoring, and scintigraphy (DaDalt et al. 1989, Hathaway et al. 1993, Swischuk et al. 1988). In pH probe monitoring, a small catheter is inserted into the esophagus through the nose and left in place for 18 to 24 hours. Measurement of pH indicates the number of reflux episodes. Scintigraphy involves radionuclide scanning to evaluate gastric emptying, gastroesophageal reflux, and lung aspiration.

Treatment focuses on techniques to reduce the reflux of feedings. Cimetadine or liquid antacids are sometimes given to reduce symptoms of colic. Metoclopramide (a smooth-muscle stimulant) given before meals has been found to be beneficial (Shannon 1993). Surgery may be required in the following cases: if the infant continues to have persistent vomiting resulting in failure to thrive after two to three months of treatment; if the infant develops severe esophagitis or esophageal strictures; or if the reflux causes the infant to have apneic spells (Hathaway et al. 1993, Shannon 1993).

Nursing care includes offering the infant small, frequent feedings thickened with rice cereal (2 to 3 teaspoons per ounce of formula). Breast-fed infants should continue nursing. After feeding, the infant should be placed in a prone position with the head elevated to 30 degrees to help reduce regurgitation.

PYLORIC STENOSIS

Description. Pyloric stenosis is a congenital defect that results in an increase in the size of the circular muscle of the pylorus. This increase causes the pyloric sphincter to narrow at the outlet of the stomach. The resulting obstruction blocks the flow of food into the small intestine, Figure 39–4a.

Symptoms. Initially, the infant has symptoms of regurgitation progressing to projectile vomiting after feedings, constipation, poor weight gain or weight loss, and dehydration. The infant is hungry and breast feeds well but develops failure to thrive, apathy, and fretfulness.

Treatment. Diagnosis is made on the basis of the history, physical examination, and

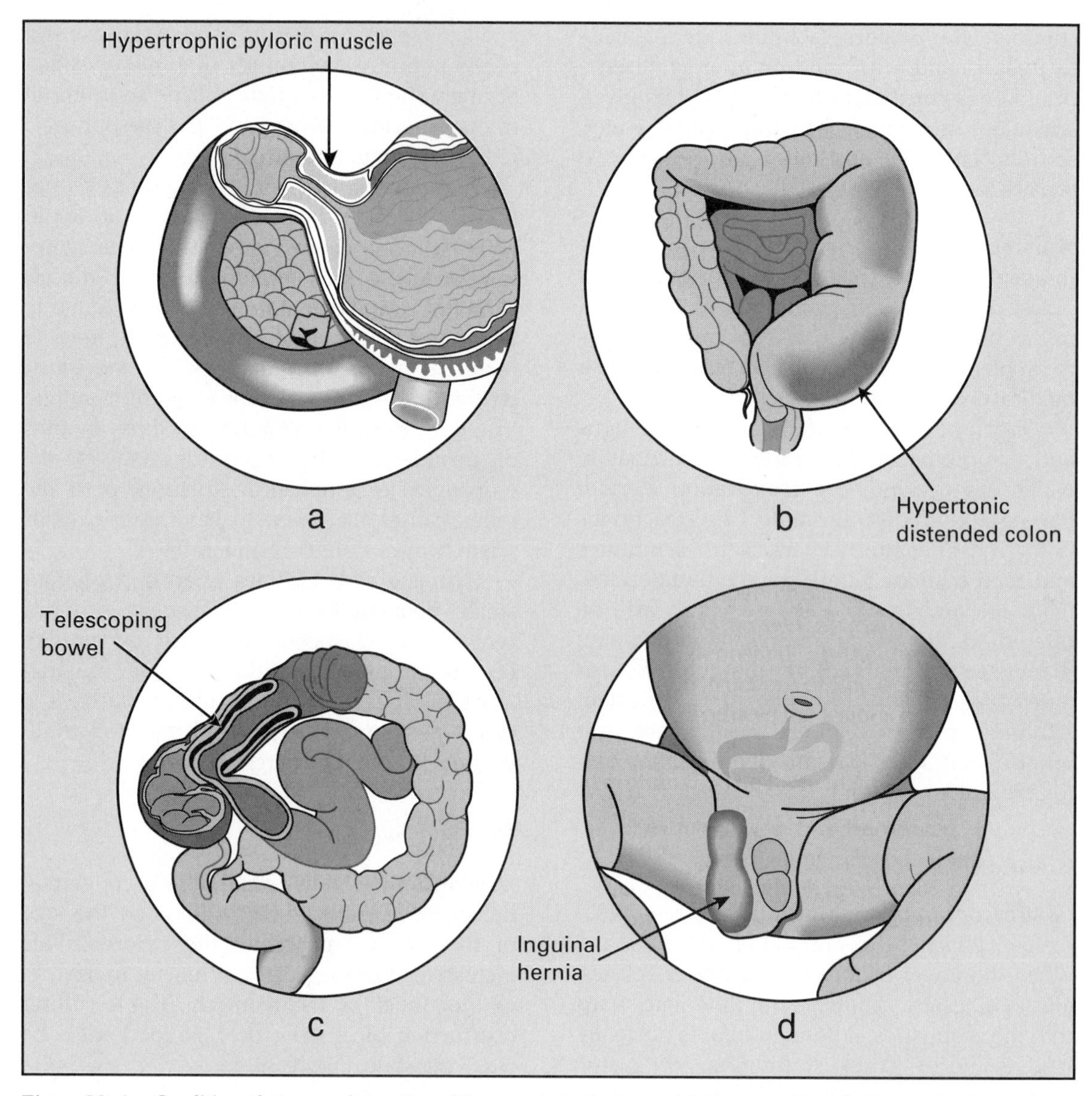

Figure 39–4 Conditions that cause obstruction of the gastrointestinal tract. (a) Hypertrophic pyloric stenosis. (b) Hirschsprung's disease. (c) Intussusception. (d) Strangulated inguinal hernia. (Used with permission of Ross Products Division, Abbott Laboratories, Columbus, OH. From Clinical Education Aid #4, *© Ross Products Division, Abbott Laboratories)*

radiological studies. Physical examination reveals a palpable olive-sized mass in the right upper quadrant of the abdomen. Gastric peristaltic waves can often be seen on the infant's distended abdomen. An upper GI series usually shows the classic "string sign" (an elongated, narrowed pyloric channel) and delayed gastric emptying. Treatment consists of surgery (pyloromyotomy) to release the constricting muscle fibers. The prognosis with surgical correction is excellent.

Nursing Care. Nursing care includes routine preoperative and postoperative care (Chapter 31).

Monitor the infant's fluid and electrolyte status and record intake and output. Monitor IV infusion rate and observe the infant for vomiting and dehydration. Provide emotional support to the parents and child.

HIRSCHSPRUNG'S DISEASE

Hirschsprung's disease is a life-threatening condition that occurs when ganglion cells fail to develop in the mucosal and muscular layers of the colon during fetal development. Ganglion cells are needed to transmit peristaltic contractions, which pass stool through the bowel. The bowel is unable to relax and becomes hypertonic, resulting in obstruction, Figure 39–4b. A small segment or the entire colon can be involved, and obstruction can be partial or complete.

In a newborn, the first clue is failure to pass meconium. Symptoms of poor feeding, irritability, vomiting, diarrhea, abdominal distention (which makes breathing difficult), and shock may develop if the condition remains undiagnosed. An older child may have symptoms of constipation, thin ribbonlike stools, abdominal distention, and failure to thrive.

Obstruction is usually diagnosed in a newborn within the first 24 to 48 hours after birth. Diagnosis is made on the basis of the history, physical examination, x-ray studies, barium enema, and biopsy.

Treatment usually involves performing a temporary colostomy. When the infant is approximately 12 months of age, the aganglionic sections of bowel are removed and corrective surgery is performed. The temporary colostomy is closed once it is determined that the distended bowel has returned to normal function.

INTUSSUSCEPTION

Intussusception is the most frequent cause of intestinal obstruction during the first 2 years of life (Hathaway et al. 1993). It occurs when a proximal portion of intestine telescopes into an adjacent distal portion of intestine, Figure 39–4c. The most common site is the distal ileum, which pushes from the cecum into the colon (Rudolph et al. 1991). Swelling, bowel incarceration, vascular flow obstruction, bleeding from the mucosa, and hemorrhage can result. Partial obstruction can lead to complete obstruction, necrosis of the bowel, perforation, peritonitis, and (if untreated) death.

Characteristically, a seemingly normal infant or toddler, 5 to 18 months of age suddenly develops severe abdominal pain (Rudolph et al. 1991). The child screams, drawing up the legs, knees, and hips. Fever and vomiting may also occur. The pain stops and recurs. Initially the child has a normal bowel movement followed two to three days later by gelatinous, bright to dark red, bloody "currant jelly" stool. Examination reveals a tender distended abdomen, and a sausage-shaped mass is felt on palpation.

A barium enema is given, which serves as a contrast hydrostatic reduction and in most cases successfully restores the telescoped bowel to the proper position. If barium enema is unsuccessful, surgery is performed.

HERNIA

A hernia occurs when an organ protrudes through an abnormal opening in the muscle wall of the cavity that normally contains it. The most common types of hernias in children are inguinal and umbilical hernias, Figure 39–4d. The hernia consists of three parts: a sac or outpouching (peritoneum), the covering of the sac (derived from the abdominal wall), and the contents of the sac (bowel, ovary, or testis) (Foster et al. 1989).

Inguinal Hernia. If the processus vaginalis does not close during fetal development, an opening exists into the inguinal canal. Abdominal contents (bowel) can protrude through this opening, creating a painless inguinal swelling. An inguinal hernia frequently occurs in conjunction with a hydrocele (Chapter 40).

COMMON PARASITIC CHILDHOOD DISEASES

Parasite	Symptoms	Treatment
Giardiasis (protozoan) *Causative organism: Giardia lamblia* (the most common parasite causing disease in the United States) *Transmission*: Person to person (especially children in day-care centers), animals (dogs, cats, beavers), food, water (contaminated reservoirs, lakes, streams)	Symptoms are variable, and children can be asymptomatic or develop severe life-threatening diarrhea, dehydration, and malabsorption (Rudolph et al. 1991). Symptoms include abdominal pain; vomiting; watery, foul-smelling diarrhea; anorexia; and fatigue.	Medications used to treat giardiasis are the anti-infective quinacrine hydrochloride (Atabrine) and the antibiotic furazolidone (Furoxone). (Metronidazole [Flagyl] is effective but not licensed in the United States to treat giardiasis.) Teach parents to use good personal hygiene. Wash hands after toileting and after changing an infant's diaper or touching stool. If a child is infected, wear gloves when handling soiled diapers or clothing. If there is any risk of contaminated water, boil water before drinking.

Figure 39–5

Treatment consists of surgical repair to prevent incarceration.

Umbilical Hernia. Incomplete fascial closure of the umbilical ring during fetal development causes a hernial protrusion near the umbilicus. Intestine and omentum protrude through the weak abdominal wall. An umbilical hernia usually looks like a soft swelling or protrusion covered by skin. If closure does not occur by 5 years of age, surgical repair is performed to prevent strangulation of the bowel. Most umbilical hernias close spontaneously by the time a child is 2 to 3 years of age.

There are many "old wives' tales" about how to cure an umbilical hernia in infants. It is important for the nurse to dispel any myths, especially the use of belly bands and the taping of a silver or half dollar over the infant's umbilicus. Both of these measures increase the risk of strangulation of the herniated bowel and infection.

TODDLER AND PRESCHOOL CHILD

INTESTINAL PARASITES

Parasitic diseases are caused by helminths (worms), protozoans, and arthropods. Although it is more common to see these diseases in tropical and subtropical climates of the world where living conditions are poor, socioeconomic status is low, and diet is inadequate, they can occur

COMMON PARASITIC CHILDHOOD DISEASES

Parasite	Symptoms	Treatment
Pinworms (helminth) *Causative organism: Enterobius vermicularis* *Transmission*: Inhaling or ingesting freshly deposited eggs. Hand to mouth transmission is common, especially when children scratch the infected anal area and then put their fingers in their mouth or bite their nails. Frequently seen in schools and day-care centers.	The most common symptom is intense perianal and perineal pruritus (especially at night). Other symptoms can include urinary tract infection and vulvovaginitis. Children frequently wake at night crying because of itching. Tiny white worms can be seen in the rectal area, stool, or vagina.	*Cellophane tape test*: The best way to diagnose pinworms is to take a tongue blade, wrap cellophane around it, and press it against the perianal area. The tape is put over a drop of toluene on a glass microscope slide and examined for pinworms. Commonly used medications to treat pinworms are mebendazole (Vermox), pyrantel pamoate (Antiminth), and piperazine citrate (Antepar). The child and everyone in the household should be treated at the same time. Treatment is usually repeated in 2 to 3 weeks. All bed sheets, bed clothing, and underwear should be washed in hot water, and the house vacuumed and damp mopped. Reassure parents that pinworms are not a result of uncleanliness.

Figure 39–5 *continued*

anywhere. Children can acquire these diseases from contact with human or animal carriers (Hathaway et al. 1993, Rudolph et al. 1991). The most common parasitic diseases of childhood are giardiasis and pinworm infestation, Figure 39–5.

Children (especially toddlers and preschoolers) are more susceptible to parasitic infestations than are adults because of their poor hygiene, frequent hand to mouth activity, and habit of playing in dirt. Nursing care centers on teaching parents appropriate treatment measures (Figure 39–5) and prevention (e.g., good hygiene practices).

FOREIGN BODY INGESTION

Foreign body ingestion is not uncommon in children (especially toddlers and preschoolers) because they frequently put a variety of objects in their mouths. Objects commonly ingested include coins, toy parts, safety pins, buttons, marbles, and button-type (disc) batteries.

If a child is suspected of having ingested a foreign body, an x-ray should be taken. An object that reaches the child's stomach has a very good chance of passing through the GI tract. Parents should be instructed to watch for the object in the child's stool. An object that does not pass and continues to be seen on x-ray may require endoscopic removal. Surgery is considered if the child develops abdominal pain, obstruction, or perforation.

If a foreign body lodges in the child's esophagus, the child can have symptoms of choking, gagging, drooling, coughing, pain, or respiratory distress. The object is removed by esophagoscopy. Of particular concern are button-type (disc) batteries, which can lodge in the esophagus and leak alkaline, causing necrosis and esophageal perforation. Prompt removal is necessary. Safety precautions should be discussed with parents to prevent future ingestions.

LEAD POISONING

Description. Lead poisoning is a preventable public health problem of children than can lead to psychological problems, mental retardation, and disorders of the neurologic, hematologic, and renal systems. Children are exposed every day to unhealthy levels of lead in the environment (Figure 39–6).

Lead enters the body through inhalation or ingestion. Children who have pica (ingestion of nonfood substances) commonly eat paint chips and are at extremely high risk for lead poisoning. Lead poisoning is most often seen in children under 5 years of age.

Lead is absorbed through the gastrointestinal tract and stored in bone, blood, and soft tissue. The tissues of the erythroid cells of the bone marrow, the nervous system, and the kidneys are most frequently affected. Lead in the body interferes with erythrocyte production and prevents hemoglobin formation, which can lead to anemia. Lead is excreted in the urine.

Symptoms. Symptoms depend on the child's age and blood lead level. A child can be asymptomatic if levels are low. Common symptoms include lethargy, anorexia, vomiting, irritability, abdominal pain, headaches, and decrease in activity level. More severe symptoms include ataxia, clumsiness, encephalopathy, seizures, and mental retardation.

Treatment. Routine screening (fingerstick) of blood lead level is performed on all children between 9 months and 6 years of age. The Centers for Disease Control and Prevention (CDC) has developed a classification system for lead poisoning based on the child's blood lead level concentration. This system enables health care providers to identify children with low, moderate, or high risk for lead poisoning and those requiring retesting.

SOURCES OF LEAD

- Lead-based paint
- Household dust
- Soil and water (contaminated from lead pipes and solder)
- Air near highways (from burning of leaded gasoline)
- Fruit tree sprays
- Ceramics made with leaded glass
- Folk remedies (e.g., powders that are used to treat fevers)

Figure 39–6

Diagnosis is made on the basis of elevated blood lead and free erythrocyte protoporphyrin (FEP) levels. If blood lead levels are elevated after fingerstick, confirmation should be made by venipuncture. X-ray studies of the long bones may be performed to identify lead lines. Abdominal x-rays are used to identify evidence of recently ingested lead.

Treatment focuses initially on identifying and removing lead sources from the child's environment, reducing the amount of lead ingested, providing dietary counseling to improve the child's diet and correct any nutritional imbalances, and encouraging a low-fat high-iron diet, which prevents lead from binding to body tissues. Children with high lead levels require chelation therapy. An agent is administered that binds with the lead to prevent its absorption by the body.

Nursing Care. Nursing care focuses on reinforcing dietary counseling, providing emotional support to parents, and providing referrals to social services or community resources for environmental clean-up.

SCHOOL-AGE CHILD AND ADOLESCENT

APPENDICITIS

Description. Appendicitis is an inflammation of the vermiform appendix (the blind sac at the end of the cecum). It is the most common cause of abdominal surgery in children.

Obstruction of the appendiceal lumen — which can occur as a result of a **fecalith** (a hard, impacted fecal mass), inflammatory changes, lymphoid tissue, parasitic infestations, or stenosis — blocks the flow of mucoid secretions, causing pressure to build up in the blood vessels of the lumen. Inflammation and ulceration of the appendiceal mucosa follow. Without treatment, necrosis and eventual rupture of the appendix occur. Rupture of the appendix can result in peritonitis from fecal and bacterial contamination of the peritoneal cavity.

Symptoms. The child usually presents with a low-grade fever, generalized abdominal pain that localizes to the right lower quadrant, and abdominal tenderness. Vomiting, diarrhea, or constipation can also occur. The child has a decreased activity level and is most comfortable lying on the side with the knees flexed. If the appendix ruptures and peritonitis develops, the child will have a sudden relief of pain followed by severe pain, abdominal distention, tachycardia, rapid shallow respirations, and restlessness.

Treatment. Diagnosis is made on the basis of the history, physical examination, and occasionally x-ray studies. On examination, the child has abdominal tenderness, pain, and guarding. An appendectomy is the treatment of choice. Before surgery, the child is kept NPO (given nothing by mouth) and an intravenous infusion is started to correct any fluid and electrolyte imbalances. If surgery is uncomplicated by perforation, the prognosis is excellent and the child is discharged within 5 days.

If the appendix ruptures before surgery, the child is started on intravenous antibiotics and nasogastric suctioning is begun. Postoperatively, the child requires a 7- to 10-day course of antibiotics, intravenous fluids, nasogastric suctioning, and dressing changes.

Nursing Care. Nursing care is the same as for any child undergoing surgery (Chapter 31). Before surgery, provide reassurance and emotional support. After surgery, check the abdominal dressing frequently for signs of increased drainage and infection. Monitor vital signs frequently, administer prescribed medications for pain and fever, and encourage the child to cough and deep breathe. It will be easier for the child to cough if a pillow is used to splint the surgical site. Provide emotional support. On discharge, instruct parents to watch for any redness or drainage from the incision. Tell parents to keep the incision clean and dry. The child should avoid contact sports and lifting any heavy objects.

DIABETES MELLITUS

Description. Insulin-dependent diabetes mellitus (IDDM), type I, previously called juvenile-onset diabetes mellitus, is a chronic metabolic condition that occurs in children as a result of a loss of pancreatic beta cell function, resulting in limited production of insulin. The deficiency of insulin leads to a decreased availability of glucose in the cells and to a buildup of glucose in the blood. Because carbohydrates are unavailable for energy, the body metabolizes fat, instead. The breakdown of fat, however, results in an excess of ketones, which are then excreted through the lungs and urine.

Several factors are thought to influence the development of IDDM. These factors include genetic predisposition, environment, and immunological mechanisms. A child inherits a susceptibility to IDDM, not the disease itself (Rudolph et al. 1991). A viral infection of the beta cells of the islets of Langerhans is then believed to trigger an immune response that results in destruction of the beta cells.

Symptoms. The cardinal sign of IDDM is **polyuria** (excessive urine output), especially at night. Other characteristic findings include nocturnal enuresis, **polydipsia** (excessive thirst), weight loss, **polyphagia** (markedly increased food intake), glycosuria (glucose in the urine) with or without **ketonuria** (loss of ketones in urine), and hyperglycemia (elevated blood glucose).

Treatment. Diagnosis is made on the basis of the history, physical examination, and blood and urine testing. Glucose tolerance tests are usually not required to diagnose IDDM (Rudolph et al. 1991). It is not uncommon for a child with early symptoms of IDDM to be diagnosed during a routine urinalysis.

Treatment of the child with IDDM depends on the severity of the condition at the time of diagnosis. Children may be hospitalized initially or treated on an out-patient basis. Management includes restoring fluid balance, correcting electrolyte imbalances, regulating insulin dosage, monitoring and correcting acidosis and glucose levels, and diet therapy.

Insulin can be given as a single dose of intermediate-acting (Lente or NPH) insulin, as multiple doses of short-acting regular insulin at different times of the day, or as a twice-daily combined dose of intermediate- and short-acting insulin mixed and given in the same syringe (usually before breakfast and before supper). Insulin doses are regulated according to the child's levels of glucose and ketones. Blood glucose levels and urine glucose and ketones are monitored before meals and at bedtime. Diet, exercise, illness, and emotional stress may all affect insulin needs.

Injection sites are rotated in a consistent pattern to different areas of the body (e.g., upper arms, thighs, abdomen, buttocks), Figure 39–7. Rotation improves the absorption of insulin by preventing development of fat pads in the injection site area. Absorption occurs rapidly in the arm and is slowest in the thigh (Wong 1993).

An alternative to daily injections of insulin is the insulin pump, which mimics pancreatic insulin secretions by providing either a slow, steady infusion or a larger (bolus) amount of regular (short-acting) insulin when needed. The pump is a small, battery-operated device, the size of a calculator. It consists of a syringe with a mechanized plunger connected by a catheter to a needle inserted in the subcutaneous tissue, usually in the abdomen (Clark and Plotnick 1990).

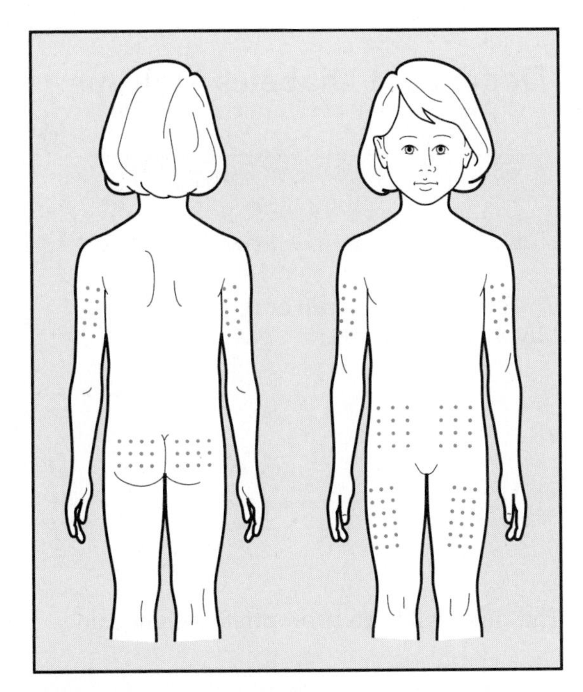

Figure 39–7 Insulin injection sites

Diet therapy is an important element in the overall management of the child with IDDM. A well-balanced diet is required that meets the caloric needs of the child and supplies the necessary nutrients to promote growth, while avoiding concentrated sugars. The child's total caloric intake should be distributed over three meals and three snacks, consumed at consistent intervals throughout the day. The American Dietetic Association food exchange lists can be used to provide a carefully measured diet for the diabetic child. To ensure compliance with dietary therapy, a dietician should help the child and family plan an exchange diet based on the foods that the child likes.

Long-term medical management of IDDM focuses on maintaining normal growth and development and preventing episodes of hypoglycemia and ketoacidosis. Hypoglycemia (low serum glucose concentration) can result from prolonged or excessive insulin secretion or excessive body needs. Symptoms include tachycardia, sweating, flushing, shakiness, drowsiness, headache, weakness, anxiety, and behavioral changes. Children with these symptoms require immediate treatment with simple sugar. Untreated hypoglycemia may result in loss of consciousness, convulsions, brain damage, and death.

Diabetic **ketoacidosis** is a complication of IDDM that results from accumulations of ketones in the body. Symptoms include acetone (fruity) odor to the breath, dyspnea, vomiting, dehydration, weight loss, mental confusion, and, if untreated, coma. Without emergency treatment, ketoacidosis can be fatal. Treatment involves restoring fluids, administering normal saline and regular insulin (via injection or drip), and monitoring glucose level, acidosis, vital signs, serum ketones, electrolytes, and fluid intake and output.

Nursing Care. The nurse's role includes managing the child during the initial hospitalization and providing continuing education to the child and family. Nursing care of the hospitalized child depends on the child's condition at the time of admission. Initial care focuses on monitoring the child's fluid and electrolyte status, measuring intake and output, monitoring intravenous fluids, checking vital signs, checking urine and blood for glucose and ketones, and administering insulin. The child should be watched closely for signs of ketoacidosis or hypoglycemia.

The education of the child and family is as important as the medical management of the child (Rudolph et al. 1991). Teaching should include how to administer insulin, how to test the urine for ketones, how to measure blood glucose levels, how to recognize hypoglycemia, and how to manage diet. Parents should also be instructed about when to contact a health care provider (for example, if ketone levels are moderate to high). Emphasize the importance of having the child wear some type of medical identification (e.g., Medic-Alert bracelet).

NURSING CARE PLAN: Insulin-Dependent Diabetes Mellitus

PATIENT PROBLEM	GOAL(S)
Potential for injury: hypoglycemia or ketoacidosis	The child will maintain or regain normal blood glucose levels.
Inability to gain weight despite adequate caloric intake	The child will have appropriate weight gain. The child and parents will state understanding of diabetic diet.
Anxiety related to lack of knowledge about disease and its management	The child and parents will state knowledge of insulin therapy, dietary management, and symptoms to report to their health care provider.

Figure 39–8

NURSING INTERVENTION	RATIONALE
Monitor blood glucose and urine glucose and ketone levels.	Provides a guide to insulin needs. Low blood glucose levels are indicative of hypoglycemia; elevated glucose and ketones are indicative of ketoacidosis.
Administer insulin as prescribed.	Insulin promotes utilization of glucose.
Assess vital signs and level of consciousness (LOC).	Changes in vital signs and LOC indicate poorly regulated blood glucose.
Provide three meals per day and three snacks at the same time each day.	Regulating daily calories and eating food at consistent intervals help the child to gain weight.
Educate child and parents about diet therapy and relationship between diet, exercise, and insulin requirements.	Knowledge helps ensure compliance with treatment plan.
Provide information about exchange lists.	Exchange lists help to regulate dietary intake.
Explain cause, symptoms, and treatment of IDDM.	Knowledge decreases anxiety.
Provide written materials for parents and child to take home.	Written materials reinforce teaching and can be referred to after discharge.
Teach parents and child: how to recognize and treat a hypoglycemic episode; to monitor ketone levels and call the child's health care provider if levels are elevated.	Early identification allows for prompt management.
Encourage school-age child or adolescent to take responsibility for self-care (glucose testing, insulin injections, and diet).	Self-management provides a sense of control and independence.
Encourage child and parents to verbalize concerns about disease and its management. Refer to peer support groups if indicated.	Provides child and family with an outlet and an opportunity to work through concerns.

Dietary teaching should include the following points:

- The child should eat a well-balanced diet but avoid pure sugar foods.
- Meals and snacks should be eaten at about the same time every day. Snacks are necessary to prevent insulin reactions.
- The amount of fat and cholesterol in the diet should be decreased.
- Exercise is important to reduce stress and promote well-being. Vigorous exercise should be scheduled after meals to minimize the risk of a hypoglycemic episode.
- The child should always carry simple sugar (glucose tablets, sugar cubes, hard candy) to ingest in case a hypoglycemic episode occurs.

Emotional support is essential for both the child and parents to help them cope with the limitations of a chronic disease. Parents can be referred to organizations such as the American Diabetes Association, 1660 Duke Street, Alexandria, VA 22314 (800) 232-3472, for information and educational materials.

Self-management is an essential component of diabetes management. The school-age child can be encouraged to begin taking responsibility for aspects of daily care, such as testing blood glucose and injecting insulin. Self-care provides the child with a sense of control. Summer camps for children with diabetes also foster a sense of independence and responsibility. Adolescents are at particular risk for noncompliance with the daily management regimen. They may rebel against the limitations and regimentation imposed by the disease. Encouraging adolescents to discuss their feelings and helping them to learn more about the disease, how to adjust their diet so they do not feel different from peers, and how to manage reactions may be beneficial.

Nursing care of the child with IDDM is summarized in Figure 39–8 (page 652).

REVIEW QUESTIONS

A. Multiple choice. Select the best answer.

1. All of the following are common causes of diarrhea in infants except
   a. rhinovirus
   b. *E. coli*
   c. *Salmonella*
   d. rotavirus
2. Recurrent regurgitation is a characteristic sign of which of the following conditions?
   a. colic
   b. gastroesophageal reflux
   c. intussusception
   d. Hirschsprung's disease
3. Jamie, 2 weeks old, has symptoms of projectile vomiting and poor weight gain. Which of the following conditions would you suspect?
   a. colic
   b. gastroesophageal reflux
   c. pyloric stenosis
   d. Hirschsprung's disease
4. All of the following are characteristic findings in children with IDDM except
   a. polyuria
   b. polydipsia
   c. polyphagia
   d. polycythemia

5. The "string sign" is a classic finding in which of the following disorders?
   a. pyloric stenosis
   b. intussusception
   c. gastroesophageal reflux
   d. Hirschsprung's disease

6. A child with moderate dehydration has a fluid loss of approximately
   a. 3% to 5% of body weight
   b. 6% to 9% of body weight
   c. 10% to 13% of body weight
   d. 13% to 15% of body weight

B. True or false. Write *T* for a true statement and *F* for a false statement.

1. ___ Colic usually resolves by the time an infant is 3 to 4 months of age.
2. ___ Fever is the most common cause of dehydration in infants and young children.
3. ___ Intussusception commonly occurs suddenly in a previously healthy child.
4. ___ Immediate surgical repair is essential for infants with umbilical hernias.
5. ___ Intestinal parasitic diseases are common in children of all ages.
6. ___ Foreign body ingestion is most common in young infants.
7. ___ The child with appendicitis usually assumes a semi-Fowler's position.

SUGGESTED ACTIVITIES

- Interview the parents of an infant with colic. Ask parents what strategies they have used to manage the infant's symptoms. Which strategies have been successful? Which have been unsuccessful?
- Write or call the American Diabetes Association (see information provided in the chapter) to request educational materials on IDDM. Assess these materials regarding their use in parent teaching.

BIBLIOGRAPHY

Boyle, J. T. Gastroesophageal reflux in the pediatric patient. *Gastroenterology Clinics of North America* 18 (1989): 315–337.

Brazelton, T. B. Crying in infancy. *Pediatrics* 29 (1962): 579–588.

Broadwell Jackson, D., and R. B. Saunders. *Child Health Nursing*. Philadelphia: J. B. Lippincott, 1993.

Cervisi, J., M. Chapman, B. Niklas, and C. Yamaoka. Office management of the infant with colic. *Journal of Pediatric Health Care* 5, no. 4 (1991): 184–190.

Clark, L. M., and L. P. Plotnick. Insulin pumps in children with diabetes. *Journal of Pediatric Health Care* 4 (1990): 3–10.

DaDalt, L., S. Mazzoleni, G. Montini, F. Donzelli, and F. Zacchello. Diagnostic accuracy of pH monitoring in gastroesophageal reflux. *Archives of Disease in Childhood* 64 (1989): 1421–1426.

Foster, R. L. R., M. M. H. Hunsberger, and J. T. Anderson. *Family-Centered Nursing Care of Children*. Philadelphia: W. B. Saunders, 1989.

Grimes, D. *Infectious Diseases*. St. Louis, MO: Mosby-Year Book, 1991.

Hathaway, W. E., W. W. Hay, J. R. Groothuis, and J. W. Paisley. *Current Pediatric Diagnosis and Treatment*, 11th ed. Norwalk, CT: Appleton and Lange, 1993.

Rosenstein, B. J., and P. D. Fosarelli. *Pediatric Pearls: The Handbook of Practical Pediatrics*. Chicago: Year Book Medical Publishers, 1989.

Rudolph, A. M., J. I. E. Hoffman, and C. D. Rudolph. *Rudolph's Pediatrics*, 19th ed. Norwalk, CT: Appleton and Lange, 1991.

Shannon, R. S. Gastroesophageal reflux in infancy: Review and update. *Journal of Pediatric Health Care* 7, no. 2 (1993): 71–76.

Swischuk, L. E., C. K. Hayden, D. H. Fawcet, and J. N. Isenberg. Gastroesophageal reflux: How much imaging is required? *Radiographics* 8 (1988): 1137–1145.

Tucker, J. A., and K. Sussman-Karten. Treating diarrhea and dehydration with an oral rehydration solution. *Pediatric Nursing* 13, no. 3 (1987): 169–174.

Wong, D. *Whaley & Wong's Essentials of Pediatric Nursing*, 4th ed. St. Louis, MO: Mosby-Year Book, 1993.

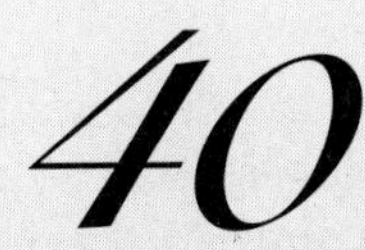

Genitourinary Conditions

Objectives

AFTER STUDYING THIS CHAPTER, THE STUDENT SHOULD BE ABLE TO:

- IDENTIFY FOUR STRUCTURAL DEFECTS OF THE GENITOURINARY SYSTEM AND DESCRIBE THEIR TREATMENT AND NURSING CARE.
- DESCRIBE THE SYMPTOMS, TREATMENT, AND NURSING CARE OF URINARY TRACT INFECTION AND IDENTIFY SEVERAL FACTORS PREDISPOSING A CHILD TO DEVELOP AN INFECTION.
- DESCRIBE THE SYMPTOMS, TREATMENT, AND NURSING CARE OF WILM'S TUMOR.
- COMPARE AND CONTRAST THE SYMPTOMS, TREATMENT, AND NURSING CARE OF NEPHROTIC SYNDROME, ACUTE GLOMERULONEPHRITIS, AND ACUTE AND CHRONIC RENAL FAILURE.
- DEFINE ENURESIS AND DESCRIBE ITS CAUSE, TREATMENT, AND NURSING CARE.
- IDENTIFY FOUR COMMON SEXUALLY TRANSMITTED DISEASES AND DESCRIBE THEIR TREATMENT AND NURSING CARE.

Key Terms

URINARY STASIS
VESICOURETERAL REFLUX
HYPOPROTEINEMIA
HYPOALBUMINEMIA
HYPERLIPIDEMIA
HYPOVOLEMIA
OLIGURIA

Genitourinary conditions in children may be congenital or acquired (a result of infection, disease, or injury). Congenital conditions include structural defects such as hypospadias, epispadias, hydrocele, and cryptorchidism. Acquired conditions include infection of the urinary tract, kidney disorders, and sexually transmitted diseases. Structural defects, if untreated, can have physical and psychological effects as the child matures. Acquired conditions, if untreated, can result in inflammation, tissue damage, and scarring. By assisting in early assessment and treatment of these conditions, the nurse can play an important role in preventing physiological and psychological complications.

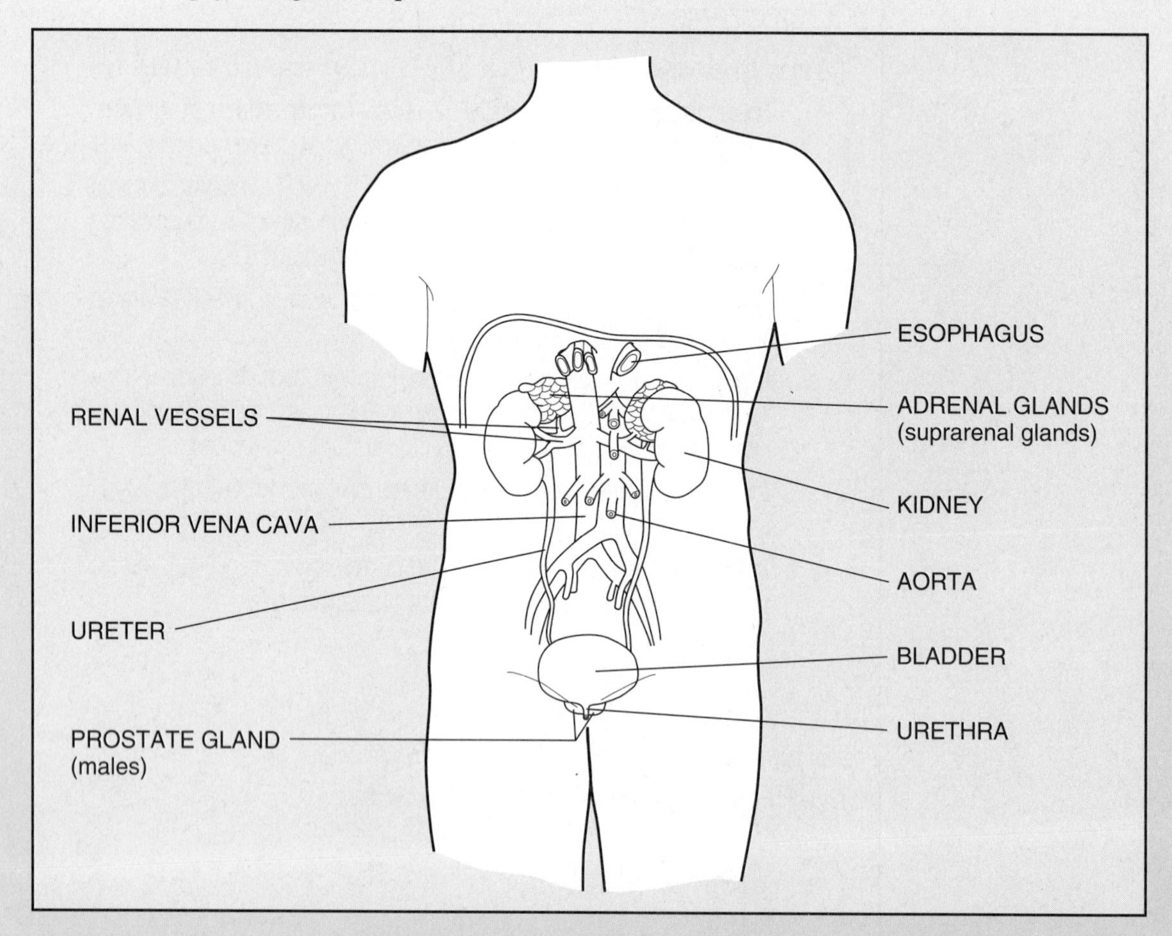

Figure 40–1 *The urinary system (Adapted from G. L. Smith, P. E. Davis, and J. T. Dennerll.* Medical Terminology: A Programmed Approach, *6th ed. Albany, NY: Delmar Publishers, 1991.)*

Overview of the System

The urinary system is made up of the kidneys, ureters, urinary bladder, and urethra, Figure 40–1. The main function of this system is to excrete nitrogenous wastes, salts, and water from the body, thus preventing the buildup of toxic wastes. The kidneys also function to regulate fluid and electrolyte balance.

Each kidney consists of an outer layer (cortex) and an inner, striated layer (medulla). The nephron is the basic structural and functional unit of the kidney, Figure 40–2. Each kidney contains over 1 million nephrons (Fong et al. 1993).

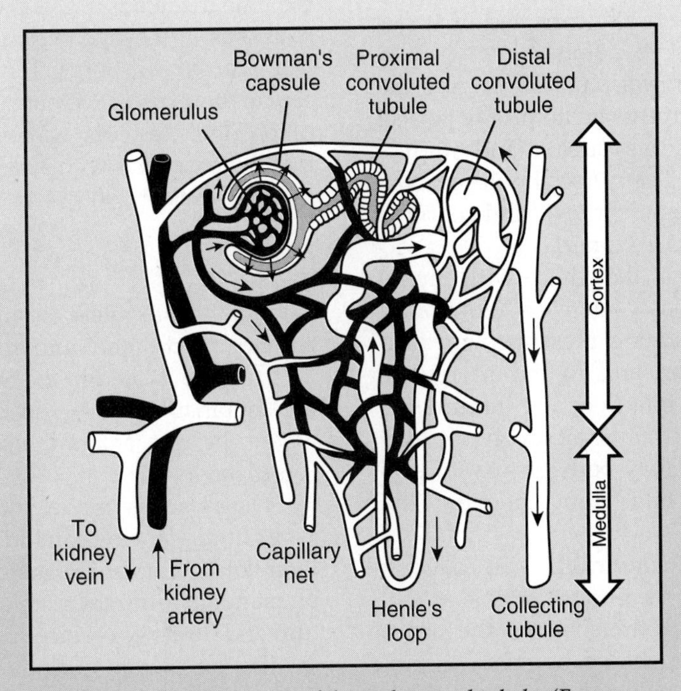

Figure 40–2 *Cross section of the nephron and tubules (From S. R. Burke.* Human Anatomy and Physiology in Health and Disease, *3rd ed. Albany, NY: Delmar Publishers, 1992.)*

INFANT AND TODDLER

HYPOSPADIAS AND EPISPADIAS

Hypospadias is a congenital anomaly of males in which the urethral meatus is located on the ventral surface of the glans penis instead of at the tip. In epispadias, the meatus is located on the dorsal surface of the penis. Epispadias is usually associated with exstrophy of the bladder.

Diagnosis is made by observation at birth, and the defect is surgically corrected in stages beginning in the first year of life.

The goal of surgical repair is to give the child a penis that appears anatomically correct with a normal voiding stream and normal sexual functioning. The nurse should encourage parents to express their fears and concerns and provide emotional support.

Nursing care of the child with hypospadias or epispadias centers on monitoring vital signs; administering prescribed medications for pain, fever, and to reduce muscle spasms; preventing infection; and limiting the child's mobility. Restraints, although not usually recommended, may be necessary to prevent the young child from touching the surgical site.

Postoperatively, the child will have a bulky dressing over the perineal area that will compress the wound, dressings on the penis, and a catheter. Care should be taken to prevent bleeding. Observe for and report immediately any increased drainage. A tent should be made from the child's sheets to prevent bed linens from touching the surgical site, penis, catheters, or dressing.

The child is kept on complete bed rest with limited mobility for 48 to 72 hours after surgery. Bed rest is usually required for 7 to 10 days. Help the parents to provide age-appropriate diversional activities for the child on bed rest (such as videos, music, computer games, puzzles, paint, books).

HYDROCELE

A hydrocele occurs as a result of failure of the processus vaginalis to close during fetal development. This condition enables fluid from the peritoneal cavity to surround the testicle.

Diagnosis is made by physical examination. Palpation of the scrotum reveals a round, smooth, nontender mass. The mass is translucent on transillumination.

A hydrocele is often associated with inguinal hernia. Most communicating hydroceles close by the time the infant is 1 year of age and the fluid reabsorbs. If the hydrocele is large, bowel may slip into the sac. Surgical intervention is necessary in these cases. Reassure parents that the condition often resolves without intervention and that the prognosis with surgical repair (if necessary) is excellent.

CRYPTORCHIDISM

Cryptorchidism refers to failure of one or both testicles to descend into the scrotal sac. The testis can be located in the abdominal cavity, in the inguinal canal, or near the external ring where the ring enters the scrotum. The cause is unclear.

Diagnosis is made by examination and x-ray findings. Cryptorchidism should be differentiated from a retractile testis, which can be manually brought back down into the scrotum and does not require surgical treatment.

Treatment can include hormone therapy (intramuscular injections of human chorionic gonadotropin [hCG] to stimulate descent) or surgery. Surgery, if it is performed, usually takes place before the child is 5 years of age. The longer an undescended testicle remains out of the scrotal sac, the greater the risk of infertility. Other complications of untreated cryptorchidism include malignancy, hernia, torsion, and the psychological effects of an "empty" scrotum.

Teach parents about the surgical procedure and discuss their concerns and fears related to their child's possible infertility. Because of the risk of testicular malignancy later in life, the importance of testicular self-examination and regular follow-up should be emphasized.

URINARY TRACT INFECTION

Description. Urinary tract infections (UTIs) are the most common genitourinary disorders and the second most common infection of childhood. These infections can be bacterial, fungal, or viral in nature. *Escherichia coli (E. coli)* is the organism responsible for 90% of first-time UTIs (Tanagho and McAninch 1992). An infection can occur in the urethra, bladder, ureters, renal pelvis, or renal parenchyma.

Conditions that may predispose a child to develop a UTI include obstruction (functional or structural), urinary stasis, and vesicoureteral reflux. **Urinary stasis** occurs when the flow of urine is interrupted, allowing bacteria to multiply. Infrequent voiding is a common cause of urinary stasis. **Vesicoureteral reflux** occurs when there is an abnormal backflow of urine from the bladder to the ureters.

Symptoms. Symptoms are variable and depend on the cause and location of the infection. Symptoms can include frequency, urgency, dysuria, enuresis, abdominal pain, fever, strong-smelling urine, flank pain, and occasionally hemorrhagic cystitis.

Treatment. Diagnosis is made on the basis of the history, physical examination, presence of characteristic symptoms (flank or abdominal pain, masses, tenderness), and laboratory data (urinalysis including culture and sensitivity). Diagnostic radiological studies can include intravenous pyelography and voiding cystourethrogram [VCUG]). A urine culture should be performed on a midstream clean-catch specimen. If the child cannot cooperate, a suprapubic bladder tap may be performed. A UTI is present when a urine culture is found to have more than 100,000 colony-forming units of a single organism per milliliter.

When no functional or structural urinary tract abnormalities are found, other possible causes should be considered. These include infrequent or incomplete voiding, poor perineal hygiene, pinworms, or constipation.

Treatment depends on a multitude of variables including whether the child is symptomatic or asymptomatic, whether this is the child's first infection or a reinfection, and whether the child has a preexisting condition or a functional or structural abnormality. A 10-day course of antibiotics (sulfisoxazole or ampicillin) is prescribed. The child should return within 48 hours of treatment for a follow-up urinalysis and culture, and again one to three weeks after treatment. Some authorities recommend follow-up cultures every one to three months for one year.

Nursing Care. It is important for the nurse to use good technique when obtaining a urine specimen from a child. Contamination frequently causes false positive results.

Teach parents to avoid putting tight nylon or silk underwear on the child. Tight underwear and synthetic materials trap moisture close to the body, providing an environment conducive to bacterial growth. Recommend the child wear cotton panties. Discourage the use of bubble bath, which can be irritating. Encourage fluids and have the parent take the child to the bathroom frequently. Teach parents the importance of good perineal hygiene. Reinforce that because the urethra is short in girls, contamination from rectal bacteria is common. Instruct parents and children to wipe the perineum from front to back. Teach sexually active teenage girls to void after intercourse.

Provide emotional support to parents and encourage them to ask questions. Reinforce to parents the importance of completing the prescribed course of medications and bringing the child back for follow-up cultures. Advise parents to call the health care provider if they have questions. Figure 40–3 summarizes nursing care for the child with a UTI.

NURSING CARE PLAN: Urinary Tract Infection

PATIENT PROBLEM	GOAL(S)
Dysuria	The child will state and show relief from pain.
Potential fluid and electrolyte imbalance (dehydration)	The child will maintain or regain normal fluid and electrolyte balance.
Lack of knowledge of preventive strategies for UTIs	The child and parents will describe strategies for preventing UTIs.

Figure 40–3

NURSING INTERVENTION	RATIONALE
Encourage frequent bladder emptying (every 3 to 4 hours).	Helps prevent urinary stasis, which encourages persistence of microorganisms.
Administer antibiotics as prescribed.	Antibiotics provide bactericidal action to kill bacteria that cause infection.
Measure pain using a pediatric pain scale (see Chapter 31).	Provides an objective measurement of a child's pain.
Provide comfort measures, such as warm baths.	Warm baths help to relieve symptoms of perineal irritation.
Encourage liberal intake of fluids. Avoid carbonated and caffeinated beverages.	Liberal fluid intake promotes normal hydration and helps prevent urinary stasis. Carbonated and caffeinated beverages may irritate the bladder mucosa in some children.
Maintain accurate intake and output records.	Enables monitoring of child's fluid status.
Administer intravenous fluids, as ordered.	IV fluids provide rapid rehydration.
Administer antipyretic medications, as indicated. Monitor vital signs frequently for evidence of recurrent fever.	Fever increases fluid loss.
Teach parents the importance of having the child: empty bladder frequently; drink adequate amount of fluids; avoid bubble baths; wear cotton underwear; perform good perineal hygiene.	These strategies help prevent recurrence of infection.
Teach girls to always wipe the perineum from front to back.	
Teach sexually active adolescent girls to void after intercourse.	

WILM'S TUMOR

Description. Wilm's tumor, also known as nephroblastoma, is the most common solid malignant renal tumor in children. The tumor occurs in both boys and girls and usually presents as an abdominal mass during the third year of life. It can occur in either kidney and occurs bilaterally in 5% of cases (Tanagho and McAninch 1992). Although the cause of Wilm's tumor is unclear, the tumor is thought to originate during embryonic development and is frequently associated with other congenital anomalies (e.g., hypospadias, ambiguous genitalia, cryptorchidism).

Symptoms. An abdominal mass is usually discovered by parents while bathing or dressing the child or by the physician or nurse during a routine physical examination. The tumor is felt as a firm nontender flank mass (Foley et al. 1993). Once the mass is detected, no further palpation should be performed. Common symptoms include abdominal pain, hypertension, hematuria, vomiting, diarrhea, and fever. Children may, however, be asymptomatic.

Treatment. Diagnosis is made by physical examination, laboratory studies (urinalysis, blood studies), ultrasonography, computed axial tomographic (CAT) scanning, and magnetic resonance imaging (MRI). Treatment is multifaceted and consists of surgery, radiation therapy, and chemotherapy. The National Wilm's Tumor Study (NWTS) has developed a clinical staging classification system based on surgical and pathological findings that is used to develop a treatment plan for the child. Prognosis depends on early diagnosis, intervention, and staging of the tumor.

Nursing Care. Nursing care of the child with a Wilm's tumor involves preoperative, operative, and postoperative care. Throughout the child's care the family and child will need emotional support and understanding. Helping the parents cope with the diagnosis of their child's cancer requires compassion and sensitivity. Provide the family with opportunities to ask questions and discuss their feelings and fears.

Preoperative teaching using anatomically correct dolls and a visit to the surgical suite can help to reduce the child's and parents' anxiety (Chapter 31). Do not massage the abdomen as it may cause the tumor to rupture. Postoperatively, close monitoring of the surgical site, vital signs, and pain threshold is required (Chapter 31). Children require both radiation and chemotherapy and should be closely monitored for adverse reactions.

PRESCHOOL AND SCHOOL-AGE CHILD

NEPHROTIC SYNDROME

Description. Nephrotic syndrome is a disorder characterized by proteinuria, **hypoproteinemia** (a decreased amount of protein in the blood), **hypoalbuminemia** (abnormally low levels of albumin in the blood), **hyperlipidemia** (an excess of lipids in the plasma), and edema. It is most common in preschool children between 2 and 3 years of age, and it is more common in boys than in girls.

In this condition, large amounts of protein are produced and excreted in the urine. The exact cause of this proteinuria is unknown. Protein loss causes hypoalbuminemia, which in turn causes interstitial fluid to accumulate. Because the child has poor renal perfusion, increased amounts of sodium and water are reabsorbed by the renal tubules, resulting in edema.

Nephrotic syndrome can occur as a result of any type of glomerular disease or as a complication of other disorders such as lupus, diabetes, or sickle cell disease.

Symptoms. The cardinal sign of nephrotic syndrome is edema, which appears gradually and spreads slowly. The periorbital area is usually affected first followed by generalized pitting edema of the hands, ankles, and feet. The child may have a protuberant abdomen and abdominal discomfort because of fluid buildup.

Treatment. A combination of corticosteroid, diuretic, immunosuppressive, and antihypertensive medications is administered. It is important to prevent infection and restrict the amount of sodium in the child's diet during the acute phase of the disease.

The prognosis depends on the cause. Children who have a favorable response to corticosteroids usually have no significant problems. Other children can have frequent relapses and progressive renal disease.

Nursing Care. Nursing care includes providing emotional support to the parents and child, monitoring the child's fluid intake and output, checking urine for protein, preventing infection by keeping the child in reverse isolation, and administering medications as ordered.

On discharge from the hospital, the nurse should reinforce to parents the importance of completing the prescribed course of medications and of keeping follow-up appointments. Teach parents that the child can return to a normal diet without sodium restrictions except during edematous periods, if allowed by the physician.

ACUTE GLOMERULONEPHRITIS

Description. Glomerulonephritis is a disease that causes inflammation of the glomerulus in the kidney. In most children, acute glomerulonephritis follows an infection of the pharynx, tonsils, or skin with group A beta-hemolytic streptococci. This form of the disease is referred to as poststreptococcal acute glomerulonephritis. Children between the ages of 3 and 10 years are most commonly affected.

In poststreptococcal acute glomerulonephritis, antigens localize in the kidney on the capillary wall. The kidney becomes edematous and enlarged. Inflammation, obstruction, and injury to the tissue occur, and glomerular filtration rate is impaired.

Symptoms. Approximately 50% of children are asymptomatic. The disease is usually discovered during routine urinalysis (Rudolph et al. 1991). In severe cases, which develop approximately 10 to 14 days after an acute streptococcal infection, the child can have a low-grade fever, headache, malaise, periorbital edema, proteinuria, decreased urine output, and hematuria. The child often has brown or tea-colored urine. The child may also be hypertensive.

Treatment. Treatment involves administration of antihypertensive and diuretic medications and a low-sodium, low-protein diet. Bed rest is advised during the acute phase. Antibiotics may be prescribed if the streptococcal infection is still present.

Follow-up visits for blood pressure monitoring and urinalysis should occur for at least one year after treatment.

Nursing Care. Nursing care is similar to that provided for the child with nephrotic syndrome. Provide emotional support to the parents and child. Monitor fluid intake and output and help the child pick foods that he or she likes, while maintaining the low-sodium, low-protein diet. Test urine frequently for the presence of blood and protein. Provide diversional activities such as video tapes, games, puzzles, and audio books while the child is on bed rest.

RENAL FAILURE

Renal failure occurs when the kidneys are unable to excrete enough water, electrolytes, and waste products to maintain normal body fluid homeostasis (Rudolph et al. 1991). Renal failure can be either acute or chronic. Acute renal failure develops suddenly and can result from impaired renal perfusion, acute renal disease, or obstructive uropathy. Early recognition and treatment are important. Chronic renal failure is a progressive deterioration in renal function that develops as a result of an underlying kidney or urinary tract condition.

ACUTE RENAL FAILURE

Description. Acute renal failure is classified as prerenal, renal, or postrenal failure, depending on the underlying cause. Prerenal failure occurs when **hypovolemia** (diminished blood flow) develops, usually as a result of dehydration, blood loss, complications of surgery, hypotension, shock, burns, or trauma. Prerenal failure is generally reversible with treatment and prognosis is usually good. Renal failure occurs when the kidneys themselves are damaged by disease or toxins. Prognosis is poor. Postrenal failure occurs when an anatomical abnormality or functional barrier (congenital anomaly) obstructs urine flow from the kidneys to the urethral meatus. This obstruction is usually correctable and the prognosis, with surgery, is good.

Symptoms. The presenting symptoms are variable and depend on the cause of the renal failure. The classic and most common symptom is **oliguria** (decreased urine output). The urine may appear dark in color. Other symptoms include dehydration, edema, pallor, and hypertension.

Treatment. Diagnosis is made on the basis of the history, physical examination, and diagnostic studies (including blood studies, urinalysis, and x-rays of the chest and abdomen). Obstructions are frequently diagnosed by scan and biopsy (Broadwell Jackson and Saunders 1993).

Treatment is supportive until renal function returns and the kidneys are able to function normally. The underlying cause of the failure and any complications must be treated. Treatment includes preventing fluid overload and electrolyte imbalance (hyperkalemia, hypocalcemia, acidosis), preventing hypotension or hypertension, maintaining adequate caloric intake, and preventing infection (Rudolph et al. 1991). Dialysis is frequently required, Figure 40–4.

Nursing Care. Nursing care of a child in acute renal failure is multifaceted. The nurse must provide physical care and close monitoring of the child's condition while at the same time providing psychosocial support to the parents and child. Nursing care includes recording intake and output and weighing the child every day on the same scale. Monitor the child's blood pressure and administer antihypertensive drugs. Encourage adequate nutrition and help the child to choose a diet that is low in sodium, potassium, and protein and high in carbohydrate, fats, and vitamins. A dietician is frequently involved in diet planning.

INDICATIONS FOR DIALYSIS

- Severe hyperkalemia
- Metabolic acidosis
- Fluid overload with or without hypertension
- Uremia

Figure 40–4

If the child requires dialysis, the nurse will explain the procedure to the child and family, monitor the child closely for any adverse effects, and provide emotional support to the child and family. (Refer to the discussion of chronic renal failure, following.)

Other nursing responsibilities include preventing infection, caring for the child if surgery is indicated, and educating the child and family about the disease, medications, diet and home care, and long-term management.

CHRONIC RENAL FAILURE/END-STAGE RENAL DISEASE

Description. Chronic renal failure occurs when a disease or abnormality of the kidneys or urinary tract results in a progressive destruction of nephrons, decreasing the ability of the kidneys to excrete metabolic wastes from the body. Causes of renal failure include developmental abnormalities of the kidney or urinary tract, inherited disorders, and acquired glomerular disease.

Chronic renal failure progresses through several stages. In the initial stages, the kidney is still able to compensate for the loss of nephrons. As more nephrons are destroyed, however, the decrease in renal function results in the buildup of metabolic wastes in the blood (Broadwell Jackson and Saunders 1993). End-stage renal disease occurs when the kidneys are no longer able to maintain fluid and electrolyte balance.

Symptoms. Symptoms depend on the stage of renal failure. Initial symptoms may be vague and nonspecific. With more advanced disease, symptoms can include fatigue, reduced exercise tolerance, decreased appetite, headache, anemia, electrolyte imbalance, metabolic acidosis, hypertension, and uremia.

Treatment. The goal of treatment is to help the child maintain the best quality of life possible by promoting normal growth and development and encouraging independence. Specific treatment centers on maintaining adequate nutrition by providing a diet with enough calories and protein for growth, limiting demands on the kidney, and preventing complications (bone disease, neurological abnormalities, and anemia). Antihypertensive, immunosuppressive, and antibiotic medications are frequently prescribed. Children with end-stage renal disease require dialysis or renal transplantation.

Nursing Care. Nursing care of the child with chronic renal failure is similar to care of the child with acute renal failure. However, the nurse needs to keep in mind the chronic nature of the disease, the effect of the disease on all body systems, and the psychological effects on the child and family of coping with a long-term and potentially terminal disease.

Specific nursing care includes monitoring fluid and electrolyte balance, recording intake and output, administering medications, helping the child and family with diet management, and providing psychosocial support.

Assist the family to arrange for home health care of the child by making referrals to appropriate agencies for visiting nurses, therapists, and equipment. Families should also be referred to social services, clergy, support groups, and for home teaching if appropriate.

ENURESIS

Enuresis is involuntary urination that occurs beyond the age when bladder control is expected to have been attained (usually 4 to 5 years of age), including either daytime or nighttime wetting. The condition is more common in boys than in girls.

Enuresis is classified as either primary or secondary. Children with primary enuresis have never been dry. Those with secondary enuresis have achieved control for months or years and then regress. Primary nighttime wetters represent the largest group of children.

Enuresis can be the result of a functional or structural problem, a symptom of an organic disease, or emotionally based. Common causes are urinary tract infections, small bladder capacity, diabetes, sexual abuse, and emotional problems. Before a treatment plan is devised, it is important that a detailed history, physical examination, and urinalysis (including culture) be performed to rule out any structural or organic causes.

Treatment involves counseling parents in the management of enuresis and providing emotional support to the parent and child, Figure 40–5. Occasionally children are treated with medications. Referral should be made for counseling if indicated.

ADOLESCENT

SEXUALLY TRANSMITTED DISEASES

Adolescents represent a population at risk for developing sexually transmitted diseases (STDs) because they tend to have multiple sexual partners, fail to use protection, wait to seek medical attention, and do not tell their partners when they develop symptoms (Rudolph et al. 1991). The most common sexually transmitted diseases seen in children and adolescents are syphilis, gonorrhea, chlamydia, and genital herpes, Figure 40–6. Acquired immunodeficiency syndrome (AIDS), which can also be transmitted through unprotected sexual intercourse, is discussed in Chapter 34.

The nurse can play an important role in prevention, treatment, and education of teenagers about STDs, Figure 40–7 (shown on page 671). During routine history taking or assessment, be sure to ask about sexual activity and knowledge about STDs. If a teenager is diagnosed with an STD, discuss not only the treatment of the disease, but also the importance of prevention. Discuss methods of protection against STDs and complications (possible infertility, ectopic pregnancy, and risk of transmission to a fetus). Explain the importance of treating sexual partners to avoid spread of the disease and reinfection.

Nurses have a responsibility to report cases of STDs in young children to local authorities. Always keep in mind the possibility of molestation or sexual abuse by an infected adult or adolescent when a preadolescent child is diagnosed with an STD.

GUIDELINES FOR PARENTS OF ENURETIC CHILDREN

- Restrict the child's fluids after dinner.
- Take the child to the toilet before he or she goes to bed, then again before the parent goes to bed, and once during the night hours.
- Work with the child to perform bladder-stretching exercises. For example, have the child drink large quantities of fluids and then hold the urine as long as possible.
- Use enuresis alarms that ring when the child has a full bladder but has not wet.
- Devise reward systems in which the child receives a sticker, star, or small favor when he or she is dry.

Figure 40–5

COMMON SEXUALLY TRANSMITTED DISEASES

Disease	Symptoms	Treatment
Syphilis *Causative organism: Treponema pallidum* *Incubation period:* 3 weeks	Primary syphilis manifests as a single lesion (chancre) at the site of contact. The characteristic chancre is a painless ulcer with a smooth base and indurated borders. The ulcer can appear in the genital area on the glans penis, labia, within the vagina, or in the perineal or rectal area. Painless, firm, enlarged inguinal lymph nodes can develop 1 to 2 weeks after the chancre appears. The chancre heals spontaneously in 1 to 5 weeks. (Bondi et al. 1991; Grimes 1991; and Habif 1990). Secondary syphilis appears as the primary lesion resolves. A diffuse, nonpruritic rash develops. Macular, papular, papulosquamous, or bullous lesions may be present. Mucous patches appear on mucosal surfaces. Broad- based, flat mucoid lesions (condylomata) appear on the genitals. The child develops flulike symptoms: sore throat, fever, malaise, lymphadenopathy.	Benzathine penicillin G or doxycycline is the antibiotic of choice. For children allergic to penicillin, erythromycin or tetracycline is given. Topical lesions can be treated with saline compresses followed by the application of a topical antibiotic (Polysporin) (Bondi et al. 1991).

Figure 40–6

continues

COMMON SEXUALLY TRANSMITTED DISEASES

Disease	Symptoms	Treatment
Gonorrhea *Causative organism: Neisseria gonorrhoeae* *Incubation period:* 3 to 5 days	Symptoms associated with gonorrheal infections usually appear within 1 week of infection. Symptoms are varied and can include vulvovaginitis, urethritis, pharyngeal infections, anorectal gonorrhea, and pelvic inflammatory disease (PID). Preadolescent girls have a vaginal discharge that is thick, green, or creamy. Preadolescent and adolescent boys will have a yellow puslike urethral discharge associated with frequency, dysuria, and an erythematous meatus. Teenage girls frequently develop cervicitis, purulent vaginal discharge, and PID.	Antimicrobial therapy is the treatment of choice. Drugs recommended are ceftriaxone or cefotaxime given IV or IM. Children under the age of 8 years of age should also be given doxycycline.
Chlamydia *Causative organism: Chlamydia trachomatis* *Incubation period:* unknown	*C. trachomatis* is the most common cause of nongonococcal urethritis. Symptoms in adolescent girls include endocervicitis, mucopurulent yellow-green endocervical discharge, and PID. Adolescent boys can develop dysuria, urethritis, discharge, epididymitis, and proctitis.	Recommended medications include doxycycline or tetracycline, erythromycin, or sulfisoxazole.

Figure 40–6 *continued*

Common Sexually Transmitted Diseases

Disease	Symptoms	Treatment
Genital Herpes *Causative organism:* Herpes simplex virus (HSV-2) *Incubation period:* unknown	Manifestations of herpes are varied and range from no symptoms to systemic involvement. Systemic symptoms include headache, fever, malaise, and myalgia. Small clusters of papules appear that develop into vesicles, pustules, and then ulcers. The lesions itch initially but when the ulcers break, there is pain. Ulcerations can appear on the external genitalia, between the vaginal folds and posterior cervix, or on the anus, buttocks, and thighs. Enlarged lymph nodes usually accompany the lesions.	Acyclovir is the drug of choice given orally and also applied topically to lesions. It is important to tell teenagers to wear a glove when applying ointment to lesions to prevent infecting other areas of the body and other people (Rosenstein and Fosarelli 1989).

Figure 40–6 *continued*

Preventive Teaching: STDs

- Abstain from intercourse completely.
- Maintain a monogamous relationship.
- Limit the number of sexual partners.
- Use condoms for vaginal and anal intercourse.
- Do not have oral sex if partner has mouth sores or sores on the penis or vagina.

Figure 40–7

REVIEW QUESTIONS

A. Multiple choice. Select the best answer.

1. Placement of the urethral meatus on the dorsal surface of the penis is characteristic of which of the following conditions?
   a. hypospadias
   b. epispadias
   c. hydrocele
   d. cryptorchidism

2. Roberto, 7 years old, complains to his mother of urgency, enuresis, dysuria, and abdominal pain, and has a mild fever. These are characteristic signs and symptoms of
   a. urinary tract infection
   b. nephrotic syndrome
   c. acute renal failure
   d. acute glomerulonephritis

3. Ultrasonography, CAT scanning, and MRI may be used to diagnose which of the following conditions?
   a. hydrocele
   b. urinary tract infection
   c. Wilm's tumor
   d. acute glomerulonephritis

4. A child with acute glomerulonephritis should be on what type of diet?
   a. low-sodium
   b. low-sodium, low-fat
   c. low-sodium, low-protein
   d. low-protein

5. A child with nephrotic syndrome is most likely to have which of the following clinical findings?
   a. vesicoureteral reflux
   b. vomiting and diarrhea
   c. low-grade fever
   d. periorbital edema

6. Brown urine is a common finding in children who have
   a. urinary tract infection
   b. nephrotic syndrome
   c. acute glomerulonephritis
   d. enuresis

B. True or false. Write *T* for a true statement and *F* for a false statement.

1. ___ A UTI is present when a urine culture reveals less than 100,000 colony-forming units of a single organism per milliliter.

2. ___ Wilm's tumor usually presents in children during the third year of life.

3. ___ Hyperproteinemia is a characteristic finding in children with nephrotic syndrome.

4. ___ Acute glomerulonephritis is most common in toddlers between the ages of 1 and 3 years.

5. ___ Acute renal failure involves a progressive destruction of the nephrons of the kidney.

6. ___ Initial symptoms in chronic renal failure are often nonspecific.

SUGGESTED ACTIVITIES

- Make a poster or other teaching tool identifying strategies to prevent UTIs in children and adolescents.
- Interview a child with nephrotic syndrome and his or her parents. Identify concerns that each one has about the condition. What strategies would you use to address their concerns?
- Visit a dialysis center that provides treatment to children with chronic renal failure. Discuss with nursing staff and parents the impact of this disease on the child's and family's lifestyle.
- Interview parents of an enuretic child. What problems or concerns did they experience related to their child's condition? What strategies did they use to manage the condition in their child?

BIBLIOGRAPHY

Bondi, E. E., B. V. Jegasothy, and G. S. Lazarus. *Dermatology*. Norwalk, CT: Appleton and Lange, 1991.

Broadwell Jackson, D., and R. B. Saunders. *Child Health Nursing*. Philadelphia: J. B. Lippincott, 1993.

Foley, G. V., D. Fochtman, and K. Hardin Mooney. *Nursing Care of the Child with Cancer*, 2nd ed. Philadelphia: W. B. Saunders, 1993.

Fong, E., A. S. Scott, E. Ferris, and E. G. Skelley. *Body Structures and Functions*, 8th ed. Albany, NY: Delmar Publishers, 1993.

Grimes, D. *Infectious Diseases*. St. Louis, MO: Mosby-Year Book, 1991.

Habif, T. P. *Clinical Dermatology: A Color Guide to Diagnosis and Therapy*, 2nd ed. St. Louis, MO: Mosby-Year Book, 1990.

Hathaway, W. E., W. W. Hay, J. R. Groothuis, and J. W. Paisley. *Current Pediatric Diagnosis and Treatment*, 11th ed. Norwalk, CT: Appleton and Lange, 1993.

Kutz, M., C. Rudy, and S. Walsh. Daytime incontinence. *Journal of Pediatric Health Care* 7, no. 2 (1993): 92, 99–100.

Last, J. M., and R. B. Wallace. *Public Health and Preventive Medicine*, 13th ed. Norwalk, CT: Appleton and Lange, 1992.

McGuire, P., and K. Moore. Recent advances in childhood cancer, advances in oncology nursing. *Nursing Clinics of North America* 25, no. 2 (1990): 447–460.

Rosenstein, B. J., and P. D. Fosarelli. *Pediatric Pearls: The Handbook of Practical Pediatrics*. Chicago: Year Book Medical Publishers, 1989.

Rudolph, A. M., J. I. E. Hoffman, and C. D. Rudolph. *Rudolph's Pediatrics*, 19th ed. Norwalk, CT: Appleton and Lange, 1991.

Tanagho, E. A., and J. W. McAninch. *Smith's General Urology*, 13th ed. Norwalk, CT: Appleton and Lange, 1992.

Wong, D. *Whaley & Wong's Essentials of Pediatric Nursing*, 4th ed. St. Louis, MO: Mosby-Year Book, 1993.

CHAPTER

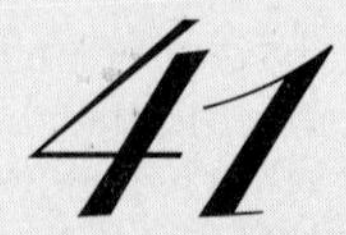

Musculoskeletal Conditions

Objectives

After studying this chapter, the student should be able to:

- Name four musculoskeletal conditions that affect infants and toddlers and describe their causes, symptoms, treatment, and nursing care.
- Name four musculoskeletal conditions that affect preschool and school-age children and describe their causes, symptoms, treatment, and nursing care.
- Identify three common sports injuries of children.
- Identify the most common type of childhood fracture requiring hospitalization.
- Describe nursing care for the child in a cast, traction, or brace.
- Name two musculoskeletal conditions that affect adolescents and describe their causes, symptoms, treatment, and nursing care.

Key Terms

pseudohypertrophy	stress fracture
lordosis	fracture
Gower's sign	traction
strains	scoliosis
sprains	limb salvage

Musculoskeletal conditions of children may be congenital or a result of disease or injury. These conditions can have a significant impact on growth and development, resulting in altered motor function and impaired mobility. Through accurate assessment, nurses can help ensure early diagnosis and treatment of these conditions, thus maintaining mobility and preventing complications.

Overview of the System

The skeletal system is composed of more than 200 bones. Along with the musculoskeletal system, it protects and supports the body and facilitates coordinated movements.

There are four classifications of bones, based on their form and shape: long, short, flat, and irregular, Figure 41–1. Both the diameter and length of the bone change as it grows. Growth in diameter occurs on the external surface of the bone as new bone is created. Growth in length occurs at the epiphyseal plates, located at the ends of the long bones. Injury to this area in a growing child is always potentially serious, because it may stop or alter the child's growth (Scoles 1988).

Joints connect the bones of the skeleton, permitting movement and flexibility. Joints are classified as fibrous, cartilaginous, or synovial, Figure 41–2. Skeletal muscles provide contour and shape over bones and are directly responsible for movement.

Types of Bones

Type of Bone	Example	Function
Long	Femur	Provide support to the body
Short	Tarsals, metatarsals	Facilitate motion within parts of the body
Flat	Sternum, skull	Provide protection to the internal organs
Irregular	Vertebrae	Vary in size and shape and accommodate other structures

Figure 41–1

Types of Joints		
Type of Joint	**Example**	**Movement**
Fibrous	Bones of the skull in childhood	Very limited
Cartilaginous	Epiphyseal plates, symphysis pubis	Slightly movable
Synovial	Elbow, shoulder, fingers	The most movable type of joint

Figure 41–2

Infant and Toddler

Congenital Hip Dysplasia

Congenital hip dysplasia, also called congenital dislocated hip, is one of the most common congenital anomalies. It occurs in about 1 in 500 to 1,000 births. The degree of dysplasia varies from acetabular dysplasia to subluxation to complete dislocation. In acetabular dysplasia, the acetabulum is shallow, but the femoral head remains in place in the acetabulum. In subluxation, incomplete dislocation occurs. The head of the femur stays in contact with the acetabulum but is partially displaced. The most severe form of dysplasia is complete dislocation, in which the femoral head loses contact with the acetabulum and is displaced.

Assessment of the hips is performed as part of the routine newborn assessment. In an infant under 3 weeks of age, hip stability can be assessed by placing the infant supine with hips and knees flexed while abducting and lifting the femurs. If a click is heard or felt as the femur enters the acetabulum, the infant is said to have a positive Ortolani's sign. Other indicators of hip dysplasia include uneven gluteal folds and uneven knee height (Schaming et al. 1990).

Treatment should begin as soon as possible after diagnosis. On an infant or toddler, three or more cloth diapers pinned front to back or some type of abduction device may be used to abduct the hip area. This treatment may be all that is needed to maintain proper alignment until the hip is stabilized, usually within about three to six months. The older child may need to be placed in traction for gradual reduction of hip and flexor muscles, and then placed into a hip spica cast for approximately four to six months.

Parent education is an important part of the treatment plan. Explain to parents using drawings and demonstration how the hips must be kept abducted and flexed. If the child is in a hip spica cast, a thorough explanation must be given regarding cast care, positioning, and handling, as well as proper diapering and skin care.

Clubfoot

Clubfoot, or talipes, is a congenital deformity in which the foot is twisted out of its normal position. Specific deformities are differentiated depending on the specific malposition of the ankle and foot. Unilateral clubfoot is more common than bilateral, and the condition occurs twice as often in boys as in girls.

Treatment involves manipulation and casting to reposition the foot and ankle. Casting is performed in a series of steps to gradually stretch and contract structures around the foot. Casts are changed every few days for one to two weeks and then every one to two weeks. Correction usually occurs by six to eight weeks. Corrective shoes and nightly splinting are used for an additional three months. Follow-up and reevaluation are necessary to prevent recurrence (Kyzer 1991).

Teach parents how to care for the infant in a cast and how to identify potential problems. The developing infant needs stimulation and comfort while in the cast. Parents are encouraged to hold and cuddle the infant.

TORTICOLLIS

Torticollis, a disorder that occurs as a result of a shortened sternocleidomastoid muscle, is usually diagnosed in the newborn period. The infant's head is tilted to the affected side, with the neck flexed and the chin rotated toward the opposite shoulder.

When diagnosed early, torticollis is treated with passive stretching exercises. If the child has sufficient normal muscle, the muscle will stretch as the child grows (Brewer 1990). An operation to release the muscle may be performed if exercises are unsuccessful. Nursing care includes observing the newborn for normal range of motion of the neck and teaching parents how to perform exercises and activities that stimulate the infant to turn the head.

RICKETS

Rickets is a disorder of bone formation that results from a deficiency of vitamin D, calcium, or phosphorus. It may be caused by inadequate dietary intake, poor absorption of nutrients, or lack of exposure to sunlight. Bones commonly affected include those of the legs and skull. Bones are weakened and bent out of shape, so bowlegs and knock knees are often seen. The child may have deformed bone shaping, delayed calcification of teeth, and vague symptoms of apathy, irritability, shortened attention span, and pain.

Rickets can be treated by exposure to sunlight and by a diet with milk and milk products, enriched cereals and breads, and fish products (cod liver oil, herring, mackerel, salmon, tuna, and sardines). Nursing care includes teaching parents about the importance of dietary intake of vitamin D, calcium, and phosphorus.

PRESCHOOL AND SCHOOL-AGE CHILDREN

DUCHENNE'S MUSCULAR DYSTROPHY

Description. Duchenne's muscular dystrophy is an X-linked genetic disorder that causes a progressive degeneration and weakening of skeletal muscles, eventually leading to death. It is the most common form of muscular dystrophy and affects boys almost exclusively.

Symptoms. Indications of muscle weakness are usually seen in the preschool child between the ages of 3 and 5 years. The child may have a history of delays in motor development, especially in beginning to walk. Initial symptoms include frequent falls and difficulty in climbing stairs, running, or riding a bicycle.

One of the classic signs of Duchenne's muscular dystrophy is **pseudohypertrophy** (seeming enlargement) of the muscles, particularly those of the calf. The muscles appear large, but the muscle fibers are replaced by fatty deposits, leaving nonfunctioning tissue. As the disorder continues, the child becomes progressively weaker. Signs of increasing muscle weakness include a waddling gait, pronounced **lordosis** (abnormal increased curvature of the lumbar spine), and **Gower's sign**, a characteristic self-climbing movement in which the child uses the arm muscles to compensate for weak hip extensor muscles in rising to an upright position.

Treatment. The disorder is incurable and most children die of respiratory complications, usually during adolescence. The goal is to maintain muscle function for as long as possible. Range of motion is maintained through exercises that are performed several times a day and by activities of daily living. Bracing and surgery to release contractures may help maintain muscle functioning.

Nursing Care. Nursing care involves helping the child and family to cope with a progressive, fatal disease; intervening to delay and reduce disabilities; maximizing the child's potential; and assisting the family to deal with the effects of the disease on all family members.

JUVENILE RHEUMATOID ARTHRITIS

Description. Juvenile rheumatoid arthritis (JRA) is a chronic inflammatory disease that affects primarily the joints but may also occur in a systemic form, affecting internal organs. The disease usually occurs in children under the age of 16 and gradually subsides by adulthood. Inflammation of the joint muscle leads to destruction of cartilage and bone in the joints.

Symptoms. The child with JRA has periods of exacerbation and remission of symptoms. Common symptoms include morning stiffness, swollen joints, a limp, increased fatigue, fever, irritability, anorexia, and failure to grow at expected rates (if the epiphyseal plates of the long bones are damaged). The knee, ankle, wrist, and finger joints are most often affected (Page-Goertz 1989).

Treatment. Treatment consists of anti-inflammatory drugs, splinting to prevent flexion contractures, and physical therapy to maintain maximum strength and motion. Nonsteroidal anti-inflammatory drugs are prescribed to decrease inflammation and relieve pain. Immunosuppressive drugs and corticosteroids may be prescribed for children with severe disease (Mosca and Sherry 1990, Reilly 1992).

Physical therapy is important to maintain range of motion and prevent deformities. Activities performed in water are more easily tolerated, so pool activities are encouraged. Heat (from tub baths, showers, heating pads, or electric blankets) may help to decrease stiffness in the joints.

Nursing Care. Nursing care includes helping the child maintain as many normal activities as possible. The nurse promotes the general well-being of the child by encouraging good posture and body mechanics, weight control to prevent undue strain on the joints, and school attendance to maintain contact with friends. The nurse also provides the child and family with information about ways to relieve inflammation, exercises to maintain joint functioning and strength, methods to relieve pain, and support groups that provide help in coping with a chronic illness.

LEGG-CALVÉ-PERTHES DISEASE

Description. Legg-Calvé-Perthes disease is a disorder that occurs when circulation to the femoral head is disrupted, resulting in necrosis of the femoral head. The disease is most often diagnosed in children between the ages of 4 and 9 years and affects boys more often than girls (Hensiger and Fielding 1990).

Symptoms. Symptoms may develop over a period of weeks to months. The child may complain of pain in the hip or other areas of the leg, such as the groin, thigh, or knee. Movement of the hip increases the pain and rest decreases it. The child may limp occasionally on the affected side and have limited motion in the affected hip.

Treatment. The goal of treatment is to decrease or prevent deformity of the femoral head by keeping it within the acetabulum. Initial treatment is rest to decrease inflammation and restore motion. Traction may be used to stretch the hip muscles and increase the range of motion of the hip. Other treatment measures include use of nonweight-bearing devices (such as abduction braces, leg casts, and harness slings) or surgical reconstruction of the hip joint. Early diagnosis and treatment improve the child's prognosis (Dunst 1990, Thompson and Salter 1987).

Nursing Care. Nursing care involves teaching family members about the use and care of nonweight-bearing devices and how to carry out activities of daily living with these devices. Children on initial bed rest can be encouraged in activities or hobbies that do not require movement (coloring, puzzles, reading, and drawing, among others).

Osteomyelitis

Description. Osteomyelitis is an infection of the bone, usually caused by *Staphylococcus* organisms. The long bones of the legs are the most common sites of infection. Bacteria may migrate to the bone through the bloodstream or enter the bone directly through a lesion or open fracture.

Within the closed space of the bone, edema and inflammation cause severe and constant pain in the affected area. An abscess may form, increasing pressure within the bone and causing the death of bone tissue. Without treatment, the infection may spread throughout the body.

Symptoms. The child may be irritable, anorexic, and weak, with a fever and localized edema and warmth in the extremity. Severe, localized pain is common with movement of the extremity. The child may avoid moving the extremity, holding it in a semiflexed position.

Treatment. Blood cultures are obtained, and intravenous antibiotics prescribed. Initially the child requires comfort measures such as bed rest, analgesics, and immobilization of the extremity with splints or casts. If the child does not improve, surgery may be required to remove areas of dead bone. Early diagnosis and treatment can help to prevent permanent damage to the bone and extremity.

Nursing Care. Nursing care includes giving analgesics for pain and positioning the extremity to maintain comfort. Assess circulation in the extremities and monitor vital signs at least every four hours. Encourage sedentary play and diversional activities to help the child deal with immobilization. A diet high in calories, protein, vitamin C, and calcium helps to promote bone healing. Figure 41–3 summarizes nursing care for the child with osteomyelitis.

Sports Injuries

Contact sports often produce acute musculoskeletal injuries, such as tears in ligaments and tendons or bone fractures. Injuries to the knee are common among children of all age groups. A blow to the side of the knee can result in ligament injury or long bone fracture. Because the epiphyseal plates of young athletes have not closed, the plates are more easily injured than are the surrounding ligaments. These injuries have the potential to affect the child's overall growth.

Overuse may produce **strains** (pulling of a ligament) and **sprains** (muscle injury caused by overstretching). Early treatment for sprains and strains depends on the extent and type of injury and consists of rest, ice, compression, and elevation for 24 to 36 hours after the injury occurs. Complete tears require surgical intervention (Mourad and Droste 1993).

NURSING CARE PLAN: Osteomyelitis

PATIENT PROBLEM	GOAL(S)
Pain	Child states and shows relief of pain.
Lack of diversional activities	Child participates in play appropriate to age.
Risk for infection	By discharge, the child maintains vital signs within normal limits, and wound is free from purulent discharge.

Figure 41–3 Nursing care plan for the child with osteomyelitis

NURSING INTERVENTION	RATIONALE
Observe for crying, statements of pain, and guarding behavior.	Information is needed for baseline data.
Assess pain using a pain scale (see Chapter 31).	Provides an objective measurement.
Administer prescribed analgesics and monitor effectiveness.	Analgesics help control pain.
Support and maintain proper body alignment.	Reduces stress on the limb and prevents trauma.
Avoid unnecessary handling of the extremity.	Moving the limb can cause increased pain.
Provide toys and activity appropriate to child's age.	Play is a child's way of expressing him- or herself.
Encourage visits by parents and siblings and parental involvement in the child's care.	Helps prevent disruption of the family structure.
Encourage the child to maintain contact with peers.	Maintaining contact is important to prevent isolation.
Monitor vital signs every 4 hours and as needed.	Changes in vital signs are signs of infection.
Assess for pain, redness, swelling, or drainage at the site every 4 hours.	Any change may indicate further infection.
Maintain good handwashing technique.	Prevents the spread of bacteria.
When indicated, change dressing according to hospital policy.	Proper skin care is the key to preventing infection.
Administer antibiotics as ordered.	Antibiotics provide bacteriocidal action.
Maintain nutrition with a diet high in protein, calories, and vitamin C.	Diet helps promote bone healing.

Stress fractures are fractures caused by repeated, prolonged stress on a bone. They rarely occur in very young children, but are more frequent in children 10 years of age or older. Most stress fractures can be prevented by proper conditioning and preseason training. Stress fractures usually occur after a rapid increase in a training activity over a short period of time. The pain of a stress fracture is usually worse during and immediately after activity but eventually becomes constant. In most cases, stress fractures are treated with immobilization and restricted activity until symptoms decrease and x-rays show evidence of new bone formation (Smrcina 1992).

FRACTURES OF THE EXTREMITIES

A **fracture** is a break that occurs in a bone, usually as a result of injury. Fractures are a common injury at any age but are more likely to occur in children as a result of traumatic injury from everyday activities. Most fractures are the result of a forceful blow. Fractures that occur in a bone weakened by disease processes are called pathological or spontaneous fractures (Campbell and Campbell 1991).

Because children's bones are still growing, they heal much more quickly than adults' bones. A fracture of the femur in a newborn heals completely in three to four weeks. In an adult, the same fracture would take six to eight weeks or longer to heal (Scoles 1988).

Types of Fractures. Fractures are described as open or closed, depending on whether a break also occurs in the skin (Barrett and Bryant 1990). Fractures may be further classified in terms of appearance:

- greenstick (incomplete)
- complete
- bend
- buckle
- comminuted
- spiral

Fracture of the Femur. A fracture of the femur is the most common type of childhood fracture treated in the hospital. Children who are involved in automobile accidents or fall from substantial heights may suffer a fractured femur. A fractured femur in an infant is uncommon and may be the result of child abuse (Cunningham 1991).

When the femur is fractured, strong tendon spasms occur, causing poor alignment of the fragments. Casting at this time is not possible. The child under 2 years of age and 40 pounds (18 kg) is placed in Bryant's traction for 7 to 14 days to restore alignment, Figure 41–6. A young child is then placed in a cast for three to four weeks. The child is positioned with hips flexed and both knees extended in a vertical position. The child's buttocks should be raised far enough off the bed that a nurse's hand can be placed beneath them. An older child is placed in 90-90 traction for four to six weeks and then casted for three to four weeks. In 90-90 traction, the lower leg is placed in a boot cast, and a skeletal pin or wire is placed through the distal fragment of the femur, Figure 41–7. Traction is maintained so that the femur is at a 90-degree angle to the bed.

Casting. A simple fracture of the limb may be treated by setting the bone and applying a cast. Casts are constructed from plaster of paris or, more commonly, from synthetic, lighter-weight, water-resistant materials such as fiberglass. A plaster of paris cast takes several hours to days to dry. Synthetic materials take only a few hours to dry. Synthetic casts come in several colors and designs.

A wet cast must be handled gently and supported with the flat of the hand or on pillows to avoid indentations that may cause pressure on the skin and lead to altered circulation and skin impairment. Turning the child frequently aids in the drying process. Use of cool-air dryers and regular fans to circulate air may help dry the cast. Heated dryers are not used because they cause the cast to dry from the outside in, weakening the cast.

A protective barrier must be formed over the rough cast edges to prevent abrasion of the underlying skin. After the cast is dry, the raw edges can be protected by a "petaled" edge. "Petals" can be made from adhesive tape or mole skin cut approximately 1½ inches wide. These are placed over the edge of the cast, with each petal overlapping the next to form a smooth edge, Figure 41–4 (Skale 1992).

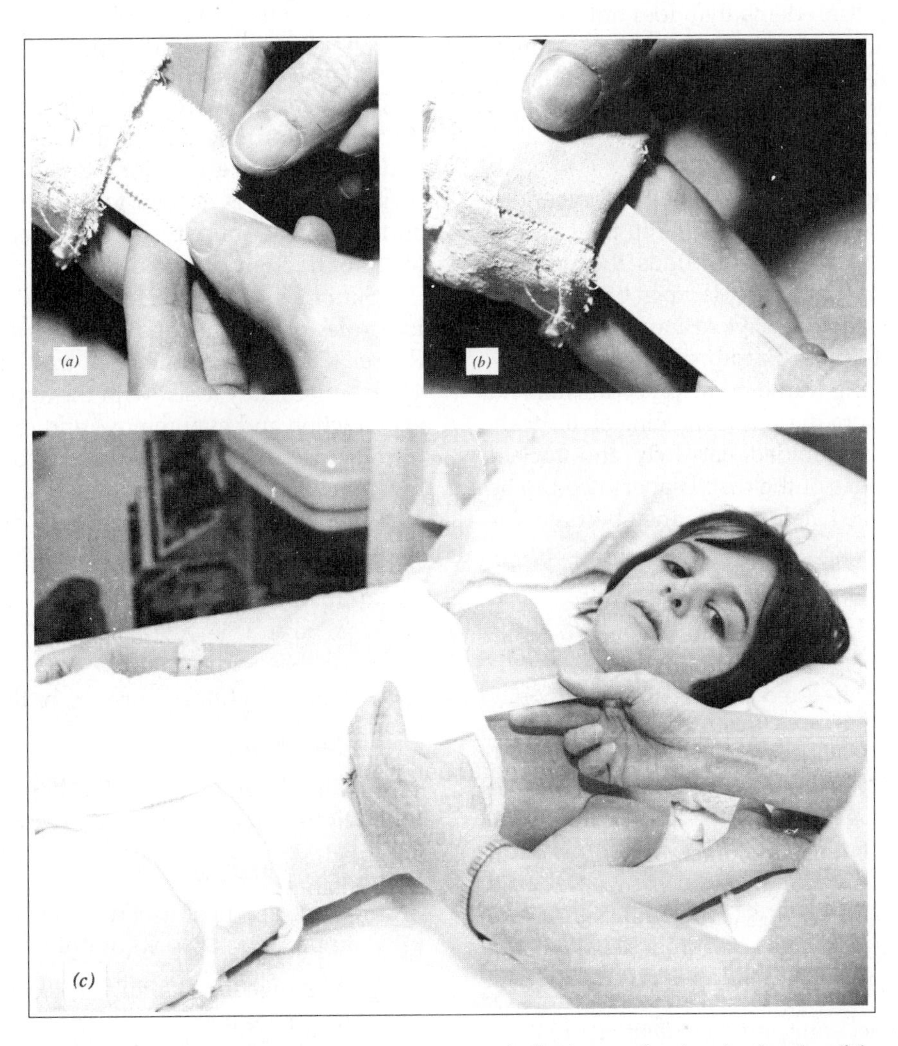

Figure 41–4 *Petaling a cast after it is clean and dry (a) Strips of adhesive are placed under the edge of the cast. (b, c) Adhesive strips are held in place with a tongue blade, and the upper edge is folded over the cast edge. After the edges are covered, the outer edges of the adhesive are covered with an encircling piece of adhesive to keep them in place. (From L. A. Mourad and M. M. Droste.* The Nursing Process in the Care of Adults with Orthopaedic Conditions, *3rd ed. Albany, NY: Delmar Publishers, 1993)*

Swelling of the extremity may continue in the first few hours after cast application. If pressure is not relieved, the cast may become a tourniquet, reducing circulation and causing neurovascular damage. Keeping the extremity elevated helps prevent further swelling. Signs of impaired neurocirculatory function include blueness or coldness of a distal part, lack of a peripheral pulse, edema that does not improve with elevation, uncontrolled pain, and numbness or tingling of the affected extremity. Any of these symptoms requires immediate follow-up.

Nursing Care. Several nursing interventions may be implemented to help keep the cast dry and clean. If the cast surrounds the perineal area, cover the cast with plastic in order to prevent urine saturation. Occasionally, the child may be placed in a Bradford frame, a canvas-covered turning frame, to help keep urine and feces away from the cast (Schaming et al. 1990). Diapers can be folded narrowly and tucked under the edges of the cast. Diapers need to be changed immediately, before they become saturated with urine. A urine collection bag may be used for the infant. Plastic pants tend to hold moisture and should not be used. Keeping the child in a semi-Fowler's position helps prevent soaking of the back of the cast. Educating parents about home cast care is essential. Figure 41–5 provides an example of home cast care instructions for parents.

Traction. **Traction** involves the use of weights and pulleys to realign bone fragments, reduce dislocations, immobilize fractures, provide rest for an extremity, help prevent contracture deformities, and allow preoperative and postoperative positioning and alignment. Significant pull is needed to restore alignment and overcome muscle spasms. There are two forms of traction: skin and skeletal.

Skin traction is applied to the skin surfaces. Examples of skin traction are Bryant's, Buck's, Russell's, and cervical halter traction, Figure 41–6. Nurses may assist with the application of skin traction and may remove and reapply skin traction according to physician's orders and institutional policies, provided that someone manually maintains the traction during the rewrapping process (Morris et al. 1988a).

HOME CAST CARE INSTRUCTIONS

- Keep the casted extremity elevated on pillows as directed by the physician.
- *Do not* allow the child to put anything inside the cast. Small items that might be placed inside the cast should be kept away from the child.
- If desired, clean the cast with a damp cloth and a dry, nonchlorine bleach cleanser if it becomes soiled.
- Contact your physician *immediately* if you note any of the following in or around the cast:
  - Pain, numbness, burning, or tingling
  - Foul odor
  - Discoloration of skin (darker or lighter than a comparable extremity)
  - Swelling (fingers or toes)
  - Cold fingers or toes not relieved by application of socks or mittens
  - A change in the ability to move the fingers or toes
- Notify the physician if the cast becomes loose and allows movement.

Figure 41–5 *(Adapted from* Information Sheet: Cast Care. *Sioux Valley Hospital, Sioux Falls, SD)*

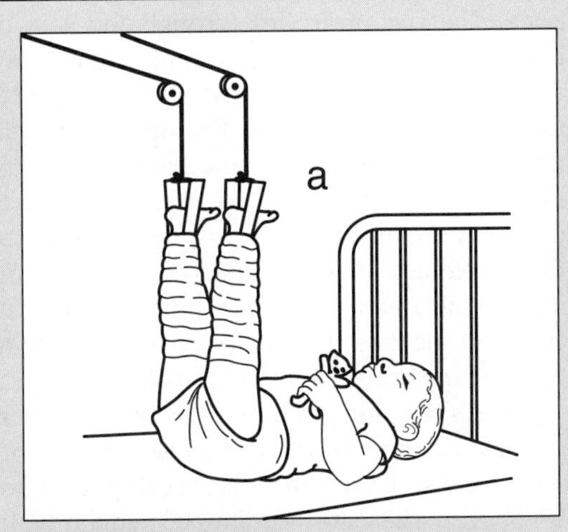

Bryant's Traction

Used for fractured femur in children under 2 years of age and under 18 kg (40 pounds). Also used as preparation for surgical repair of congenital hip deformities.

The child is positioned with hips flexed and both knees extended in a vertical position. The child's buttocks should be raised far enough off the bed that a nurse's hand can be placed beneath them.

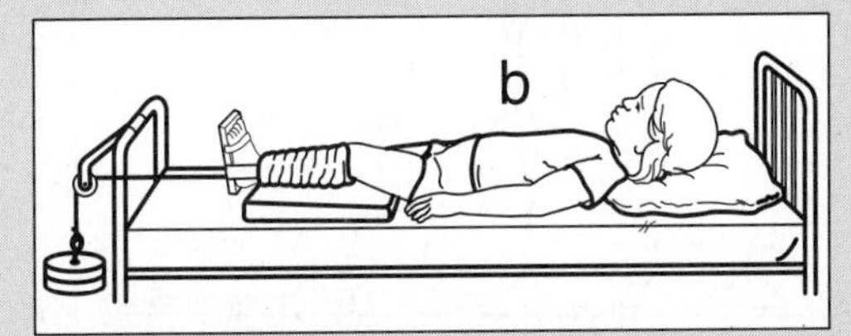

Buck's Traction

Used for arthritic conditions and as a temporary measure to provide support to a fracture before surgery.

A foam rubber boot is applied on the lateral surfaces of one or more extremities. The boot is held in place with elastic bandages. Weights are then attached to a spreader bar connecting the distal end of the boot.

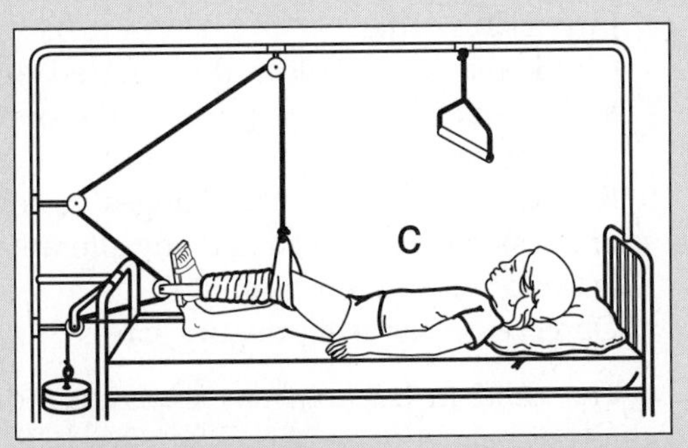

Russell's Traction

A modification of Buck's traction, with the addition of a sling under the affected leg. Allows more movement in bed and permits flexion of the knee joint.

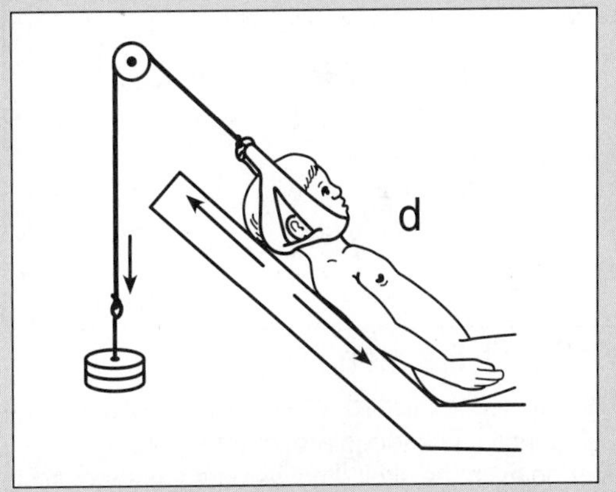

Cervical Halter Traction

Used to treat arthritic conditions of the cervical vertebrae and muscles.

A halter is fitted over the head and chin. Straps are attached to a spreader bar with ropes and weights attached to the spreader.

Figure 41–6 *Types of skin traction. (Illustrations from D. B. Broadwell Jackson and R. B. Saunders.* Child Health Nursing. *Philadelphia: J. B. Lippincott, 1993)*

Skeletal traction is applied directly to the bone by inserting a stainless steel pin or wire called a Steinmann pin or Kirschner wire (K-wire) through the end of the fractured long bone. The pin protrudes through the skin on both sides of the extremity, and weights are attached to a rope that is tied to a spreader bar for the purpose of traction. Examples of skeletal traction are 90-90 traction and Crutchfield tongs, Figure 41–7. Once initiated, traction must be maintained over long periods of time to be effective. Weights cannot be lifted or removed and must hang freely. Release of the weight could cause an increase in muscle spasms, displacing the fracture fragments (Morris et al. 1988b).

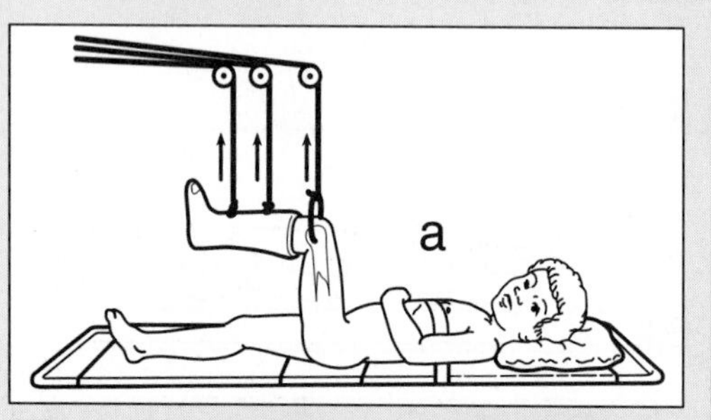

Ninety-Ninety Skeletal Traction

The most common type of skeletal traction. The lower leg is placed in a boot cast and a skeletal pin or wire is placed in the distal fragment of the femur. Traction is maintained so that the femur is positioned at a 90-degree angle to the bed.

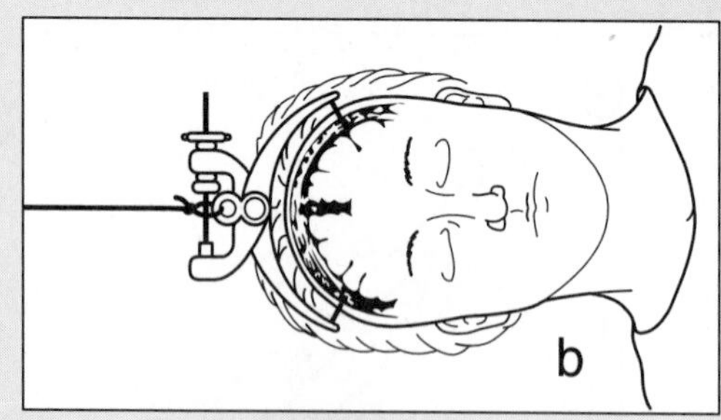

Cervical Traction

Usually accomplished with the use of Cruchfield tongs. The tongs are inserted through burr holes in the skull, and weights are attached to the hyperextended head. Immobilization of the fracture until healing takes place is essential.

Figure 41–7 *Types of skeletal traction (*a *adapted from D. B. Broadwell Jackson and R. B. Saunders.* Child Health Nursing. *Philadelphia: J. B. Lippincott, 1993;* b *adapted from Stein, A. M. and Jacobson, N. H.* NCLEX-RN Review 1991. *Albany, NY, 1991)*

The site of the pin or wire insertion is prone to infection and must be cleansed to remove secretions and prevent infection (Jones-Walton 1991). The sites are monitored frequently for signs of infection and for loosening or slippage of the pins. The tips of the pins are covered with protective material to prevent puncture of other parts of the body.

Nursing Care. Nursing interventions for children in traction include the following measures:

- Keep the child's body in proper alignment.
- Ensure that weights hang freely from the bed and are never removed without the physician's order.
- Check the pulse below the affected area and compare with the pulse in the opposite extremity.
- Report immediately any changes in color of the skin and nail bed and any alterations in sensation and motor ability.
- Observe for signs of pressure sores.

The child in traction may experience discomfort or pain because of muscle spasms. Pain relief is provided with muscle relaxants and analgesics. Limited mobility and forced confinement pose challenges to the child's care. Play, participation in self-care, encouragement with school work, and opportunities to socialize all stimulate the child and promote normal growth and development. Maintaining contact with peers is extremely important and is encouraged.

ADOLESCENT

SCOLIOSIS

Description. **Scoliosis** is a lateral S-shaped curvature of the spine that occurs most often in adolescent girls. It is classified as structural or functional in origin. Structural scoliosis may be idiopathic, congenital, or secondary to other disorders such as muscular dystrophy. It results in loss of flexibility of the spine and deformity. Functional scoliosis results from poor posture, and treatment of the underlying problem usually corrects the misalignment.

Symptoms. The lateral curvature of the spine results in uneven height of the shoulders and hips, which may be identified when the child bends forward at the waist, Figure 41–8. Pain is usually not present (Brosnon 1991).

Treatment. Treatment involves straightening and realigning the spine through conservative measures, surgery, or a combination of both approaches. Conservative measures include exercises and bracing. The Milwaukee brace is one of the most successful types of braces for scoliosis. This brace is individually fitted from the neck to the hips and initially is worn continually except when bathing. The child wears the brace for six months to two years and should continue to perform normal activities of daily living while wearing the brace. In addition, exercises should be performed daily to maintain spinal and abdominal muscle tone. The brace is adjusted regularly as the child grows, and wearing time is gradually decreased as the bone matures.

Curvatures also may be corrected with casts or halofemoral traction. This form of traction consists of weights attached by a halo device to

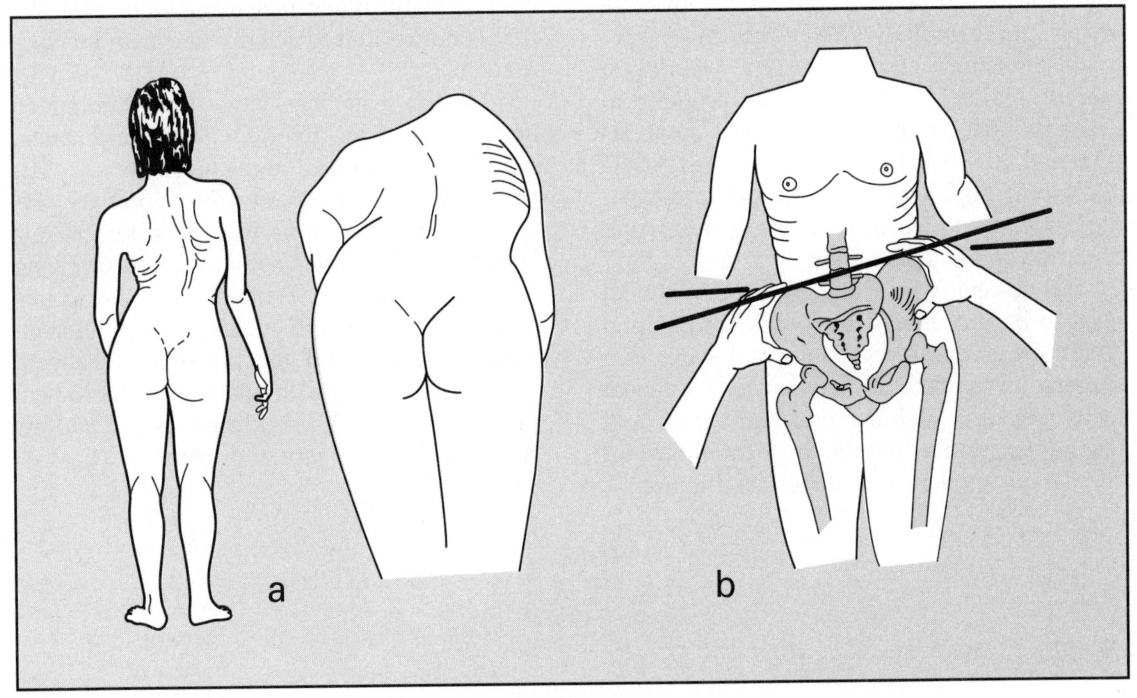

Figure 41–8 *Scoliosis (a) Lateral S-shaped curve with right rib hump on forward flexion and noticeable shoulder obliquity (b) Pelvic obliquity (From L. A. Mourad and M. M. Droste.* The Nursing Process in the Care of Adults with Orthopaedic Conditions, *3rd ed. Albany, NY: Delmar Publishers, 1993)*

the skull with counterweights attached to the femur. Surgical treatment is used to realign and straighten the severely curved spine. During surgery, a Harrington rod or other device is inserted to correct the curve, and the spine is fused. The Harrington rod is a metal rod with clips that are attached to vertebrae to permanently fuse them. After surgery, the child is placed in a body cast or brace, which is worn for several months (Cotton 1991). More recently the Luque rod has been used. This rod is a flexible L-shaped metal rod attached with wires to the spinous process of the vertebrae. After surgery, the child does not have to be immobilized and may be up and walking within a few days (Cotton 1991).

Nursing Care. Scoliosis is a slowly progressive condition that may not be diagnosed until adolescence. Supportive care is needed to help the adolescent cope with concerns about body image and comply with the treatment program. Encourage the adolescent wearing a brace to maintain correct posture and perform exercises that strengthen the back muscles (Olsen et al. 1991). Teach both parents and the adolescent how to properly apply and wear the brace and to watch for signs of skin irritation from rubbing or chafing.

Adolescents who require surgical treatment need to be prepared with specific information about the surgical procedure and care after surgery. Postoperative nursing assessment focuses special attention on neurological and respiratory status. Assess the extremities for circulation, motion, and sensation frequently. Encourage coughing and deep breathing at least every two hours. Surgery can be very painful and frequent administration of analgesics may be necessary. Physical therapy is begun as soon as possible after surgery, using range-of-motion exercises. Providing diversional activities and encouraging participation in decision making are important components of care of the adolescent patient (Mason 1991).

OSTEOSARCOMA

Osteosarcoma, also called osteogenic sarcoma, is a rapidly growing tumor of the bone that usually occurs in adolescent or young adult males. The primary tumor site is usually in an area of active bone growth, commonly the distal femur. The adolescent may complain of bone tenderness and increasing pain at the site that is not related to activity and may increase at night.

Treatment involves either limb amputation or removal of the tumor without amputation, called **limb salvage**, and chemotherapy. The prognosis depends on treatment, primary site, and whether metastasis has occurred. Overall, 50% of children with osteosarcoma survive long term. Nursing care centers on assisting the patient and family as they deal with a life-threatening condition and the potential for altered body image. Provide emotional support to help the family cope with the diagnosis and address concerns about surgery and treatment (Caswell and Ehland 1989).

REVIEW QUESTIONS

A. Multiple choice. Select the best answer.

1. Which of the following assessment data would indicate a properly applied cast?
   a. pallor, cyanosis, or discoloration of the skin
   b. edema of the toes
   c. warm, dry toes
   d. loss of pedal pulse
2. An appropriate nursing intervention for a child in skeletal traction would be to
   a. reapply traction as needed
   b. observe pin sites for infection
   c. remove traction weights when repositioning the child
   d. rest weights on bed frame
3. Which of the following statements best describes Duchenne's muscular dystrophy?
   a. It is inherited as an autosomal dominant disorder.
   b. It is characterized by remissions and exacerbations.
   c. Symptoms include a waddling gait and lordosis.
   d. Onset is usually in late childhood or adolescence.
4. Stress fractures are commonly caused by
   a. a rapid increase in a training activity over a short period
   b. excessive training activities over a long period of time
   c. jogging over rough terrain
   d. sudden change in weight distribution on impact with the ground
5. A muscular condition resulting from abnormal contraction or injury of the sternocleidomastoid muscle is
   a. brachial plexus palsy
   b. lordosis
   c. rickets
   d. torticollis

B. True or false. Write *T* for a true statement and *F* for a false statement.

1. ___ The purpose of the Harrington rod in scoliosis treatment is to straighten the spine.
2. ___ The Milwaukee brace is worn up to 16 hours a day until the spine stops growing.
3. Which of the following statements is (are) true about Legg-Calvé-Perthes disease?
   a. ___ It is more likely to occur in girls than in boys.
   b. ___ It requires long-term treatment.
   c. ___ It can result in permanent disability.
   d. ___ It is treated initially with rest.
4. ___ Osteomyelitis is an infection of the bone caused by bacterial infection.
5. ___ Musculoskeletal dysfunction can adversely affect the child's self-concept.

SUGGESTED ACTIVITIES

- Visit an orthopedic clinic to see how casts and braces are applied.
- Discuss ways to help parents provide care for children who are immobilized in casts or traction.
- Plan age-appropriate play activities for a child in a cast or traction.
- Invite a child with a musculoskeletal condition to the classroom to discuss his or her perception of the particular condition. Have students prepare their questions in advance and include a discussion of what nurses can do and say to make hospital stays easier for children with these conditions.

BIBLIOGRAPHY

Barrett, J. B., and B. H. Bryant. Fractures: Types, treatment, perioperative implications. *AORN Journal* 52 (1990): 755–771.

Brewer, K. Identifying and treating torticollis. *Clinical-Management* 10, no. 4 (1990): 19–21.

Broadwell Jackson, D., and R. B. Saunders. *Child Health Nursing*. Philadelphia: J. B. Lippincott, 1993.

Brosnon, H. Nursing management of the adolescent with idiopathic scoliosis. *Nursing Clinics of North America* 26, no. 1 (1991): 17–31.

Campbell, L. S., and J. D. Campbell. Musculoskeletal trauma in children. *Critical Care Nursing Clinics of North America* 3, no. 3 (1991): 445–456.

Caswell, L. J., and J. M. Ehland. Don't bump my bed, don't touch my feet. *Journal of Pediatric Oncology Nursing* 6, no. 4 (1989): 111–120.

Cotton, L. A. Unit rod segmental spinal instrumentation for the treatment of neuromuscular scoliosis. *Orthopaedic Nursing* 10, no. 5 (1991): 17–23.

Cunningham, N. Physical abuse in children: Recognition and management. *Emergency Pediatrics* 4, no. 1 (1991): 13–15.

Curry, L. C., and L. Y. Gibson. Congenital hip dislocation: The importance of early detection and comprehensive treatment. *Nurse Practitioner* 17, no. 5 (1992): 49–55.

Dunst, R. M. Legg-Calvé-Perthes disease. *Orthopaedic Nursing* 9, no. 2 (1990): 18–27.

Hensinger, R. N., and J. W. Fielding. The lower limb. Pp. 741–766 in R. T. Morrissy, ed. *Lovell and Winter's Pediatric Orthopaedics*, 3rd ed. Philadelphia: J. B. Lippincott, 1990.

Hiller, L. B., and C. K. Wade. Upper extremity functional assessment scales in children with Duchenne muscular dystrophy. *Archives of Physical Medicine and Rehabilitation* 73, no. 6 (1992): 523–534.

Jones-Walton, P. Clinical standards in skeletal traction pin site care. *Orthopaedic Nursing* 10, no. 2 (1991): 12–16.

Kyzer, S. Congenital idiopathic clubfoot. *Orthopaedic Nursing* 10, no. 4 (1991): 11–18.

Mason, K. J. Congenital orthopedic anomalies and their impact on the family. *Nursing Clinics of North America* 26, no. 1 (1991): 1–16.

Morris, L., S. Kraft, S. Tessem, and S. Reinisch. Nursing the patient in traction. *RN* 51, no. 1 (1988a): 26–31.

Morris, L., S. Kraft, S. Tessem, and S. Reinisch. Special care for skeletal traction. *RN* 51, no. 2 (1988b): 24–29.

Mosca, V. S., and D. D. Sherry. Juvenile rheumatoid arthritis. Pp. 298–324 in R. T. Morrissy, ed. *Lovell and Winter's Pediatric Orthopaedics*, 3rd ed. Philadelphia: J. B. Lippincott, 1990.

Mourad, L. A., and M. M. Droste. *The Nursing Process in the Care of Adults with Orthopaedic Conditions*, 3rd ed. Albany, NY: Delmar Publishers, 1993.

Olsen, B., L. Ustanko, and S. Warner. The patient in a halo brace: Striving for normalcy in body image and self-concept. *Orthopaedic Nursing* 10, no. 1 (1991): 44–50.

Page-Goertz, S. S. Even children have arthritis. *Pediatric Nursing* 15 (1989): 11–16.

Reilly, P. Juvenile rheumatoid arthritis. Pp. 336–354 in P. L. Jackson and J. Vessey, eds. *Primary Care of the Child with Chronic Conditions*. St. Louis, MO: C. V. Mosby, 1992.

Rudolph, A. M., J. I. E. Hoffman, and C. D. Rudolph. *Rudolph's Pediatrics*, 19th ed. Norwalk, CT: Appleton and Lange, 1991.

Schaming, D., et al. When babies are born with orthopedic problems. *RN* 53, no. 4 (1990): 62–66.

Scoles, P. V. *Pediatric Orthopedics in Clinical Practice*. Chicago: Year Book Medical Publishers, 1988.

Skale, N. *Manual of Pediatric Nursing Procedures.* Philadelphia: J. B. Lippincott, 1992.

Smrcina, C. M. Stress fractures in athletes. *Nursing Clinics of North America* 27, no. 1 (1992): 159–166.

Thompson, G. H., and R. B. Salter. Legg-Calvé-Perthes disease: Current concepts and controversies. *Orthopedic Clinics of North America* 18, no. 4 (1987): 617–635.

Wilkins, K. E. Changing patterns in the management of fractures in children. *Clinical Orthopaedics and Related Research* 232 (1991): 136.

CHAPTER

42

Neurological Conditions

Objectives

After studying this chapter, the student should be able to:

- Identify three types of neural tube defects.
- Compare and contrast the types of cerebral palsy and describe their treatment and nursing care.
- Describe the typical behaviors associated with seizures and discuss their treatment and nursing care.
- Describe the cause, symptoms, treatment, and nursing care of meningitis.
- Discuss the cause, symptoms, treatment, and nursing care of neuroblastoma.
- Differentiate between the types of head injury and discuss their treatment and nursing care.
- Describe the cause, symptoms, treatment, and nursing care of brain tumors.
- Describe the cause, symptoms, treatment, and nursing care of encephalitis.
- Discuss the cause, symptoms, treatment, and nursing care of Reye's syndrome.
- Describe the treatment and nursing care of a child in a coma.

Key Terms

- PARESIS
- EPILEPSY
- AUTOMATISM
- STATUS EPILEPTICUS
- NUCHAL RIGIDITY
- BRUDZINSKI'S SIGN
- KERNIG'S SIGN
- COMA

The neurological system is a complex system that is responsible for the control and coordination of body function. Changes in the neurological system may result from trauma, disease, or congenital anomalies. Early diagnosis of these potentially devastating conditions requires a complete history, good observation skills, and a thorough neurological assessment. By observing changes and recognizing differences, the nurse assists in early diagnosis and treatment of these conditions in infants and children.

Overview of the System

The major structures of the nervous system are the spinal cord, spinal nerves, and brain, Figure 42–1. The spinal cord functions as a conductive pathway to and from the brain. Within the cord, connections are made between incoming and outgoing nerve fibers. Thirty-one pairs of nerves are connected to the cord.

The nervous system performs three general functions: (1) a sensory function (conveying information to the brain), (2) a conscious or integrative function (translating information into sensation, perception, thought, and memory), and (3) a motor function (stimulating muscle activity). Nervous system functioning thus enables us to see, hear, feel, respond, think, remember, and move.

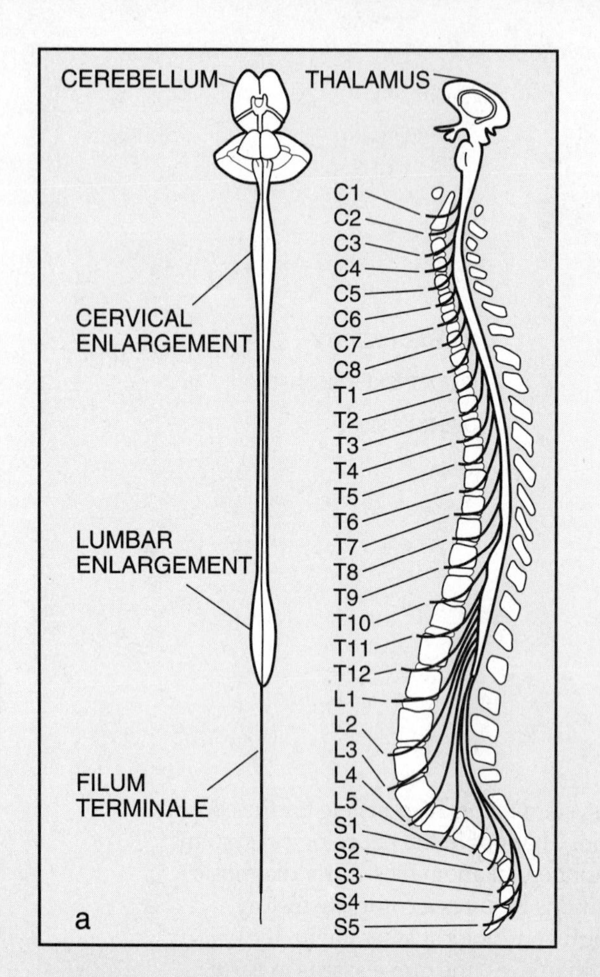

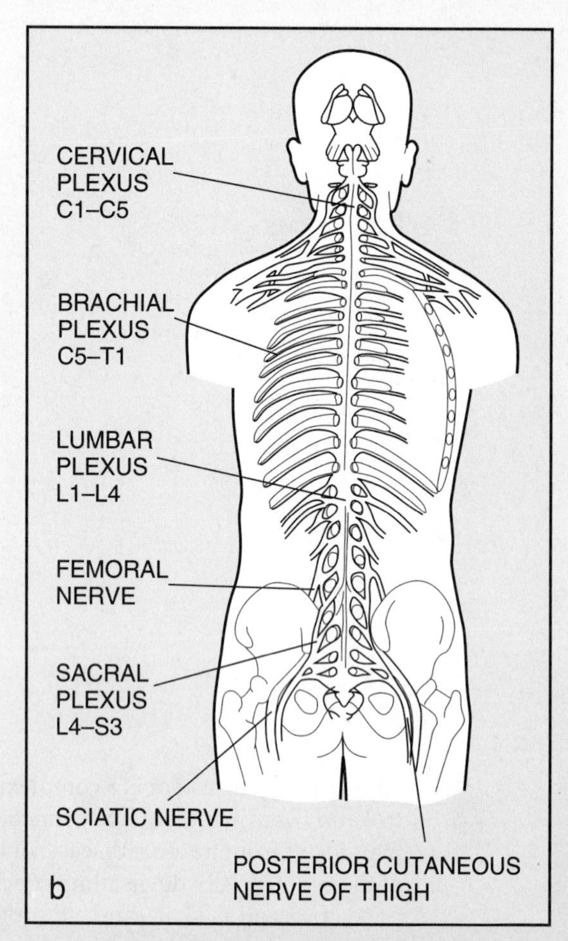

Figure 42–1 *(a) The spinal cord. (b) Spinal nerves. (c) Cross section of the brain. (Adapted from G. L. Smith, P. E. Davis, and J. T. Dennerll.* Medical Terminology: A Programmed Approach, *6th ed. Albany, NY: Delmar Publishers, 1991.)*

Infant and Toddler

Neural Tube Defects

Neural tube defects are malformations that occur when the neural tube fails to close during fetal development. Another name for this malformation is spina bifida.

Neural tube defects may be further subdivided into spina bifida occulta, meningocele, and myelomeningocele. Spina bifida occulta involves a defect of the vertebrae, only. In a meningocele, a sac containing meninges and spinal fluid protrudes through an opening in the spinal column. In a myelomeningocele, the sac contains meninges, spinal fluid, and neural tissue.

A comprehensive, coordinated, interdisciplinary approach is necessary to provide care for children with neural tube defects. Infants

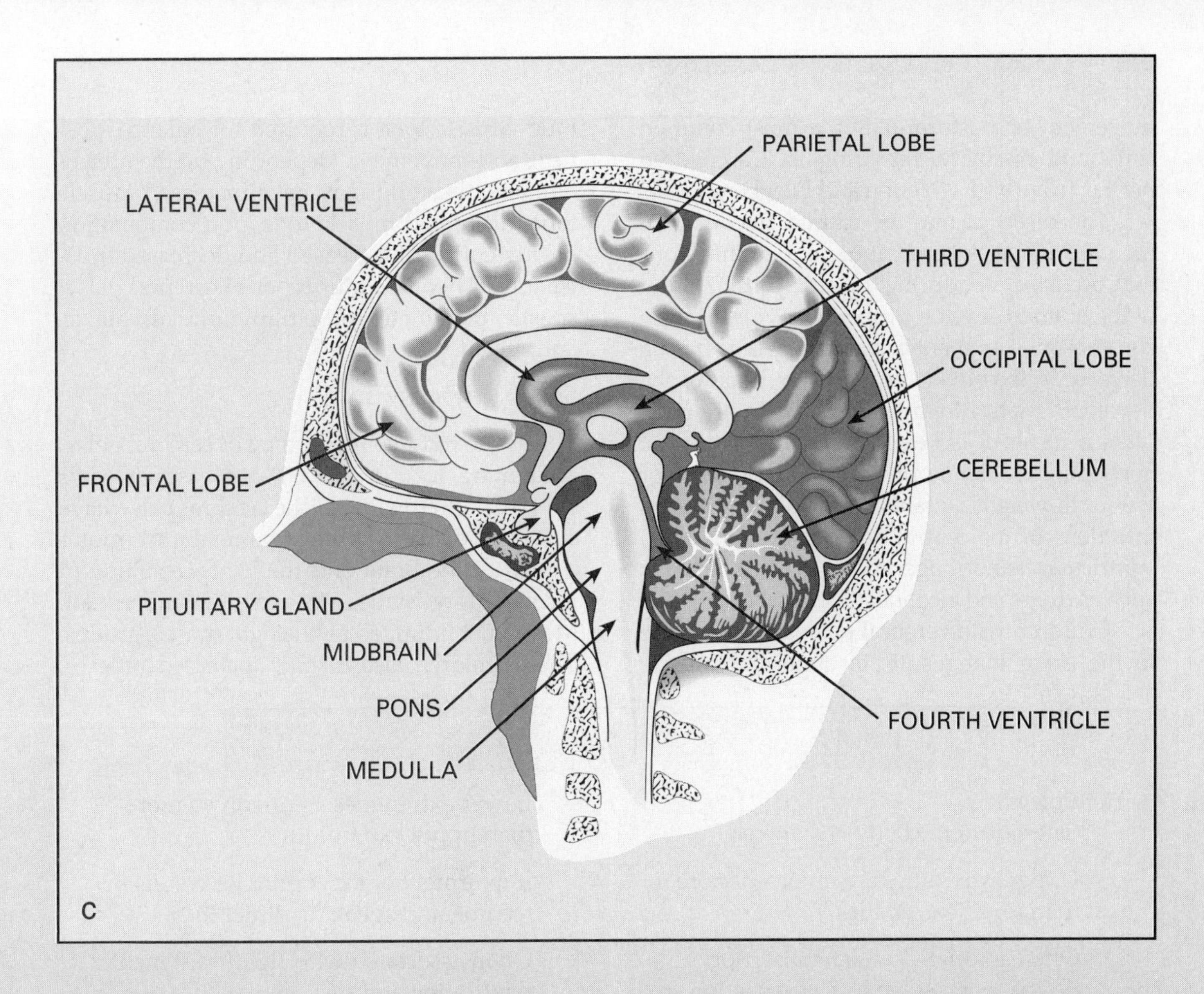

Figure 42–1 *continued*

with myelomeningocele often are born with or develop hydrocephalus. Surgical placement of a shunt is necessary to drain the extra fluid from the brain. These children also require meticulous skin care because they lack or have limited feeling below the lesion. Bowel and bladder dysfunction is common. Management involves intermittent catheterization and a bowel stimulation program coupled with a nutritional program (Smith 1990). Depending on the type and location of the lesion, the child may be able to ambulate with assistive devices or may require a wheelchair.

Refer to Chapter 20 for additional discussion of spina bifida defects and their care.

Cerebral Palsy

Description. Cerebral palsy is a broad term for a nonprogressive neurological disorder that affects movement or posture. It is the most common childhood disability, occurring in 1.2 children per 1,000 live births (Nelson and Ellenberg 1978).

The disorder may be caused by developmental anomalies, cerebral trauma, or infections that occur before, during, or after birth. Failure of the brain to develop properly may result from chromosomal or genetic abnormalities or from a decrease in the blood supply to the brain of the developing fetus. Injuries to the brain are most often a result of ischemia and cerebral anoxia. Such injuries commonly occur in preterm or low-birth-weight infants, difficult deliveries, infections of the central nervous system, intraventricular hemorrhage, and as a result of toxins such as drugs and alcohol.

Children with cerebral palsy have damage to the brain that results in abnormal muscle tone. Muscle tone is required for balance, posture, and movement. Depending on the area of damage, the child may have increased muscle tone, decreased muscle tone, or a combination or fluctuation of increased and decreased muscle tone. There are four types of cerebral palsy: spastic, dyskinetic (or extrapyramidal), ataxic, and mixed.

Spastic Cerebral Palsy

This is the most common type of cerebral palsy, accounting for 50% to 60% of cases (Geralis 1991). Children with spastic cerebral palsy have sustained damage to the pyramidal tract (motor cortex) of the brain and the joints, resulting in increased resistance to passive movement. Movement is limited by the tight muscle groups. These children also display increased reflexes,

PATTERNS OF DISABILITY IN CEREBRAL PALSY

Hemiplegia
- One side of the body is involved
- Upper extremities are involved more than lower extremities
- Often associated with hemisensory deficit, a one-sided loss of sensation on the same side as the paralysis **(paresis)**
- Occurs in one-third of children with cerebral palsy

Diplegia
- Both sides of the body are involved
- Lower extremities are involved more than upper extremities
- Often associated with apraxia, inability to initiate voluntary movements

Quadriparesis
- All four limbs are involved
- Lower extremities are involved more than upper extremities
- Impairment of facial muscles results in feeding and speaking difficulties
- Often associated with significant mental retardation and seizures

Monoplegia
- Only one extremity is involved
- Usually mild and often goes away with time
- Rare

Paraplegia
- Only the legs are involved

Triplegia
- Three extremities are involved

Figure 42–2

persistent primitive reflexes, and a positive Babinski sign after 2 years of age. The signs and symptoms of spastic cerebral palsy are further defined by the pattern of disability, Figure 42–2.

Dyskinetic Cerebral Palsy

Dyskinetic, or extrapyramidal, cerebral palsy occurs when there is damage to the basal ganglia and cranial nerve VII (Whaley and Wong 1991). This damage causes abnormal involuntary and uncontrolled movements, especially in the face, tongue, neck, arms, and trunk, Figure 42–3. These abnormal movements often make speaking, eating, reaching, and holding objects very difficult. Muscle tone often is decreased, and thus maintaining posture for sitting and walking is difficult. The movements usually disappear in sleep and are worsened by stress.

Ataxic Cerebral Palsy

This is the least common form of cerebral palsy and is caused by a problem with coordination of voluntary movements. Children with ataxic cerebral palsy lose coordination in standing, walking, and balance and have a characteristic wide-based gait. The child has difficulty reaching for objects and performing rapid repetitive movements. There is delayed development during the first 3 to 5 years of life.

Mixed-Type Cerebral Palsy

Children with mixed-type cerebral palsy have spastic muscle tone and involuntary movements. Spasticity is often the first sign, followed by involuntary movements between 9 months and 3 years of age.

Treatment. Mild cases of cerebral palsy may not be diagnosed until a delay or absence of a gross motor skill such as standing or walking is seen. Diagnosis is made on the basis of the neurological examination and history. Physical assessment signs in neonates include decreased activity, poor suck and swallow reflexes, abnormal muscle tone (increased or decreased), periods of apnea, temperature instability, and seizures. Assessment signs in older infants and toddlers include leg extension and adduction when the child is lifted by the axillae, presence of the Moro reflex after 6 months of age, hand

MOVEMENTS ASSOCIATED WITH CEREBRAL PALSY

Type	Movement	Location
Athetosis	Slow, writhing, wormlike	Wrists, fingers, face
Choreic	Abrupt, quick, jerky	Head, neck, arms, legs
Dystonia	Slow, rhythmic twisting or abnormal postures	Trunk or entire arm or leg
Hemiballismus	Flailing, circular movements	Arms, legs
Rigidity	Extremely high muscle tone in any position	Anywhere

Figure 42–3

dominance before 1 year of age, prolonged tonic neck reflex, toe walking, and hypotonia with brisk deep tendon reflexes.

The child is evaluated and treated by an interdisciplinary team consisting of the family, physician(s) (neurologist, pediatrician, rehabilitation physician), nurse, physical therapist, occupational therapist, psychologist, speech therapist, audiologist, nutritionist, social worker, teacher, and child life specialist.

The goal of treatment is to improve motor skills and minimize adverse effects. Independence is fostered by encouraging mobility, communication, education, and self-help skills to maximize the child's potential, Figure 42–4. Specific treatment approaches are listed in Figure 42–5.

Nursing Care. Nursing care focuses on observation, education of child and family, home care, psychosocial support, and referral of the family to support groups and community resources. Early recognition of developmental delays or failure to reach developmental milestones enables health care providers to begin therapy and teach the family how to care for the child. Education of the family is essential as they will need to carry out a detailed home program involving feeding, exercises, positioning for play, dressing, and bathing. Referral to support groups and other resources can benefit both parents and siblings of the child with cerebral palsy. Encourage the family to express their frustrations and concerns.

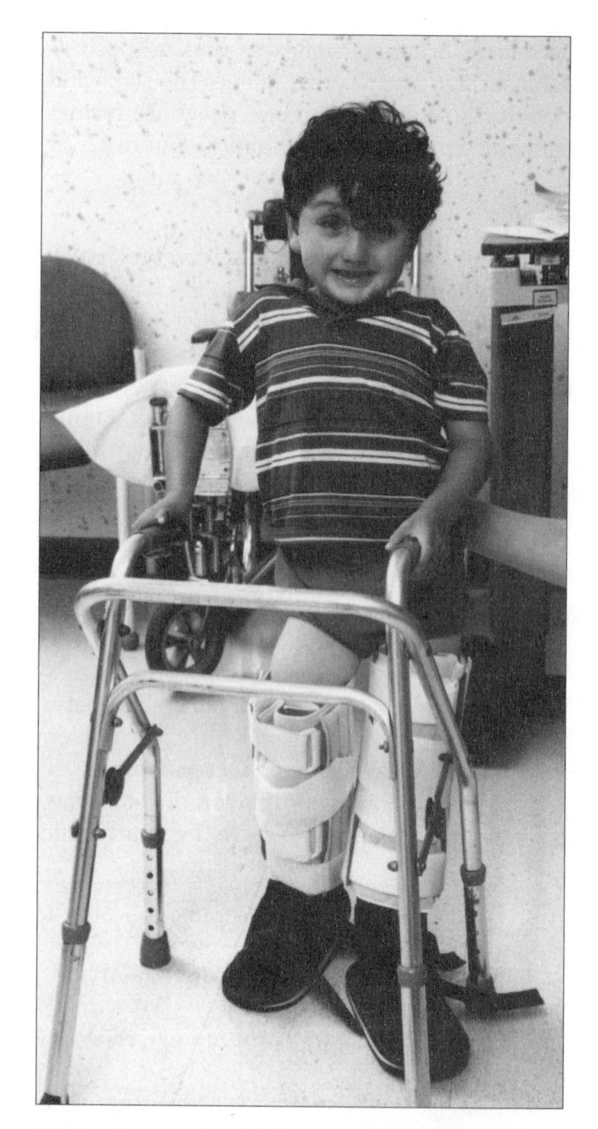

Figure 42–4 *This child with cerebral palsy has had surgery to improve muscle function. A walker assists with mobility.*

SEIZURES

Description. A seizure is a sudden, uncontrolled episode of excess electrical activity in the brain. The excess electrical activity can produce a change in behavior, consciousness, movement, perception, or sensation. **Epilepsy** is the term given to recurrent seizures. Seizures may be idiopathic or a result of trauma, injury, or metabolic alterations such as hypoglycemia or hypocalcemia. A febrile seizure is transient and occurs with a rapid rise in fever over 101.8°F (38.8°C). Febrile seizures occur in children between 6 months and 5 years of age.

Symptoms. There are many types of seizures. Classification is based on the changes pro-

TREATMENT APPROACHES FOR CEREBRAL PALSY

Approach	Use
Casts and braces	Assist with positioning and mobility.
Mobility devices (scooter boards, wheelchairs)	Allow the child freedom of movement.
Orthopedic surgery	Improves function by lengthening tendons or releasing spastic muscles.
Medications (diazepam, dantrolene, baclofen) to modify and decrease spasticity	Of limited use. Diazepam frequently will relax muscle tone but has a tranquilizing effect. Dantrolene (Dantrium) and baclofen may also be used as skeletal muscle relaxants.

Figure 42–5

duced by the excess electrical activity and on the electroencephalogram (EEG), which shows the part of the brain involved. Seizures may be generalized (that is, the excess electrical activity affects the brain as a whole) or partial (confined to a certain area of the brain), Figure 42–6. **Status epilepticus** (a series of generalized tonic-clonic seizures in which the child does not regain consciousness between seizures) is an emergency situation that is life-threatening.

Treatment. The goal of treatment is to control recurrent seizures and reduce the frequency of occurrence. Complete control is possible in 50% to 75% of children. Medical management is based on using as few antiepileptic drugs as possible with the least amount of side effects (Santilli and Sierzant 1987). Medications are started slowly and increased gradually to desired levels that are measured by a blood test. Patient compliance is very important in treatment. Once a child is seizure-free for 2 to 3 years, the medication is tapered and discontinued. If drugs are unsuccessful and the electrical discharge is limited to one place in the brain, surgical removal of the irritable brain tissue or lesion may be considered.

Nursing Care. Nursing care consists of observation skills, documentation of the seizures, and support and education of the child and family. Careful documentation of when and where the seizure began, what the child was doing, and how long the seizure lasted will help with diagnosis and treatment. Figure 42–7 outlines seizure first aid.

Educate the child and family about diagnostic tests and medications. It is essential that they understand the importance of the medication schedule and how to administer the medication. Parents also need to understand what happens during a seizure and how to help the child during a seizure. Encourage parents to allow the child to lead a regular life and not restrict activities. Teachers, babysitters, grandparents, and friends need the same information.

TYPES OF SEIZURES

Type	Description
Generalized Seizures	Consciousness is impaired (may be brief and unnoticed).
Tonic-clonic seizure (Grand mal)	Characterized by a sudden fall to the ground with possibly a shrill cry. In the tonic phase, the body is rigid and the child is not breathing and may become cyanotic. This phase lasts about 10–20 seconds. In the clonic phase, the body begins to jerk and the child may lose control of bowel and bladder function and foam at the mouth. This phase lasts from 30 seconds to 30 minutes. After the seizure, the child is semiconscious and hard to arouse. The child may sleep for up to several hours, have a headache, or vomit, and has no memory of the seizure.
Absence seizure (petit mal)	A brief period when the normal activity of the brain stops with minimal or no changes in muscle tone; may be mistaken for daydreaming or inattention. The child has no memory of the seizure, but must catch up with the activity in which he or she was involved. These seizures may occur frequently during the day and interfere with school performance.
Myoclonic seizure	Sudden, brief jerks of a muscle or muscle group; may be mild or throw the child to the ground. These seizures are usually associated with worsening neurological conditions.
Atonic seizure	Drop attacks that involve a sudden loss of muscle tone, causing the child to slump and be unable to maintain an upright position. Injuries to the face and head are common, and children prone to these seizures often wear helmets for protection.
Partial Seizures	Confined to one hemisphere. Consciousness may or may not be impaired.
Simple partial seizure	The child remains conscious. If the discharge is located in the motor part of the brain, the leg may jerk.
Complex partial seizure	Like a simple partial seizure, except the child is not conscious. May be the result of a simple partial seizure that spreads to the part of the brain that determines consciousness. The child may manifest **automatisms** (involuntary movements that look purposeful), such as fumbling with clothes or chewing.

Figure 42–6

SEIZURE FIRST AID

Although a seizure cannot be stopped once it has begun, the following measures can be taken to protect the child from injury:

- Cushion the head and remove objects that could injure the child.
- *Do not* place anything in the child's mouth. (It is impossible to swallow your tongue.)
- Do not try to hold the child or stop the limbs from jerking.
- If possible, turn the child or the child's head to the side to let excess saliva drain from the mouth. This position helps to maintain a patent airway.
- After the seizure, stay with the child and offer reassurance. Tell other children who witnessed the seizures what happened to allay their fears.

Figure 42–7

There are many misconceptions about epilepsy, and the nurse can help encourage a healthy attitude toward the disorder. The Epilepsy Foundation of America (4351 Garden City Drive, Landover, MD 20785, 301-459-3700) is a resource for information and support. Many states have local chapters that provide educational programs and offer support groups.

Figure 42–8 summarizes nursing care for a child with seizures.

MENINGITIS

Description. Meningitis is an acute inflammation of the meninges (the surrounding membranes of the brain and spinal cord) that usually occurs in infants between 6 and 12 months of age. There are three main types: bacterial, tuberculous, and viral, Figure 42–9.

The central nervous system is at risk for infection by the same organisms that affect the other organs of the body. In 95% of children over 2 months, meningitis is caused by one of three bacterial organisms. Beta-streptococci and *Escherichia coli* are the prevalent organisms in neonates. *Hemophilus influenzae* is the predominant organism in children from 3 months to 3 years of age.

The most common route of infection is vascular spread from an infection located elsewhere (most often the nasopharynx). Bacteria can also enter the body through skull fractures, penetrating head wounds, lumbar puncture, or surgical procedures (Wong 1993).

Symptoms. Symptoms vary depending on the age of the child. In neonates the symptoms are vague. The neonate usually appears healthy for a few days and then develops symptoms of poor suck, weak cry, vomiting, diarrhea, jaundice, irritability, and lack of movement. In infants and young children, symptoms include seizures, irritability, fever, poor feeding patterns or loss of appetite, and vomiting. In infants under the age of 18 months, bulging fontanel is the most significant sign. Parents may report a resistance to diaper changes and to being held or cuddled.

In older children and adolescents, the illness is usually abrupt and the child appears very ill. Fever, chills, headache, vomiting, and sensory changes are usually present.

NURSING CARE PLAN: Seizures

PATIENT PROBLEM	GOAL(S)
Possible injury resulting from seizure	The child will not experience injury during a seizure.
Anxiety (child's and parents') about home management of seizures	The child (at appropriate age) and family will be able to state information about seizure disorder. Anxiety will lessen as knowledge about the disorder increases. The parents will be able to list prescribed medication(s), dosages, frequency of administration, and side effects. The parents will be able to state first aid for seizures (see Figure 42–7). The child and parents will contact appropriate support groups.

Figure 42–8

NURSING INTERVENTION	RATIONALE
Initiate seizure first aid (see Figure 42–7).	Seizure first aid helps to prevent injury and maintain a patent airway.
Avoid placing anything in the child's mouth.	Injury can occur when objects are placed in the mouth. Teeth may be knocked out, the object may be bitten, or it may injure the child's mouth.
Do not try to restrain or stop movement.	A seizure cannot be stopped and must be allowed to run its course.
Explain to child and family (in terms they can understand) the cause of seizures. Provide written information and brochures about the disorder.	Knowledge of the disorder and its management will enable child and family to return to normal routine and patterns of activity.
Explain medications and provide a list including purpose, dose, frequency, and side effects. Help parents develop a system or chart for administering medication.	Medications must be given as ordered to obtain a therapeutic blood level of drug(s).
Explain first aid for seizures and provide written instructions or brochures.	Knowledge of how to manage a seizure makes the family more comfortable and able to encourage the child to lead an unrestricted life.
Provide name and telephone number of local support group. If one does not exist, arrange for parents to talk to parents of another child with epilepsy.	Support group and other parents of epileptic children provide ongoing support to parents once the child has been discharged.

COMMON TYPES OF MENINGITIS

Bacterial: Caused by pus-forming bacteria:

Hemophilus influenzae (*H. influenzae* meningitis)

Neisseria meningitidis (meningococcal meningitis)

Streptococcus pneumoniae (pneumococcal meningitis)

H. influenzae occurs from autumn to early winter; *N. meningitidis* and *S. pneumoniae* occur from late winter to early spring.

Tuberculous: Caused by the tubercle bacillus *(Mycobacterium tuberculosis)*

Viral or aseptic: Caused by a wide variety of viruses.

Figure 42–9

Treatment. A lumbar puncture to examine cerebrospinal fluid is required for diagnosis of meningitis. A culture and gram stain are used to identify the causative organism. A blood culture, computerized axial tomographic (CAT) scan, and EEG may also be obtained.

Treatment depends on the causative organism. Intravenous antibiotics are administered for 10 to 14 days. In addition, the child is usually placed in respiratory isolation for 24 to 48 hours after initiation of antibiotic therapy.

Nursing Care. Specific nursing care depends on the neurological status of the child. For the child who is placed in respiratory isolation, nursing care should be organized in order to provide minimum stimulation to the child. Keep the room darkened and quiet. The child will be most comfortable without a pillow, with the head of the bed slightly raised, and in a side-lying position. Care should be taken not to move the child's head and neck because moving them is very painful.

Mild analgesics such as acetaminophen are used to decrease pain and irritability. Stronger medications are not used because they can change the neurological status of the child. Fluids are restricted initially to reduce central blood volume and intracranial pressure. It is important to maintain a strict record of intake and output. Maintain the IV line at all times. In the infant, head circumferences should be measured every 8 hours to identify the early signs of developing hydrocephalus. Because of the decreased level of consciousness, all children with meningitis are at increased risk for injury. Children must also be observed for seizures.

The child's disease and symptoms should be explained to the parents. Parents also require emotional support during the initial phase of the illness. The child may be irritable and in pain, and parents may have difficulty comforting the child. Encourage them to bring the child's "security items," such as a blanket or teddy bear, from home.

Visitors should be kept to a minimum during the initial phase of the illness. Advise parents that the risk of an adult contracting meningitis is slight. There is some risk, however, to children and siblings exposed to the infected child, and prophylactic treatment may be suggested.

During recovery, encourage diversional activities and visits by parents and siblings to help prevent the effects of long-term hospitalization, such as regression, dependence, and boredom.

Parents often have many questions and fears related to the prognosis. The age of the child and the speed with which the diagnosis is made affect outcome. Complications that can occur as a result of meningitis include mental retardation, learning disabilities, physical or motor disabilities, and alterations in vision and hearing.

Figure 42–10 summarizes nursing care for the child with meningitis.

NEUROBLASTOMA

Description. Neuroblastoma, the most common malignant tumor of infancy, occurs in 1 child per 1,000 and slightly more often in boys than in girls. Half of all cases occur in children under 2 years of age, and one-quarter in children under 4 (Whaley and Wong 1991). Because these tumors arise from cells that, in the embryo, make up the adrenal glands and part of the sympathetic nervous system, they are usually located in the abdominal cavity. Other sites include the pelvis, chest, and neck.

Symptoms. Symptoms depend on the primary tumor site. A tumor in the abdomen causes a mass, pain, decrease in appetite, and bladder and bowel changes. A tumor in the chest may cause pain, cough, and shortness of breath. A tumor in the neck may cause pain and difficulty in swallowing. Metastases are often present at diagnosis and account for joint and bone pain. In infants, the presenting symptoms are hepatomegaly, anemia, poor feeding patterns, and dyspnea. Children may have weight loss, fever, and anemia.

A clinical staging classification system has been developed to establish an appropriate treatment plan for the child with a neuroblastoma. Tumors are classified into four stages, ranging from stage I (no metastasis) to stages IV and IV-S (metastases to other body sites).

Treatment. Prognosis and treatment are based on the stage of the tumor. Children younger than 2 years and those with localized disease (stage I or II) have the best prognosis. The goal of treatment is to remove the tumor. In half of the cases, however, metastasis is present and total surgical removal is impossible. Radiation and chemotherapy may also be used.

Nursing Care. Nursing care includes supportive care, preparing the child and family for diagnostic tests and treatment, and planning for a return to normal activities upon discharge. Analgesics are used judiciously with the realization that they may alter neurological functioning. Provide a quiet room with dim lights, limit visitors, and avoid sudden movements. Ice compresses may provide comfort and relieve pain, especially if edema is present.

If possible, the nurse should be present during physician visits to reinforce and clarify information presented. Encourage the family to verbalize fears and questions. Parents and siblings will need emotional support. The nurse and other interdisciplinary team members (social worker, psychologist, child life specialist, and clergy) can help the family discuss the illness with the child and siblings.

HEAD INJURY

Head injury — an injury of the scalp, skull, or brain — is one of the most common causes of disability and death of children (Patterson et al. 1992). Each year, 200,000 children sustain head injuries, 4,000 of which are fatal (Patterson et al. 1992).

Common head injuries include concussions, contusions and lacerations, vascular injuries, skull fractures, and coma. Falls and motor vehicle crashes are the primary causes of head injuries. Other causes are child abuse, unhelmeted biking accidents, diving accidents, and sports injuries.

Hitting the head is a common occurrence in childhood. In infants and very young children, the head is large in proportion to the rest of the body. Infants often fall from beds and high chairs, landing on their heads. Toddlers, who are unsteady on their feet, often bump their heads.

NURSING CARE PLAN: Meningitis

PATIENT PROBLEM	GOAL(S)
Irritability, altered consciousness, and disorientation	The child's neurological status will remain stable and/or improve each day.
Pain and discomfort	The child will state or demonstrate comfort.

Figure 42–10

NURSING INTERVENTION	RATIONALE
Assess neurological status and vital signs as ordered. Maintain a quiet environment in room and hallway. Keep the lights low. Avoid jarring the bed, and group nursing care activities to avoid unnecessary disturbances.	A quiet environment with minimal disturbances facilitates recovery.
Approach the child in a calm manner and limit the number of caregivers. Tell the child who you are and what you are going to do. Have parents bring the child's favorite toys and objects from home.	Reorientation helps the child adjust to the new environment.
Encourage parents to limit visitors until the child's neurological status improves.	Limiting visitors helps maintain a quiet environment.
Administer analgesics or antipyretics as ordered and assess effectiveness and side effects.	Medications should be given on schedule and monitored for effectiveness and side effects.
Avoid moving the child, and minimize movements of the head and neck. Do not use pillows, and keep the head of the bed elevated 30 degrees. Assist the child to avoid straining, coughing, or nose blowing.	Sudden movements cause pain and discomfort.
Provide age-appropriate diversional activities.	If distracted, the child may relax and feel more comfortable.

The skull serves as protection to the brain. When the head is hit, the skull accelerates, causing the brain to move. When the head stops, the skull decelerates, and the brain strikes sharp edges of the skull, causing damage. The technical term for this type of injury is coup-contrecoup injury, Figure 42–11. Rotational injury is also possible from twisting of the brain within the skull.

Concussion. In a concussion (the most common head injury), acceleration-deceleration produces a loss of consciousness that lasts for seconds to hours. There is no structural damage to the brain, Figure 42–12. Amnesia is common but normally disappears by 24 hours after the injury. Postconcussion syndrome occurs when the amnesia lasts longer than 24 hours or the loss of consciousness is prolonged. Symptoms of postconcussion syndrome include vertigo, visual disturbances, light-headedness, memory and concentration problems, mood alterations, and fatigue. These symptoms may last for days to months, but usually resolve.

Contusion and Laceration. A contusion is a bruising or hemorrhage of the brain, Figure 42–12. In a serious injury, there may be many sites of hemorrhage, causing changes in motor, sensory, or visual functioning. A laceration is a traumatic tearing of the brain that causes bleeding that leads to a more severe injury and often permanent disability. Contusions and lacerations are usually caused by blunt trauma and penetrating injuries to the head.

Vascular Injuries. Hemorrhage occurs in about 7% of all head injuries (Whaley and Wong 1991). Bleeding may result in an intracranial, epidural, or subdural hemorrhage.

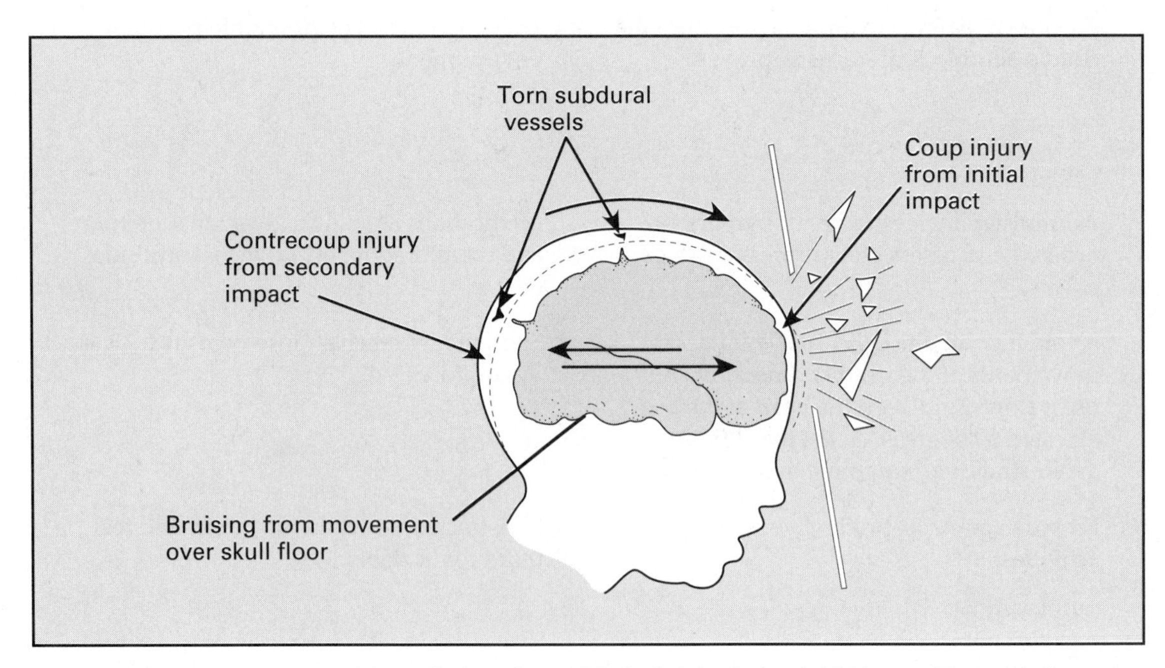

Figure 42–11 *Coup-contrecoup injury. The frontal area of the brain is bruised on initial impact. The occipital area of the brain is bruised as the brain bounces back and strikes the back of the skull. (From M. R. Eichelberger, J. W. Ball, G. S. Pratsch, and E. Runion.* Pediatric Emergencies: A Manual for Prehospital Care Providers. *Reprinted by permission of Prentice-Hall. Englewood Cliffs, NJ: Brady/Prentice-Hall, 1992.)*

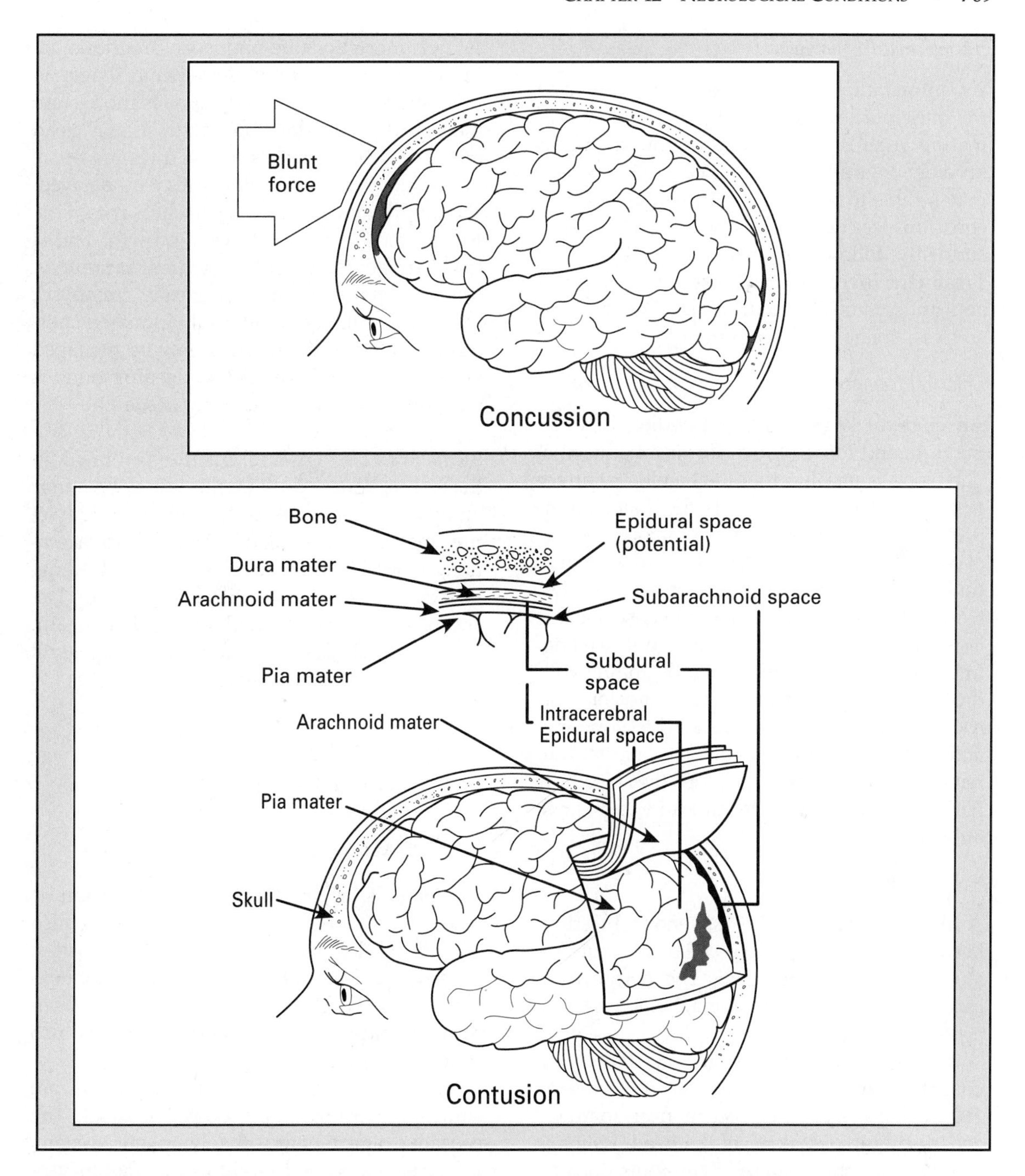

Figure 42–12 *Concussion and contusion injuries. A concussion involves no detectable brain damage. A contusion involves bruising or rupturing of the brain tissue and vessels at any of the identified levels. (From M. R. Eichelberger, J. W. Ball, G. S. Pratsch, and E. Runion.* Pediatric Emergencies: A Manual for Prehospital Care Providers. *Reprinted by permission of Prentice-Hall. Englewood Cliffs, NJ: Brady/Prentice-Hall, 1992.)*

Intracranial Hemorrhage

An intracranial hemorrhage is bleeding into the intraventricular space. It may occur in premature infants as a result of trauma or in severely injured children. The child initially may be able to respond to commands, but then consciousness deteriorates. Seizures may begin suddenly, followed by respiratory difficulties. Treatment involves cardiorespiratory support and anticonvulsive medications. The prognosis in severe hemorrhage is poor.

Epidural Hemorrhage

An epidural hemorrhage is bleeding between the dura and the skull that forms a hematoma. The blood is usually from the meningeal artery or vein. As the blood expands, the brain is compressed. The child usually has a momentary loss of consciousness, followed by a return to normal consciousness for a few hours or several days. How long the period of normal consciousness lasts depends on the rapidity of bleeding. Impaired consciousness follows, beginning with drowsiness that progresses to confusion and coma. There may also be headache, vomiting, and seizures. Treatment involves surgery to remove the clot and to stop the bleeding. Early diagnosis and treatment lead to a positive outcome.

Subdural Hemorrhage

A subdural hemorrhage is venous bleeding between the dura and the cerebrum that creates pressure on the brain. The hemorrhage causes a subdural hematoma, which can be acute or chronic.

In an acute hemorrhage, an underlying contusion or laceration usually is present. Hemorrhage also may occur from damage caused by rapid shaking of the head, which is common in child abuse. Symptoms include headache, drowsiness, agitation, confusion, and fixation and dilation of the ipsilateral pupil (the pupil on the same side as the hematoma). A high mortality rate and poor prognosis are associated with acute subdural hemorrhage.

Chronic subdural hematoma is more common and may develop from minor head injuries. If the fontanels and sutures are open, the occurrence of symptoms may be delayed. The child may exhibit headache, irritability, full fontanel, increased head growth, and a low hematocrit. In older children, large subdural hematomas are surgically removed, whereas in infants, a subdural tap may be performed. A small hematoma may be managed without surgery because the bleeding often is reabsorbed by the surrounding tissue.

Skull Fracture. A skull fracture is a break in the cranial bones. Skull fractures may be minor or life-threatening. A child with a skull fracture may have an accompanying scalp laceration, which can be a major source of bleeding. In fact, a skull fracture with a major scalp laceration can cause a child to bleed to death. Figure 42–13 describes four common skull fractures and their management.

PRESCHOOL AND SCHOOL-AGE CHILD

ENCEPHALITIS

Encephalitis, an inflammation of the brain, is most often caused by viruses but may also be caused by bacteria, fungi, or parasites. Ingestion of lead, inhalation of carbon monoxide, certain vaccines, and complications from measles, mumps, rubella, and rabies may also produce encephalitis.

Signs and symptoms of encephalitis are similar regardless of the causative agent. The causative agent enters the lymphatic system, infects the blood, and produces an inflammatory response that results in cellular damage, cerebral edema, and temporary neurological dysfunction. The child presents with a headache, fever,

COMMON SKULL FRACTURES

Type	Description	Treatment
Linear (or simple) skull fracture	A line or crack in the skull.	Usually heals on its own in 3–4 months.
Depressed skull fracture	Involves a broken bone with fragments that are pushed in and toward the brain. The skull is indented, and brain tissue below the indentation is injured. The bone may be broken in several places or comminuted.	If the depression is very deep, surgery is necessary.
Compound skull fracture	A laceration of the scalp with a depressed skull fracture that allows access to the cranium. Debris may enter the cranium.	Requires surgery and antibiotics.
Basilar skull fracture	The most serious type of skull fracture. Occurs at the base of the skull and may be linear, depressed, or comminuted. Cerebrospinal fluid is often noted leaking from the child's nose or ear. "Raccoon eyes," caused by blood leaking into the frontal sinuses, often are present. Bruising behind the ear may also be present because of blood leaking into the mastoid sinus. This bruising is called the battle sign.	Children with a basilar skull fracture are at risk for meningitis. Frequent neurological assessment is required. Safety must also be considered because the child may be disoriented and restless. The room should be kept dim and quiet, and visitors should be limited.

Figure 42–13

irritability, gastrointestinal distress, and often mild respiratory symptoms. The onset of symptoms may be sudden or gradual. In severe cases, the child has a high fever, seizures, disorientation, and possibly lapses into a coma. Other symptoms include alterations in motor function, such as inability to walk or changes in balance and coordination.

Diagnosis is made on the basis of the history, physical examination, lumbar puncture, and laboratory tests, including cultures of cerebrospinal fluid (CSF) and blood. The child is hospitalized for neurological assessment and supportive care. Cerebral symptoms are managed as for a child with meningitis. Nursing care is also similar.

REYE'S SYNDROME

Reye's syndrome is a multisystem disease that is damaging to the liver and brain. The liver fails to convert ammonia to urea, resulting in toxic uremia. Diagnosis is made by liver biopsy, which shows hepatic fatty degeneration. Children between the ages of 5 and 10 years are at greatest risk. Public education about the disorder and its symptoms has resulted in a decline in the number of reported cases.

Most cases of Reye's syndrome occur during the winter flu season. The disease usually follows a viral illness (most often influenza or varicella). The child is usually ill with flu-like symptoms for a week, is healthy for several days, and then experiences prolonged vomiting for 2 to 3 days. The child's level of consciousness decreases each day. Symptoms progress to include persistent or continuous vomiting, listlessness, personality change, disorientation, delirium, convulsions, and coma. Infants with Reye's syndrome may have diarrhea or respiratory distress but no vomiting. Because of the possible link between aspirin use and Reye's syndrome, aspirin should not be given to children less than 18 years of age to relieve symptoms of cold, flu, or varicella.

At the onset of symptoms, the child should be evaluated by a health care provider. Medications to reduce fever or pain should not be given, because they may mask the symptoms of the disease. Recovery depends on early diagnosis and treatment to control cerebral edema, reverse metabolic injury, and prevent respiratory compromise. Symptoms may progress rapidly without intervention and treatment.

Treatment for mild symptoms is supportive, involving return to normal acid-base balance, control cerebral edema, and decreasing the risk of intracranial pressure. More severe symptoms require aggressive management in a pediatric intensive care unit. Measures to maintain a patent airway and control cerebral edema are necessary to prevent irreversible brain damage.

Prognosis and sequelae are based on the amount of cerebral edema. The child may recover completely or have slight to severe brain damage. If the child has a rapid progression of symptoms or becomes comatose, the prognosis is worse. Neurological sequelae include speech and language disorders, fine and gross motor skill problems, and problems with memory, concentration, and attention.

BRAIN TUMOR

Brain tumors originate in the neural tissue and are the most common type of solid tumors in children (Shiminski-Maher 1990). They account for 20% of childhood cancers and occur in 1,000 to 1,500 children each year (Shiminski-Maher 1990). Most brain tumors occur in children between 5 and 10 years of age. The prognosis depends on the age of the child, and the type, anatomical location, and size of the tumor. Figure 42–14 lists common pediatric brain tumors.

Accurate diagnosis of a brain tumor can be difficult because symptoms often are vague. In infants, the sutures and fontanels are open, and early signs of increased intracranial pressure are not noticeable. In older children, the symptoms may resemble those of other common illnesses.

Classic symptoms are a recurrent and progressive headache that is present in the morning and projectile vomiting. Other symptoms include muscular disturbances such as clumsiness, unsteady gait, and a decrease in fine motor coordination. The child's personality may also change, and vision and speech changes and seizures may occur.

Diagnosis is based on a detailed history combined with CAT scan or magnetic resonance imaging (MRI). Nursing care for children undergoing these tests includes patient and family education as well as administration of any medication that may be needed for sedation.

Treatment options include surgery, radiation therapy, and chemotherapy, all of which have risks.

COMMON PEDIATRIC BRAIN TUMORS

Type	Description
Medulloblastoma	Fastest-growing, malignant brain tumor. Located in the cerebellum.
Cerebellar astrocytoma	Cystic or benign and slow-growing tumor.
Brain-stem glioma	Often grows very large before resulting in symptoms. Hard to resect surgically because of location.
Ependymoma	Grows at varying rates. Located in the ventricles.
Craniopharyngioma	Located near the pituitary. Removal may necessitate hormone replacement.

Figure 42–14

- *Surgery*: The tumor needs to be removed as completely as possible without causing residual neurological damage.
- *Radiation*: Children undergoing radiation treatment receive treatment twice a day for eight weeks. It is important to orient children to the procedure so they will not be frightened during the treatment. Side effects include nausea and vomiting, decreased oral intake, fatigue, hair loss, skin sensitivity, and possible loss of cognition.
- *Chemotherapy*: The goal of chemotherapy is to destroy tumor cells and spare healthy cells. The types, amounts, and frequency of chemotherapy vary with the particular hospital and pediatric oncologist, but the side effects of nausea, vomiting, and immunosuppression remain the same.

Regardless of the treatment, nurses play a major role in the support, education, and discharge planning of children with brain tumors. The goal is for the child to return to a normal routine, activities, and school as soon as possible.

COMA

Coma is a state of unconsciousness in which the child cannot open the eyes, speak, obey commands, or be aroused by any measure. The Glasgow Coma Scale (GCS) is a well-known scale used to assess the neurological responses of patients with head injuries. The scale relies on the best response to eye opening, motor, and verbalization requests, and the score can range from 3 points to 15 points. Because the original GCS does not take into consideration the developmental levels of children, many hospitals use a modified GCS for pediatric patients, Figure 42–15. Neurological assessments are performed frequently. Nurses who care for a child in a coma must work closely with parents to identify the child's normal behaviors. These behaviors provide a measure for assessing return to normal functioning.

Family support is essential to the nursing care of the child in a coma. Parents exhibit a wide range of feelings and emotions intensified by the uncertain prognosis for the child.

NEUROLOGIC ASSESSMENT

Pupils	Right	Size	
		Reaction	
	Left	Size	
		Reaction	

++ = Brisk
+ = Sluggish
− = No reaction
C = Eye closed by swelling

Pupil scale (mm): 1, 2, 3, 4, 5, 6, 7, 8

GLASGOW COMA SCALE

Eyes open	Spontaneously	4			
	To speech	3			
	To pain	2			
	None	1			
Best motor response	Obeys commands	6			
	Localizes pain	5			
	Flexion withdrawal	4			
	Flexion abnormal	3			
	Extension	2			
	None	1			
Best response to auditory and/or visual stimulus	>2 years			<2 years	
	Orientation	5		5 Smiles, listens, follows	
	Confused	4		4 Cries, consolable	
	Inappropriate words	3		3 Inappropriate persistent cry	
	Incomprehensible words	2		2 Agitated, restless	
	None	1		1 No response	
	Endotracheal tube or trach	T			
COMA SCALE TOTAL					

Usually record best arm or age-appropriate response

HAND GRIP:
Equal
Unequal
R____L
Weakness

LOC:
Alert/oriented ×4
Sleepy
Irritable
Comatose
Disoriented
Combative
Lethargic
Awake
Sleeping
Drowsy
Agitated

MUSCLE TONE:
Normal
Arching
Spastic
Flaccid
Weak
Decorticate
Decerebrate
Other ________

EYE MOVEMENT:
Normal
Nystagmus
Strabismus
Other ________

FONTANEL/ WINDOW:
Soft
Flat
Sunken
Tense
Bulging
Closed
Other ________

MOOD/AFFECT:
Happy
Content
Quiet
Withdrawn
Sad
Flat
Hostile

Figure 42–15 *Pediatric coma scale (From D. Wong,* Whaley & Wong's Essentials of Pediatric Nursing, *4th ed. St. Louis, MO: Mosby-Year Book, 1993.)*

Fear of death, and physical and mental disability are foremost. If the child dies, the family needs support to cope with the loss. If the child remains comatose, parents must decide whether to place the child in a long-term care facility or care for the child at home.

Parents of a child in a coma face many difficult decisions. The brain may be damaged so severely that life is maintained only through life-support systems. On the other hand, the coma may resolve, but the child may be physically or mentally disabled and require long-term care and rehabilitation.

Nurses can help parents during this decision-making process by listening and providing information. Regardless of the outcome, parents should be encouraged and taught to provide physical care for the child through bathing, skin care, and range-of-motion exercises. Parents should also be encouraged to bring items from home (such as toys and blankets) and to talk with, read to, and touch the child. When parents or siblings cannot visit, they should be encouraged to send tapes to be played for the child.

REVIEW QUESTIONS

A. Multiple choice. Select the best answer.

1. Children with cerebral palsy usually
   a. die before the age of 2
   b. have progressive worsening of symptoms
   c. have developmental problems
   d. get better over time with therapy

2. A child with cerebral palsy who has quadriparesis will not have
   a. limited function in all four extremities
   b. impairment of facial muscles
   c. mental deficits or delays
   d. disappearance of symptoms over time

3. Which of the following best describes the appearance of a child experiencing a tonic-clonic seizure?
   a. is confused and sleepy after the seizure
   b. is initially flaccid followed by jerking motions
   c. stares blankly into space
   d. has unimpaired consciousness

4. First aid for a seizure involves which of the following actions?
   a. placing an object in the mouth to protect the tongue
   b. attempting to stop the seizure
   c. loosening tight clothing and turning the head to the side
   d. putting your fingers in the mouth to keep the child from biting the tongue

5. Nursing care for the child with meningitis includes
   a. elevating the head with two pillows
   b. restricting fluids
   c. encouraging visitors
   d. administering strong sedatives to alleviate pain

6. Children who are at risk of developing Reye's syndrome have usually
   a. taken acetaminophen to treat cold, flu, or varicella
   b. been healthy before developing Reye's syndrome symptoms
   c. taken aspirin to treat cold, flu, or varicella
   d. been exposed to bacteria
7. A child with a brain tumor may have which of the following symptoms?
   a. projectile vomiting
   b. a recurrent and progressive pain behind the ears
   c. increasing difficulty in being awakened in the morning
   d. constipation
8. Treatment for brain tumors may include all of the following except
   a. chemotherapy
   b. antibiotic therapy
   c. radiation therapy
   d. surgery
9. Which of the following is true of neuroblastoma?
   a. usually involves metastases
   b. cannot be treated with surgery
   c. commonly presents in the brain
   d. is always fatal
10. Damage from a head injury may result from
    a. rapid acceleration followed by rapid deceleration
    b. seizures
    c. being in a coma
    d. lack of nutrition

SUGGESTED ACTIVITIES

- Contact a local outpatient facility or infant intervention program and arrange to observe a child with cerebral palsy during physical therapy, occupational therapy, and speech therapy.
- Call the Epilepsy Foundation of America (1-800-EFA-1000) and request brochures about children with epilepsy. Investigate an area such as school issues, psychosocial issues, or first aid.
- Call a local school system and make arrangements to observe in a classroom with disabled students.
- Arrange a tour of a pediatric intensive care unit. Talk with the nursing staff about management issues for children with meningitis or brain tumors.

BIBLIOGRAPHY

American Association of Neuroscience Nursing. *Core Curriculum for Neuroscience Nursing*, 3rd ed. Chicago: Chicago University Press, 1990.

Avery, M., and L. First, eds. *Pediatric Medicine.* Baltimore: Williams and Wilkins, 1989.

David, R. *Pediatric Neurology for the Clinician.* Norwalk, CT: Appleton and Lange, 1992.

Foster, R. L., M. M. Hunsberger, and J. J. Anderson. *Family-Centered Nursing Care of Children.* Philadelphia: W. B. Saunders, 1989.

Geralis, E., ed. *Children with Cerebral Palsy: A Parent's Guide.* Kensington, MD: Woodbine House, 1991.

Hazinski, M. *Nursing Care of the Critically Ill Child.* St. Louis, MO: C. V. Mosby, 1987.

Hockenberry, M., D. Coody, and B. Bennett. Childhood cancers: Incidence, etiology, diagnosis, and treatment. *Pediatric Nursing* 16, no 3 (1990): 239–246.

Lovejoy, F., A. L. Smith, M. J. Bresnan, J. M. Wood, D. I. Victor, and P. C. Adams. Clinical stages in Reye's syndrome. *American Journal of Diseases of Childhood* 128, no. 2 (1974): 36–41.

Maheady, D. Reye's syndrome: Review and update. *Journal of Pediatric Health Care* 3, no. 5 (1985): 246–250.

National Reye's Syndrome Foundation. *Be Wise about Reye's*, Awareness Bulletin. Bryan, OH: National Reye's Syndrome Foundation, 1983.

Nelson, K., and J. Ellenberg. Epidemiology of cerebral palsy. *Advances in Neurology* 19, no. 3 (1978): 421–435.

Patterson, R., G. Brown, M. Salassi-Scotter, and D. Middaugh. Head injury in the conscious child. *American Journal of Nursing* 92, no. 8 (1992): 22–27.

Peacock, W., L. Arens, and B. Berman. Cerebral palsy, spasticity and selective posterior rhizotomy. *Pediatric Neuroscience* 13, no. 2 (1987): 61–66.

Reisner, H., ed. *Children with Epilepsy: A Parent's Guide.* Kensington, MD: Woodbine House, 1988.

Santilli, N., and T. Sierzant. Advances in the treatment of epilepsy. *Journal of Neuroscience Nursing* 19, no. 3 (1987): 141–157.

Shiminski-Maher, T. Brain tumors in childhood: Implications for nursing practice. *Journal of Pediatric Health Care* 14, no. 3 (1990): 122–130.

Smith, K. A. Bowel and bladder management of the child with myelomeningocele in the school setting. *Journal of Pediatric Health Care* 4, no. 4 (1990): 175–180.

United Cerebral Palsy. *What Everyone Should Know about Cerebral Palsy.* Boston: Channing L. Bete, 1992.

Whaley, L., and D. Wong, eds. *Nursing Care of Infants and Children*, 4th ed. St. Louis, MO: Mosby-Year Book, 1991.

Wong, D. L. *Whaley & Wong's Essentials of Pediatric Nursing*, 4th ed. St. Louis, MO: Mosby-Year Book, 1993.

CHAPTER

43

Conditions of the Blood and Blood-Forming Organs

Objectives

After studying this chapter, the student should be able to:

- Describe the components of blood and their functions.
- Identify the cause, symptoms, treatment, and nursing care of iron deficiency anemia.
- Identify the cause, symptoms, treatment, and nursing care of sickle cell anemia.
- Define hemophilia and discuss its treatment and nursing care.
- Identify the cause, symptoms, treatment, and nursing care of leukemia.
- Define idiopathic thrombocytopenia purpura and discuss its treatment and nursing care.
- Identify the cause, symptoms, treatment, and nursing care of Hodgkin's disease.

Key Terms

plasma

erythrocytes

leukocytes

thrombocytes

granulocytes

leukopenia

agranulocytes

petechiae

ecchymosis

The blood and blood-forming organs (hematologic system) help to regulate, directly or indirectly, all other body functions. Thus, changes in this system may compromise the functioning of many other body systems and organs. Because signs of altered hematologic functioning are often subtle, a careful history and thorough physical assessment are essential for accurate diagnosis. Nurses can play an important role in ensuring prompt diagnosis and treatment of these conditions, and in providing necessary teaching and emotional support to children with these conditions and their parents.

Overview of the System

Blood is composed of two parts, a liquid and a solid portion. The liquid portion, called **plasma**, contains protein, clotting factors, and electrolytes. The solid portion is made up of red blood cells **(erythrocytes)**, white blood cells **(leukocytes)**, and platelets **(thrombocytes)**. The plasma transports the solid elements of the blood throughout the body. Plasma also aids in distributing heat throughout the body.

Red blood cells (RBCs) are responsible for transporting oxygen to the tissues of the body. They do this by synthesizing hemoglobin, which then binds with oxygen and carbon dioxide to carry gases to and from the tissues. Mature RBCs live approximately 120 days. Because they are destroyed at approximately the same rate at which they are produced, the number of circulating RBCs remains relatively constant. This number, however, varies according to the age of the child.

White blood cells (WBCs) are responsible for fighting infection. There are two major classifications of WBCs: granulocytes and agranulocytes. The **granulocytes** consist of neutrophils, which are responsible for fighting bacterial and fungal infections, and eosinophils. The exact function of eosinophils is unknown, although they are elevated in parasitic infections as well as in allergic conditions. **Leukopenia**, a reduction in WBCs, decreases the ability of the body to fight infection.

The **agranulocytes** consist of lymphocytes and monocytes. Lymphocytes, which are divided into B-cells and T-cells, are necessary for the maintenance of the immune system. Monocytes serve as "back-up" to the neutrophils when the body is faced with an infection.

Platelets are necessary for clotting. When the body is injured, platelets form a "plug" at the site of the injury. Platelets alone, however, cannot stop bleeding; blood coagulation factors also are necessary. (Deficiencies of factors VIII and IX are discussed later in the section on hemophilia.) Children with low platelet counts may develop **petechiae** (pinpoint hemorrhages) and **ecchymoses** (bruises).

INFANT AND TODDLER

IRON DEFICIENCY ANEMIA

Description. Iron deficiency anemia is a reduction in RBCs that occurs as a result of inadequate dietary intake of iron. It is the most common type of anemia in children and usually occurs between 6 months and 3 years of age. Young children are at higher risk for this disorder because of their proportionately higher need for iron compared with adults as well as their high consumption of milk (which decreases absorption of iron). The incidence of iron deficiency anemia is also higher in adolescent girls. This higher incidence is due to the combination of the increased need for iron once menstruation begins and the often poor dietary habits of teenagers.

Symptoms. Children with iron deficiency anemia may have few or no symptoms until their anemia is quite profound. On physical examination, the conjunctiva appear pale. Parents may also comment on the child's decreased activity level. Children with mild anemia usually compensate so effectively that few other symptoms are seen (Stockman 1992). If the anemia has been present for some time, cardiomegaly, splenomegaly, and tachycardia may be present. The definitive diagnosis is made using laboratory data. A complete blood count, serum iron, and iron-binding capacity will probably be ordered.

Treatment. The best treatment is prevention. All breast-fed infants should receive iron supplementation. Formula-fed infants should receive iron-rich formula. When the child is started on solids, iron-enriched cereals and other foods high in iron should be encouraged. Parents should be advised to decrease the amount of formula or breast milk ingested as the child moves into the second year. Children with iron deficiency anemia are given iron supplements such as ferrous sulfate. Occasionally intramuscular iron is prescribed. There is no indication, however, that response is any more complete with parenteral iron than with oral iron (Stockman 1992).

Nursing Care. The primary focus of nursing care is education. Teach parents about good dietary sources of iron (see Figure 43–1) and about side effects of the iron medication. In particular, parents should be told that iron can turn the child's stools green or black and that this color is not a sign that something is wrong with the child. Other side effects include nausea and diarrhea or constipation.

Teach parents to give iron between meals with a source of vitamin C (such as orange juice) to enhance absorption. Liquid iron should be given with a straw or dropper to avoid staining the teeth.

Treatment and nursing care for adolescents with iron deficiency anemia are similar to treatment and care for young children: iron supplementation or improved dietary intake of iron, or both.

IRON-RICH FOODS	
Apricots	Poultry
Eggs	Prunes
Fish	Raisins
Iron-fortified cereal	Red meat
Liver	Spinach
Oysters	

Figure 43–1

SICKLE CELL ANEMIA

Description. Sickle cell anemia is an autosomal recessive disease that occurs primarily in black children. Both parents must be carriers for the disease to be present in the child. There is a one in four chance with each pregnancy that the child will have the disease, a one in two chance of being a carrier, and a one in four chance of being neither a carrier nor an affected individual.

In sickle cell anemia, the red blood cell is elongated and sickle-shaped. This configuration decreases its oxygen-carrying capacity. From 80% to 95% of the hemoglobin may be sickled. This percentage increases when the cells are hypoxic (Stockman 1992). Once sickled, the cells are more fragile and more easily destroyed. The life span of the sickled cell averages only 10 to 20 days, as compared with a normal cell life span of 120 days. The altered shape also

SICKLE CELL CRISES

Crisis	Symptoms	Treatment
Vasoocclusive crisis Clumped RBCs occlude (or block) the vessels, resulting in tissue death. May be caused by infection, dehydration, acidosis, stress, or exertion.	Severe pain (due to hypoxia distal to the occlusion); fever; swelling; respiratory distress; priapism (prolonged painful erection of the penis)	Alleviate underlying cause of the occlusion. Relieve pain. Antibiotics. Blood transfusion may be necessary to correct anemia. Supplemental oxygen is given to severely hypoxic children.
Splenic sequestration crisis Occurs when large volumes of blood are sequestered (trapped) in the spleen. May result in death.	Splenomegaly (enlarged spleen); shock; decreased hemoglobin	Blood transfusion. Splenectomy (removal of the spleen), if indicated. Supportive care.
Aplastic crisis Occurs rarely, but may be life-threatening. Bone marrow shuts down despite increased destruction of RBCs.	Anemia; rapid heart rate; weakness	Blood transfusions are given until the marrow begins to function.

Figure 43–2

increases the chances of the cells' becoming caught in the capillaries, causing decreased circulation distal to the site of the occlusion.

Sickle cell anemia can be diagnosed in utero or during the newborn period. An infant will not, however, be symptomatic until 4 to 6 months of age (when fetal hemoglobin is replaced by adult hemoglobin).

Symptoms. Symptoms vary depending on the severity of the disease and the age at which the diagnosis is made. In infants, symptoms may include pallor, irritability, and jaundice. In older children splenomegaly, hepatomegaly, and cardiomegaly may occur. Children may also present with anemia or bacterial infections. Leg ulcers are a characteristic finding in adolescents.

Treatment. Treatment will vary according to the symptoms that are present. Sickle cell disease is a chronic disease, and children usually require hospitalization only for acute crises. Three different types of sickle cell crises may occur: splenic sequestration crisis, aplastic crisis, and vasoocclusive crisis, Figure 43–2. The most common is vasoocclusive crisis; however, aplastic crisis may be life-threatening. Infection, dehydration, and acidosis are the most common factors precipitating vasoocclusive crises.

Nursing Care. Nursing care focuses on the immediate problems of relieving the child's pain and replacing lost fluids. An intravenous line is started for rehydration and to administer pain medication. Replacement of fluids helps to decrease viscosity of blood, decreasing occlusion of the blood vessels by the sickled cells. Morphine is usually the drug of choice for pain management. Older children may be able to use patient-controlled analgesia pumps; whereas younger children may receive a continuous morphine drip or IV push morphine at regularly scheduled intervals. Guided imagery (the use of mental images and imagination to reduce pain) and heat may also be helpful in managing pain.

The nurse should monitor intravenous fluids, intake and output, and urine specific gravity, and should weigh the child daily. Remember that the baseline urine specific gravity in these children will be lower than normal because of their inability to concentrate urine.

After the child is stabilized, attention should be paid to educating the child and family about the disease as well as establishing a home health maintenance program. Long-term management includes nutritional counseling and education about the need for increased fluid intake. Maintaining adequate hydration is of prime importance in preventing further complications. Figure 43–3 presents several topics to be addressed in teaching parents of children with sickle cell anemia.

HEMOPHILIA

Hemophilia is inherited as an X-linked recessive trait. Women are carriers who transmit the disease to their sons. Refer to Chapter 3 for information on sex-linked traits and genetic inheritance.

The two most common types of hemophilia are hemophilia A (or classic hemophilia), which results from a deficiency of factor VIII, and hemophilia B, which is a deficiency of factor IX. Although there are differences in diagnostic criteria and replacement therapy depending on the type of hemophilia, the nursing care for the two types is virtually the same.

The diagnosis is usually made when the child has prolonged bleeding from a minor injury. Bleeding may occur when the infant is circumcised or when the child becomes more mobile and sustains one of the many injuries that occur in toddlerhood. Typically, these children bleed into the joints. The joint appears swollen, and the child keeps the joint flexed.

PARENT TEACHING: SICKLE CELL ANEMIA

- Encourage parents to offer children fruit juice, flavored ices, frozen slushes, gelatin desserts, broth, soup, and fruits with a high fluid content, such as oranges and grapefruit, to increase fluid intake.
- Caution parents to keep the child away from persons with known infections and from large crowds, and to keep the child's immunizations up to date.
- Children with asplenia (a nonfunctioning spleen) or who have had their spleen surgically removed should receive the pneumococcal vaccine. These children are often placed on prophylactic antibiotics. Emphasize the importance of taking antibiotics at the designated times to child and parents.
- Teach parents to monitor the child for signs of infection, such as temperature elevation, cough, or change in behavior. If any of these occur, parents should take the child to a health care provider promptly.
- Counsel parents that the child should avoid high altitudes and unpressurized aircraft; these can cause increased sickling. Activities that result in hypoxia — for example, strenuous exercise or surgery — should be monitored carefully. Caution is needed in the summer months, in particular, because high temperatures combined with increased activity heighten chances of dehydration.

Figure 43–3

The definitive diagnosis is made when the child's activated partial thromboplastin time is prolonged and specific clotting factors are found to be deficient.

Nursing care focuses on educating parents to care for the child at home. Parents must learn many skills, including home infusion of replacement factors and manipulation of the environment to prevent additional injuries to the child. Parents must also learn appropriate first-aid techniques, including the application of ice and elastic bandages to an affected joint, and they must know when to seek help from the health care team. As children become older, they can be taught to perform self-infusion, Figure 43–4.

Genetic counseling should be offered so parents can make informed decisions about future pregnancies.

PRESCHOOL AND SCHOOL-AGE CHILD

LEUKEMIA

Description. Leukemia is marked by the rapid growth of immature white blood cells, called blasts. Because the blast cells are unable to carry out the usual functions of the mature white blood cells, children with leukemia are prone to repeated infections. The immature white blood cells also crowd out the other elements of the bone marrow, causing the child to exhibit symptoms of anemia and thrombocytopenia (for example, fatigue and easy bruising). The peak incidence of leukemia is in children between 3 and 5 years of age.

Leukemia may occur as an acute or chronic disease. Chronic leukemia is rare in children,

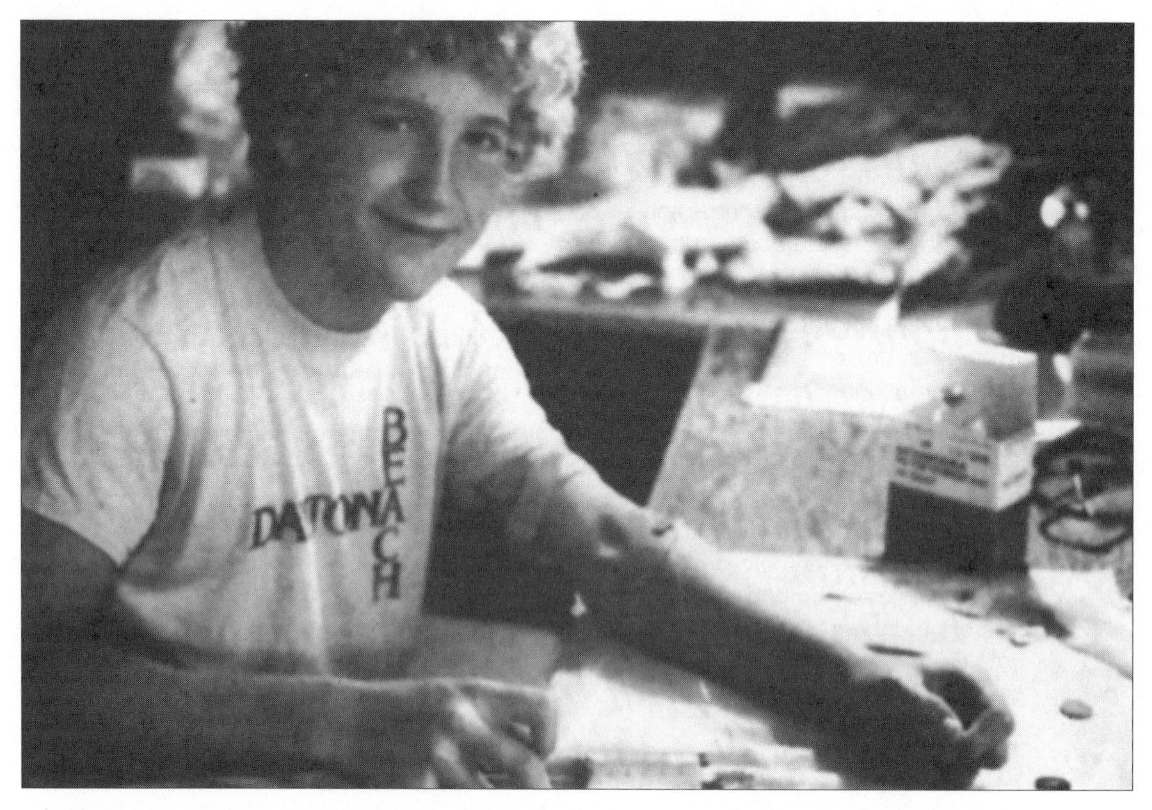

Figure 43–4 *Self-infusion helps to promote positive self-esteem. (From R. L. Foster, M. M. Hunsberger, and J. J. Anderson.* Family-Centered Nursing Care of Children. *Philadelphia: W. B. Saunders, 1989.)*

accounting for only 1% to 5% of all leukemias. Acute leukemia has a more rapid onset and is, without treatment, fatal. There are two main types of acute leukemia: acute lymphocytic leukemia (ALL) and acute nonlymphocytic leukemia (ANLL). ALL is the most common type, but ANLL is more deadly.

The cause of leukemia is unknown. Children with chromosomal defects or immunologic deficiencies, however, are at increased risk for ALL.

Symptoms. Children with leukemia often present with very subtle symptoms. Parents may report repeated infections or bruising, but because these signs also occur in well children, they may be ignored. When leukemia is suspected, a complete blood count is ordered. The WBC count may be low or elevated. The child is anemic and thrombocytopenic, and may have enlarged lymph nodes, spleen, and liver. Bone marrow aspiration and lumbar puncture confirm the diagnosis.

Treatment. Treatment includes chemotherapy and, occasionally, radiation. Bone marrow transplantation may also be performed. The long-term prognosis for children with ALL has improved dramatically with the advent of aggressive chemotherapy. Chemotherapy is administered to induce remission. There are three phases of chemotherapy: induction-remission, sanctuary therapy (or central nervous system prophylaxis), and maintenance.

Induction-Remission

The actual drugs used will vary according to the type of leukemia and chemotherapy protocol (treatment plan), but almost all protocols include prednisone. Parents should be educated about the possible side effects of chemotherapy, including the cushingoid features (moon face) and alopecia, Figure 43–5, increased appetite, and growth retardation.

Sanctuary Therapy (CNS Prophylaxis)

The goal of sanctuary therapy is to prevent leukemic cells from seeking sanctuary in the central nervous system (CNS). At one time both intrathecal (into the spinal canal) methotrexate and CNS irradiation were used to prevent this occurrence. Because of the link between learning disabilities and CNS irradiation, however, most facilities now give only intrathecal drugs except for high-risk patients (Leventhol 1992).

Maintenance

During the maintenance phase, the child continues to receive chemotherapy as well as periodic bone marrow examinations to monitor for recurrence of the disease.

Nursing Care. Nursing care varies depending on the specific drugs used and the family's response to the disease. All families need emotional support as they learn more about the disease and its treatment. Families need to be made aware of other problems that could occur in response to chemotherapy and its side effects, which may include increased bleeding tendencies, infection, and anemia. Changes in body image resulting from alopecia and cushingoid features present problems, particularly for older children. Figure 43–6 summarizes nursing care for the child with leukemia.

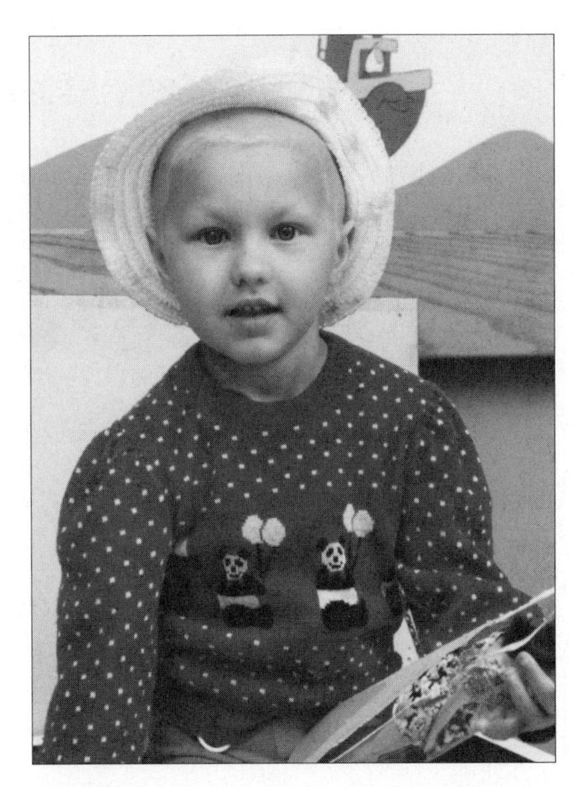

Figure 43–5 *This child has alopecia resulting from chemotherapy.*

IDIOPATHIC THROMBOCYTOPENIA PURPURA

Idiopathic thrombocytopenia purpura is a commonly occurring blood disorder characterized by a decrease in thrombocytes. In approximately 30% of cases, the onset can be traced to medications or a viral infection. In most cases, however, the cause is unknown.

Many cases resolve spontaneously, but some are treated with prednisone or intravenous gamma globulin. Splenectomy is performed in chronic cases that do not respond to therapy.

Nursing care focuses on protecting the child from injury and on education. Children should be cautioned to avoid contact sports, to brush their teeth with a soft-bristled toothbrush, and to avoid drugs such as aspirin, which can damage platelets.

NURSING CARE PLAN: Leukemia

PATIENT PROBLEM	GOAL(S)
Anxiety (child) caused by invasive diagnostic procedure (bone marrow aspiration)	Before bone marrow procedure, the child will understand the need for diagnostic tests.
Anxiety (parents) caused by potentially life-threatening condition of child	The parents will be able to explain treatment for leukemia and hoped-for response.
Immunosuppression due to chemotherapy and disease process	The child will remain infection-free. The parents will be able to identify signs of infection.

Figure 43–6

NURSING INTERVENTION	RATIONALE
Before each procedure, explain exactly what is happening and what the child's role will be.	Knowledge decreases anxiety, which in turn decreases pain.
Discuss use of Lidocaine patch. Let child put Lidocaine cream on arm and feel the effect. Teach guided imagery techniques and breathing exercises.	Lidocaine decreases pain perception. Control over what is happening increases child's ability to manage pain.
Explain cause and common symptoms of leukemia. Give parents written information on leukemia and its treatment. Identify usual side effects of treatment.	Knowledge decreases anxiety. Written information gives parents something to refer to.
Introduce parents to parents of other children with leukemia and to resources such as chaplain and social worker.	Provides support and comfort.
Instruct child and parents on the need to wash hands frequently and the need to limit visitors, particularly those with infections.	Handwashing and limitation of visitors decrease child's contact with organisms, which decreases chance of developing an infection.
Teach parents to monitor child for signs of infection, such as cough, fever, or earache.	Early identification of infection allows for prompt treatment.

continues

PATIENT PROBLEM	GOAL(S)
Side effects of chemotherapy (e.g., constipation and oral ulcers)	The child will maintain a normal stool pattern. The child's mouth will be kept clean, and child will experience minimal oral ulcers.
Change in body image caused by hair loss and cushingoid appearance	The child will cope with changed appearance.
Weight loss caused by nausea and vomiting associated with chemotherapy	The child will: maintain current weight during hospitalization; gain 1 lb per month when home; eat a nutritious diet high in protein and complex carbohydrates.
Potential for hemorrhage caused by decreased platelets as a result of chemotherapy	The child will not sustain injury or hemorrhage.

Figure 43–6 *continued*

NURSING INTERVENTION	RATIONALE
Keep a record of daily stool pattern. Encourage 8 glasses of preferred beverage daily. Encourage fruits and vegetables.	Increasing fluid and fiber intake will increase bowel motility.
Instruct child to brush teeth with soft-bristled toothbrush after eating, before bed, and on awakening.	A clean mouth decreases the chance of oral ulcers developing.
Teach parents to inspect child's mouth daily for oral ulcers.	Early identification allows for prompt treatment.
Reassure child that hair loss is temporary. Suggest use of hats or scarves if child wants to cover head. If child wants to wear a wig, advise parents to purchase it before hair loss occurs.	Knowing that hair loss is temporary decreases child's concern. Hats and scarves are colorful and cheaper than wigs. If a wig is worn, child should start wearing it before loosing all hair so that the contrast is not so apparent.
Premedicate child with antiemetic before chemotherapy.	Prevention is the best treatment for nausea and vomiting related to therapy.
Keep room odor-free.	Noxious stimuli can cause nausea.
Offer preferred foods. Encourage parents to bring favorite foods from home.	Child is more apt to eat favorite foods than hospital food.
Provide parents with handouts identifying foods high in protein and complex carbohydrates. Encourage high-calorie foods such as milk shakes, cheese cake, ice cream, and eggnog.	Gives parents information they can refer to. Milk-based foods are packed with calories and protein.
Discourage rough play or contact sports.	Unintentional injury causes bleeding.
Teach first aid for bleeding (ice, pressure, elevation).	Minor bleeding may be managed at home.
Administer platelets per physician's order.	When platelets fall to predetermined level, replacement must be given.

ADOLESCENT

HODGKIN'S DISEASE

Description. Hodgkin's disease, or cancer of the lymphatic system, occurs most often in late adolescence or young adulthood and is twice as common in boys as in girls.

Symptoms. Symptoms initially include painless lymphadenopathy, followed by shortness of breath, cough, and splenomegaly. The diagnosis is made by lymph node biopsy. Exploratory laparotomy is often performed to assess the extent of the disease.

Treatment. Once the diagnosis has been made and the extent of disease (staging) determined, the child is treated with either short-term radiation or, for more advanced disease, with a combination of chemotherapy (such as MOPP — mustargen, Oncovin, procarbazine, and prednisone) and radiation. Children with less-advanced disease (stage I or II) have an excellent prognosis.

Nursing Care. Nursing care for the child with Hodgkin's disease is similar to that for the child with leukemia. Because children with Hodgkin's disease are older, they may have more difficulty with problems of body image as well as difficulty facing their own death. The adolescent who is diagnosed with advanced (stage III or IV) disease may benefit from counseling resources. Oncology nurses, clinical nurse specialists, social workers, members of the clergy, or the hospital chaplain may provide support to the child and family. It is important that the adolescent and family be kept informed of the child's progress and prognosis at all times.

REVIEW QUESTIONS

A. Multiple choice. Select the best answer.

1. Johnny is a 2-year-old diagnosed with iron deficiency anemia. His mother states that he loves milk, and since "milk is nature's most nearly perfect food" she sometimes allows him to drink milk in place of meals. What will you tell Johnny's mother?
   a. "Milk is an excellent food for children Johnny's age. I cannot understand why Johnny is anemic."
   b. "Milk is an excellent source of calcium, but not iron. Let's review some iron-rich foods."
   c. "Whatever made you think that milk could be used in place of meals? Johnny needs to eat from the basic food groups every day."
   d. "The amount of milk Johnny drinks each day should be limited to no more than 12 ounces."

2. Shamiqua is admitted to the hospital in sickle cell crisis. She is 4 years old and was diagnosed with sickle cell anemia at age 2. This is Shamiqua's third hospitalization in 6 months. Her mother asks what she can do to decrease the chance that Shamiqua will be hospitalized again in the near future. What will you tell her?
   a. "There really isn't much you can do about sickle cell crisis. It just happens."
   b. "You must feel bad about Shamiqua's hospitalizations. Do you attend a support group?"
   c. "The two most common reasons for hospitalization are dehydration and infection. If you can see to it that Shamiqua avoids crowds and drinks plenty of fluids you may see a decrease in her hospitalizations."
   d. "Is Shamiqua up-to-date on all of her immunizations? If you can prevent some of these infections, she should be able to stay out of the hospital."

3. The child with idiopathic thrombocytopenic purpura usually does not receive intramuscular injections or venipunctures unless absolutely necessary. Why?
   a. The child's blood does not clot properly. Intrusive procedures are avoided because of the danger that blood will ooze from the puncture site and the increased risk of bruising.
   b. The child already has bruising and it is difficult to identify anatomical landmarks, so it is difficult to find an appropriate site.
   c. The child has already had so many injections that an attempt is made to avoid any more.
   d. The child is at risk for bleeding. Therefore, injections are avoided to decrease the danger of a fatal hemorrhage.

4. Jonathan is a 10-year-old with hemophilia A. His mother states, "I don't understand how this happened. Neither his father nor I have hemophilia." What will you tell them about the disease?
   a. "Hemophilia occurs randomly, and there is no way to predict who will have it."
   b. "Hemophilia is usually transmitted genetically from father to son."
   c. "This must be confusing for you. I'll tell the doctor that you have some questions."
   d. "The most common method of transmission is from a carrier mother to her son."

5. The child with an infection normally has an increase in
   a. RBCs
   b. WBCs
   c. platelets
   d. hemoglobin

6. The white blood cells that are responsible for fighting infection are the
   a. neutrophils
   b. eosinophils
   c. lymphocytes
   d. monocytes
7. Which of the following orders should you question when your patient has a diagnosis of idiopathic thrombocytopenia purpura?
   a. oral acetaminophen
   b. platelet count
   c. oral aspirin
   d. oral prednisone

B. True or false. Write *T* for a true statement and *F* for a false statement.

1. ___ Iron deficiency anemia is common in preschoolers.
2. ___ Hemophilia is equally common in boys and girls.
3. ___ A good source of iron is dried apricots.
4. ___ Children with acute lymphocytic leukemia have an invariably poor prognosis.
5. ___ Hodgkin's disease is cancer of the lymphatic system.

SUGGESTED ACTIVITIES

- Arrange to observe a pediatric hematology clinic. Note how the children cope with painful procedures.
- Plan to spend a day with a pediatric oncology clinical nurse specialist or clinician. Make careful note of his or her role on the pediatric oncology team.
- Role play the necessary explanation and teaching to a parent of a child with a disorder of the blood or blood-forming organs.

BIBLIOGRAPHY

Diamond, C. A., and K. K. Matthay. Childhood acute lymphoblastic leukemia. *Pediatric Annals* 17 (1988): 156.

Dudek, S. *Nutrition Handbook for Nursing Practice.* Philadelphia: J. B. Lippincott, 1993.

Fochtman, D., G. V. Foley, and K. Mooney, eds. *Nursing Care of the Child with Cancer*. Boston: Little, Brown, 1993.

Foster, R. L., M. M. Hunsberger, and J. J. Anderson. *Family-Centered Nursing Care of Children.* Philadelphia: W. B. Saunders, 1989.

James, S. R., and S. R. Mott. *Child Health Nursing*. San Francisco: Addison-Wesley, 1988.

Leventhol, B. Neoplasms and neoplasm-like structures. In R. E. Behrman and V. C. Vaughan, eds. *Nelson's Textbook of Pediatrics*, 14th ed. Philadelphia: W. B. Saunders, 1992.

Morrison, R. A., and D. A. Vedro. Pain management in the child with sickle cell disease. *Pediatric Nursing* 15, no. 5 (1989): 595–599, 613.

Shapiro, B. S. The management of pain in sickle cell disease. *Pediatric Clinics of North America* 36, no. 4 (1989): 1029–1043.

Stockman, J. Diseases of the blood. In R. E. Behrman and V. C. Vaughan, eds. *Nelson's Textbook of Pediatrics*, 14th ed. Philadelphia: W. B. Saunders, 1992.

CHAPTER 44

Emotional and Behavioral Conditions

Objectives

After studying this chapter, the student should be able to:

- Describe behaviors and responses of an infant or toddler with failure to thrive.
- Formulate a basic plan of care for the infant with failure to thrive that will nurture the infant and promote attachment.
- Briefly describe attention deficit hyperactivity disorder and discuss its symptoms, treatment, and nursing care.
- Discuss the cause, symptoms, and treatment of school phobia.
- Name three eating conditions that affect school-age children and adolescents and describe their causes, symptoms, and treatment.
- Describe symptoms of depression and suicidal behavior in adolescents and discuss treatment and nursing care for these patients.
- Identify causes and symptoms of substance abuse and describe treatment and nursing care for the substance-abusing adolescent.

Key Terms

FAILURE TO THRIVE
ATTACHMENT
BONDING
PHOBIA
SEPARATION ANXIETY
BINGING
PURGING
DYSPHORIA
ANHEDONIA
PSYCHOACTIVE

As the health care provider who first establishes rapport with a child and family in the health care system, the nurse needs to be able to use basic communication skills as a tool to gather assessment data. The nurse must also be knowledgeable about general norms of behavior, stages of growth and development, and signs and symptoms of disease. Finally the nurse needs to know when and where to refer a patient for further assessment and treatment.

It is not always clear whether an individual's responses or symptoms have a physiological (organic) cause or are related to emotional and psychological factors. It is not unusual for symptoms of the infant, child, and adolescent to present as a physical problem, at least initially.

The conditions discussed in this chapter are considered to be primarily behavioral and emotional problems. For some conditions, however, there is a strong physiological component. The nurse must be constantly aware of this component and address physiological needs while responding to and being supportive of emotional and psychological needs and behavioral responses.

Overview of Emotional and Behavioral Conditions

For a newborn infant to become an integrated and emotionally healthy person, the infant must be perceived as an individual, with separate needs who, through his or her behavior, tells the parents what those needs are. Parents must, in turn, observe and interpret the infant's cues to find out what the infant is "telling" them through these sounds and behaviors.

Before an infant is born, parents may plan for the infant's characteristics — gender, personality, talent — sometimes going so far as planning a role the infant will play in life. This role may be one that parents believe will correct for disappointments in their own lives. Each child, of course, has his or her own way of responding to life. Some children may accept and respond more or less comfortably to the role given by their parents; others may be unsuited for the chosen role. These children may be at risk for behavioral or emotional problems.

When parents are unable to relate to the infant as a separate person, they may respond in ways that interfere with the infant's emotional well-being. Such a response may create difficulties as the child matures, ranging from emotional "hang-ups" to pervasive childhood behavioral conditions.

Figure 44–1 presents general principles that may assist the nurse in relating to and gathering information about a child with an emotional or behavioral condition.

General Assessment Principles

- Be knowledgeable about the norms for each stage of growth and development.
- Remember that each child and each situation is unique.
- Show willingness and patience to listen to the child's story. Often stories are "told" through emotions and behavior. Many important messages are transmitted by the way we sit, stand, walk, and respond, as well as by how we say things (tone, affect) and what we say (words). Because the child's vocabulary is not well developed, it is essential to pay attention to other cues.
- Be willing to see the problem through the child's eyes.
- Demonstrate a belief that the child has the ability to solve his or her own problem.
- Show willingness and patience to help parents make the changes needed to lessen the difficulty the child is experiencing. (Helping the parents to change may be particularly difficult if they are embarrassed, angry, protective, or refuse to or cannot separate themselves from the child and the child's needs.)
- Be aware of cultural differences that can cause misinterpretations of cues (e.g., stoicism, hysteria).

Figure 44–1 *General principles in assessment of children with emotional and behavioral conditions*

INFANT AND TODDLER

FAILURE TO THRIVE

Description. **Failure to thrive** (FTT) is a condition of infants and children under 2 years of age characterized by a weight for age that is below the third percentile. (Because National Center for Health Statistic growth charts do not give values below the fifth percentile, some authorities use weight below the fifth percentile as the criterion for FTT.) Failure to thrive may have an organic or nonorganic basis. This discussion focuses on children with nonorganic FTT. In these cases, the infant, parents, and environment interact in a way that results in emotional deprivation and, often, an accompanying lack of food. Sometimes an infant is offered sufficient food, but the emotional interaction and environment are not conducive to well-being. Sometimes the infant is too lethargic to eat. At other times, parents do not feed the infant properly because they lack knowledge about nutritional needs or feeding techniques, are unconcerned, or are neglectful.

The period immediately following birth has been described as the maternal sensitive period (Olds et al. 1992, Wong 1993). Certain predictable behaviors occur when mothers (as well as fathers) are with their infants soon after birth. These include: touching the infant, examining the infant with the fingers, observing, and having direct eye contact while holding the infant in front of them, Figure 44–2. The infant responds to these behaviors, creating a reciprocal interaction. This interaction results in **attachment** (the emotional ties from infant to parent) and **bonding** (the ties from parent to infant).

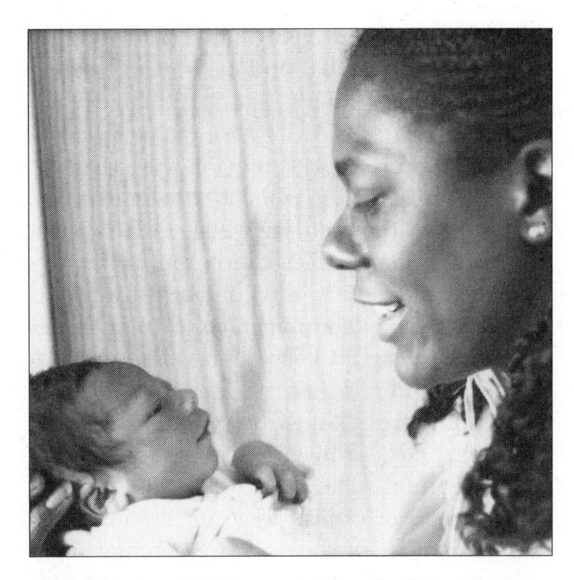

Figure 44–2 *Attachment and bonding behaviors occur in the period immediately after birth. (Courtesy Carol Toussie Weingarten)*

Neglect of the infant and a lack of attachment and bonding can result in poor parent-child relationships in the future. When care is irregular, inconsistent, or mostly absent, attachment and bonding do not occur. The infant does not learn to trust or may perceive the world as confusing and unstable. As the child matures, this perception may give rise to difficulties in trusting himself or herself and problems with self-esteem. These children may also demonstrate social and behavioral delays and cognitive difficulties.

Symptoms. Infants with FTT may be listless, apathetic, and passive, or hyperalert to the environment. They may avoid (or have minimal) eye contact and demonstrate a lack of stranger anxiety (do not cry when they see a stranger). Sucking responses, cooing, and crying may be minimal or absent. Older infants may demonstrate reluctance to reach, crawl, or pull themselves to standing. A lack of interest in toys or play is common. Toddlers or preschool children may demonstrate delayed speech.

Treatment. The goals of treatment are to ensure adequate nutrition, provide support to parents, encourage parental involvement in care of the child, and teach the parents about developmental patterns and nutritional needs of infants and children. Continued support by health care providers and family counseling may be necessary.

Nursing Care. Assess the infant's behavior for cues to determine whether attachment and bonding have occurred, Figure 44–3. Assessment of the infant or toddler can be performed by observing the mother and child at feeding and visiting times to determine interaction patterns. Assessment should include several observations to avoid basing conclusions on random and isolated behavior. Observe the infant for approach and responses to the parent and others. Abnormal attachment behaviors include listlessness, lack of interest in the environment and parent, lack of cooing and eye contact, and lack of crying. The assessment must also include data on the weight and height of the infant and a comparison with norms and the infant's own growth rate.

Observe the parent(s) for affect (feeling state), ability to give care, concerns (voiced or not), and ways of relating and responding to the infant. Negative comments — including disappointments about the infant, not looking at the infant, not wanting to hold the infant, not asking questions about the infant, and general lack of interest and withdrawal — are all possible signs of impaired bonding to the infant.

Many factors have an effect on the bonding process. Cultural and ethnic differences may influence the ways in which mothers relate to their infants. Determine whether the behavior of the mother is related to a lack of knowledge about care of the infant, fear of hurting the infant, or anxiety over being a parent. Other barriers to the bonding process are physical illness of either the mother or infant, drug abuse (of parents or withdrawal in the infant), AIDS, premature birth, and the parent's feelings of guilt and failure (Olds et al. 1992, Pillitteri 1992, Wong 1993).

Nursing care includes giving parents information about the infant, telling them what is normal, helping them to interpret the infant's cues, listening to expressions of concern and feelings, and teaching parents how to care for the infant.

The infant is placed on a diet specific for his or her needs. Parents are incorporated into the plan of care and encouraged and assisted as necessary to care for their infant. Some parents may need continuing support or counseling to become effective parents. Figure 44–4 summarizes nursing care for an infant with failure to thrive.

ATTACHMENT BEHAVIORS

Newborns	Infants (1–12 months)	Toddlers (2–3 years)
• Visually follow the caregiver • Smile • Reach • Grasp	• Imitate (imprint) • Need visual or tactile contact with the parent while exploring an unfamiliar environment • Fear of strangers (cry when looking at strangers)	• Curious • Cooperative • Responses indicate separation anxiety (cry when parent leaves) • Adapt to changes, even when the parent is out of sight

Figure 44–3

SCHOOL-AGE CHILD

ATTENTION DEFICIT HYPERACTIVITY DISORDER

Description. Attention deficit hyperactivity disorder (ADHD) is characterized by excessive and constant motor activity with little or no ability to concentrate. The condition occurs in boys more often than girls and affects approximately 3% of the school-age population (Townsend 1993). The cause is unknown but may be linked to biochemical or genetic factors.

Symptoms. Although symptoms usually appear before the child is 7 years of age (Rudolph et al. 1991), hyperactivity is often first observed by the child's teacher and reported to the school nurse, counselor, or parent because of difficulties in the classroom. The following behaviors may be seen:

- exaggerated muscle activity
- unfocused or aimless motion
- interruption of and intrusion on others
- impulsive and unpredictable behavior
- fidgeting
- squirming
- difficulty finishing a task or remaining seated when asked to do so

Symptoms can result in impaired emotional and psychological development, as parents often become frustrated with the child, which in turn can affect the child's self-esteem and ability to cope.

Cognitively, children with ADHD have difficulty concentrating, do not seem to listen when spoken to, blurt out information, and often have difficulty with space perception (right-left and front-back), which may be revealed by difficulty in turning faucets on or off, turning doorknobs to open or close, or by reaching beyond an object and tipping the object over. Written work may be messy, with poorly formed and reversed letters (b/d, g/p/q). These children may have difficulty putting words in sequence and using conjunctions and prepositions. They have difficulty learning to read and learning rules of math and language because they cannot remember the information (for example, a child will be unable to remember two numbers in order to add them to a third number and find the total). Environmental stimuli seem to compound these difficulties. Children with ADHD seem to be less able than "normal" children to filter out irrelevant stimuli to concentrate on a task.

Treatment. Diagnosis includes a medical workup (neurological examination, electroencephalogram) to rule out a physical problem, psychological testing, and testing for learning disabilities. A safe, nonstimulating, structured though relaxed, and consistent environment is essential.

Management is directed toward enhancing self-esteem and self-control and decreasing anxiety. Care of the child with ADHD requires patience, warmth, and discipline mixed with love. Parents need support both in managing their feelings (often anger and frustration, sometimes a sense of failure) and in maintaining consistency.

Nursing Care. In order to best support and meet the child's needs, all the people who have responsibility for the child's development should be involved in the treatment plan. Frequent meetings allow for verbalization of feelings and concerns, communication of changes, and maintenance of consistency. Limits for the child will need to be set and adhered to. Instructions should be given clearly and concisely. Choices need to be limited and distractions minimized. Reminders, preparation for changes in routines, and planned periods of exercise enhance the child's well-being, as do praise, promotion of self-control, and immediate discipline when warranted (e.g., when the child deliberately does something wrong).

NURSING CARE PLAN: Failure to Thrive

PATIENT PROBLEM	GOAL(S)
Body weight below third percentile for age, height, and gender	Infant receives adequate oral intake and experiences weight gain of 1 to 2 oz. daily.
Altered growth and development (listless, absence of cooing, diminished sucking response)	Infant's responses are within normal range for chronological age.

Figure 44–4

NURSING INTERVENTION	RATIONALE
Select one caregiver to care for child.	Encourages development of trust and attachment.
Model positive parenting techniques: cuddle, talk with, and have eye contact with infant during feeding.	These techniques stimulate interaction and relating, promote bonding, and stimulate development.
Establish consistent caregiving routine.	Consistency provides structure, lessens anxiety, and promotes trust (infant knows what to expect).
Avoid interruptions and minimize environmental stimulation during care and feeding.	Minimizes unwanted stimuli that might distract from the feeding process.
Give prescribed formula. Record schedule, intake, daily weight, and responses to staff, parent, and environment.	This information provides a baseline for evaluating progress and determining whether to continue or change approach and management of care.
Have the same caregiver provide care to the infant.	Frequent contacts with the same caregiver help establish a relationship of trust and promote attachment.
Encourage play times and use of developmentally appropriate stimuli.	Play and stimulation encourage development and growth.
Handle the infant gently, lovingly, with confidence, and with consistency: cuddle, soothe, coo, talk with, and make eye contact with infant.	These types of contacts will promote a sense of safety, comfort, and belonging in the infant.

continues

PATIENT PROBLEM	GOAL(S)
Inappropriate parenting practices	Parents are able to state feelings and concerns related to care of the infant.
	Parents request information about proper care of the infant.
	Parents participate in care of the infant.

Figure 44–4 *continued*

NURSING INTERVENTION	RATIONALE
Set aside time during each visit to listen to parents' concerns.	A consistent and designated time period allows parents to express feelings and concerns and promotes interaction and formation of a trusting relationship with the caregiver.
Encourage parents to discuss concerns, frustrations, and fears; acknowledge parental difficulties and frustrations.	Expressing feelings (especially negative) and receiving acknowledgment of feelings lessens anxiety and resentment and promotes the expression of positive feelings.
Nurture and give emotional support to parents.	Providing emotional support will enhance parents' self-esteem and confidence.
Identify needs and determine readiness to receive information.	Before any health teaching takes place, it is necessary to identify what information is needed and determine learner readiness.
Encourage questions by parents about infant.	Parents may be reluctant to admit they don't know how to care for the infant; encouraging parents' questions helps to provide this information.
Provide information and guidance about normal infant development and growth; teach parenting skills (for example, holding, touching, talking, physical care techniques, feeding, etc.).	Be clear with information given. Provide information at a level geared to parents' level of understanding; do not overload parents with too much information at one time (more sessions are better than too much information at one time). Provide diagrams and written information that parents can refer to at a later time. Follow up the next day to assess understanding and retention by having parents repeat information.
Model appropriate parenting behaviors; encourage parental caregiving; assist parents to recognize infant cues and interpret these cues when necessary.	Giving encouragement, feedback, positive comments, and helpful hints promotes confidence in parents and reinforces their efforts.

continues

PATIENT PROBLEM	GOAL(S)
Inappropriate parenting practices *(continued)*	Parents participate in care of the infant.
	Identify and contact appropriate referral resources for follow-up support, as appropriate.

Figure 44–4 *continued*

SCHOOL PHOBIA

School phobia is a condition in which a child has a traumatic aversion to school, characterized by the development of physical symptoms before or at school in an attempt to be allowed to stay home or be sent home. (The word **phobia**, from the Greek word for fear, refers to an excessive or unfounded fear of someone or something.) It is thought that about 3% of children have school phobia, and the condition is three to nine times more common in boys than in girls (Pillitteri 1992).

School phobia may be a form of **separation anxiety** in which the child has fear of separation from or has not successfully dealt with separation from the parent (usually the mother). Factors associated with school phobia include difficulty in making the adjustment to school and doing school tasks; difficulty with the teacher; feelings of ridicule, humiliation, or embarrassment; fear of having to speak in front of others; fear of tests; feelings of losing the parent's attention to younger siblings; and parental fears of "losing" the child or overprotectiveness, which may be imparted to the child.

Symptoms may include irritability, nausea, abdominal pain, headache, leg pain, or dizziness. In class, the child may be tense, tremulous, and perspire. Symptoms are absent on weekends and holidays and often decrease if the parent is present in the class. A behavioral description by teacher and parent is important because children with school phobias may be anxious and timid away from home and controlling and obstinate in the home. Tests are performed to rule out physical causes for the child's symptoms.

Treatment includes listening to the child's story and being consistent with responses. It may be that this behavior is the child's way of breaking away from conformity or a rigid mold or of dealing with family problems by displacing

NURSING INTERVENTION	RATIONALE
Assess parental and infant responses and behaviors to determine whether attachment and bonding are occurring.	Continual assessment by the nurse assists in evaluating progress and determining whether any changes in the management plan are needed.
Assess (discuss) home environment (situation, stressors) and support system. Identify resources available to parents for support after discharge.	Knowledge about the home environment and resources for support when infant is discharged and parents are on their own will often help parents continue to give the care learned in the hospital or other structured setting.

them to the school setting. Treatment approaches might include a modified systematic desensitization plan in which a therapist works with the child in the classroom or counseling with the child and parents or family.

EATING DISORDERS

Eating disorders are conditions in which a person uses food in a dysfunctional way, most often as a source of emotional nurturance. These disorders are most likely to occur during crisis periods when the person feels overwhelmed or during periods of significant change. Eating disorders may be linked to an underlying depression. They may also represent a person's attempt to gain some control over changing and extraordinary events by engaging in behaviors that he or she, and no one else, can control (McCoy 1985).

Early diagnosis and treatment of these disorders is important to minimize or prevent harmful effects on the body and address self-esteem and body-image issues.

Obesity. Obesity is a condition in which a person's weight is 20% to 30% or more above his or her "ideal" weight for sex, height, and age (Haber et al. 1992, Townsend 1993). Overweight, in contrast, is described as a condition in which the person is 10% over the ideal weight. Because the height and weight of children vary, obesity and overweight are often difficult to define. In addition, a person can be overweight and at the same time malnourished because the foods consumed lack nutritional value.

Various factors have been proposed as causes of obesity, including genetic predisposition, excessive numbers of fat cells, and body build. Obesity often begins in infancy when a parent overfeeds the infant. Cultural influences, misconceptions such as "a fat baby is a healthy baby," attempts to quiet an infant, and lack of knowledge are some of the reasons given for overfeeding at this age. Because needs and habits developed in infancy continue for a lifetime, prevention during this period is important.

Boys tend to be overweight during the school-age years; girls after puberty. (Girls also tend to try to control their weight through fad diets and dysfunctional eating patterns; see later discussion of anorexia nervosa and bulimia nervosa.) Physiological complications of obesity in school-age children and adolescents include hypertension and elevated total cholesterol, along with poor self-esteem and body-image disturbances. Obese children are often excluded from activities or even taunted about their appearance and may become withdrawn and socially isolated as a consequence.

Treatment focuses on dietary planning to meet the nutritional needs of the growing child while ensuring necessary caloric restrictions. School-age children should be encouraged to achieve short-term dietary goals and to engage in preferred physical exercises and activities. The child's dietary program should be supervised by a physician and dietician who understand the metabolic and psychological impact of weight loss (Rudolph et al. 1991). Parents play an important role in the treatment success of the child. Having obese parents makes it more difficult for the child to succeed. Consistency of approach, support, and acknowledgment of the child's successes in meeting goals are important aspects of the treatment plan.

ADOLESCENT

EATING DISORDERS

Anorexia Nervosa. Anorexia nervosa is a condition of self-starvation based on an unrealistic fear of being fat. The disorder occurs predominantly in adolescent and young adult females. Total body weight is 20% to 40% below normal, Figure 44–5 (Pillitteri 1992, Varcarolis 1990). Death may occur in prolonged, severe cases from self-starvation itself or as a result of complications such as electrolyte imbalances, cardiovascular problems and arrhythmias, and renal impairment.

The typical adolescent with anorexia is described as a compliant, "model" child and a high achiever who receives attention for these behaviors. The parents are demanding (usually the father, regarding expectations for achievement) and controlling (usually the mother). The adolescent attempts to control the environment, body, and other people, but does not truly succeed at having control over his or her own self.

The adolescent is obsessed with food, although often giving the appearance of not being interested in eating. Symptoms usually include amenorrhea, lanugo, dry skin, and bruising. Body image is distorted, so that the excessively thin adolescent looking in the mirror sees a reflection that is fat. Characteristically, the adolescent refuses to admit that anything is wrong and does not think treatment is necessary.

Treatment requires a multidimensional, coordinated, and consistent approach. An approach that facilitates trust is an essential part of treatment. Establishing trust may not be easy because of the often manipulative behavior of the anorexic patient. Staff may have difficulty coping with mixed feelings that are often generated by working with these patients.

Depending on the severity of the illness, the adolescent may be hospitalized to manage physiological aspects of the disorder. The treatment plan may include short-term separation from the family, a prescribed dietary regimen, psychotherapy that includes individual and family counseling, weighing several times weekly (observing for extra clothing or hiding of objects that might increase the weight), observance of mealtimes, limitation of exercise and activity, and providing opportunities for the adolescent to verbalize loss, fears, and anxiety. Long-term management is required to

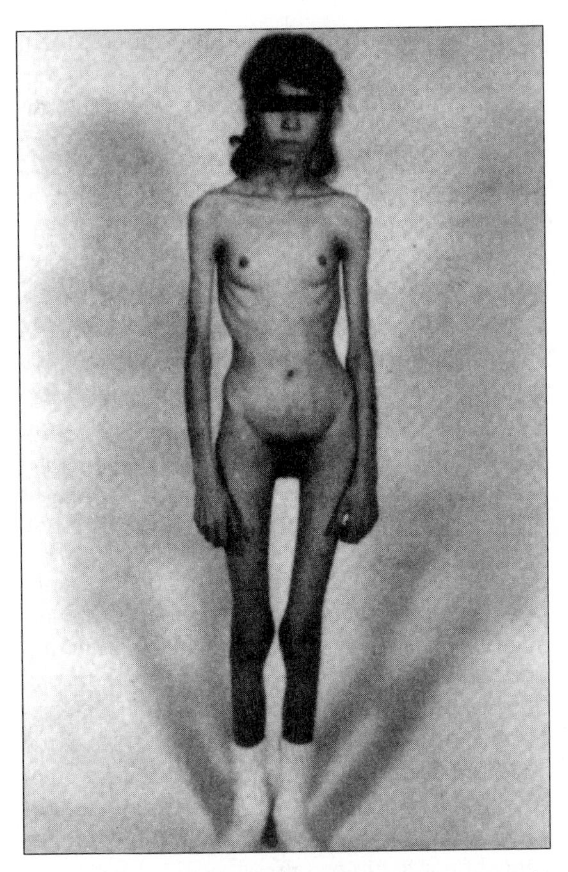

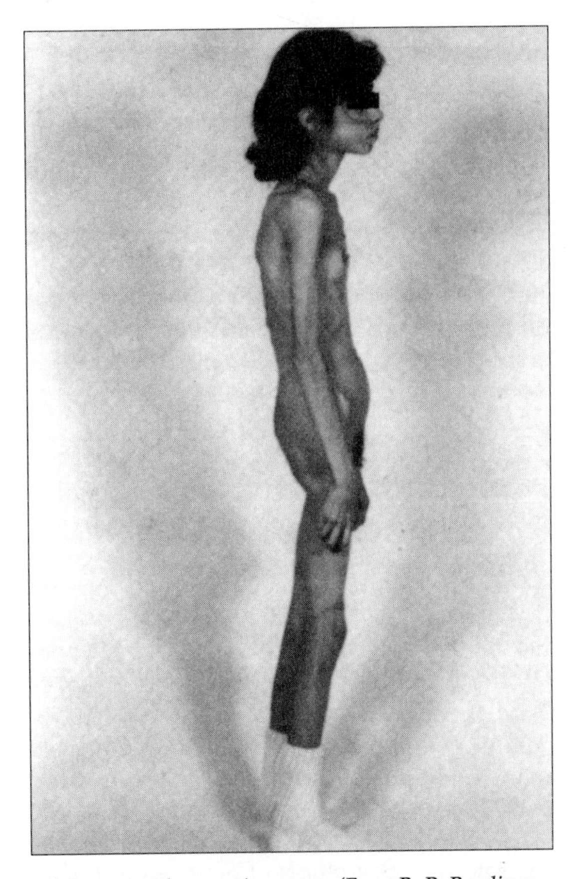

Figure 44–5 Physical manifestations of extreme wasting in an adolescent with anorexia nervosa (From R. P. Rawlings, S. R. Williams, and C. K. Beck. Mental Health-Psychiatric Nursing, *3rd ed. St. Louis, MO: Mosby-Year Book, 1992)*

monitor the success of behavioral modification and weight gain.

Bulimia Nervosa. Bulimia nervosa is characterized by a cycle of abnormal consumption of food (**binging**) — as much as 3,000 to 5,000 calories at one time — followed by self-induced vomiting or use of diuretics or laxatives (**purging**). Like anorexia, bulimia affects primarily adolescent and young adult females. The adolescent has an overconcern about weight and attempts to maintain weight through the binge-purge behaviors. Psychological factors associated with bulimia include a belief of not "measuring up," feeling inadequate, and not feeling accepted by the peer group.

Because the adolescent with bulimia usually maintains a weight within normal limits, the disorder is often difficult to diagnose. The adolescent may hide food, be dishonest or lie about the behavior, and eat normally in front of others. Symptoms include muscle wasting, dark circles under the eyes, and dental caries or loss of dental enamel caused by vomiting of stomach acids. The adolescent may be unable to stop eating once binging starts, with the cycle ending in depression and sleep. As behavior interferes with normal daily activities, the adolescent becomes more isolated. Cardiovascular complications as well as gastrointestinal problems (such as parotitis, gastritis, ulcers, hernias, and bowel and liver problems) may result. The stomach may become very large, distended, and even rupture (Mitchell 1989). In severe cases, the disorder may be fatal.

Treatment focuses on increasing the adolescent's self-esteem and, through a long-term process, changing the bulimic lifestyle and thinking patterns. The treatment program requires a consistent approach; supportive environment; and multidisciplinary team to address the physiological, emotional, and behavioral components of the disorder.

DEPRESSION

Description. Depression can occur in children of any age but is most common in adolescents. Teenagers who suffer from feelings of low self-esteem, pronounced **dysphoria** (anguish), and distorted and disturbed thinking are at greatest risk for depression. Contributing factors in adolescent depression are a sense of loss (of childhood, of love), feelings of failure or lack of control, and threats to self-esteem. Other factors may include a family move, separation, divorce, death, or loss of a boyfriend or girlfriend.

Symptoms. Symptoms of depression in children and adolescents include listlessness and **anhedonia** (absence of pleasurable feelings; lack of interest in activities); impaired school work; preoccupation with morbid thoughts; irritability and even hostility; and somatic symptoms such as headaches, stomach aches, muscle aches, and changes in eating and sleeping patterns. The adolescent may act out these feelings, sometimes in the form of delinquency. At other times, there may be withdrawal and isolation. The use and abuse of substances (alcohol and drugs, both prescription and illegal) may occur. The adolescent may also engage in high-risk activities that result in frequent injuries. Thoughts of suicide are always a possibility.

Treatment. The treatment program includes providing a safe, predictable, controlled, and controllable (by the individual) environment for the adolescent. Promotion of self-esteem and the development of coping skills, including learning to make choices, are essential parts of the treatment plan. Continued assessment of behavior changes and suicide risk is necessary.

Open communication allows for expression of feelings and assists the adolescent to express feelings, learn to cope, and to understand himself or herself. Many parents have difficulty understanding that adolescents go through stages, such as being tired or sleeping much of the time (related to physiological changes) and need to be with peer groups in order to become healthy, functioning adults.

Nursing Care. The nurse needs to be supportive of the adolescent as well as understanding and supportive of parents. Listening and providing information about the normal development and expected tasks of adolescence may be helpful for both parents and the adolescent. Knowledge of what to expect often eases the pressures that parents feel about their child and their insistence that the adolescent should act in certain ways.

SUICIDE

Suicide has become the second leading cause of death in adolescents and young adults aged 15 to 24 years, after accidents (Townsend 1993). Since the early 1960s, suicides in this age group increased 300% (Townsend 1993). Among suggested underlying causes are: increased life stresses (related to the assumption of adult responsibilities), factors such as those discussed above for depression, feelings of rejection, confusion about life and personal circumstances, failure to meet self and parental expectations, lack of purpose, and lack of coping skills to deal with these situations.

Adolescents at risk for suicide may demonstrate warning signs such as sleep and eating disorders (often with severe weight loss in a short amount of time); behavioral changes (often abrupt); changes in mood (including abrupt elevation of mood after a depressed mood and affect); changed or lack of interest in friends, family, school, and life; expressed feelings of helplessness, hopelessness, and worthlessness; expressed intent to commit suicide; giving away valued possessions; increased use of illegal drugs or substances; and high-risk activities.

A thorough assessment of the adolescent's symptoms, feelings, thoughts, and behaviors is necessary. Assessment must include environmental aspects, such as recent changes in the adolescent's or family's life; relationships; impulsivity and decision-making capability; and risk factors such as previous attempts, attempts by other family members, and suicide of a peer. Children and adolescents are often impulsive and may act on their feelings and thoughts without regard to the consequence (that death is permanent). *These symptoms must be taken seriously!* The adolescent should be asked directly whether he or she is considering suicide and then asked if he or she has a plan. This approach does not create thoughts of suicide; in fact, the adolescent may be relieved that someone is inquiring.

Depending on the seriousness of the threat, treatment of an adolescent at risk for suicide may include hospitalization. Adolescents with suicidal symptoms and risk factors require immediate intervention and referral to a mental health care professional with expertise in this area. Probably the single most important factor in reducing the possibility of suicide is the formation and continuation of a relationship with a supportive, concerned person.

SUBSTANCE ABUSE

Description. Substance abuse is the use of any **psychoactive** (mind-altering) substance in a manner other than that prescribed by cultural standards or in ways that impair a person's ability to function. Psychoactive substances include alcohol, prescription drugs (amphetamines, barbiturates), and illicit drugs (marijuana, cocaine/crack, heroin, phencyclidine [PCP], and LSD).

Many adolescents experiment with drugs or alcohol; experimentation is not considered abuse. It may occur or be precipitated by the need to be a part of a group, for "kicks," because of peer pressure ("Just try it"), to test one's own capabilities, or as an escape from problems and overwhelming stress. Continued experimentation, however, may lead to regular use, resulting in physical and psychological dependency, tolerance, habituation, and addiction. Regular substance use has many long-term implications, including unexpected overdose and possible death.

Symptoms. Symptoms depend on the particular substance abused. Characteristic physical findings include reddened eyes, euphoria, loss of appetite and weight loss, wearing long sleeves (to hide needle marks), blackouts, sweating, nervousness, and lethargy. Long-term effects of commonly used drugs and substances are listed in Figure 44–6.

Treatment. An important part of the treatment of the adolescent is to provide an environment that is safe and supportive of the individual. Chemical dependency programs for adolescents that provide a structured, predictable environment and assist the adolescent to learn new coping skills, behaviors, and attitudes while encouraging the development of self-esteem have the best long-term results. Trusting relationships with staff are most important. The recovery process is slow, requiring long-term management. Health care team members need to be nonjudgmental and caring.

Support groups (Tough Love for parents, Alcoholics Anonymous for teens [Al-anon, Alateen], Cocaine Anonymous, Narcotics Anonymous) and family counseling can provide a support system for the adolescent and family. Prevention education programs such as

EFFECTS OF SUBSTANCE ABUSE

Drug/Substance	Effects of Long-Term Use
Alcohol	Gastritis; peptic ulcer disease; increased risk for depression, suicide, and automobile accidents; blackouts; cirrhosis
Cocaine Crack	Chronic sinus and upper respiratory congestion; nose bleeds; chronic cough; anorexia or weight loss
Inhalants	Liver or kidney damage (depends on substance abused)
LSD	Flashbacks; psychoses, depression, and personality changes
Marijuana	Apathy, passivity, and decreased motivation; impaired ability to concentrate and memorize new information; increased risk for respiratory cancers
PCP	Psychotic states; increased capacity for aggressive and violent behavior

Figure 44–6 *(Based on information in E. G. Bennett and D. Woolf.* Substance Abuse: Pharmacologic, Developmental and Clinical Perspectives, *2nd ed. Albany, NY: Delmar Publishers, 1991, and A. D. Hoffman and D. E. Greydanus.* Adolescent Medicine, *2nd ed. Norwalk, CT: Appleton and Lange, 1989)*

D.A.R.E. (Drug Abuse Resistance Education), M.A.D.D. (Mothers Against Drunk Driving), and S.A.D.D. (Students Against Driving Drunk) that focus on drug and alcohol awareness have been implemented in schools and communities. The goals of these programs are to provide general education about drugs, teach antidrug attitudes, stress the importance of personal values, teach decision-making skills, and teach social skills (Bennett and Woolf 1991).

Nursing Care. The role the nurse plays in providing care to children and adolescents who are substance abusers will depend on the hospital or facility in which he or she is employed. Nurses who care for adolescent substance abusers must become familiar with (1) their own feelings about the use of psychoactive substances and (2) their feelings about the use and abuse of substances by children and adolescents.

It is most important for the nurse to be nonjudgmental and understanding while being able to: (1) identify the problem, (2) communicate about the problem, (3) educate the adolescent and family, (4) counsel the adolescent and family, and (5) refer the adolescent and family for treatment.

Areas for assessment include parental substance abuse, family dynamics, availability of prescription drugs and alcohol in the home, support systems, and ways of handling problems and conflicts. Always be alert to behaviors that could indicate potential substance abuse and report them to nursing managers and physicians.

REVIEW QUESTIONS

A. Multiple choice. Select the best answer.

1. Which characteristics suggest that an infant is experiencing failure to thrive syndrome?
   a. stomach aches, high-pitched crying, uneven growth spurts
   b. apathy, avoidance of eye contact, delayed development
   c. stranger anxiety, rocking motions, sucking reflexes
   d. muscle tension, cooing, eye contact with parent

2. Nursing interventions to increase parent bonding might include:
   a. encouraging parents to talk to the infant
   b. showing parents what is wrong with their parenting skills
   c. feeding the infant when the parents visit
   d. showing parents how to weigh the infant

3. When parents ask the nurse what to do about their hyperactive child, the most helpful response would be:
   a. indulge the child when the behavior begins to be unmanageable
   b. discuss the child's behavior with the child to help the child decide how to stop the activity
   c. limit environmental stimuli, distractions, and choices given the child
   d. tell the child he or she is overstimulated and out of control

4. A mother whose child has school phobia might be advised to
   a. ignore complaints and expressions of fear by the child
   b. keep the child at home when there are physical symptoms
   c. have the child walk to school with another child
   d. work with school staff to desensitize the child's anxiety

5. Parents of a 14-year-old girl who has been diagnosed with anorexia nervosa would most likely tell the nurse:
   a. "We found her to be such an active, impish child."
   b. "She's always made us so proud of her until now."
   c. "We had trouble getting her to eat the right foods as a child."
   d. "She had difficulty getting along in grade school."

6. The highest priority for treatment of an adolescent hospitalized with anorexia nervosa related to extremely low weight is to
   a. establish rapport with the patient and family to gain their trust
   b. teach the patient the basics of good nutrition
   c. follow the prescribed plan to restore nutritional balance
   d. discuss the importance of adhering to the treatment plan

7. Which question would elicit the most information about the status of an adolescent who has been treated for bulimia nervosa?
   a. "What's happening in your life with people and activities?"
   b. "How are you managing your diet since you began the treatment program?"
   c. "What have been the fluctuations in your weight over the past three to six months?"
   d. "Are you continuing to follow the treatment plan developed when you were hospitalized?"
8. An 11-year-old middle-school child doesn't want to go to school, isn't interested in school or after-school activities, and admits that when she watches television she doesn't remember the programs. This is an example of
   a. morbid preoccupation
   b. listlessness
   c. isolation
   d. anhedonia
9. Tim, a 15-year-old high school sophomore, has been engaging in reckless behaviors since he broke up with his girlfriend last month. Which of the following questions is essential for assessment at this time?
   a. "Why are you doing all of these activities?"
   b. "What have you been doing since the breakup with your girlfriend?"
   c. "How are you doing?"
   d. "Are you thinking about suicide?"
10. Joan, a 13-year-old freshman whose parents have recently divorced, has been seen smoking marijuana cigarettes and says she "had a few beers" over the weekend. An intervention plan for Joan would include
    a. monitoring symptoms daily to determine if there is substance abuse
    b. finding out what her perceptions are about her family situation
    c. reporting her behavior and comments to the school psychologist for testing
    d. calling the parent with whom Joan lives to find out whether the parent is aware of the situation

SUGGESTED ACTIVITIES

- Review the characteristics of a child with attention deficit hyperactive disorder, and normal growth and development responses. Then observe a 3-year-old, a 5-year-old, and a 7-year-old child. According to data given, are the children hyperactive or normal?
- Given the importance of being direct and, at the same time, sensitive to an adolescent, formulate questions to ask regarding substance use. An example might be, "When you are with friends, do you drink alcohol or use drugs?" Or, being more direct (and assuming that an adolescent experiments with drugs), "What drugs have you tried?"
- Investigate resources in your community that an adolescent might turn to for help with (1) feelings of distress or despair, (2) suicidal thoughts, and (3) use or abuse of alcohol and other substances (drugs). (One place to begin is in the telephone book.) Which would you give as a resource or referral?

BIBLIOGRAPHY

American Psychiatric Association. *Diagnostic and Statistical Manual of Mental Disorders*, 3rd ed, revised (DSM-III-R). Washington, D.C.: American Psychiatric Association, 1987.

Bennett, E. G., and D. Woolf. *Substance Abuse: Pharmacologic, Developmental and Clinical Perspectives*, 2nd ed. Albany, NY: Delmar Publishers, 1991.

Bouchard, C. Genetic influences on body composition and regional fat distribution. *Contemporary Nutrition* 15, no. 10 (1990).

Carpenito, L. *Nursing Diagnosis: Application to Clinical Practice*, 4th ed. Philadelphia: J. B. Lippincott, 1992.

Davies, J., and E. Janosik. *Health and Psychiatric Nursing*. Boston: Jones and Bartlett, 1991.

Haber, J., A. McMahan, P. Price-Hoskins, and B. Sideleau. *Comprehensive Psychiatric Nursing*. St. Louis, MO: Mosby-Year Book, 1992.

Hoffman, A. D., and D. E. Greydanus. *Adolescent Medicine*, 2nd ed. Norwalk, CT: Appleton and Lange, 1989.

Jacques, J., and N. Snyder. Newborn victims of addiction. *RN* (April, 1991): 47–53.

Levy, G., and J. Hickey. Fighting the battle against drugs. *RN* (April, 1991): 44–47.

Lucas, A. Update and review of anorexia nervosa. *Contemporary Nutrition* 14, no. 9 (1989).

McCoy, K. *Coping with Teenage Depression*. New York: Dutton, 1985.

McEnany, G. Managing mood disorders. *RN* (September, 1990): 28–33.

Mitchell, J. Bulimia nervosa. *Contemporary Nutrition* 14, no. 10 (1989).

Olds, S., M. London, and P. Ladewig. *Maternal-Newborn Nursing*, 4th ed. Redwood City, CA: Addison-Wesley, 1992.

Pillitteri, A. *Maternal and Child Health Nursing*. Philadelphia: J. B. Lippincott, 1992.

Roth, G. *When Food Is Love*. New York: Plume Books, 1991.

Rudolph, A. M., J. I. E. Hoffman, and C. D. Rudolph. *Rudolph's Pediatrics*, 19th ed. Norwalk, CT: Appleton and Lange, 1991.

Smith, M., and F. Lifshitz. Failure to thrive. *Contemporary Nutrition* 15, no. 5 (1990).

Townsend, M. *Psychiatric Mental Health Nursing: Concepts of Care*. Philadelphia: F. A. Davis, 1993.

Varcarolis, E. *Foundations of Psychiatric and Mental Health Nursing*. Philadelphia: W. B. Saunders, 1990.

Wong, D. *Whaley & Wong's Essentials of Pediatric Nursing*, 4th ed. St. Louis, MO: Mosby-Year Book, 1993.

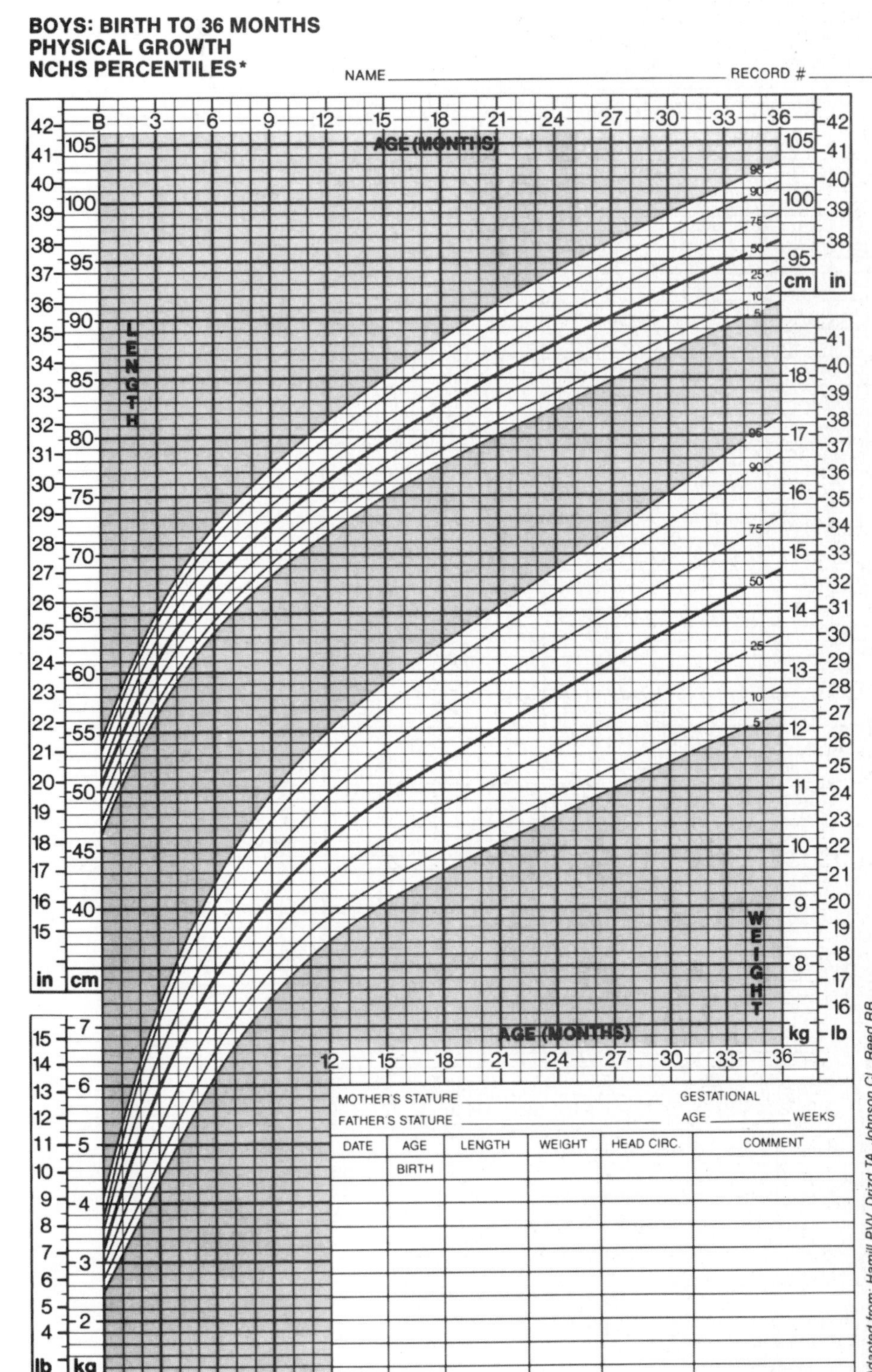

*Adapted from: Hamill PVV, Drizd TA, Johnson CL, Reed RB, Roche AF, Moore WM: Physical growth: National Center for Health Statistics percentiles. AM J CLIN NUTR 32:607-629, 1979. Data from the Fels Longitudinal Study, Wright State University School of Medicine, Yellow Springs, Ohio.

BOYS: BIRTH TO 36 MONTHS
PHYSICAL GROWTH
NCHS PERCENTILES*

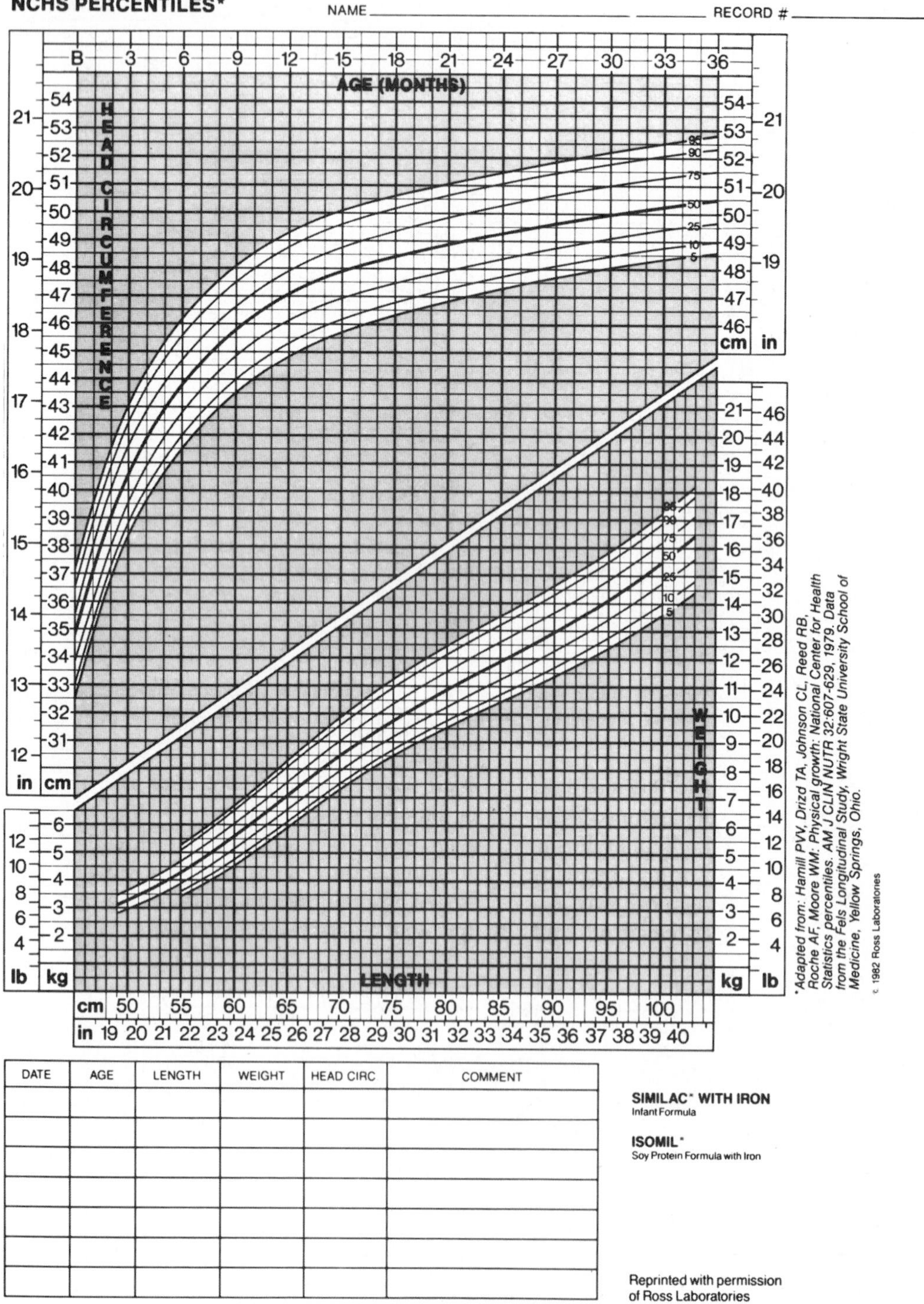

DATE	AGE	LENGTH	WEIGHT	HEAD CIRC	COMMENT

Reprinted with permission of Ross Laboratories

GIRLS: BIRTH TO 36 MONTHS PHYSICAL GROWTH NCHS PERCENTILES*

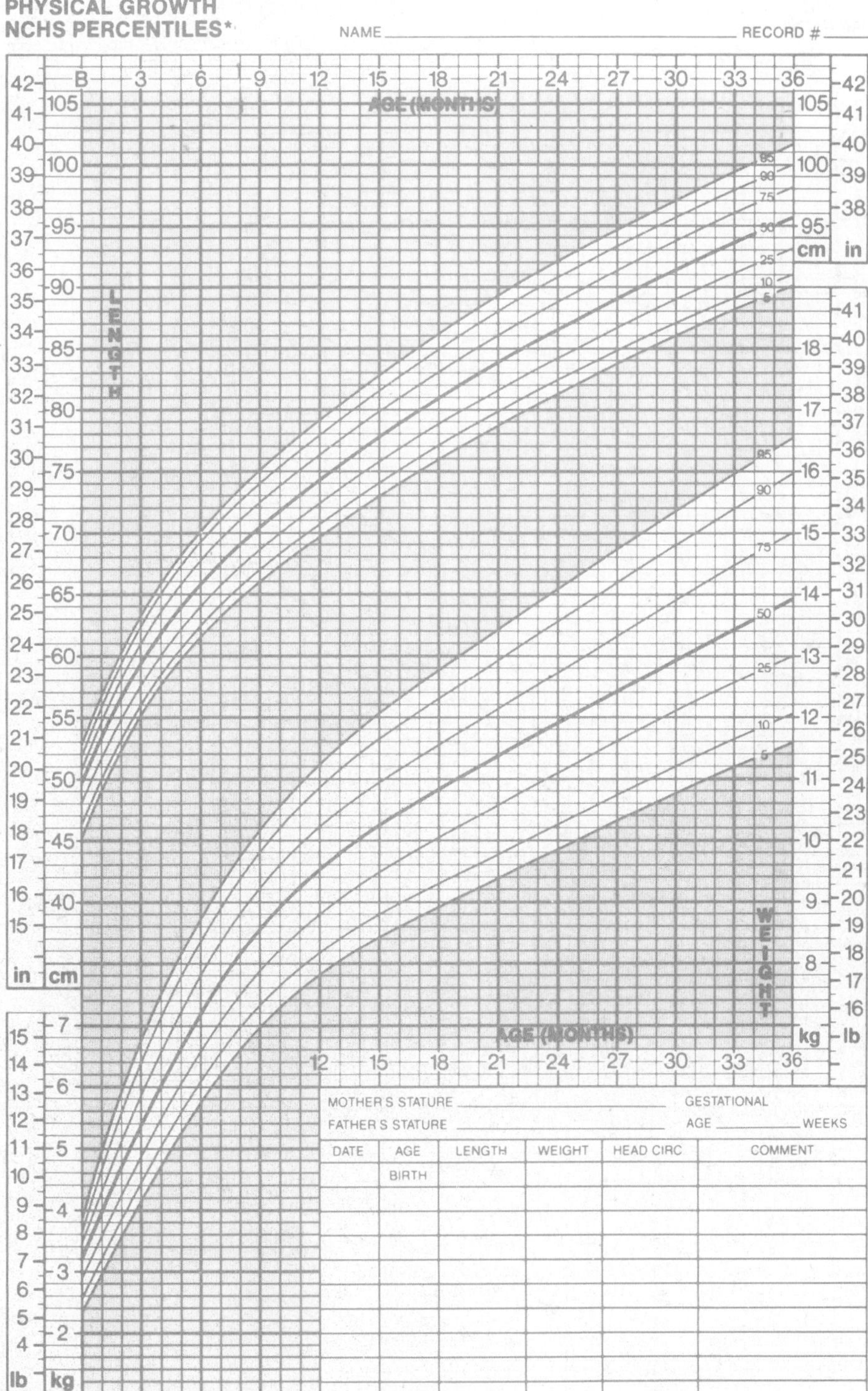

*Adapted from: Hamill PVV, Drizd TA, Johnson CL, Reed RB, Roche AF, Moore WM: Physical growth: National Center for Health Statistics percentiles. AM J CLIN NUTR 32:607-629, 1979. Data from the Fels Longitudinal Study, Wright State University School of Medicine, Yellow Springs, Ohio.

GIRLS: BIRTH TO 36 MONTHS PHYSICAL GROWTH NCHS PERCENTILES*

NAME ____________________ RECORD # ____________

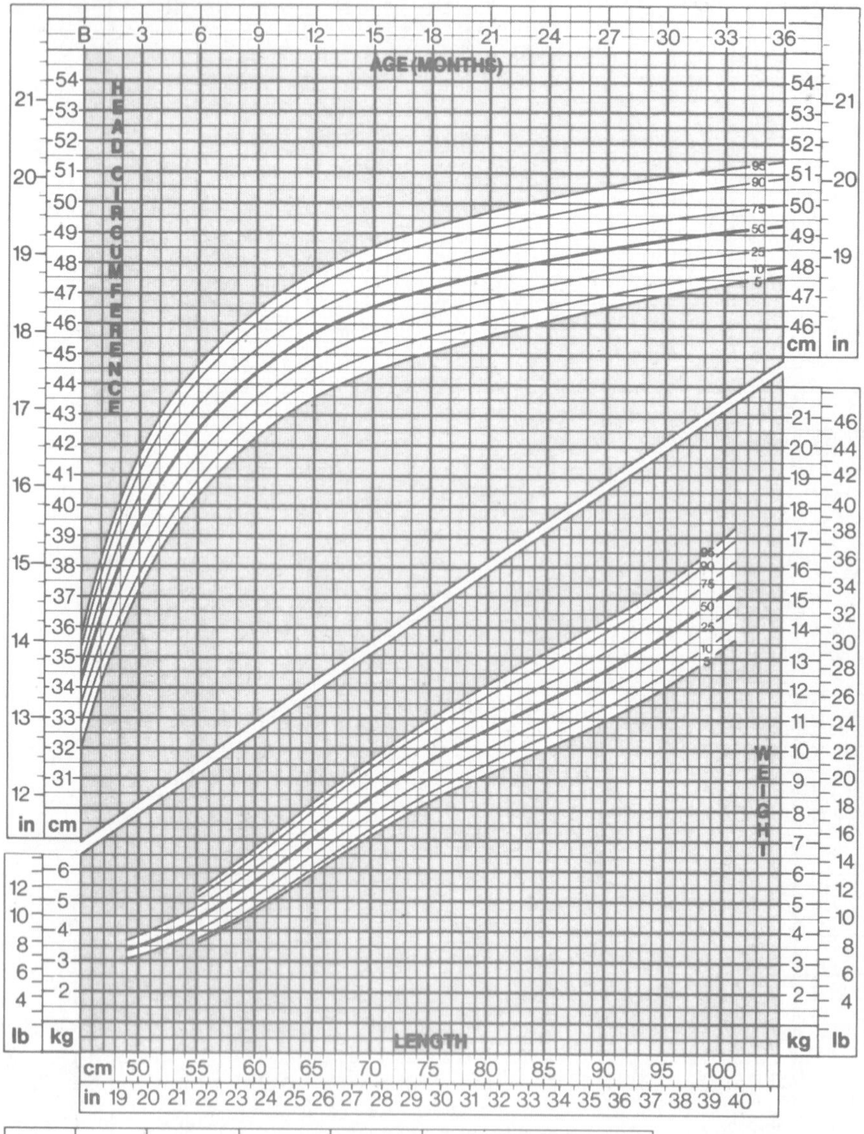

DATE	AGE	LENGTH	WEIGHT	HEAD CIRC	COMMENT

* Adapted from: Hamill PVV, Drizd TA, Johnson CL, Reed RB, Roche AF, Moore WM: Physical growth: National Center for Health Statistics percentiles. AM J CLIN NUTR 32:607-629, 1979. Data from the Fels Longitudinal Study, Wright State University School of Medicine, Yellow Springs, Ohio.

SIMILAC® WITH IRON
Infant Formula

ISOMIL®
Soy Protein Formula with Iron

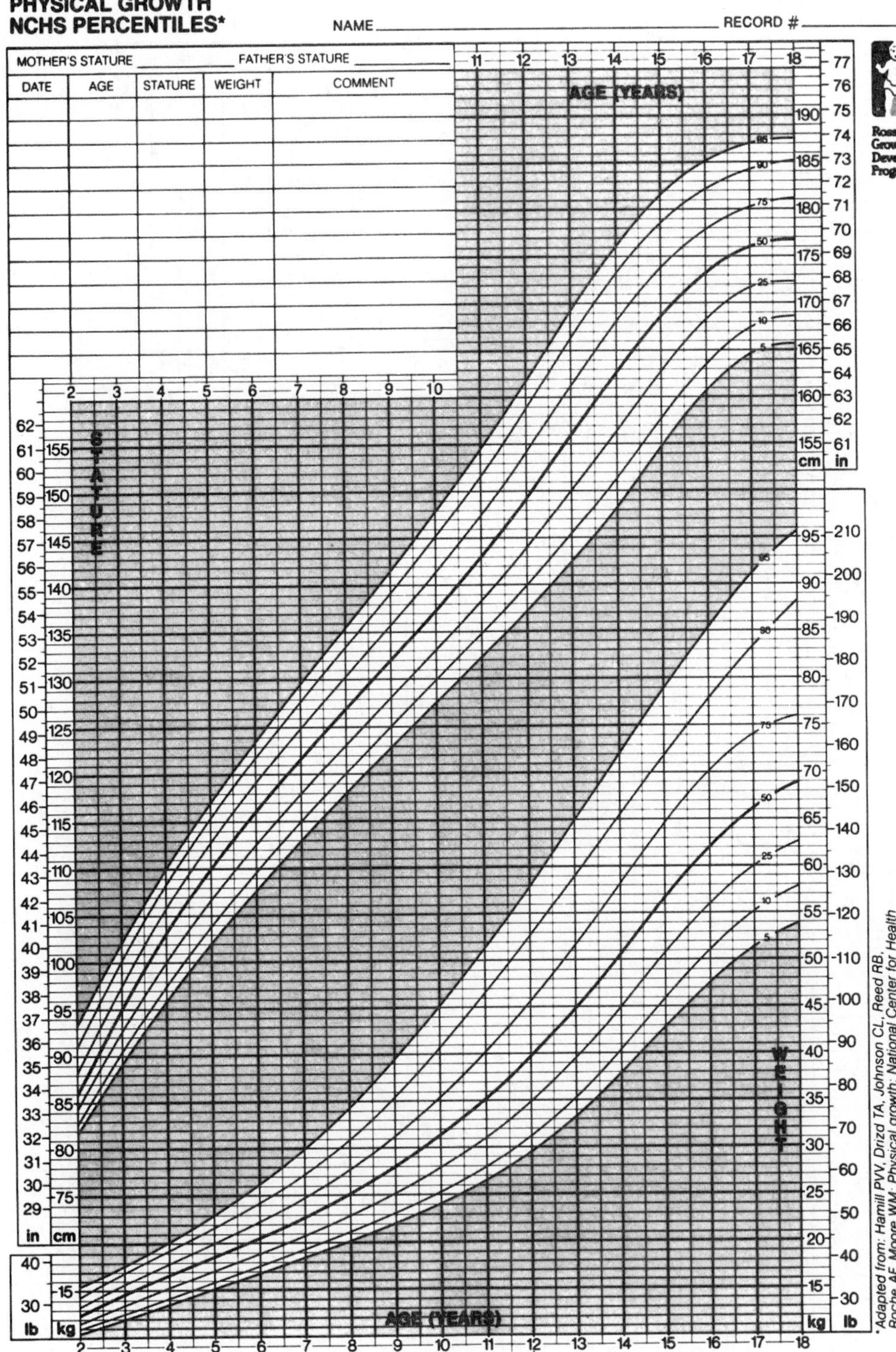
BOYS: 2 TO 18 YEARS
PHYSICAL GROWTH
NCHS PERCENTILES*
NAME
RECORD #
MOTHER'S STATURE
FATHER'S STATURE
DATE
AGE
STATURE
WEIGHT
COMMENT
AGE (YEARS)
STATURE
WEIGHT
in
cm
lb
kg
Ross
Growth &
Development
Program
*Adapted from: Hamill PVV, Drizd TA, Johnson CL, Reed RB, Roche AF, Moore WM: Physical growth: National Center for Health Statistics percentiles. AM J CLIN NUTR 32:607-629, 1979. Data from the National Center for Health Statistics (NCHS), Hyattsville, Maryland.
© 1982 Ross Laboratories

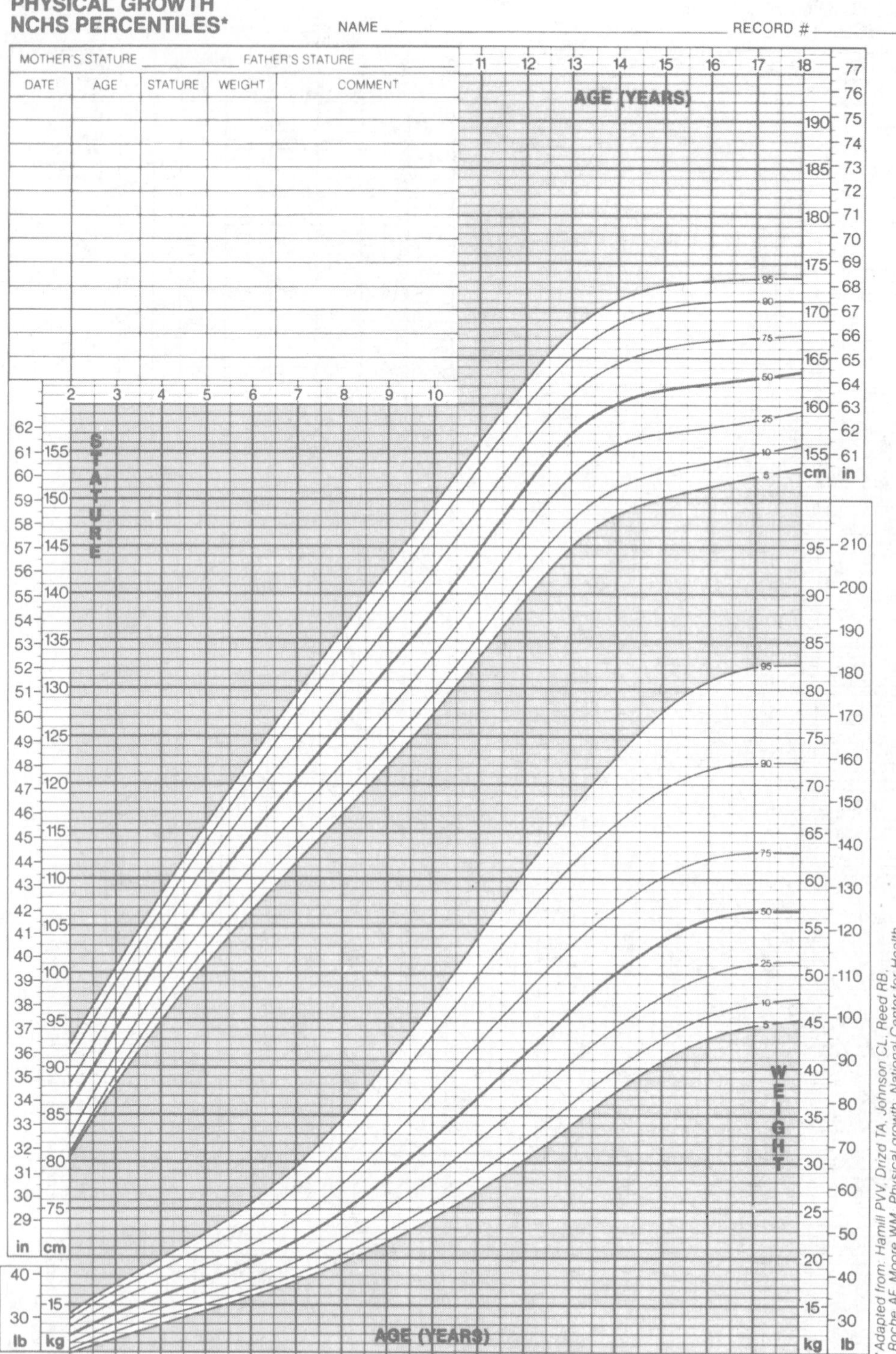
GIRLS: 2 TO 18 YEARS
PHYSICAL GROWTH
NCHS PERCENTILES*
NAME
RECORD #
MOTHER'S STATURE
FATHER'S STATURE
DATE
AGE
STATURE
WEIGHT
COMMENT
AGE (YEARS)
STATURE
WEIGHT
cm
in
kg
lb
95
90
75
50
25
10
5
*Adapted from: Hamill PVV, Drizd TA, Johnson CL, Reed RB, Roche AF, Moore WM: Physical growth: National Center for Health Statistics percentiles. AM J CLIN NUTR 32:607-629, 1979. Data from the National Center for Health Statistics (NCHS), Hyattsville, Maryland.

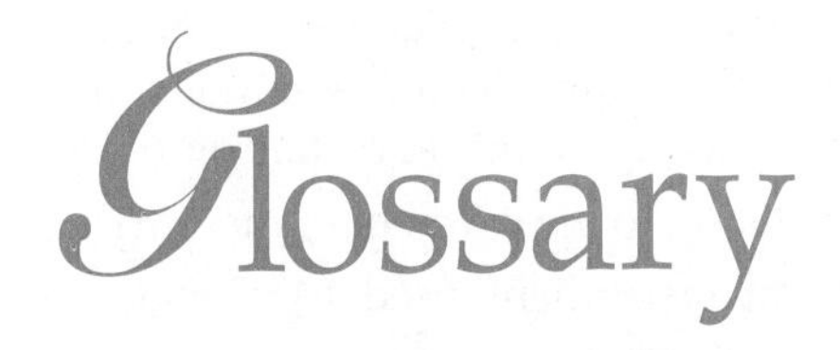

abdominal palpation: a means of determining the position and presentation of a fetus by examining the abdomen with the hands

ABO incompatibility: a hemolytic disease caused by the presence of naturally occurring antigens of blood group A and B

abortion: the termination of a pregnancy at any time before the fetus has obtained a stage of viability

- **complete:** an abortion in which the entire product of conception is expelled
- **habitual:** a condition in which three or more successive pregnancies have ended in spontaneous abortion
- **incomplete:** an abortion in which part of the product of conception is passed but part remains in the uterus
- **induced:** the termination of a pregnancy with the aid of mechanical or medical agents
- **missed:** an abortion in which the fetus dies in utero but the product of conception is retained
- **spontaneous:** the termination of a pregnancy through natural causes

abruptio placenta: *see* placenta abruptio

accelerated phase: phase in the first stage of labor with cervical dilatation measuring from 5 to 7 cm

acceleration: quickening; increase in speed

acidosis: depletion of the alkaline reserve in the blood and body tissues

acini: milk-producing cells lining the alveoli in the breast tissue

acme: the most intense phase of a contraction

acquired heart disease: a heart condition that occurs after birth as a result of complications of another disease

acquired immune deficiency syndrome (AIDS): a multisystem disorder characterized by cellular immunodeficiency that results from infection with human immunodeficiency virus; transmitted by intimate sexual contact or through direct contact with blood or blood products of someone with AIDS

active immunity: an immune response that occurs when an individual forms antibodies or antitoxins against specific antigens, either by exposure to the infectious agent or by introduction of the antigen; also called humoral immunity

actual effectiveness rate: the percent of pregnancies that are prevented with any given method of contraception when that method is used with expected misuse or noncompliance

acyanotic heart disease: condition usually associated with defects that increase the flow of blood to the lungs

adolescence: the period of increased physical growth and development, characterized by the development of primary and secondary sex characteristics, occurring between the ages of 12 and 19 years

adolescent growth spurt: a period of accelerated growth affecting practically all skeletal and muscular growth in an adolescent; typically lasts about 2 years

afterbirth: the placenta and membranes

afterbirth pain: discomfort caused by uterine contractions that continue for a period of time after delivery; also called afterpain

afterpain: *see* afterbirth pain

agranulocytes: a type of white blood cell; specifically, lymphocytes and monocytes

AIDS: *see* acquired immune deficiency syndrome

albuminuria: albumin in the urine

alkaloidal cocaine: also known as "crack"; an illegal drug that can adversely affect the fetus if used during pregnancy

allergen: a substance capable of inducing hypersensitivity

allergic shiner: dark circles under the eyes or discolorations greater than usual; a symptom of allergic rhinitis

alpha fetoprotein (AFP): a substance made by the fetal liver and concentrated in the fetal spinal fluid; if a neural tube defect is present, large amounts of AFP leak into the amniotic fluid and then into the mother's blood, where it can be measured

alternative birthing centers (ABC): homelike accommodations for the birth process for low-risk pregnancies outside of a hospital

alternative birthing choices: alternatives from which a woman may choose regarding her labor and delivery; birthing room versus labor room; baby kept in the nursery during the hospital stay versus rooming-in; medication versus unmedicated birth; and so on

alveoli: anatomical nomenclature to designate small saclike dilatation; clusters of lobules in the breast, lined with milk-producing cells

amenorrhea: permanent or temporary suppression of menstruation

American Academy of Pediatrics: governing board responsible for recommendations for health care involving infants and children

amnesiac: relating to impairment of memory

amnihook: an instrument used to artificially rupture the amniotic sac

amniocentesis: a procedure whereby the amniotic sac is punctured with a needle and amniotic fluid is withdrawn

amnion: the innermost of the two fetal membranes; forms the amniotic sac, or bag of waters, that encloses the fetus

amnioscope: device for looking inside the amniotic cavity

amniotic fluid: fluid filling the amniotic sac and surrounding the fetus; slightly alkaline and about 98% water

amniotic fluid bilirubin: a prenatal test to measure liver maturity

amniotic fluid creatinine: a test prenatally to assess fetal muscle mass and renal function

amniotic membrane: the innermost fetal membrane

amniotic sac: bag of waters; a sac or bag in which the embryo is suspended; formed by fusion of the amnion and chorion

amniotomy: artificial rupture of the amniotic sac

analgesia: relief from pain

anaphylaxis: the generalized systemic response of a sensitized individual to a specific antigen; can result in life-threatening symptoms, including respiratory distress and shock

android pelvis: heart- or wedge-shaped pelvis less suitable to childbearing than gynecoid pelvis

anemia: a decrease in the erythrocyte or hemoglobin content or both of the blood

anesthesia: absence of sensibility to pain

anhedonia: absence of pleasurable feelings in acts that normally give pleasure; lack of interest in activities

anomalies: deviations from normal

anovulatory menstruation: a failure of the ovary to release an ovum

anoxia: reduction of oxygen in body tissue

anteflexion: the bending of an organ so that its top is thrust forward

antepartum: occurring before childbirth

anthropoid pelvis: pelvis shape with greater anteroposterior diameter than other shapes; narrow in its transverse plane

anticipatory grieving: the process by which parents begin to work through their grief in accepting the loss of their child; increases in intensity until the child's death

anticipatory guidance: a form of teaching that provides information to help parents understand their children's behavior and improve their parenting skills

antigen: any substance that, when introduced into the blood or tissues, incites the formation of antibodies

anus: the opening of the rectum

aorta: the main trunk from which the systemic arterial system proceeds

apathy: lack of feeling of emotions

Apgar scoring system: guide to evaluation of the infant's condition at birth

apical pulse: the pulse heard at the apex of the heart

apnea: cessation of respirations

areola: the darkened ring surrounding the nipple of the breast

asphyxia: suffocation

asphyxia neonatorum: imperfect breathing in newborn infants

atony: lack of muscle tone

atrial contraction: contraction of the atrium of the heart; represents the first phase of the fetal heart rate pattern

atrophy: decrease in size of an organ or tissue that is normally developed

attachment: an enduring affectional tie one person forms for another; the emotional ties from infant to parent

attitude: state of flexion or extension of the fetus

augmentation: increasing

auscultation: listening for sounds within the body

automatic walking: reflex of newborn where legs move reciprocally, imitating walking, when supported upright

automatisms: involuntary movements that look purposeful

AV valve closure: the second phase of the fetal heart pattern when the atrial-ventricular valve closes

bacterial endocarditis: a bacterial infection of the valves or the inner lining of the heart

bacterial vaginosis: a chalky white or gray-green vaginal discharge and a foul odor caused by bacteria *(Gardnerella vaginalis)* that live in the vagina

bag of waters: amniotic sac, which contains the fetus during pregnancy

ballottement: a term used in an examination when the fetus can be pushed about in the uterus

barbiturate: drug used as a central nervous system depressant

barrier: a method to prevent exposure to infectious agents in blood or other body fluids of patients; involves use of gloves, gown, mask, and protective eyewear

Bartholin's glands: pair of small compound glands situated on either side of the posterior vaginal opening that secrete a mucoid material upon sexual arousal

basal temperature: a measurement of body temperature when first awakening after at least six hours of sleep

basal temperature method: method of contraception that relies on documenting basal temperature changes to determine fertile days

baseline FHR: the range of a normal fetal heart rate; 120 to 160 beats per minute; the range reflects autonomic control

benign: tending not to progress or recur

bikini cut: skin incision made horizontally just above the pubic bone for delivery of the baby

bilateral tubal ligation: surgical procedure that blocks off the fallopian tubes

bilirubin: a red bile pigment from the hemoglobin of erythrocytes

binging: abnormal consumption of food

biophysical profile: a means of evaluating fetal well-being in the last weeks of pregnancy by looking at the amount of amniotic fluid, fetal breathing movements, fetal movement, fetal heart tones, and fetal reaction

birthing bed: a bed that converts into various positions appropriate for the delivery process

birthing chair: a supportive chair that easily changes positions to accommodate the delivery process

bladder: a storage receptacle for urine

blastocyst: the developing ovum during the second week after fertilization when it is a small hollow ball of cells

blastoderm: stage of development of the embryo; a disc of cells from which the primary germ layers are derived

blastomere: cells that result from the first division of the fertilized ovum

bonding: a gradually unfolding emotional attachment to another person; the emotional ties from parent to infant

Bradley: a method of prepared childbirth using relaxation and breathing techniques to facilitate childbirth. Known as husband-coached childbirth

bradycardia: abnormal slowness of the heartbeat; fewer than 120 beats per minute

BRAIDED: acronym for benefits, risks, alternatives, inquiries, decision, explanation, and documentation; informed consent

Braxton-Hicks contractions: painless uterine contractions occurring periodically throughout pregnancy thereby enlarging the uterus to accommodate the growing fetus

breech presentation: the presentation in which the buttocks precedes the head; can be footling, complete, or frank

broad ligaments: two structures that extend from the walls of the uterus to the pelvic wall and to which the ovaries and fallopian tubes are attached

brow presentation: the brow or forehead of the fetus presents at the cervix; partial extension

Brudzinski's sign: flexion of the hips when the neck is flexed from a supine position

bulbourethral glands: two small glands located below the prostate gland on either side of the urethra; add secretions to the semen through ducts that open into the urethra; also called Cowper's glands

bulb syringe: a manual instrument used to suction secretions from the newborn's airway

candidiasis: infection with fungi of the genus *Candida*

canthus: the angle at the junction of the eyelids at either corner of the eye

caput: the head

caput succedaneum: soft tissue of the scalp becomes swollen as a result of delivery

carcinogen: a substance that causes cancer

carcinoma: malignant tumor

cardiomegaly: enlargement of the heart

cardiopulmonary resuscitation (CPR): a technique that provides basic life support to a victim who is unable to breathe or pump sufficient blood through the body

cataract: an opacity of the crystalline eye lens

caudal anesthesia: injection of a local anesthetic into the caudal space in the sacrum

causative agent: an organism that causes a disease; also called a pathogen

cephalic: pertaining to the head

cephalic presentation: presenting part of the fetus is the head

cephalocaudal: the process in which maturation begins at the head and moves toward the toes

cephalocaudal disproportion: refers to the fact that the circumference of the neonate's head is usually 1 to 2 in. larger than the circumference of the chest

cephalohematoma: soft tissue of the scalp becomes swollen as bloody fluid collects under the covering layer of the skull bone and is located within the bone structure

cephalopelvic disproportion: the head of the baby is of such size, shape, or position that it cannot pass through the mother's pelvis

cerebral injury: damage to brain tissue

cervical cap: latex thimble-shaped device with soft dome that stays firmly in place on the cervix with suction making an airtight seal against sperm

cervix: the narrow lower portion of the uterus

cesarean section: delivery of the baby through abdominal surgery

Chadwick's sign: the violet color on the mucous membrane of the vagina just below the urethral orifice that is seen after the fourth week of pregnancy

chain of infection: the process by which infectious diseases are transmitted in human beings

chest retractions: see-saw type of respiration typical of infant with respiratory distress syndrome

child abuse: the intentional physical or emotional maltreatment or neglect of children

childbirth preparation: instruction with information about pregnancy, labor, and delivery; physical conditioning, relaxation techniques, and breathing patterns to be used during labor; and information about breast feeding, postpartum experiences, and infant care

chlamydia: a sexually transmitted disease caused by *Chlamydia trachomatis*; it lives in the vagina and urethra and is sometimes asymptomatic in the female; can cause PID

chloasma gravidarum: various pigmentary discolorations of the skin during pregnancy

chorea: ceaseless occurrence of involuntary, rapid, purposeless movements of the muscles of the face and limbs

chorioamnionitis: inflammation of fetal membranes caused by bacterial infection

chorion: the outermost of fetal membranes

chorionic gonadotropin: a hormone secreted by the fertilized ovum that enables the corpus luteum to continue to secrete progesterone during the first three months of pregnancy

chorionic membrane: the outermost fetal membrane that fuses with the amnion to become the sac that contains the embryo

chorionic somatotrophin: hormone produced by the placenta that stimulates fetal growth

chorionic villi: fingerlike projections from the chorion that contain blood vessels communicating with the fetus and developing early in pregnancy

chorionic villi sampling: samples of placenta cells for examination of chromosomes to detect some genetic abnormalities

chromosome: the structure that carries the gene in the nucleus of a cell

cilia: hairlike projections that help carry the ovum along the fallopian tubes with their waving actions

circumcision: excision of the foreskin of the penis

cleavage: the early splitting of a fertilized ovum into smaller cells by mitosis

cleft lip: failure of the soft or bony tissue in the lip to unite during fetal development

cleft palate: failure of the soft or bony tissue in the palate to unite during fetal development

clitoris: elongated mass of tissue, nerves, and muscle richly supplied with blood; synonymous with the male penis

coccyx: small triangular bone made up of four vertebrae fused together; found at the end of the spine

cognitive: intellectual development encompassing a wide variety of mental abilities, including learning, language, memory, reasoning, and thinking

coitus: intercourse; sexual union

coitus interruptus: withdrawal of the penis from the vagina before ejaculation; a method of contraception

colostrum: the thin yellowish fluid released by the breasts during the latter part of pregnancy and for the first few days after delivery, before milk is released

coma: a state of unconsciousness in which a person cannot open the eys, speak, obey commands or be aroused by any measure

combined oral contraceptives: estrogen and progesterone birth control pill taken daily for 21 out of 28 continuous days to prevent pregnancy

comedones: accumulation of keratin and sebum within the opening of a hair follicle; commonly called black heads or white heads

communicable diseases: diseases spread from one person to another either directly or indirectly

complete breech: the position of the fetus when the buttocks and feet present at the cervix with the knees drawn up

conception: union of the sperm and ovum; fertilization

condom: male, a contraceptive sheath that may be put on the erect penis before entering the vagina; female, contraceptive barrier pouch inserted into the vagina

condylomata acuminato: pedunculated, elongated, and fleshy raised lesions that are in the genital region

congenital: existing at birth as a result of heredity or some other factor occurring during intrauterine development

congenital heart disease: a heart condition that arises during fetal development and is present at birth

congestive heart failure: a condition in which the blood supply to the body is insufficient to meet metabolic demands

consolability: the ability of the newborn to be calmed when irritable

continuous positive airway pressure (CPAP): a treatment to assist ventilation of an infant with respiratory distress syndrome

contraception: prevention of conception

contraceptive: that which prevents conception

contraction: involuntary tightening of the uterine muscle

contraction ring: the internal os of the cervix

Coombs test: test done on Rh-negative mothers to measure the presence of Rh antibodies

copulation: the sexual act whereby sperm is delivered to the female uterus by the erect penis

cord prolapse: *see* prolapsed cord

corpus luteum: yellowish mass formed in the graafian follicle after the ovum has been released

cot death: *see* sudden infant death syndrome

cotyledons: any one of the subdivisions of the uterine surface of the placenta

Cowper's glands: *see* bulbourethral glands

cradle hold: a method of holding infant in which the infant's head rests in the bend of the nurse's elbow, with the back supported; the infant's thigh is held by the carrying arm

creatinine: a basic substance in the urine

Crede treatment: instillation of 1% silver nitrate solution in the eyes of the newborn infant

crib death: *see* sudden infant death syndrome

crowning: stage at which the fetal head can be seen at the vaginal orifice

cyanosis: bluish discoloration of the skin due to insufficient oxygen in the blood

cyanotic heart disease: condition associated with defects that result in the mixing of unoxygenated blood with oxygenated blood; skin has bluish tint because of the unoxygenated blood circulating through the body

cystitis: infection of the bladder

cytomegalovirus (CMV): one of a group of highly host-specific viruses that affect humans; a viral infection that can be passed to the fetus through the placenta, the vagina, or the breast milk

dartos: involuntary muscle fibers that allow the scrotum to contract or relax with temperature changes

D&C: *see* dilation and curettage

D&E: *see* dilation and evacuation

deceleration: decrease in speed

decidua basalis: a portion of the endometrium that is directly beneath the embedded ovum in the uterus

deciduous: temporary or falling out

decrement: the amount by which a quantity is decreased; phase of a contraction in which intensity decreases

DeLee aspirator: a machine to help remove secretions from the newborn's airway

delivery: expulsion or extraction of a child at birth

demand feeding: feeding a baby when the infant signals hunger rather than on a time schedule

dental caries: cavity; decay of the teeth

Denver II Developmental Screening Test: a screening test given to children between 1 month and 6 years of age to assess gross motor skills, fine motor skills, personal and social development, and language development

Depo-Provera (DMPA): injectable progestin which will give three months of continuous contraceptive protection

despair: the second phase in an infant's response to hospitalization, characterized by sadness, withdrawal, anger, and increasing protest

desquamated: peeled off; separated

detachment: the third phase in an infant's response to hospitalization, usually occurring after prolonged separation, characterized by an apparent loss of interest in the parent

development: the qualitative, continuous process in which the child's level of functioning and progression of skills become more complex

diaphragm: soft, dome-shaped device with a flexible rim that is inserted into the vagina and covers the cervix; spermicide is necessary for effectiveness

Dick-Read method: a method of childbirth that uses specific exercises and relaxation techniques

differentiation: development into a more specialized or complex form; the progression from general and simple responses to more specific and complex responses as children mature

diffusion: the movement of a substance from an area of high concentration to one of lower concentration until both areas are of equal concentration

dilatation: stretching of an opening as in the cervix during labor

dilation and curettage (D&C): the opening of the cervical os and the gentle manual removal of the lining from the walls of the uterus

dilation and evacuation (D&E): the procedure to remove the products of conception between 13 and 16 weeks gestation by opening the cervical os and removing the uterine lining and the developing fetus and placenta

diplopia: double vision

direct contact: transmission of infection to a susceptible host through physical contact (person to person, body to body)

direct method: a way of monitoring a fetus using various ECG electrodes attached directly to the fetus

disbelief: inability of parents to believe (or admit) that their child has a serious disease or disability; often coupled with anger or guilt

DNA: deoxyribonucleic acid; nucleic acid that contains all the genetic information passed from parents to offspring

dominant trait: a trait or characteristic that appears in the offspring even though it is present in only one of the parents; carried by a dominant gene

Doppler: ultrasonic transducer used to monitor fetal heart rate by detecting the fetal heart movements

dorsal position: pertaining to the back

Down syndrome: congenital disorder characterized by brain and body damage

ductus arteriosus: the fetal blood vessel that joins the aorta and pulmonary artery

ductus venosus: a fetal blood vessel that connects the umbilical vein and the inferior vena cava

duration: length of time a contraction lasts; timed from beginning to end of one contraction; measured in seconds

dysmenorrhea: painful menstruation

dysphoria: a disorder of affect characterized by extreme anguish

dyspnea: difficult breathing

dystocia: excessively painful, difficult, or slow labor or delivery

early deceleration: a decrease in fetal heart rate early in a contraction, suggesting head compression

ecchymosis: a bruise

eclampsia: an acute toxemia of pregnancy causing coma and convulsions, proteinuria, edema, and hypertension

ectoderm: the outermost layer of the three primary germ layers of the embryo

ectopic pregnancy: a pregnancy in which the fertilized ovum begins to develop outside the uterus

EDC: expected date of confinement or expected delivery date

effacement: thinning and shortening of the cervix

ego: according to Freud, the aspect of the personality that represents reason or common sense; its goal is to find a way to gratify the id

ejaculation: forcible release of seminal fluid from the penis

electrode: a conductor through which electrical current enters or leaves a cell, apparatus, or body

embolus: any material that is carried by the blood to another part of the body and obstructs a blood vessel

embryo: a new organism during the first eight weeks of development

emotional abuse: any interaction over time that causes a child unnecessary psychological pain; can include excessive demands, verbal harassment, excessive yelling, belittling, teasing, or rejection

endoderm: the innermost of the three primary germ layers of the embryo

endometritis: inflammation of the endometrium

endometrium: the mucous lining of the uterus, the thickness and structure of which vary with the phase of the menstrual cycle and pregnancy

engagement: presenting part of fetus descends and fully enters the pelvis

engorgement: excessive fullness of any organ or passage

epididymis: coiled tube located on the testes; the storehouse for sperm; adds a secretion to the semen that activates the spermatozoa

epilepsy: recurrent seizures, which may be idiopathic or a result of trauma, injury, or metabolic alterations

episiotomy: surgical incision of the perineum toward the end of the second stage of labor to facilitate delivery

epispadias: the urethra opens on the upper surface of the penis

Erb's palsy: partial paralysis of the arm due to injury to the brachial plexus

erectile: turgid and upright

erection: the enlarging and stiffening of the penis caused by the cavernous bodies in the penis filling with blood; generally occurs from sexual excitement

erythroblastosis fetalis: a hemolytic disease of the newborn

erythrocytes: red blood cells

eschar: the tough, leathery scab that forms over severely burned areas

essential amino acids: amino acids that cannot be manufactured by the body and must be provided in food

estrogen: the female hormone responsible for female sexual changes; instrumental in the menstrual cycle

expiratory grunt: noisy expulsion of air from the lung

expulsion: expelling or pushing out

exstrophy of the bladder: the interior of the bladder lies completely exposed through the abdominal opening

extension: fetal head becomes unflexed; pushes upward out of vaginal canal

external os: the opening from the cervix into the vagina

extrauterine: outside the uterus

face presentation: the face of the fetus presents at the cervix; complete extension

failure to thrive: a disorder of infants and children under 2 years of age, characterized by a weight for age that is below the third percentile

fallopian tubes: two tubes that extend from the upper corners of the uterus to the abdominal cavity; transport the ovum from the ovary to the uterus

false labor: abdominal discomfort resembling labor contractions, but no marked change in the cervix occurs

family-centered concept: idea that a laboring woman should remain in the same room for labor and delivery, surrounded by the support people of her choice

family-centered units: homelike atmosphere in hospital birthing room

fascia: bands of connective tissue that help to support organs in the pelvis

fatty acids: straight-chain monocarboxylic acids; classified as saturated or unsaturated

fear-tension-pain syndrome: a condition where pain is intensified by tension and fear of the unknown outcome of an event

fecalith: a hard, impacted fecal mass

fertilization: the union of the sperm and the ovum

fetal alcohol syndrome (FAS): a possible consequence if an expectant mother consumes alcohol during her pregnancy; symptoms include prenatal and postnatal growth retardation, neurological abnormalities, developmental delay, and facial dysmorphology

fetal blood sampling: a method of determining fetal distress by analyzing a small sample of blood taken from the presenting part of the fetus

fetal heart rate (FHR): number of beats per minute of the fetus's heart

fetal heart tones (FHT): the heartbeat of the fetus heard with a fetoscope or Doppler

fetal monitoring: a method used to gather data about fetal condition

fetal scalp electrode: a small electrode attached to the fetal scalp to directly monitor the heart rate of the fetus

fetone: an instrument that can detect fetal heart tones as early as the 12th week

fetopelvic disproportion: the head of the baby is of such size, shape, or position that it cannot pass through the mother's pelvis

fetoscope: an obstetrical stethoscope worn on the examiner's head, used to detect fetal heartbeat

fetus: the developing individual in the uterus after the eighth week of pregnancy

FHR: *see* fetal heart rate

FHT: *see* fetal heart tones

fifth disease: a flu-like illness with a rash caused by human parvovirus B19; contagious; puts a pregnant woman at an increased risk for miscarriage if she contracts the disease in the first or early second trimester

fine motor skills: ability to coordinate the small muscle groups

first stage of labor: stage of labor that begins with the start of cervical dilatation and effacement and ends when they are complete

flaccid: limp

flatulence: excessive formation of gas in stomach or intestine

flexion: act of bending

floating: term used to describe presenting part of fetus in utero that is freely movable above the brim of the pelvis

follicle-stimulating hormone (FSH): hormone in the female partly responsible for control of ovarian function

follicular phase: early phase in the menstrual cycle where follicles enlarge and migrate toward the surface of the ovary; also called preovulatory phase

fontanel: unossified space or soft spot between two or more sutures of the fetal skull

food pyramid: guide for daily food planning, published by the U.S. Department of Agriculture

football hold: a method of holding infant in which the infant's body is supported on the nurse's forearm, with the infant's head and neck resting in the nurse's palm; the rest of infant's body is securely held between the nurse's body and elbow

footling breech: the position of the fetus when one or both feet are the presenting part

foramen ovale: opening between the auricles of the fetal heart

forceps: an instrument with two blades and handles for pulling, grasping, or compressing

forces: uterine dysfunction

foremilk: breast milk stored directly under the nipple and not as rich in fats and calories as hindmilk

foreskin: *see* prepuce

fourchet: the posterior junction of the labia majora

fourth stage of labor: the first few hours after delivery

fracture: a break in a bone, usually as a result of injury

frank breech: the position of the fetus when the buttocks present at the cervix with the legs extended up and pressed against the abdomen and chest

frequency: rate of contractions; timed from beginning of one contraction to beginning of next; measured in minutes

fundus: the upper rounded end of the uterus

funic souffle: a soft flowing or whistling sound produced by the blood flowing through the umbilical cord; synchronizes with the fetal heart sounds

Galant reaction: if the newborn's back is stroked on one side while he is lying on his stomach his trunk will curve toward that side

gastric lavage: instillation of large amounts of warm normal saline through an orogastric tube into the patient's stomach until the return is clear

gavage feeding: feeding by means of a stomach tube

gene: the biological unit of heredity contained in the chromosome; each gene controls the inheritance of one or more characteristics

general anesthesia: a state of unconsciousness produced by anesthetic agent with absence of pain sensation over the entire body and a greater or lesser degree of muscular relaxation

genetic abnormalities: inherited problems transmitted through faulty genes

geneticist: a student of genetics, the study of heredity

genotypical: the fundamental hereditary constitution of an individual

gestation: the period of development of a new individual within the uterus from conception to birth

gestational diabetes: a metabolic disorder occurring in the latter half of pregnancy in which the ability to oxidize carbohydrates is faulty

glands of Montgomery: small nodular follicles or glands on the areola around the nipple

glans penis: slightly enlarged structure at the end of the penis that contains the orifice of the urethra

glycogen: a chief carbohydrate storage material in humans formed by and largely stored in the liver; animal starch

gonadotropic hormone: any hormone that acts on the gonads

gonadotropin-releasing hormone (GnRH): hormone secreted by the hypothalamus; helps to control ovarian function

gonorrhea: a sexually transmitted disease caused by *Neisseria gonorrhea* that causes a purulent vaginal discharge

Goodell's sign: softening of the cervix; a presumptive sign of pregnancy

Gower's sign: self-climbing movement in which a child uses arm muscles to compensate for weak hip extensor muscles in rising to an upright position; characteristic symptom of Duchenne's muscular dystrophy

graafian follicle: microscopic sac in which the ovum develops

granny midwives: untrained, illiterate, and often superstitious women who delivered babies

granulocytes: a type of white blood cell; specifically, neutrophils and eosinophils

grasp reflex: the newborn will firmly grasp a finger placed in his palm

gravida: pregnant woman

gross motor skills: ability to control the large muscle groups

growth: the continuous and complex process in which the body and its parts increase in size

gynecoid pelvis: round or transverse oval pelvis that accommodates childbirth well

gynecomastia: breasts of a newborn (male or female) enlarge and secrete tiny amounts of fluid

hCG: *see* human chorionic gonadotropin

head circumference: size of head, measured at its greatest circumference, slightly above the eyebrows and pinna of the ears and around the occipital prominence at the back of the skull; usually measured in all children up to 3 years of age

heartburn: burning sensation in the epigastrium

Hegar's sign: softening of the lower uterine segment; a sign of pregnancy

Heimlich maneuver: method of dislodging food or other material from the throat of a choking victim; uses subdiaphragmatic abdominal thrusts to forcefully expel the material

HELLP syndrome: *h*emolysis, *e*levated *l*iver enzymes, and *l*ow *p*latelets

hemoglobin: the oxygen-carrying pigment of human blood

hemolysis: disintegration of elements of red blood cells

hemophilia: a condition characterized by impaired coagulability of the blood and a strong tendency to bleed

hemorrhoids: dilation of the veins in the lower rectum and anus

heparinized: to render blood coagulable with heparin

heredity: transmission of characteristics from parent to offspring

hermaphrodite: condition in which a newborn possesses gonadal tissue typical of both sexes

herpes genitalis: a herpes simplex infection involving the genital mucosa; an inflammatory skin disease characterized by the formation of small vesicles in clusters

herpes simplex: a contagious sexually transmitted infection characterized by the formation of small vesicles in clusters

heterozygote: the product of two unlike genes in regard to a given characteristic

heterozygous: hybrid; having one or many pairs of unlike genes in regard to characteristics as a result of cross-breeding

Hill-Burton Act: 1946, supplied funds for construction of hospitals in rural areas to meet the need for safer hospital births

hindmilk: breast milk stored in the alveoli and milk-producing cells of the breast; rich in fats and calories

histone: a simple protein found in cell nuclei that interferes with coagulation

HIV: *see* human immunodeficiency virus

Homans' sign: pain or discomfort behind the knee or in the calf due to an inflammation of a vein resulting from a blood clot

homozygote: the product of two like genes in regard to a given characteristic

homozygous: pure-bred; having like genes

hospice care: provides holistic care and support for the patient with a terminal illness; goal is to enable the person to live life as fully as possible, free of pain, and with respect, choices, and dignity

host: person who harbors or nourishes an infectious organism

human chorionic gonadotropin (hCG): a hormone produced by the developing embryo that signals the corpus luteum to continue stimulating progesterone production for the maintenance of the pregnancy for the first three months; hormone that signals a positive pregnancy in serum and urine tests

human immunodeficiency virus (HIV): third T-lymphocyte virus renamed in 1986 to HIV; the virus that causes AIDS

hyaline membrane disease: *see* respiratory distress syndrome

hyaluronidase: enzyme that dissolves the layer of cells surrounding the ovum

hydatidiform mole: an abnormal condition in which the fertilized ovum degenerates and dies and the chorionic villi convert into a mass of transparent cysts

hydramnios: amniotic fluid in amounts greater than 2,000 mL at the time of delivery

hydrocephalus: a condition characterized by abnormal accumulation of fluid in the cranial vault; accompanied by enlargement of the head, prominence of the forehead, atrophy of the brain, mental weakness, and convulsions

hymen: fold of mucous membrane that protects the vaginal opening

hyperbilirubinemia: excessive bilirubin in the blood

hyperemesis gravidarum: excessive vomiting during pregnancy

hyperglycemia: an excess of sugar in the blood

hyperlipidemia: an excess of lipids in the plasma

hypertension: high blood pressure

hypoalbuminemia: an abnormally low level of albumin in the blood

hypoglycemia: a deficiency of sugar in the blood

hypoproteinemia: a decreased amount of protein in the blood

hypospadias: the urethra terminates on the under side of the penis

hypotension: diminished tension; low blood pressure

hypovolemia: diminished blood flow

id: according to Freud, the aspect of the personality that represents one's desires; is present at birth and seeks immediate gratification under the pleasure principle

Identabands: identification bands attached to wrist or ankle with name and other important information

ilium: the lateral, flaring portion of the pelvis

immune response: occurs when the body's lymphocytes are stimulated to produce antibodies that react with antigens

impacted shoulder: shoulder of the fetus is unable to pass through the maternal pelvis

imperforate anus: the anal opening is abnormally closed

impetigo: skin infection caused by staphylococcal organism

implantation: attachment of the blastocyst to the endometrium

impotent: term used when a man cannot have an erection or an ejaculation

increased titers: a rise in a substance required to react with another substance

increment: the amount by which a quantity is increased; phase of a contraction in which intensity increases

incubator: an apparatus for maintaining a premature infant in an environment of proper temperature and humidity

indirect contact: transmission of infection to a susceptible host by means of an animate or inanimate object, which becomes a common source and can infect many people

indirect method: a way of monitoring a fetus without direct contact with fetus; external monitoring

induced labor: labor that is artificially started or enhanced

infancy: the period of rapid growth and development occurring between birth and 1 year of age

infectious diseases: diseases caused by microorganisms that invade the body and then reproduce and multiply

inhalation agent: anesthetic administered by the respiration of a gaseous agent

innominate bones: three bones that make up the pelvis — the ilium, the ischium, and the pubis

insomnia: inability to sleep

integration: the process of combining simple movements or skills to achieve complex tasks

internal os: the innermost opening of the cervix as it leads into the uterus

intrauterine: within the uterus

intrauterine device (IUD): a contraceptive device that is inserted by a physician and remains within the uterus

intrauterine transfusion: the injection of Rh-negative erythrocytes into the peritoneal cavity of the fetus while in utero

intubation: the insertion of a tube; especially the introduction of a tube into the larynx through the glottis

intussusception: telescoping of the bowel

involution: return of the uterus to its normal size after childbirth

ischium: the posterior heavy portion of the pelvis

isolation: separation of infected individuals from those uninfected for the period of communicability of a particular disease; purpose is to interrupt the chain of infection by preventing the transmission of microbes

jaundice: yellowish discoloration of the skin and eyes from bile pigments

Kegel exercise: perineal squeeze or tightening of the pelvic floor muscles

kerion: a boggy, pustular inflammation that usually develops in association with tinea infections

kernicterus: a severe form of icterus neonatorum with involvement of brain and spinal cord (jaundice)

Kernig's sign: inability to fully extend the legs when in supine position

ketoacidosis: accumulation of ketones in the body, causing acidosis

ketonuria: loss of ketones in the urine

killed inactivated virus: form of vaccine in which the virus has been killed and therefore inactivated

labia: lips surrounding the vagina for coverage and protection

labia majora: two heavy outer lips of the vulva

labia minora: two smaller lips of the vulva that lie inside the labia majora

labor: the function by which a new individual is expelled through the vagina to the outside world

Lact-Aid: a device consisting of a pouch for formula with a tube that can be placed in the baby's mouth alongside the breast nipple; baby's sucking efforts bring in milk from the pouch for nourishment as well as stimulate the mother's breast to produce a greater quantity of milk

lactose: a complex carbohydrate (disaccharide) obtained from milk

Lamaze: early founder of childbirth preparation methods for the expectant mother and her support person to deal with the pain of childbirth without the use of medication using psychoprophylactic methods

lanugo: fine hair covering the body of the fetus

laryngospasm: involuntary vibrating contractions of the muscles of the larynx

late deceleration: decreased fetal heart rate after a contraction ends; suggests utero-placental insufficiency

latent phase: early phase in the first stage of labor with cervical dilatation measuring between 1 and 4 cm

Leboyer method: an approach to childbirth that emphasizes gentle, controlled delivery

lecithin-sphingomyelin (L-S) ratio: a prenatal test to measure fetal lung surfactant phospholipids to determine fetal pulmonary maturity

Leopold's maneuvers: a way to determine the fetal position in the uterus by sliding hands down the sides of the mother's abdomen

let-down reflex: a release of milk from alveoli to the main sinuses under the nipple in the breast

leukocytes: white blood cells

leukopenia: decrease in the number of white blood cells in the body

leukorrhea: a whitish discharge from the vagina and uterine cavity

levator ani: powerful muscle that helps support the organs in the pelvis

lie: the relationship of the long axis of the baby to that of the mother

lightening: dropping of the uterus caused by the settling of the fetal head into the pelvis in the last weeks before delivery

limb salvage: removal of a tumor without amputation

linea nigra: a dark line appearing on the abdomen and extending from the pubis toward the umbilicus

lingual: pertaining to the tongue

lipid: any one group of substances that include the fats, oils, and fat-like substances called sterols

lithotomy position: a position the woman assumes to have a pelvic exam; the woman is lying on her back with her legs out to the sides supported by either calf or foot stirrups

live attenuated virus: form of vaccine in which the virus has been weakened

LMP: the date of the first day of a woman's last menstrual period; an important date to help determine an expected delivery date

local anesthesia: anesthesia confined to one part of the body

lochia: vaginal discharge following delivery

lochia alba: from the 14th day of the postpartum period to the end of the puerperium, the vaginal secretion is less profuse than earlier and whitish

lochia rubra: uterine and vaginal discharge after delivery; red from the first to fourth day

lochia serosa: when the vaginal discharge changes from red to dark brownish red and then to yellowish brown, from the 4th to the 14th postpartum day

longitudinal lie: when the long axis of the baby is parallel to the long axis of the mother

lordosis: abnormal increased curvature of the lumbar spine

L-S ratio: *see* lecithin-sphingomyelin ratio

lumbar epidural block: anesthesia produced by injection of the anesthetic agent into the epidural space of the lumbar region

lunar month: a period of approximately 28 days; from one cycle of the moon to the next

luteal phase: phase of the menstrual cycle after the mature follicle ruptures and the corpus luteum stimulates production of the hormone progesterone

luteinizing hormone (LH): a hormone of the anterior pituitary gland that stimulates formation of the corpus luteum

maceration: the softening of a solid by soaking

magical thinking: belief that thoughts and deeds can cause an event to occur; characteristic of preschool children

malnutrition: condition resulting from inadequate intake of essential nutrients

mask of pregnancy: chloasma; a pigmentary discoloration of the face during pregnancy

mastitis: inflammation or infection of the breast

masturbation: stimulation of the sex organs by means other than sexual intercourse

maternal xiphoid: female breast bone or lowest segment of the sternum

mechanism of labor: the series of movements the fetus goes through to exit through the mother's pelvis during delivery

meconium: dark green, tarlike substance in the intestines of a full-term fetus

meconium-stained fluid: amniotic fluid that has evidence of meconium in it; may indicate fetal distress

meiosis: the process in the maturation of the germ cells by which the chromosome number is reduced from two sets to one set of chromosomes

menarche: the beginning of the menstrual function

meningocele: hernial protrusion of the meninges through a defect in the skull or vertebral column

meningomyelocele: hernial protrusion of a part of the meninges and substance of the spinal cord through a defect in the vertebral column; also called myelomeningocele

menopause: cessation of menstruation

menorrhagia: prolonged or excessive bleeding during the menstrual period

menses: the periodic discharge of blood from the uterus, occurring at approximately four-week intervals

menstruation: cyclic, physiological discharge of blood from a nonpregnant uterus, occurring at about four-week intervals

mentum: chin, face

mesoderm: the middle layer of the three primary germ layers of the embryo

metrorrhagia: vaginal bleeding at a time other than the normal menstrual period

microcephaly: condition in which the head is abnormally small

midline incision: a vertical incision between the navel and the pubic bone for the delivery of the baby

milia: small whitish nodules in the skin, especially of the face; usually retention cysts of sebaceous glands

miliaria rubra: prickly heat or heat rash

minipill: progestin-only birth control pill taken every day to prevent pregnancy

miniprep: small amount of pubic hair is removed around the anal and perineal area in anticipation of an episiotomy

miscarriage: expulsion of fetus before the stage of viability

mitosis: indirect cell division

molar pregnancy: *see* hydatidiform mole

monilial vaginitis: vaginal infection caused by fungi

mons veneris: pad of fat covering pubic area

Montgomery tubercles: small nodular follicles or glands on the areolae around the nipple

Moro reflex: a startle reflex with stimulation in which the infant's arms are suddenly thrown out in an embrace attitude

morula: the solid mass of blastomeres formed by cleavage of the fertilized ovum, filling all the space occupied by the ovum before cleavage

multigravida: a woman who has been pregnant more than once

multipara: a woman in labor with or having borne her second child and subsequent children

multiple pregnancy: more than one fetus present in the uterus during the same pregnancy

myometrium: the smooth muscle coat of the uterus that forms the main mass of the organ

myringotomy: surgical incision of the eardrum

NAACOG: Nurses Association of the American College of Obstetricians and Gynecologists

Naegle's rule: a method used for calculating the expected delivery date by adding seven days to the first day of the last menstrual period, subtracting three calendar months from the new date, and adding one year

narcosis: unconscious state caused by drugs

narcotic: an agent that produces insensibility or stupor

naris: (plural, nares) nostril

nasal salute: wiping the nose with the heel of the hand; a symptom of allergic rhinitis

natural family planning (NFP): a contraceptive method that relies on the natural menstrual cycle and abstinence or barrier protection during the fertile time in the cycle

NBAS (neonatal behavioral assessment scale): an assessment scale for the purpose of obtaining more exact knowledge of the developing neurological functions as early as possible

neglect: deliberate or unintentional lack of care for a child's basic needs that places the child's life or health in danger

neonatal hypoglycemia: a deficiency of sugar in the blood of the newborn

neonatal period: the first four weeks of life

neonate: a newborn in his first four weeks of life

neural tube defect: a specific malformation of the nervous system in the infant including brain, spinal cord, and nerves

nevi: local anatomic alterations of the cellular and vascular components of the skin

Nile blue sulfate: rarely used test for fetal maturity

nonessential amino acids: amino acids that can be manufactured by the body

nonoxynol-9: a chemical in a spermicidal that destroys sperm

nonstress test (NST): a means of determining fetal well-being by measuring fetal heart tones in correlation with fetal movement

Norplant system: six silicone matchstick-sized capsules filled with progesterone that are inserted beneath the skin in the upper inside arm; prevent pregnancy for up to five years by continuous release of progesterone

nuchal cord: umbilical cord wrapped around the neck of the fetus

nuchal rigidity: stiff neck

nullipara: a woman who has not borne children

nursing care plan: written guidelines that direct nursing care: assessment, plan of action, and rationale are included

nursing process: framework upon which nursing care is based; includes assessing the problem, formulating a care plan, implementing the plan, and evaluating its effectiveness

nutricius: to nourish, to protect, to foster

nutrients: foods or their components that are necessary for proper body function, including carbohydrates, protein, fats, minerals, and vitamins

OB-GYN: obstetrics and gynecology — a branch of medicine dealing with pregnancy, birth, and women's health care

oblique lie: the fetus lies in a diagonal position; situated at a 45° angle to the long axis of the mother

obstetrics: branch of medicine that deals with childbirth and that which precedes and follows it

occiput: back part of the skull

occlusion therapy: closure or obstruction to prevent or improve a condition (e.g., wearing a patch over the stronger eye in strabismus and ambylopia)

oligohydramnios: the presence of less than 300 mL of amniotic fluid at term

oliguria: decreased urine output

omentum: a double fold of the peritoneum attaching the stomach to adjacent organs

ophthalmia neonatorum: eye infection in the newborn

osmosis: the diffusion of solvent molecules through a semipermeable membrane, going from the side of lower concentration to that of higher concentration

ossification: formation of bone; conversion of other tissue into bone

ovaries: sex glands of the female; discharge ova and produce hormones necessary to the process of reproduction

oviducts: the tubelike structures that carry the ovum from the ovary to the uterus

ovulation: the maturation and release of the ovum from the ovary

ovulation method: a method of contraception that relies on observing and understanding vaginal secretions that indicate ovulation

ovum: the female reproductive cell, which is capable of becoming a new individual after being fertilized by a sperm

oxytocic: an agent that promotes uterine contractions

oxytocin: a posterior pituitary hormone that stimulates uterine contractions

oxytocin challenge test (OCT): a means of evaluating how well the placenta is nourishing and supplying oxygen to the fetus

pain management: control of pain through administration of medications at regular intervals and/or nonpharmacological methods such as distraction, hypnosis, imagery, and application of heat and cold

Pap (Papanicolaou) smear: a cervical smear for cancer cytology test

-para: refers to the number of previous pregnancies that have gone to the period of viability

paracervical block: a regional anesthetic administered into the region around the cervix to reduce the pain caused by cervical dilatation

parasympathetic: part of the autonomic nervous system that controls many internal functions of the body (heart, lungs, organs of the abdomen)

parenteral: administration of fluids, food, or drugs by means other than through the intestinal canal

paresis: paralysis

parturition: expulsion or delivery of the fetus

passive immunity: an immune response that occurs when an individual receives ready-made antibodies from a human or animal that has been actively immunized against the disease

pathogen: *see* causative agent

pediatric technician: an allied health professional with basic understanding of normal childhood development and common childhood illness to help the health care team deliver care to children

penis: the male organ of copulation

perimetrium: the serous coat of the uterus

perineal preparation: cleansing and otherwise preparing the perineal area for a vaginal delivery

perineal squeeze: tightening of the pelvic floor muscles

perineum: the area of skin, connective tissue, and muscle that lies between the vulva and anus

peritoneum: the membrane lining of the abdominal walls

permeable: able to be passed through

personality: the pattern of characteristic thoughts, feelings, and behaviors that distinguishes one person from another

petechiae: pinpoint hemorrhages

phagocytosis: the ingestion of solid particles by living cells

phenotypical: the outward visible expression of the hereditary constitution of an organism

phenylketonuria (PKU): rare metabolic abnormality in which phenylketones are excreted in the urine and can cause retardation

phobia: an excessive or unfounded fear of someone or something

phocomelia: fetus with hands and feet but no legs or arms

phonotransducer: a combination of mechanical and electrical filtering of fetal heart activity

photophobia: extreme sensitivity to light

phototherapy: treatment of disease by light rays; used to treat jaundice

physical abuse: deliberate physical maltreatment that causes injury to the body

physiological jaundice: mild yellowing of the newborn's skin and eyes occurring the first few days after birth and self-resolving

pica: craving for nonfood substance

PID: pelvic inflammatory disease; an infection in the uterus or the fallopian tubes or both

pigmentation: the deposit of a coloring matter in the skin

PIH: pregnancy-induced hypertension; categorized as hypertension, preeclampsia, and eclampsia

pitocin: a synthetic oxytocin that stimulates uterine contractions

pituitary gland: a gland at the base of the brain divided into anterior and posterior lobes

placenta: a fleshy organ that develops from embryonic and maternal tissue; it serves as a respiratory, nutritive, and excretory organ for the fetus

placenta abruptio: a premature separation of a normally implanted placenta

placenta previa: placenta is implanted in the lower segment of the uterus and either wholly or partially covers the cervix

placental souffle: a soft murmur produced by the blood flow in the placenta synchronized with the mother's pulse

placing reaction: when the newborn's shins are placed against an edge, the baby steps upward to place his feet on top of the surface

plasma: the liquid portion of blood, containing protein, clotting factors, and electrolytes

platypelloid pelvis: flattened pelvis shape that does not accommodate childbearing well

polydipsia: excessive thirst

polyphagia: markedly increased food intake

polyuria: excessive urine output

portal of entry: the method by which an infectious organism enters a host; may occur through breaks in the skin or mucous membranes, ingestion, inhalation, or across the placenta in utero

portal of exit: the method by which an infectious organism leaves the reservoir; occurs through bodily secretions

position: pertaining to the presenting part of the fetus to the right or left side of the mother

positive signs of pregnancy: conclusive evidence of a positive pregnancy

postoperative care: physical and emotional care that occurs in the postanesthesia room and the nursing unit during recovery from a surgical procedure

postoperative exercises: actions performed after surgery, such as coughing, deep breathing, and ambulating, to stimulate circulation and respiration, thereby preventing atelectasis and blood stasis

postpartum: the period following childbirth

postpartum depression: an absence of cheerfulness or hope following the birth of a baby

postpartum hemorrhage: loss of more than 500 mL of blood during the first 24 hours after delivery

precipitate delivery: a very rapid delivery process

precipitous labor: a spontaneous labor that progresses very rapidly and usually lasts less than three hours

precocious dentition: early eruption of teeth

preeclampsia: a toxemia of pregnancy shown by elevated blood pressure, edema, and albuminuria

pregnancy: the state of developing a fertilized ovum within the uterus

pregnancy-induced hypertension: *see* PIH

premature infant: infant born before 37 weeks' gestation or that weighs less than 5½ lb (2,500 g)

premature labor: labor that begins before 37 weeks' gestation

preoperative care: emotional and physical care given in preparation for upcoming surgery

preoperative checklist: steps of the preoperative process, used in preparing a patient for surgery

preoperative teaching: teaching before surgery, designed to reduce preoperative anxiety and promote a positive outcome

prepared childbirth classes: *see* childbirth preparation

prepubertal growth spurt: a growth spurt that begins at about age 7, preceding the true growth spurt of adolescence

prepubescent period: period ranging from 10 to 12 years for girls and 12 to 14 years for boys

prepuce: a fold of skin sometimes called the foreskin, that encloses the glans penis in the male; a partial hood that covers the clitoris in the female

preschool: a period in which physical growth slows and stabilizes, occurring between 3 and 6 years of age

presentation: the part of the fetus, such as the head, face, buttocks, or shoulder that first enters the pelvis (presents)

presenting part: the part of the fetus that lies nearest the internal opening of the cervix

presumptive signs of pregnancy: presumed but not proven indication of a pregnancy

previable fetus: a fetus that is not sufficiently developed to live outside the uterus

primary irritant: an agent that produces irritation (contact dermatitis) on the first exposure to it

primary standing: if supported upright, the newborn will support some of his body weight

primary (deciduous) teeth: first teeth; children have 20 primary teeth, usually by age 33 months

primigravida: a woman pregnant with her first child

primipara: a woman in labor with or having borne her first child

probable signs of pregnancy: likely signs of pregnancy but not definite

prodromal phase: the earliest phase of a developing disease or condition

progesterone: a hormone secreted by the corpus luteum that prepares the endometrium for the reception and development of the fertilized ovum and causes uterine secretions

projectile vomiting: vomitus ejected with force

prolactin: a hormone secreted by the anterior pituitary that stimulates milk production

prolapsed cord: the umbilical cord lies beside or below the presenting part; premature expulsion of the cord

proliferative phase: phase of the menstrual cycle in which the glands of the uterine lining are stimulated to thicken

PROM: premature rupture of membranes

prostaglandin: a substance, naturally found in semen, that causes strong contraction of smooth muscle and dilation of certain vascular beds

prostate gland: gland that surrounds the urethra at the base of the bladder; adds an alkaline secretion to semen that neutralizes the acid fluid from the testes

protective reflex: blinking, coughing, sneezing, yawning, swallowing with stimulation

proteinuria: albumin in the urine

protest: the initial phase in an infant's response to hospitalization in which the infant cannot be consoled and refuses any attention except from the parent

proximodistal: the process in which development proceeds from the center of the body outward toward the extremities

pseudohermaphrodite: condition in which a newborn has the external sex organs of one sex and the gonads of the other sex

pseudohypertrophy: seeming enlargement

psychoactive: affecting the mind or behavior; mind-altering, as in psychoactive drugs

psychoprophylaxis: a method of childbirth in which the discomfort of labor and delivery is controlled by mental and physical means rather than chemical ones

puberty: period of time between the ages of 9 and 14 years; an increased amount of sex hormones is usually released into the bloodstream at this time as secondary sex characteristics develop

pubis: the anterior portion of the pelvis

pudendal block: anesthesia produced by injection of a regional anesthetic into the pudendal nerves, numbing the perineum and vagina

puerperal infection: postpartum infection of the pelvic organs

puerperal sepsis: postpartum infection of the pelvic organs

puerperal thrombosis: formation of a blood clot during childbirth

puerperium: period of time from delivery to complete involution of the organs; about six weeks

purging: self-induced vomiting or use of diuretics or laxatives to rid the body of ingested food

pyelitis: inflammation of the kidney with special involvement of the renal pelvis

pyloric stenosis: a constriction at the junction of the stomach and the small intestine

quickening: the mother's first perception of the movement of her fetus

radiography: x-ray exam will show bones, including fetal skeleton

RDS: *see* respiratory distress syndrome

recessive trait: a trait that can be masked by another (dominant) trait; appears in offspring only when a pair of recessive genes is present

Recommended Dietary Allowances: guidelines for the intake of essential nutrients from infancy through adulthood

rectum: distal portion of the large intestine

reflex: an automatic action or movement; any particular involuntary activity

regional anesthesia: the production of insensibility of a part of the body by interrupting the sensory nerve conductivity from that region of body

regurgitation: abnormal backward progression of fluids or undigested food from the stomach; vomiting

renal: pertaining to the kidney

rescue breathing: breathing for a victim who is unable to breathe on his/her own because of unconsciousness or airway obstruction; part of CPR procedure

reservoir: the place where an organism grows and reproduces; serves as a source from which others can be infected; can be someone with the disease, someone carrying the disease, an animal, or the environment

respiratory distress syndrome (RDS): condition in which alveoli of lungs fail to expand due to lack of surfactant (phospholipid); also called hyaline membrane disease

restitution: after the delivery of the head, rotation of the fetus back to align the head and shoulders

resuscitation: restoration to life

retraction: a visible drawing in of the soft tissues of the chest, often a sign of severe distress

Rh factor: a term applied to an inherited antigen in the human blood

RhoGAM: solution of gamma globulin containing Rh antibodies

rickets: a deficiency disease of infancy and childhood that causes abnormalities in structure and shape of bones

ritualistic behavior: repetitive actions, often connected with mealtime, especially in toddlers

rituals: a series of repetitive acts performed as part of daily living for the child (e.g., story before bedtime, afternoon nap, snack time); provide comfort and stability for the child

RNA: ribonucleic acid; the nucleic acid that is responsible for transferring genetic information within a cell

rooming-in: newborn infant remains in the postpartum room with the mother throughout her hospital stay

rooting reflex: newborn's head turns toward direction of touch on the cheek in search of the nipple

round ligaments: structures that help support the pelvic organs; attached to the side walls of the uterus and the mons veneris

RU-486: a drug being tested for various treatments; a progesterone antagonist that will effectively produce an abortion

rubella: German measles; an acute infectious disease that can cause serious anomalies in the developing fetus if the mother contracts the disease in the first three months of pregnancy

rugae: small folds or ridges within the mucous membrane lining the vagina

sacrum: lower back (triangular bone between lumbar vertebra and coccyx), formed of five unified vertebrae

saddle block: a form of low spinal anesthesia

scapula: shoulder

scarlet fever: an infection caused by group A hemolytic streptococci

school age: a period of slow, steady growth occurring between 6 and 12 years of age

scoliosis: a lateral S-shaped curvature of the spine, occurring most often in adolescent girls

scrotum: pouch of loose skin and superficial fascia that contains the testes

scurvy: a disease due to deficiency of ascorbic acid; characterized by bone deformities

second stage of labor: stage of labor that begins with the full cervical dilatation and ends with the delivery of the baby

secondary (permanent) teeth: permanent teeth that emerge starting at about age 6 years and continuing through childhood and early adulthood

secretory phase: the phase of the menstrual cycle that prepares the uterus to receive a fertilized ovum

sedative: a drug that allays activity and excitement

semen: fluid in which the sperm is carried; consists of secretions from the epididymis, the prostate gland, the seminal vesicles, and the bulbourethral gland

semilunar valve opening: the second phase of the fetal heart pattern being monitored

seminal ducts: transport sperm from the testes

seminal vesicle glands: two saclike structures located behind the prostate gland that secrete a fluid that makes up a part of the semen

seminiferous tubules: structures within the testes that produce sperm

sensorium: any sensory nerve center

separation anxiety: responses of distress and apprehension in a child on being removed from parents, home, or familiar surroundings; common in toddlers

sex-limited characteristics: traits that appear in one sex only

sex-linked characteristics: physical traits that are associated with the genes in the sex chromosomes

sexual abuse: sexual contact between a child, aged 16 years or younger, and another person in a position of authority, no matter what the age, in which the child's participation has been obtained through force, threats, bribes, or gifts; can include intercourse, masturbation, fondling, exhibitionism, sodomy, or prostitution

sexual maturity: stage reached after the adolescent growth spurt ends; principal sign in girls is menstruation; principal sign in boys is presence of sperm in urine

sexually transmitted disease (STD): an infection transmitted through sexual contact; also called venereal disease

shake test: a prenatal test to determine fetal pulmonary maturity that can be obtained quickly but may not be as reliable as other tests

shoulder dystocia: a difficult delivery due to the size or position of the shoulders as they attempt to rotate through the pelvis

shoulder presentation: the shoulder is the presenting part of the fetus and the infant lies crosswise

show: mucus plug; pink vaginal discharge consisting of thick stringy mucus streaked with blood

Silverman-Anderson Index: a means of continuous evaluation of an infant's respiratory status

sinus arrhythmia: normal cycle of irregular heart rhythm associated with respiration; heart rate is faster on inspiration and slower on expiration

sleep apnea: cessation of breathing for brief periods during sleep

SOAP notes: medical notes with subjective information, objective information, assessment of the problem, and a plan for patient care

spectrophotometer: instrument used to measure the intensity of various wavelengths of light transmitted

sperm: *see* spermatozoa

spermatogenic: sperm-producing

spermatozoa: sperm; mature male sex cells that are formed in the testes

spermicidal: a chemical that produces a reaction destructive to spermatozoa; spermicide

spina bifida occulta: malformation of the spine in which the posterior portion of the laminae of the vertebrae fails to close; defect only in the vertebrae

spinal anesthesia: injection of a regional anesthetic into the subarachnoid space around the spinal cord

spinal headache: a headache and associated symptoms following puncture of spinal canal and leakage of cerebrospinal fluid

sponge: a small, pillow-shaped polyurethane sponge that contains nonoxynol-9 spermicide that is placed within the vagina before intercourse

sprains: injuries caused by overstretching of a muscle

stasis: maintaining a constant level

station: degree of engagement above or below the ischial spines

status epilepticus: series of generalized tonic-clonic seizures in which child does not regain consciousness between seizures

STD: *see* sexually transmitted disease

steatorrhea: presence of fat in the stool

sterility: the inability to bring about conception; the lack of viable sperm

sterilization: the process of making conception impossible

stillbirth: a fetus that is born dead

strains: injuries caused by pulling of a ligament

stressors: adverse physical, mental, or emotional stimuli that cause anxiety for the child or parents, often creating situations beyond their ability to cope

striae gravidarum: streaks on the sides of the abdomen, breasts, and thighs caused by stretching of the skin; stretch marks

stridor: high-pitched, noisy sound or wheezing created by narrowing of the airway, often caused by foreign-body aspiration

subcutaneous: beneath the layers of the skin

sucking reflex: newborn's ability to grasp nipple and areola with his mouth

sudden infant death syndrome (SIDS): the sudden death of an infant under 1 year of age that remains unexplained after a complete autopsy investigation and review of the history; leading cause of death in children aged 1 to 12 months in the United States

superego: according to Freud, the aspect of the personality that incorporates "shoulds" and "should nots" into one's personal value system; the conscience

supply and demand: the woman's ability to manufacture an adequate milk supply to meet the baby's growing and changing needs

surfactant deficiency: an insufficiency of the agent that stabilizes alveolar sacs by lowering surface tension; this agent is necessary for normal respiratory function

susceptible host: a person at risk for contracting an infectious disease

suture: junction between bones of the skull; also refers to sewing together an incision

sweat test: diagnostic test that analyzes the sodium and chloride content of a child's sweat; used to diagnose cystic fibrosis

symphysis pubis: line of fusion between the pubic bones

symptothermal method: a contraceptive method that relies on the body's basal temperature changes and symptoms that signal ovulation

syphilis: a contagious sexually transmitted disease leading to many structural and cutaneous lesions; untreated syphilis in the mother can adversely affect the fetus

tachycardia: abnormally rapid heartbeat; more than 160 beats per minute in the fetus

tachypnea: excessively rapid respirations

talipes: clubfoot; a foot or feet may turn in any abnormal direction

temperament: a person's style of approaching other people and situations

teratogen: having the ability to cause abnormal development

testes: (singular, testis) primary sex organs of the male; produce sperm and testosterone

testosterone: primary male sex hormone; contributes to the development of secondary sex characteristics

tetany: a nervous disorder characterized by sharp flexion of the wrist and ankle joints, muscle twitching, cramps, and convulsions

tetonic: prolonged uterine contractions lasting over 90 seconds

theoretical effectiveness rate: the percent of pregnancies that are prevented with any given method of contraception when that method is used correctly at all times and there is no product failure

third stage of labor: the stage of labor that begins with the birth of the baby and ends with the expulsion of the placenta

thrombocytes: platelets

thrombophlebitis: inflammation of a vein that results in a blood clot

thrombus: blood clot that remains at the place it was formed

thrush: fungal infection in the mouth

titer: the quantity of a substance required to react with a given amount of another substance

tocolytic treatment: medication given to stop premature labor

tocotransducer: monitors uterine activity by detecting external geometrical changes

toddlerhood: a period of slower growth occurring between 1 and 3 years of age

tonic neck reflex: postural reflex of newborn

tonus: tone or contraction of skeletal muscles

torticollis: condition in which neck tilts to one side; caused by shortening of the sterocleidomastoid muscle

toxemia: a disorder encountered during gestation or early in the puerperium; characterized by one or more of the following signs: hypertension, edema, albuminuria, and, in severe cases, convulsion and coma

toxoid: form of vaccine in which the agent has been treated to destroy its toxic qualities

toxoplasmosis: infection caused by a parasite *(Toxoplasma)* that lives in some mammals, such as cats, and can be passed to humans who eat raw or undercooked meats or who come in contact with feces from a cat who harbors the parasite

TPAL: abbreviation for the number of term pregnancies, premature births, abortions, and living children a woman has had

traction: use of weights and pulleys to realign bone fragments, reduce dislocations, immobilize fractures, provide rest for an extremity, help prevent contracture deformities, and allow preoperative and postoperative positioning and alignment

trait: a distinguishing quality or feature

tranquilizer: a drug used to reduce anxiety and relax the patient

transducer: electronic equipment used to convert one form of energy into another form of energy

transition phase: latter phase in the first stage of labor with cervical dilatation measuring from 8 to 10 cm

transmission: spread of pathogens, either by direct or indirect contact, by airborne spread, by inanimate objects, or by vectors

transverse lie: the fetus is in a crosswise position; situated at right angles to the long axis of the mother

transverse presentation: shoulder is the presenting part

Trichomonas vaginalis: a sexually transmitted microorganism that lives in the vagina and urethra that produces a profuse discharge

trichomoniasis: profuse irritating vaginal discharge caused by *Trichomonas vaginalis*

trigger: stimulus (substance or condition) that precedes an asthmatic episode or allergic reaction

triglycerides: compounds consisting of three fatty acids combined with glycerol

trimester: a three-month period during gestation

trophoblast: the rim of the blastocyst; becomes the placenta and the chorion, which nourish and protect the developing fetus

true labor: rhythmic increasingly intense uterine contractions with changes in the cervix

tubal ligation: a form of sterilization for a woman whereby the fallopian tubes are cut and tied off

tubal pregnancy: fertilized ovum implanted within the fallopian tube

tympanometry: measurement of internal ear pressure

tyrosine: amino acid in the body

ultrasonography: a form of sound waves that can be used to visualize a fetus in utero and pelvic organs

umbilical cord: a structure, approximately 20 in. long, containing two arteries and one vein, that attaches the fetus to the placenta

umbilical hernia: protrusion of part of an organ (usually intestine) through the wall of the umbilical ring

umbilicus: navel

upright hold: a method of holding infant in which the infant is held upright against the nurse's chest and shoulder; infant's buttocks are supported by one of the nurse's hands, with the other hand and arm supporting the infant's head and shoulders

ureter: tube carrying urine from the kidneys to the bladder

urethra: tube leading from the bladder to an opening in the vulva

urinary estrogens: test for fetal-placental assessment

urinary meatus: the opening in the vulva through which urine is voided

urinary stasis: condition in which flow of urine is interrupted

uterine activity transducer: tocotransducer; a monitor that responds to the muscle tone in the abdominal wall and measures uterine activity

uterine atony: lack of muscle tone in the uterus

uterine dysfunction: weak, irregular, uncoordinated uterine contractions; the forces

uterine ligaments: supporting structures of the uterus

uterogestation: gestation (development of life) in the uterus

uterosacral ligaments: extend from posterior cervical portion of the uterus to the sacrum, and support the cervix

uterus: female organ that holds the fetus during pregnancy

vaccine: an active immunizing agent that incorporates an infectious antigen

vacuum curettage: the gentle suctioning of the uterine cavity evacuating the lining and the products of conception if present

vacuum extractor: an instrument that applies a gentle suction used for drawing out, pulling, or extracting

vagina: a tubelike passage leading from the vulva to the uterus

variable deceleration: FHR pattern slows to less than 100 bpm at various times with no consistent relationship to contractions. Usually due to compressed umbilical cord

variability: degree of deviation from the baseline fetal heart rate

varicose vein: a vein that has become abnormally painful and swollen as a result of prolonged increased pressure

vas deferens: slim muscular tube, about 45.7 cm (18 in.) long, that carries semen to the urethra

vasectomy: the cutting of the vas deferens to keep sperm from being ejaculated and reaching the ovum

VBAC: vaginal birth after cesarean

vena cava: the vessel that conveys blood toward the heart

venereal disease: *see* sexually transmitted disease

venous thrombosis: blood clots in the legs

vernix caseosa: a cheeselike substance that covers the skin of the fetus for protection

version: altering of the fetal position in utero

vertex: the crown or top of the head

vesicoureteral reflux: abnormal backflow of urine from the bladder to the ureters

visual acuity: clarity or clearness of sight; refractive ability

visual field: an area within which stimuli will produce the sensation of sight

vital signs: temperature, pulse, respirations, and blood pressure

vulva: labia majora and external structures contained within them

weaning: discontinuing the breast feeding of an infant with substitution of other feeding methods

Wharton's jelly: a mucoid substance that surrounds the umbilical cord and protects the blood vessels inside the cord

zygote: a cell produced by genetic union; one cell with one nucleus containing all the necessary elements for future development of the offspring

Index

Note: Page numbers in **bold** type reference nontext material.